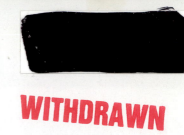

Comprehensive Perinatal & Pediatric

RESPIRATORY CARE

Fourth Edition

Comprehensive Perinatal & Pediatric
RESPIRATORY CARE

Fourth Edition

KENT B. WHITAKER, MEd, PA-C
Clinical Assistant Professor
Physician Assistant Program
Idaho State University
Pocatello, Idaho

PAUL G. EBERLE, PhD, RRT
Professor and Chair/Department of Respiratory Therapy
Weber State University
Ogden, Utah

LISA TRUJILLO, DHSc, RRT
Assistant Professor
Director of Clinical Education
Weber State University
Ogden, Utah

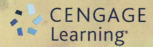

CENGAGE
Learning®

Australia • Brazil • Japan • Korea • Mexico • Singapore • Spain • United Kingdom • United States

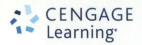

Comprehensive Perinatal and Pediatric Respiratory Care, Fourth Edition
Kent Whitaker, Paul Eberle, Lisa Trujillo

Vice President, Careers & Computing:
Dawn Gerrain

Director of Learning Solutions: Steve Helba

Product Manager: Christina Gifford

Director, Development-Career and
Computing: Marah Bellegarde

Product Development Manager: Juliet Steiner

Senior Content Developer: Darcy M. Scelsi

Market Development Manager: Michele
McTighe

Senior Production Director: Wendy Troeger

Production Manager: Andrew Crouth

Content Project Manager: Brooke
Greenhouse

Senior Art Director: David Arsenault

Cover image(s): Background:

   © Sideways Design/shutterstock.com

Boy: © David Buffington/Getty Images

Girl: © Inga Marchuk/shutterstock.com

For product information and technology assistance, contact us at
Cengage Learning Customer & Sales Support, 1-800-354-9706

For permission to use material from this text or product,
submit all requests online at **www.cengage.com/permissions**.
Further permissions questions can be e-mailed to
permissionrequest@cengage.com

Library of Congress Control Number: 2014934990

ISBN-13: 978-1-4390-5943-2

Cengage Learning
200 First Stamford Place, 4th Floor
Stamford, CT 06902
USA

Cengage Learning is a leading provider of customized learning solutions with office locations around the globe, including Singapore, the United Kingdom, Australia, Mexico, Brazil, and Japan. Locate your local office at: **www.cengage.com/global**

Cengage Learning products are represented in Canada by Nelson Education, Ltd.

To learn more about Cengage Learning, visit **www.cengage.com**

Purchase any of our products at your local college store or at our preferred online store **www.cengagebrain.com**

Notice to the Reader
Publisher does not warrant or guarantee any of the products described herein or perform any independent analysis in connection with any of the product information contained herein. Publisher does not assume, and expressly disclaims, any obligation to obtain and include information other than that provided to it by the manufacturer. The reader is expressly warned to consider and adopt all safety precautions that might be indicated by the activities described herein and to avoid all potential hazards. By following the instructions contained herein, the reader willingly assumes all risks in connection with such instructions. The publisher makes no representations or warranties of any kind, including but not limited to, the warranties of fitness for particular purpose or merchantability, nor are any such representations implied with respect to the material set forth herein, and the publisher takes no responsibility with respect to such material. The publisher shall not be liable for any special, consequential, or exemplary damages resulting, in whole or part, from the readers' use of, or reliance upon, this material.

Printed in the United States of America
1 2 3 4 5 6 7 18 17 16 15 14

Contents

Preface

Respiratory care practitioners working with pediatric and perinatal populations are presented with unique challenges in today's rapidly changing health care environment. Respiratory diseases represent a significant and increasing portion of pediatric and perinatal disorders. *Comprehensive Perinatal and Pediatric Respiratory Care*, fourth edition, has been updated and expanded to provide students with the theory and clinical expertise necessary to embark on their careers and meet these changing needs.

In this new edition, we believe that we have responded to the market's need for current and updated information on ventilators and monitors as well as new modes of ventilation. In this rapidly changing and dynamic specialty area, today's special procedures quickly become tomorrow's common techniques, and we have remained steadfast in our desire to provide students with information on equipment and procedures with which they will be working as they enter their careers.

We also understand that students need their textbooks' content to correlate with information that they will find on their certification exams. To that end, the information in the text is designed to correspond with the NBRC content outline for the perinatal/pediatric specialty exam. As in the previous edition, we have incorporated clinical laboratories and checklists directly into the text. Students will continue to have all the necessary tools and visual aids at hand while conducting laboratory exercises. Clinical competencies are included in the text as well and allow students to assess their proficiency with specific skills.

New to This Edition

- **Now in full color**.
- Reorganized into units—content related to neonatal and infant care is grouped in one unit; content related to and pediatric care is in another; general care of all pediatric populations is grouped together; ventilation and oxygenation is one unit; and the final unit focuses on specialized practice areas. All content has been updated with current accepted practices.

Chapter 1

- Expanded discussion of fertilization and conception
- Expanded discussion of the saccular and alveolar stages of lung development
- Added discussion of transition in fetal circulation to extrauterine life

Chapter 2

- Updates where appropriate

Chapter 3

- Added description of medical terminology used during pregnancy
- Expanded discussion of risk factors for premature labor

Chapter 4

- Thoroughly revised and updated to the latest resuscitation standards including a review of S.T.A.B.L.E training.
- Content focused on the neonate. Content for older children is covered in Unit 2.

Chapter 5

- Content focuses on the neonate. Content for older children is covered in Unit 2.

Chapter 6

- Formerly Chapter 7.

Chapter 7

- Formerly Chapter 10.
- Updates throughout where appropriate to treatment and diseases discussed

Chapter 8

- Formerly Chapter 11.
- Discussion of TORCH complex
- Thoroughly updated discussion of HIV
- Expansion of discussion of *Pneumocystis jirovecii*
- Update of the discussion on prevention of infection
- Deleted discussion of diaphragmatic hernia

Chapter 9

- New chapter
- Focuses on resuscitation techniques of the pediatric patient—following American Heart Association standards
- Discusses management of various traumatic injuries common to children and stabilization of those injuries
- Content moved to this chapter from former Chapter 12 includes: epiglottitis, croup, smoke inhalation, chlorine inhalation, and sudden infant death syndrome.

Chapter 10

- Former Chapter 5 was divided into two chapters: one focusing on the assessment of the neonate (now Chapter 5) and one focusing on assessment of the pediatric patient (now Chapter 10)

Chapter 11

- New chapter focusing on the continuing care needs of the pediatric patient.

Chapter 12

- Content moved from this chapter to Chapter 9 includes: epiglottitis, croup, smoke inhalation, chlorine inhalation, and sudden infant death syndrome

Chapter 13

- Formerly Chapter 6

Chapter 14

- Formerly Chapter 8
- Discussion of newer types of drugs on the market has been added

Chapter 15

- Formerly Chapter 9
- Includes discussion of respiratory rate, color, work of breathing, breath sounds, and tactile fremitus

Chapter 16

- Formerly Chapter 13

Chapter 17

- Formerly Chapter 14

Chapter 18

- Formerly Chapter 15

Chapter 19

- Formerly Chapter 16
- Chapter is completely rewritten to discuss the most current ventilators in use today

Chapter 20

- Formerly Chapter 17

Chapter 21

- Formerly Chapter 18

Chapter 22

- Formerly Chapter 19

Chapter 23

- Formerly Chapter 20

The Clinical Case Studies, formerly in Chapter 21, have been adapted into an interactive supplement for the text. This supplement aims to hone the student's critical thinking and problem-solving skills in real-world applications.

Reviewers

Dee Arkell, BS, RRT, CPFT
Director Clinical Education, Respiratory Care
Spokane Community College
Spokane, Washington

Melissa Dearing, BS, RRT-NPS
Professor of Respiratory Care
Lone Star College
Kingwood, Texas

Faye Mathis, RRT, M.Ed.
Program Director
Okefenokee Technical College
Waycross, Georgia

Daneen Nastars, BS, RRT
Clinical Instructor
University of Texas Medical Branch
Galveston, Texas

Ralph Webb, BAS, RRT, RCP
Program Chair Respiratory Therapy
Edgecombe Community College
Rocky Mount, North Carolina

UNIT ONE

The Neonatal Patient

Life is a flame that is always burning itself out,
but it catches fire again every time a child is born.

—*George Bernard Shaw*

Embryologic Development of the Cardiopulmonary System

OBJECTIVES

Upon completion of this chapter, the reader should be able to:

1. Describe the embryology of the morula, blastocyst, blastoderm, and trophoblast.
2. Identify the three germ layers and the body structures that evolve from each.
3. Describe the development of the placenta and umbilical cord and identify the major anatomical structures of each.
4. Explain the function of amniotic fluid and define the following:
   a. Polyhydramnios
   b. Oligohydramnios
5. Identify the five periods of embryonic lung growth and describe the features of each period.
6. Define surface tension and describe the following:
   a. How it is developed
   b. Laplace's law
   c. Application to alveolar mechanics
7. With regard to surfactant, describe the following:
   a. Function and purpose
   b. The approximate gestational age at which immature and mature surfactant appears
   c. Components and methods to detect its presence
   d. How lung maturity is determined
8. Regarding fetal lung fluid, describe the following:
   a. Composition
   b. Function
   c. The hazards of lung fluid retention
9. Describe the embryologic development of the heart including:
   a. Development of the cardiac chambers
   b. Formation of major vessels and cardiac valves

10. With regard to fetal circulation, describe and explain:
    a. The cause of pressure differences between the right and left heart
    b. The flow of blood from the placenta through the body and back to the placenta
    c. Each shunt that is encountered
    d. Transition from fetal to adult circulation
11. Describe the location and function of the baroreceptors and chemoreceptors.

KEY TERMS

amnion	ectoderm	oligohydramnios
baroreceptor	embryo	ovum
blastocyst	endoderm	phosphatidylglycerol
blastoderm	fertilization	phospholipid
blastomere	fetus	polyhydramnios
chemoreceptor	foramen ovale	septum primum
choana	functional residual	sinus venosus
chorionic villi	capacity (FRC)	sphingomyelin
cotyledon	intervillous space	surfactant
dichotomy	mesoderm	transition
ductus arteriosus	morula	trophoblast
ductus venosus	neonate	truncus arteriosus

INTRODUCTION

The purpose of this chapter is to discuss the growth of the fetus from conception to delivery, to explain the physiologic changes that occur throughout this development, and to understand when and why abnormalities may develop during this process. An understanding of embryologic development, allows the respiratory therapist to be better prepared to respond to the needs of the neonate at birth regardless of the gestational age.

BRIEF OVERVIEW OF EMBRYOLOGIC DEVELOPMENT OF THE FETUS

Fertilization, or the union of the sperm cell and the mature ovum, occurs in the outer third of the fallopian tube. From the time of conception, the fetus begins a 40-week process of growth and development that leads to a fully developed baby. In the first month alone, the fetus grows in weight by nearly 3000%.

The duration of human pregnancy is referred to as either 10 lunar months of 4 weeks each, 9 calendar months in which there are 3 trimesters of 3 months each, or 40 weeks, which is the most common time reference in the clinical setting. In this text, gestational age refers to the time since conception.

Development and growth are divided into three distinct stages. The first stage is the period from conception to the completion of implantation or about 12 to 14 days. During this stage of growth and development, the developing organism is called an **ovum**. The first division or cleavage results in two identical cells. Further cleavage of the two cells results in four cells, eight cells, and so forth. The cells that are produced during this rapid cleavage are called **blastomeres** and are surrounded by a transparent tissue envelope, the zona pellucida.

The newly fertilized ovum advances quickly through various stages of growth. Cellular division begins as the ovum travels through the fallopian tube toward the uterus. Entrance into the uterus, roughly a 10 to 13 cm distance, occurs around the fourth or fifth day. Soon, the cells have grown substantially in number and now form a ball, called a **morula**. It is at this stage of growth that the ovum, consisting of 16 to 50 cells, enters the uterus. The zona pellucida is now replaced by an outer layer of cells, called the **trophoblast**. With the loss of the zona pellucida, the trophoblast attaches itself to the lining of the uterus, the endometrium, to receive nourishment. At this point of development, the cells are called a **blastocyst**. This attachment, or implantation, normally occurs in the upper portion of the uterus. Following implantation, the blastocyst becomes completely covered by the endometrium. The trophoblast grows into the endometrial tissue, forming what will become the placenta. The various stages of development up to implantation are illustrated in Figure 1–1.

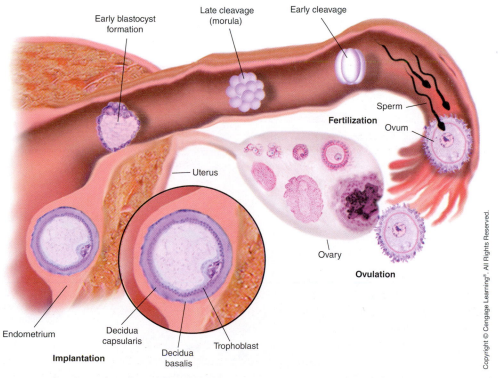

FIGURE 1–1. Stages of embryologic development through implantation.

During the second stage of growth and development, the organism is called an **embryo**. This stage occurs from the end of the ovum stage to the time it measures roughly 3 cm from head to rump or around 54 to 56 days. As the blastocyst continues to expand, some of the cells gather toward one end forming what is known as the **blastoderm** or embryonic disc. The embryonic disc, at this point, includes two layers of cells, the **ectoderm** and the **endoderm**. They are named according to their location, the ectoderm being the outer and thicker layer, and the endoderm being the innermost layer. The third cell layer, known as the **mesoderm**, forms between the other two layers shortly thereafter (Figure 1–2). It is during this stage and from these primary germ layers that all tissues, organs, and organ systems will differentiate. The structures that arise from the three primary germ layers are listed in Table 1–1. The embryo is extremely vulnerable to the effects of drugs, infections, and radiation. Exposure to any of these agents during this period can lead to severe congenital malformations.

During the third stage of growth and development, the organism is called a **fetus**, which is what it will remain until the end of the pregnancy. The major organs have developed and now proceed to grow during this period. Because the organ systems are mostly developed, they are less susceptible to drugs, infections, and radiation. However, exposure may lead to an interruption of normal functional development of the organ systems.

Following delivery, developmental stages in this text are identified by the following terms:

- **Neonate** is used from delivery through the first month of life.
- Infant is used for the period from 1 month to 1 year of life,
- Child identifies the patient above 1 year of age.

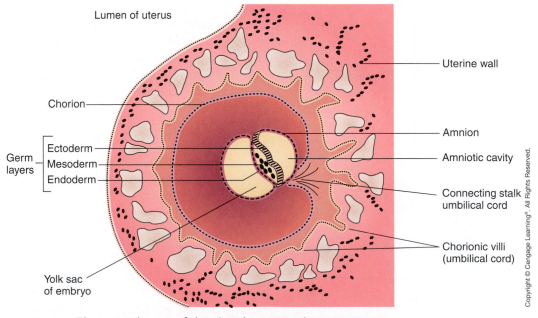

FIGURE 1–2. The germ layers of the developing embryo.

Table 1–1

STRUCTURES ARISING FROM THE THREE GERM LAYERS

Endoderm	Mesoderm	Ectoderm
• Respiratory tract • Epithelium of the digestive tract, bladder, thyroid • Primary tissue of the liver and pancreas	• Dermis • Muscles • Bone, connective tissue, lymphoid tissue • Reproductive organs • Cardiovascular system	• Epidermis • Hair, nails • Lens of the eye • Central and peripheral nervous system • Skin glands

DEVELOPMENT AND FUNCTION OF INTRAUTERINE STRUCTURES

The intrauterine structures include the placenta, the umbilical cord, the amnion, and the amniotic fluid.

Placenta

During the 40 weeks of gestational development, the placenta acts as the organ of respiration for the fetus. It is through the placenta that the growing fetus receives nutrients and oxygen and rids itself of CO_2 and other wastes. Soon after the embryo implants itself in the wall of the uterus, small projections of the trophoblast begin invading the endometrium, not unlike a seed sending roots into the soil. These projections, known as **chorionic villi**, are the beginning of the placenta. The anatomy of the term placenta is illustrated in Figure 1–3.

The villi continue to branch and develop, embedding themselves deeply in the endometrium. Each villus has an outer epithelial layer and an internal connective tissue core that contains the fetal vessels. As the villi continue to expand and grow, the endometrium begins to erode, creating pockets around the villi that will contain the maternal blood. These irregular spaces are known as the **intervillous spaces**.

At term, the normal placenta is round, occupies about one third of the uterine surface, and weighs around 1 pound, or 15% to 20% of the fetal weight at term. The maternal surface contains 15 to 28 segments, known as **cotyledons**. Each cotyledon contains the chorionic villus and an intervillous space.

Blood coming from the fetus follows the two umbilical arteries to the placenta, at which point they branch into smaller and smaller vessels. This branching supplies each cotyledon with a portion of the fetal blood. Upon reaching the cotyledon, the fetal blood advances throughout the branches of the chorionic villi. It is here that the exchange of nutrients, oxygen, CO_2, and waste takes place between maternal and

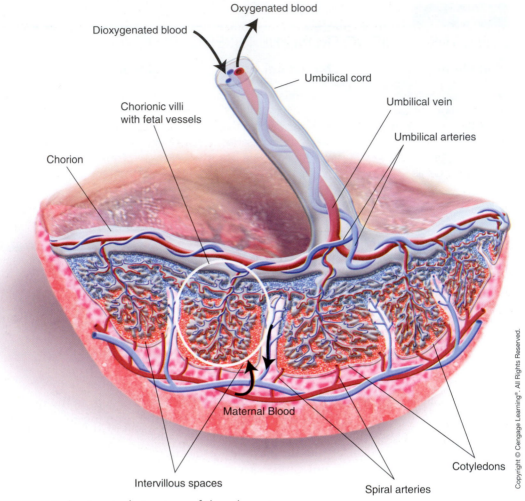

Oxygenated blood

Dioxygenated blood

Umbilical cord

Chorionic villi
with fetal vessels

Umbilical vein

Umbilical arteries

Chorion

Maternal Blood

Intervillous spaces

Spiral arteries

Cotyledons

FIGURE 1–3. Anatomical structurs of the placenta.

fetal blood. There is no contact between the two blood supplies. They are separated by the thin epithelial layer of the villus. This allows passive exchange to proceed quite easily.

The maternal blood enters at the base of the intervillous space by way of spiral-arteries. The maternal arterial blood completely surrounds the chorionic villus, allowing a tremendous surface area for exchange. The fetal blood has high levels of CO_2 and waste materials but is low in oxygen and nutrients. In contrast, the maternal blood has high levels of oxygen and nutrients but is low in CO_2 and waste materials.

Following gradients of high to low concentrations, the fetal blood gets its needed oxygen and nutrients, while giving up the CO_2 and waste to the maternal blood. Maternal blood returns to the mother's venous system by way of venous openings in the chorionic villi, which drain into larger vessels and eventually reach the maternal vena cava.

Fetal blood, now carrying needed oxygen and nutrients, exits the villi through small veins. These veins collect the fetal blood from each cotyledon and return it to the fetus by way of the umbilical vein.

Umbilical Cord

The umbilical cord is the lifeline between mother and fetus. To perform this vital role, the umbilical cord has a unique makeup. A cross section of the umbilical cord (Figure 1–4) reveals three vessels surrounded by a tough, gelatinous material, called Wharton's jelly. Wharton's jelly insulates and protects the umbilical vessels. The three vessels consist of two smaller arteries and one large floppy vein. The umbilical arteries have relatively thick walls, whereas the vein is thin walled.

Because of the constant movement of the fetus in utero, it is possible that the umbilical cord could bend and pinch off, stopping the flow of blood to the infant. The presence of Wharton's jelly prevents this from occurring. While it is flexible enough to allow bending and movement of the cord, it is also rigid enough to prevent the cord from kinking and occluding blood flow. However, as the fetus nears term and has grown significantly in size, there is a possibility for cord compression, which can be life threatening. This is rare, and when it occurs, it is most often during the birthing process. Following delivery, ubrupt temperature changes cause the Wharton's jelly to collapse the umbilical vessels within about 5 minutes.

Amnion

The **amnion** is the sac that surrounds the growing fetus and contains the amniotic fluid. It arises from the trophoblast around the seventh gestational day. It begins as a small vesicle and develops into a sac, which covers the dorsal surface of the embryo. As gestation progresses it enlarges and surrounds the embryo.

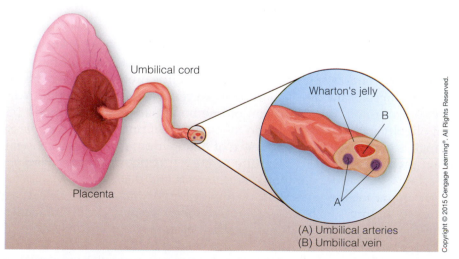

Umbilical cord

Wharton's jelly

B

Placenta

A

(A) Umbilical arteries
(B) Umbilical vein

FIGURE 1–4. Cross-sectional view of the umbilical cord.

Amniotic Fluid

Fluid fills this newly developed sac, called amniotic fluid. The amniotic fluid compartment found early in pregnancy is largely made up of maternal fluids and fluid from the amniotic membrane. The amount of amniotic fluid is greatest at about 34 weeks gestation and averages around 800 mL. The amount slowly diminishes to reach around 600 mL at full term.

Amniotic fluid is dynamic, meaning it is constantly being absorbed and replenished. There are signs that up to about 24 to 26 weeks gestation, when keratinization of the skin occurs, the fetal skin is very permeable to amniotic fluid. Once keratinization has occurred, most of the absorption of the fluid is accomplished by fetal swallowing. The fluid is replenished by a combination of fetal urination and lung fluid. The term fetus swallows around 500 mL per day and excretes about 500 mL of hypotonic urine per day.

Polyhydramnios The amount of amniotic fluid present at birth is dictated by how much the fetus swallows and urinates. Abnormally large amounts of fluid, usually over 2000 mL, indicate hydramnios or **polyhydramnios** which occurs in about 1% of pregnancies. Its presence may indicate a problem with the swallowing mechanism of the fetus. Possible anomalies that may cause hydramnios include: 1) central nervous system (CNS) malformations such as hydrocephalus, microcephaly, anencephaly, spina bifida; 2) orogastric malformations such as esophageal atresia, pyloric stenosis, cleft palate; and 3) disorders such as Down syndrome, congenital heart disease, infants of diabetic mothers, and prematurity. Frequently, the cause of polyhydramnios is undetermined.

The major complication for the fetus with polyhydramnios is the risk of premature rupture of the amniotic membranes. This condition leads to a possible prolapse of the umbilical cord and premature delivery. Other complications include maternal hypertension, maternal urinary tract infections, excessive fetal growth, and heavy bleeding following delivery due to a lack of uterine tone.

Oligohydramnios Scant or decreased amount of amniotic fluid is known as **oligohydramnios**. Causes are usually associated with a defect in the urinary system of the fetus. Often, renal dysplasia or agenesis as well as urethral stenosis are involved. A classic example of the association between renal agenesis and oligohydramnios is Potter's syndrome. Fetal adhesion of one body part to another body part may occur if oligohydramnios develops in the first part of pregnancy. Hypoplasia of the fetal lungs is often seen in the presence of oligohydramnios. Other causes include placental problems, leaking or rupture of the amniotic membranes, and maternal complications such as dehydration, preeclampsia and diabetes.

Implications for the fetus with oligohydramnios include the risk of asphyxia secondary to compression of the umbilical cord and the danger of significant skeletal deformities from intrauterine growth restriction.

Functions of Amniotic Fluid Amniotic fluid serves several important functions, outlined in Table 1–2. First, it allows the fetus to move and grow freely while within

Table 1–2

FUNCTIONS OF AMNIOTIC FLUID

- Protection from traumatic injury

- Thermoregulation

- Facilitation of fetal movement

the confines of the uterus. It offers protection to the fetus by buffering any shock or impact to the maternal abdomen. Amniotic fluid also helps in thermoregulation of the fetus. It allows the mother to go through wide changes in environmental temperature, while maintaining a fairly constant fetal temperature. During labor and delivery, the presence of amniotic fluid helps to dilate and efface the cervix. Amniotic fluid may also aid in metabolism by aiding with the water needs of the infant.

DEVELOPMENT OF THE PULMONARY SYSTEM

The development of the pulmonary system begins soon after conception and continues well into the pediatric years. Recall that there are three distinct fetal development stages, as discussed earlier in this chapter. There are five distinct pulmonary development stages, which occur consecutively throughout the three fetal development stages, as illustrated in Figure 1–5.

Embryonal Stage

The first stage of fetal lung development is called the embryonal stage. This stage of development covers the first eight weeks of gestation. At roughly 21 days, the embryonic disc elongates and becomes broad at the cephalic end and narrow at the caudad end. The endoderm forms a tube-like structure, shaping the future gastrointestinal tract. The ectoderm is also developing into a cylindrical tube, forming the future CNS.

As the primitive gut develops, the upper portion forms the early oral and nasal openings, while the lower segment forms the pharynx and the foregut. The nasal cavities now develop from the ectoderm. The connection of the primitive mouth and the foregut, which will become the alimentary tract, occurs during the fourth gestational week.

The pharynx begins development near day 21, arising from the upper portion of the primitive foregut. A small furrow, known as the laryngotracheal groove, appears at the lower end of the developing pharynx.

The earliest development of the lung begins at 24 days following conception (Figure 1–5A). At this time the lung bud appears as a small pouch, arising from the laryngotracheal groove in the developing pharynx. By day 28, the small pouch

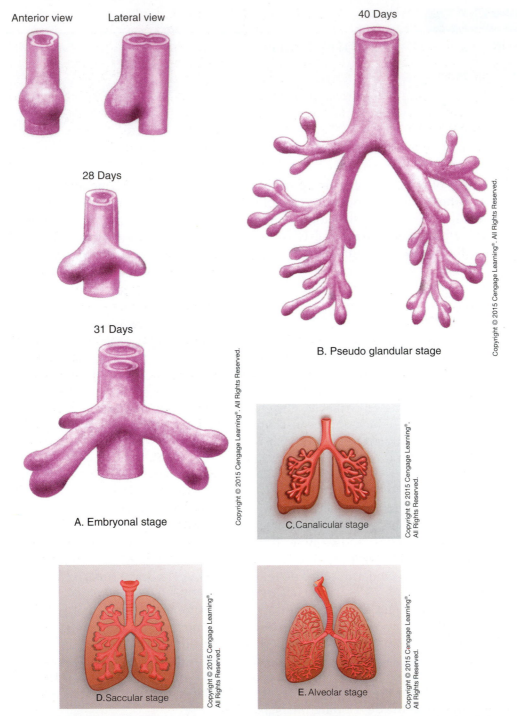

Anterior view   Lateral view

40 Days

28 Days

31 Days

A. Embryonal stage

B. Pseudo glandular stage

C. Canalicular stage

D. Saccular stage

E. Alveolar stage

FIGURE 1–5. A. The embryonal stage of lung development. B. The pseudoglandular stage of lung development. C. The canalicular stage of lung development. D. The saccular stage of lung development. E. The alveolar stage of lung development.

has grown and now branches into the right and left lung buds. As these branches develop, they will become the right and left main stem bronchi. Both the mesoderm and the endoderm develop as the primitive airways progress in their division. The mesodermic tissue becomes the smooth muscle, connective tissue, cartilage, and blood vessels in the mature lungs.

Branching continues with lobar bronchi forming around day 31, dividing into two branches on the left bud and three branches on the right bud. The primitive mesoderm begins to differentiate into its respective muscle, tissue, and vessel formation. It is during this stage that the diaphragm begins its development and is fully formed by the end of 7 weeks. Any incomplete formation of the diaphragm during this stage may result in the development of a congenital diaphragmatic hernia.

Pseudoglandular Stage

The second stage is the pseudoglandular stage, which covers weeks 7 to 16. This stage of lung development is depicted in Figure 1–5B. By week 7 of gestation, the tissue that will form the epiglottis is present. Above the epiglottal tissue, the arytenoid tissues begin developing at about the same time, eventually becoming the opening to the lower airways.

During the seventh gestational week, the membrane that separates the nasal cavity from the oropharynx disintegrates at the **choana**, opening the anterior nasal cavity to the pharynx. Failure of this membrane to disintegrate appropriately results in a blockage known as choanal atresia. Continuing at week 7 the anterior and posterior palates begin to develop, separating the oral and nasal cavities. The palates are completely developed by the end of week 12. The anterior palate eventually becomes ossified and is known as the hard palate. The posterior palate remains soft and, therefore, is known as the soft palate. The area above the soft palate is the portion of the pharynx called the nasopharynx, whereas the area above the hard palate contains the nasal cavities. The vocal cords appear during week 8 as small folds of connective tissue in the larynx and are soon fully developed.

The fetal lung resembles a gland at this point in its development, thus the name pseudoglandular. Lung development during this period results in significant branching, or **dichotomy**. This branching progresses from 4 generations at the beginning of this stage to 25 generations by the end of week 16, with the majority of branching occurring between weeks 10 and 14. Segmental bronchi are present by the end of week 6, followed by the development of the subsegmental bronchi. By week 11, cartilage begins to appear in the airways and continues to form from that time forward. The major lobes of the lungs are identifiable by week 12.

Goblet cells, those that produce airway mucus, form in the human lung during the 13th gestational week. The mucus they produce collects in the upper portion of the cell, causing it to bulge out. This bulging causes the cell to appear as a wine glass or a goblet, hence the name. The goblet cells appear to proliferate in the larger upper airways while remaining in relatively small numbers in the small distal airways.

The bronchial glands begin development during week 13 and complete their development by week 24. Bronchial glands contain mucus-producing cells and serous cells. The bronchial gland secretions appear to contribute more to respiratory tract secretions than do the goblet cells. Ciliated cells appear sometime around week 10 and at birth are found in the airways down to the level of the terminal bronchioles. It is the cilia that move the mucus blanket up the airways, removing lung debris to the point that it can be expectorated out of the system.

Canalicular Stage

The third stage is known as the canalicular stage and covers weeks 17 through 26. During the canalicular stage, the terminal and respiratory bronchioles continue to multiply, as shown in Figure 1–5C. It is during this period that the fetal lung undergoes a tremendous amount of vascularization. As the stage advances, small outpouchings begin appearing along the walls of the respiratory bronchioles, eventually becoming the true alveoli during the alveolar stage.

In these primitive alveoli, the epithelial tissue, which is now capable of producing fetal lung fluid, is beginning to differentiate into its two separate types. Type I will form the alveolar capillary membrane, while the Type II cells will produce pulmonary surfactant. Capillaries are present in proximity to the alveolar cavity during week 20 to 21, but it is not until week 24 to 25 that they are close enough to allow for adequate gas exchange. By this time, smooth muscle has developed around conducting airways and the conducting airways are capable of participating in gas exchange through the thinning air–blood barrier.

Saccular Stage

The fourth stage is termed the saccular stage covering the period from week 26 to approximately 34 to 36 weeks. By week 24 to 26, the lungs are completely formed (Figure 1–5D). However, the terminal airways do not contain true alveoli. Saccules exist where true alveoli will develop during the alveolar stage of pulmonary development. During the saccular stage, the smooth saccules begin to form structures called secondary crests. These secondary crests will eventually grow together forming true alveoli. Secondary crests are highly sensitive to hyperoxia and positive pressure through mechanical ventilation. If damaged, these secondary crests may fail to develop and may prevent further alveolar growth resulting in decreased overall surface area available for gas exchange in lung.

Alveolar Stage

It is difficult to draw a distinct separation between the saccular and alveolar stage as they overlap to some degree (Figure 1–5E). Researchers disagree when true alveoli actually exist. It is argued that true alveoli appear around 32 to 34 weeks, but they may be present as early as 29 weeks according to some researchers. Alveoli develop from a thinning of the terminal air saccules and the increased growth of secondary crests. The number of alveoli at birth ranges from 50 to 150 million and continues to increase until the approximate age of 8 years. It is during the alveolar period that mature pulmonary surfactant is produced in increasing amounts by the Type II alveolar cells.

SURFACE FORCES AND THE ROLE OF SURFACTANT

At this point in development, the lung is capable of functioning as an organ of respiration. For the lung to function properly, however, strong surface forces must be overcome. An understanding of these forces and the role of surfactant in lessening their effect will now be examined.

Surface Tension

A basic understanding of surface tension stems from the knowledge that similar molecules attract each other from all directions. An excellent example of this is to place a drop of water on a hard surface. The water molecules present inside the droplet attract one another from all directions, causing the water to bead. The molecules on the surface, while being drawn together and inward, are not being pulled outward by the air molecules. This causes the surface molecules to be pulled inward and together very tightly, forming a surface tension (Figure 1–6).

Surface tension is what allows a needle to float or a spider to walk across the water's surface. If you could suspend the droplet in mid-air, surface tension would cause the droplet to form a sphere. The constant inward pull of the molecules causes the droplet to retract to its smallest size. This inward pull can only be offset by an equal and opposite pressure from without.

This phenomenon of surface tension also occurs in the alveoli. Because the alveoli are largely liquid and they surround a gas, the same surface forces as described above are present in the alveoli. The surface molecules of the alveolus are attracted

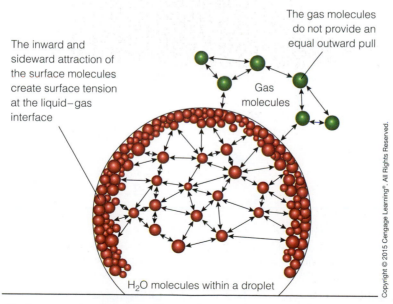

The gas molecules do not provide an equal outward pull

The inward and sideward attraction of the surface molecules create surface tension at the liquid–gas interface

Gas molecules

H_2O molecules within a droplet

FIGURE 1–6. Surface tension is created by surface molecules pulling inward and together.

inward due to the lack of attraction by the gas molecules. This shrinks the alveolus to its smallest diameter.

Laplace's Law

Pierre-Simon de Laplace was a scientist who lived during the late 1700s and early 1800s. He discovered the important relationship between the internal pressure of a sphere, its radius, and surface tension. According to Laplace's law, as the radius of the bubble, or in this case the alveoli, decreases, the surface tension increases (Figure 1–7). An excellent example of Laplace's law is found in a simple balloon. A new, deflated balloon requires a modest amount of pressure to begin inflation, but a balloon that is partially inflated requires much less pressure or force to inflate it further.

Applying this understanding to the alveoli, it should be clear that as the alveoli become smaller, as happens during exhalation, much force is required to reopen them. In this scenario, the work and energy required to inflate the lungs would quickly exhaust energy and lead to death. To overcome this collapsing force, there must be something present on the surface of the alveoli to reduce the amount of tension that develops.

The Role of Surfactant

Surfactant is the substance found on the alveolar wall that lowers surface tension. An understanding of how surfactant lowers surface tension is given in the following example. If we were to mix a surfactant with water, the molecules of the surfactant would attract the water molecules less strongly. This would cause the molecules of surfactant to gather at the surface of the water. At the surface, the weaker attractive force of the surfactant dilutes the attraction of the water molecules and thus weakens surface tension.

The physiologic importance of this is twofold. First, an alveolus that has a lower surface tension requires less counter pressure to keep it open at a smaller radius.

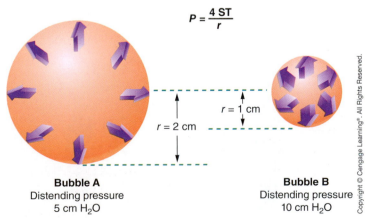

$$P = \frac{4\,ST}{r}$$

$r = 1$ cm

$r = 2$ cm

Bubble A
Distending pressure
5 cm H_2O

Bubble B
Distending pressure
10 cm H_2O

FIGURE 1–7. LaPlace's law. As the radius of the alveoli decreases, the surfance tension increases.

Therefore, less muscle effort is required to open and ventilate the lungs. Second, the effect of surfactant changes as the surface area of the alveoli changes. In the lung, there are many different sizes of alveoli. If surfactant does not change its influence as the alveoli change in size, then many different pressures would need to be present in the lungs to keep the different alveoli from collapsing.

Due to its unique composition and the fact that the amount remains stable in the alveoli, surfactant exerts varying influence on alveoli as they enlarge and shrink (Figure 1–8). As the alveoli are stretched during inspiration, the surfactant thins on the surface and tension builds. This aids in the process of passive exhalation, allowing surface tension to constrict the alveoli back down to a small size. As the alveoli become smaller, the surfactant thickens on the alveolar surface, weakening surface tension and preventing the alveoli from collapsing.

Appearance and Production of Surfactant

The first appearance of pulmonary surfactant coincides with the development of Type II pneumocytes. Surfactant is composed of **phospholipids** (mainly phosphatidylcholine [PC] and **phosphatidylglycerol** [PG]), neutral lipids, and proteins. After being produced, the surfactant is stored in the cell in what are known as lamellar

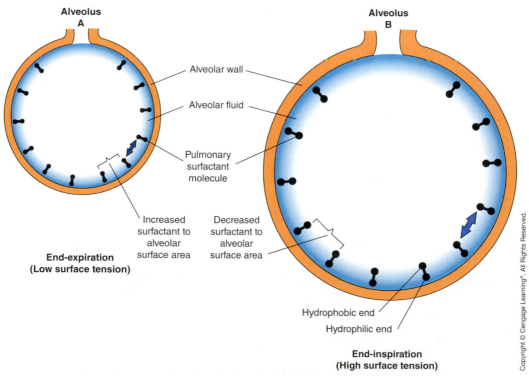

FIGURE 1–8. Effects of surfactant on surface tension of the alveoli.

inclusion bodies. The first surfactant to be produced lacks PG and is termed immature surfactant. This is first seen at approximately 24 weeks gestation.

During this early stage, surfactant production is easily inhibited by hypoxia, hypothermia, and acidosis. Babies born prematurely, especially those of less than 30 weeks, are extremely prone to both of these disorders. The result is a rapid deterioration in the respiratory status following delivery, commonly called respiratory distress syndrome (RDS). Mature surfactant is present around week 35, at which time PG appears.

Measurement of Fetal Surfactant and Determination of Lung Maturity

From the time the immature surfactant first appears, it can be measured in a sample of amniotic fluid. Fluid produced by the lungs contributes to the amniotic fluid. Some of the surface-active phospholipids excreted by the alveolar cells are carried to the amniotic fluid by the lung fluid. Lung maturity can be predicted by withdrawing a sample of amniotic fluid and comparing the level of PC (also called lecithin) to the level of **sphingomyelin** in the amniotic fluid. Sphingomyelin is another type of phospholipid produced by the fetus that remains at a fairly stable level in the amniotic fluid throughout gestation. By comparing the levels of each in the amniotic fluid, a quick determination of fetal lung maturity is possible. This comparison is called the lecithin-to-sphingomyelin ratio (L/S ratio) (Figure 1–9).

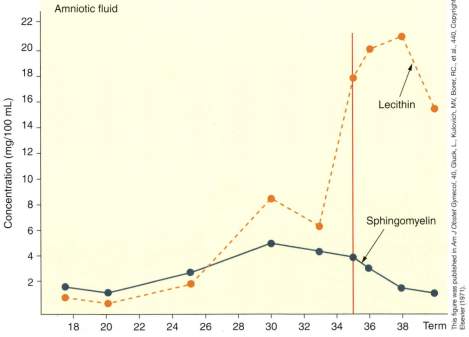

FIGURE 1–9. The comparison of lecithin-to-sphingomyelin concentrations, plotted against gestational age.

The fetal lungs are considered mature when the L/S ratio reaches 2:1; in other words, there is twice as much lecithin as sphingomyelin. This 2:1 ratio occurs near week 35 of gestation. The achievement of the 2:1 ratio usually coincides with the onset of mature surfactant production and indicates little chance of developing in RDS.

As gestation progresses, surfactant production is enhanced. As previously mentioned, PG is produced as surfactant production reaches maturity.

This fact has led to the practice of testing amniotic fluid for the presence of PG, as well as for determining L/S ratio, as a better determinant of fetal lung maturity. The combination of L/S ratio and testing for PG is called the lung profile. Studies have demonstrated that the lung profile is a better predictor of lung maturity than either the L/S ratio or PG detection when used alone. Many factors can either delay or accelerate the production of mature surfactant. Those factors are listed in Table 1–3.

Another relatively simple method of determining lung maturity is by a test known as shake or foam test. This procedure is done by mixing amniotic fluid with ethanol which is then shaken for 15 seconds. A reading is made 15 minutes later. If there is a ring of bubbles in the ethanol after 15 minutes, it shows there is enough lecithin present to create a stable foam. This technique is a fairly reliable way of

---

Table 1–3

CONDITIONS THAT DELAY OR ACCELERATE SURFACTANT PRODUCTION IN THE FETUS

Conditions that delay surfactant production:
- Acidosis
- Hypoxia
- Shock
- Overinflation
- Underinflation
- Pulmonary edema
- Mechanical ventilation
- Hypercapnia
- Infants of diabetic mothers classes A, B, and C
- Erythroblastosis fetalis
- The smaller of twins

Conditions that accelerate surfactant production:
- Infants of mothers with gestational diabetes
- Maternal heroin addiction
- Premature rupture of membranes
- Maternal hypertension
- Maternal infection
- Placental insufficiency
- Maternal administration of betamethasone or thyroid hormone
- Abruptio placentae

determining fetal lung maturity. If foam is not present following the 15-minute period, an L/S ratio should be performed.

There are several techniques that have been successful in predicting fetal lung maturity. The concentration of lamellar bodies in the amniotic fluid has compared favorably to the lung profile in its ability to predict lung maturity. Another screening test, the amniotic fluid surfactant-albumin ratio (SAR), has been shown to be accurate in clinical studies. A third test, called the TDx-FLM assay, also can be used to predict RDS with as much reliability as the lung profile. Finally, the fluorescence polarization (FP) assay has been shown to accurately predict RDS.

Studies by Liggins and Howie that were done on fetal lung surfactant led to the discovery that lung maturation can be artificially induced.[1] These studies show that the administration of glucocorticoids to women in premature labor increases the rate of lung maturity and decreases the incidence of RDS. The limitations of this method require administration of the drug when the fetus is between 27 and 34 weeks gestation, it needs to be given at least 48 hours before delivery, and delivery is recommended within 7 days of administration.

Other factors influencing lung maturation include thyroxine, thyrotropin-releasing hormone, β-adrenergic drugs, estrogen, prolactin, and epidermal growth factor.[2]

The role of surfactant is vital. Its presence enhances capillary circulation allowing for normal ventilation/perfusion ratios. It may also offer protection to the alveolar tissues against barotrauma. Through its ability to lower surface tension, increase lung compliance, and provide stable alveoli for ventilation, its presence aids in the evacuation of lung fluids.

The lack of surfactant in the lung or the deterioration of its production following birth is the leading cause of pulmonary complications in the neonate. When surfactant is not present, the lungs become stiff, noncompliant organs. Every breath requires tremendous energy. The unassisted neonate will soon deplete his or her energy stores and die from hypoxia and hypoventilation. With the disruption of the normal mechanisms of surfactant production in premature infants, the administration of surfactant results in a reduction of these lung complications. Following much trial and error, an adequate surfactant was developed. The circumstances surrounding its development and use are discussed in Chapter 20.

FETAL LUNG FLUID

The fetal lung, being a metabolically active organ and acting somewhat similar to a gland, produces and secretes its own fluid. At term, the lung is filled with about 20 to 30 mL/kg of fluid, or roughly the equivalent volume of the **functional residual capacity (FRC)**, which is the volume of air that remains in the lungs at the end of a normal, passive exhalation. The total amount of lung fluid produced per day is approximately 250 to 300 mL. During normal fetal breathing movements, fetal lung fluid moves steadily at a rate of approximately 15 mL/hour outward from the lung through the trachea and is excreted through the mouth into the amniotic fluid or it is swallowed by the fetus. It is by this mechanism that lung surfactant can be measured in an amniotic sample.

Composition

Fetal lung fluid is of a different composition than is amniotic fluid. It has lower pH, protein, and bicarbonate, but higher concentrations of sodium and chloride. Lung fluid appears early in gestation and continues to generate until shortly before delivery, at which time production ceases.

Function

It is apparent that the lung fluid has multiple functions. One of its earliest functions is to maintain the patency of the developing airways. It also appears to play an important role in the formation, size, and shape of potential air spaces. As the lungs grow and develop, it would be difficult for them to develop their complicated structures if they were collapsed. In order for ventilation to proceed unhindered in the neonate, it is important that the lung fluid be completely evacuated from the lungs at birth. This takes place by a variety of methods. If the fetus is delivered vaginally, one third of the fluid is removed by the squeezing of the thorax as the fetus descends through the maternal pelvis. Most of the remaining lung fluid is rapidly absorbed by the pulmonary lymphatic system. This absorption takes place within a few hours following delivery.

Hazards of Lung Fluid Retention

It is not uncommon for neonates delivered by cesarean section to retain a larger amount of lung fluid. This is primarily due to the lack of the squeezing action on the thorax that occurs during a vaginal delivery. In these neonates, the fluid must be rapidly absorbed in order for breathing to progress. Positive pressure ventilation has been shown to distend the interstitial spaces, possibly enhancing the absorption and uptake of the fluid. Neonates who fail to remove the lung fluid adequately are prone to a syndrome known as transient tachypnea of the newborn (TTN) or RDS type II. TTN is fairly common in babies delivered by cesarean section, for reasons outlined above. TTN is discussed in more detail in Chapter 7.

DEVELOPMENT OF THE CARDIOVASCULAR SYSTEM

The importance of the heart to the growth and development of the fetus can be shown by the speed at which it develops. The heart is the first major organ to develop and is fully formed and functional by the eighth gestational week. This rapid development is primarily due to the tremendous growth of the fetus and its nutritional needs. Any development of congenital cardiac anomalies or malformations occurs during this period. It is important to note that although the maternal blood supply provides the fetus with nutrients and gas exchange, there is no communication between maternal and fetal blood. This is discussed in greater detail later in this chapter. Figure 1–10 illustrates the development of the heart and associated structures.

Early Embryologic Development

Indistinct clumps of cells appear from the mesoderm around gestational day 21. By the end of the third week, these cells have formed two tubes surrounded by a sheath of myocardial cells. The tubes begin to fuse at their center and soon form a single, continuous chamber. As early as the fourth week, the heart begins to beat. This early embryonic heart begins a twisting and folding that will eventually form the four heart chambers.

The bottom of the fetal heart begins swelling into a small cavity and contains a pair of branches known as horns. These horns are called the **sinus venosus** and will

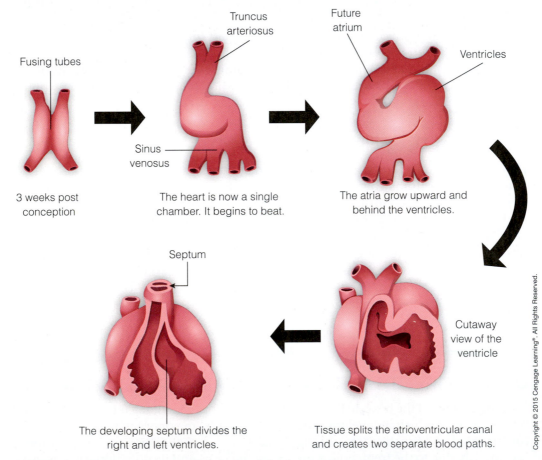

FIGURE 1–10. Embryologic development of the heart.

eventually become the inferior and superior vena cava and a portion of the right atrium. At the top of this small cavity, the primitive ventricle and atrium appear. A hollow tube of myocardium, the **truncus arteriosus**, grows from this primitive ventricle. The truncus arteriosus will develop into the pulmonary artery and the aorta. At this point, the heart appears as a bulging, hollow tube.

Development of the Cardiac Chambers

The heart now begins to bend in the middle, forming itself into a rough S shape. As the heart continues its rapid growth, the sinus venosus and the atrium are pushed upward behind the developing ventricle. The single ventricle divides into the right and left ventricles by splitting at the center of the S. The internal chambers are identified on the outer surface by the presence of grooves, called sulci.

The blood, which began flowing around the third week, now begins a one-way flow instead of its back and forth motion. The blood enters through the sinus venosus and travels through the primitive atrium, the left and right ventricles, and out through the truncus arteriosus. By the beginning of the fifth week, the embryonic heart no longer looks like an S, but now has assumed the shape of the adult heart.

In the uppermost portion of the heart, the developing veins and arteries couple the heart to the expanding circulatory system. The single atrium divides into two separate chambers by the emergence of a tissue known as the **septum primum**. During this division, tissue growth stemming from the front and back walls of the heart forms the openings between the atria and ventricles. The truncus arteriosus allows blood to exit the right ventricle and is the only outlet for blood.

Formation of Major Vessels and Cardiac Valves

During the sixth week the truncus is divided into two vessels by a thin tissue that spirals down the center of the truncus. These two vessels are the pulmonary artery and the aorta. This tissue continues to grow, eventually separating the right and left ventricles completely. The newly formed aorta is now the escape route for blood in the left ventricle, and the pulmonary artery provides the outlet for the right ventricle.

During this time, the valves begin to form between the atria and ventricles as well as in the root of both the pulmonary artery and aorta. In two short months, the heart has formed and begins pumping and circulating blood, a tiny replica of an adult heart.

FETAL CIRCULATION

Fetal circulation refers to the unique system of shunts and pressures that are found in the fetal circulatory system. It is important to understand and identify the flow of blood in the fetus. Of equal importance is to understand *why* the blood follows the peculiar fetal path.

The pressures found inside the fetal vasculature are the reverse of those found in the adult. Pressures in the right, or venous system, are higher than those in the left, or arterial system. There are two reasons for this.

First, during the development of the fetus, the growing lungs provide a very high resistance to blood flow. This high resistance is secondary to pulmonary vasculature constriction caused by the low PaO_2 in the fetal blood and also by the fact that the lungs are for the most part collapsed. The collapsed lungs exert a high external force on the pulmonary vasculature, decreasing their size and increasing resistance to blood flow. The high pulmonary vascular pressures result in increased pressures in the pulmonary artery. This increases pressure in the right ventricle, right atrium, vena cava, and so forth, throughout the venous system.

The second cause of the reversal of blood pressures is the fact that the placenta offers very little resistance to blood flow. Because of the enormous amount of vasculature in the placenta, the blood flows to the placenta with relative ease. The low resistance of the placenta causes low pressures in the aorta, left ventricle, left atrium, and the entire arterial system. The combination of these two factors causes the reversal of pressures found in the fetus. With that understanding we can now look at fetal blood flow.

Blood Flow and Shunts in Fetal Circulation

Fetal circulation is depicted in Figure 1–11. After the fetal blood has received its oxygen and nutrients from the placenta, it collects into progressively larger and larger vessels until it arrives at the umbilical vein. The umbilical vein carries the fresh blood from the placenta through the umbilical cord and into the fetus.

Ductus Venosus Soon after the blood enters the abdominal cavity, the first shunt is encountered—the **ductus venosus**. Upon reaching the liver, roughly 50% to 70% of the blood flow is directed through branches of the umbilical vein into the liver. The remaining 30% to 50% of the blood flow is diverted directly into the inferior vena cava through the ductus venosus. The ductus venosus is merely a continuation of the umbilical vein, which connects to the inferior vena cava.

The shunted blood mixes with blood returning from the lower extremities. This mixing causes a reduction in the total oxygen saturation of the blood. The venous blood from the extremities is true venous blood with a low oxygen content. The mixed blood continues toward the right atrium. Upon entering the right atrium, the blood mixes with the venous return of the superior vena cava. It is at this point that the second shunt is met.

Foramen Ovale An opening between the right and left atrium is present in the atrial septum. This opening is the second shunt, known as the **foramen ovale**. With pressures being higher in the right atrium than in the left and due to the location of where the inferior vena cava attaches to the right atrium, most of the oxygenated blood that enters the right atrium shunts through the foramen ovale into the left atrium. On the left atrial surface of the foramen ovale is a tissue flap, which acts as a

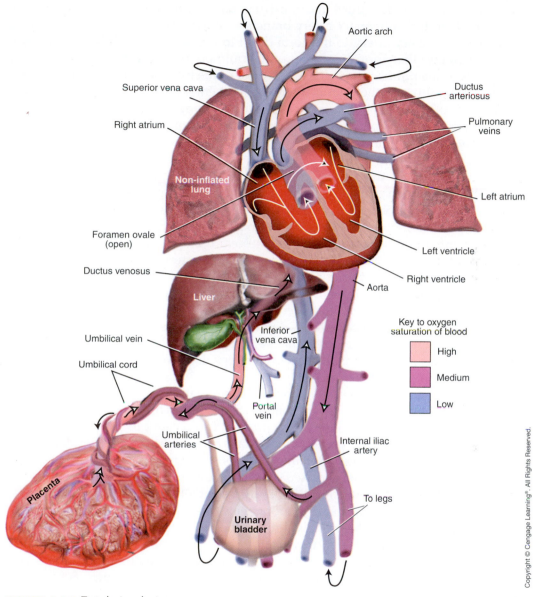

FIGURE 1–11. Fetal circulation.

one-way valve. After birth, as pressure inside the left atrium increases and becomes greater than that in the right, the flap is held closed mechanically, preventing blood from shunting back into the right atrium.

    The remaining blood, which did not pass through the foramen ovale, enters the right ventricle. Because of the anatomy of the right atrium, most of this blood comes from the superior vena cava. From the right ventricle, the blood passes through the pulmonary artery toward the lungs.

Ductus Arteriosus The third and most familiar shunt, the **ductus arteriosus**, is located where the pulmonary artery branches into the lung. The ductus arteriosus joins the pulmonary artery to the aorta distal to the aortic arch. It is a short vessel with a diameter that approaches that of the pulmonary artery. Because of the high resistance in the pulmonary vasculature, most of the blood entering the pulmonary artery passes through the ductus arteriosus and enters the aorta. This leaves only 13% to 25% of the total blood supply to perfuse the lungs, which is greater than previously thought. The blood flow to the pulmonary system at this point serves mainly to perfuse the developing lungs.

Blood Flow beyond the Heart The blood that shunts from the right to left atrium through the foramen ovale enters the left ventricle. From there it passes into the aorta, where it combines with the flow from the ductus arteriosus. As it travels through the aorta, some of the blood exits to perfuse the upper extremities, the kidneys, the gut, and other abdominal organs. Near the upper pelvic region, the aorta splits into the two common iliac arteries. The iliac arteries further divide into the external and internal iliac arteries. It is from the internal iliac arteries that the two umbilical arteries branch. Roughly 50% of fetal blood resides in the vascular surface of the placenta. Throughout fetal circulation, between 17% and 33% of blood flow passes through the umbilical arteries depending upon gestational age, returning to the placenta to participate in gas exchange, waste removal, and to pick up nutrients essential to the growing fetus. The cycle then repeats itself.

Transition to Extrauterine Life During fetal circulation, systemic blood pressure is much lower than blood pressure in adult circulation. This is due to the presence of the placenta as part of the circulatory process. Upon clamping the umbilical cord following delivery, the low-pressure placenta is removed from the circulation process. This immediately causes systemic blood pressure to rise. It also causes a drop in right heart pressures. The increased systemic pressure backs up through the aorta into the left side of the heart, resulting in increased left atrial pressure over that of right atrial pressure, thus causing the foramen ovale to close. The increase in aortic pressure also reduces the blood flow through the ductus arteriosus and forces blood flow from the right ventricle to travel into the lower pressure pulmonary system, where it will participate in gas exchange. Closure of the ductus arteriosus occurs slowly over the next 96 hours with 20% closure in the first 24 hours, 80% closure within 48 hours, and 100% closure by 96 hours (Figure 1–12). If closure of the ductus arteriosus doesn't occur as planned, medical and surgical interventions are available; this is discussed further in Chapter 9.

Simultaneously, the neonate is taking initial breaths that stimulate pulmonary changes such as the initiation of gas exchange. As the neonate inspires, pulmonary vessels respond to the oxygen that is present in the inspired gas by dilating, thus reducing pulmonary artery pressures and also reducing right heart pressures. Stretch receptors stimulate vasodilating agents that assist in pulmonary vasodilation. There are also vasoconstricting agents that exist during fetal circulation that are inhibited upon lung inflation.

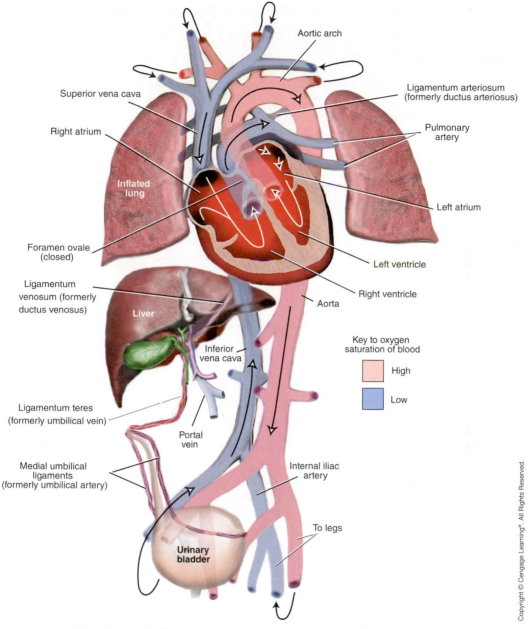

FIGURE 1–12. Newborn circulation.

This change from fetal circulation to adult circulation is referred to as **transition**. Most neonates transition very easily and without complication, however some neonates require assistance to make this transition safely. Further discussion of resuscitation will be discussed in Chapter 4.

THE DEVELOPMENT OF BARORECEPTORS AND CHEMORECEPTORS

Barorecepters, otherwise known as stretch receptors, stimulate bradycardia and hypotension, while chemoreceptors, which are sensitive to PaO_2, $PaCO_2$, and pH, play a role in regulation of ventilation.

Baroreceptors

Baroreceptors, which have the ability to detect changes in pressure, are located in the bifurcation of the carotid arteries and in the aortic arch. These receptors are actually stretch receptors and are stimulated as they are stretched or distorted in shape. Stimulation of these receptors leads to bradycardia and hypotension. Whether baroreceptors are active during fetal life or not is a subject of controversy. The progressive rise in arterial pressure during gestation, as well as the sudden increase in blood pressure and fall in heart rate that follow clamping of the cord, may show that these reflexes are present to some degree in the fetus and neonate.

Chemoreceptors

Chemoreceptors, although present in the fetus, are not generally active. Immaturity of the carotid sinus synapses found in the CNS may be one cause of this inactivity. Chemoreceptors are located in the carotid arteries and aorta and are called carotid and aortic bodies. Because of their sensitivity to PaO_2, $PaCO_2$, and pH, their role is in regulation of ventilation. They also have a function in the initiation of the first breath. This will be covered in Chapter 3.

SUMMARY

The embryologic development of the fetus is an extraordinary event that begins with two cells and finishes as a fully developed child with all of the intricacies of the body systems in place. The lungs, which develop from the endoderm, begin development at 24 days with the appearance of a small outpouching on the primitive foregut. The lungs undergo five stages of growth and development, called the embryonal stage, the pseudoglandular stage, the canalicular stage, the saccular stage and finally, the alveolar stage. While most lung structures are completely developed by 40 weeks, alveoli continue to increase in number for roughly the first 8 years of life.

Because the alveoli have a liquid-air interface, they are subject to surface tension which, if allowed to remain, would make normal breathing impossible. According to Laplace's law, surface tension increases as the size of the alveoli shrinks, making each successive breath more difficult, resulting in RDS. Surfactant, produced by Type II alveolar cells and stored in lamellar bodies, is secreted onto the surface of each alveoli and lowers surface tension to the point that breathing is not hindered. Fetal lung maturity can be detected by several methods, including the L/S ratio, the presence of PG in the amniotic fluid, the shake test, the concentration of lamellar bodies in amniotic fluid, the surfactant–albumin ratio, the TDx-FLM assay, and the fluorescence polarization assay. Certain drugs and hormones have been shown to influence lung maturation, including glucocorticoids, thyroxine, thyrotropin-releasing hormone, β-adrenergic drugs, estrogen, prolactin, and epidermal growth factor.

The placenta is the fetal organ of respiration. Maternal arterial blood enters the intervillous spaces that surround the chorionic villi carrying the fetal blood. At that point, an exchange of oxygen, carbon dioxide, and nutrients takes place following concentration gradients. Blood flows from the placenta to the fetus via a large umbilical vein and is returned to the placenta through two umbilical arteries.

Amniotic fluid is constantly being swallowed and absorbed and replenished through fetal urination and lung fluid. It serves several vital purposes for the developing fetus. It allows free fetal movement, protects the fetus from injury, and aids in thermoregulation. At delivery, it helps to dilate and efface the cervix. Too much amniotic fluid (polyhydramnios) or too little fluid (oligohydramnios) may indicate possible fetal anomalies and may expose the fetus to other risks.

The heart is the first major organ to be developed, starting to beat at roughly 4 weeks gestation and is fully formed by 8 weeks. Blood flow in the fetus follows a unique series of shunts in the fetus, known as fetal circulation. The first shunt encountered is the ductus venosus, followed by the foramen ovale and, finally, the ductus arteriosus. Blood flow is directed through the shunts due to a reversal of the typical pressures found in the cardiovascular system, that is, high pressure in the right heart, low pressure in the left heart. Following delivery and the clamping of the umbilical cord, fetal circulation transitions to extrauterine or adult circulation.

The fetal lung produces fluid throughout gestation, which helps maintain the size, shape, and patency of airways and spaces. Normally expulsed during vaginal delivery, lung fluid may be retained following delivery by cesarean section and may lead to a syndrome called TTN.

With this brief look at fetal development, the respiratory therapist is more able to understand the complex problems associated with premature delivery and is better able to treat these tiny patients.

POSTTEST

1. At what stage of embryologic development does the ovum enter the uterus?
    a. zygote
    b. morula
    c. blastocyst
    d. blastoderm

2. The respiratory system arises from which of the following germ layers?
   a. endoderm
   b. mesoderm
   c. ectoderm
   d. myeloderm
3. The earliest development of the lung begins at:
   a. conception
   b. 24 days
   c. 36 days
   d. 8 weeks
4. Dichotomy of the airways occurs during which phase of lung development?
   a. embryonic
   b. pseudoglandular
   c. canalicular
   d. alveolar
5. Which of the following statements best describes surface tension?
   a. diffusion of similar molecules following concentration gradients
   b. the inward movement of surface molecules due to kinetic energy
   c. the tendency of a liquid surface to contract
   d. the attraction of surface water molecules to gas molecules
6. Which of the following, when found in amniotic fluid, is the best indicator of fetal lung maturity?
   a. PC
   b. lecithin
   c. sphingomyelin
   d. PG
7. Which of the following does not appear to accelerate fetal lung maturation?
   a. thyroxine
   b. estrogen
   c. aternal preeclampsia
   d. prolactin
8. Which of the following are true concerning lung fluid?
   I.   There is approximately 20 to 30 mL/kg present at birth.
   II. At term, it is produced at a rate of 2 to 4 mL/kg/hr.
   III. It has lower pH, protein, and bicarbonate levels than amniotic fluid.
   IV. It has lower sodium and chloride concentrations than amniotic fluid.
   V.   It maintains the patency of the developing airways.
       a. I, III, V
       b. II, IV, V
       c. I, II, III, V
       d. I, II, III, IV
9. Which of the following may occur following Cesarean section?
   a. RDS
   b. TTN
   c. diaphragmatic hernia
   d. aspiration pneumonia

10. The heart develops from which germ layer(s)?
    a. endoderm
    b. mesoderm
    c. ectoderm
    d. myeloderm
11. The embryologic truncus arteriosus develops into:
    I. the vena cava
    II. the pulmonary artery
    III. the atria
    IV. the aorta
    V. the right and left ventricles
        a. IV, V
        b. I, III
        c. I, II, III
        d. II, IV
12. Which of the following describes the path of blood that is shunted through the foramen ovale?
    a. from the umbilical vein to the inferior vena cava
    b. from the right to left atrium
    c. from the right to left ventricle
    d. from the iliac artery to the umbilical artery
13. The ductus arteriosus shunts blood from:
    a. the pulmonary artery to the aorta
    b. the right to left atrium
    c. the umbilical vein to the inferior vena cava
    d. the right to left ventricle
14. Which of the following statements is correct?
    a. Baroreceptors are not active during fetal life.
    b. Baroreceptors sense changes in PaO_2, pH, and $PaCO_2$.
    c. Baroreceptors are actually stretch receptors.
    d. Baroreceptors are instrumental in the initiation of the first breath.
15. In the placenta, the fetal vessels are contained in the
    a. intervillous space
    b. cotyledon
    c. spiral arteries
    d. chorionic villi

16. Identify the umbilical vein(s) on the following diagram by circling the correct letter.

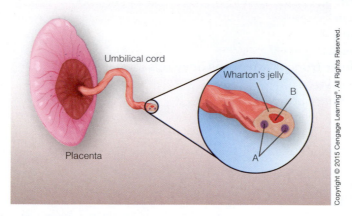

17. Polyhydramnios is defined as
    a. an absence of amniotic fluid
    b. a decreased amount of amniotic fluid
    c. infection of the amniotic fluid
    d. an excessive amount of amniotic fluid
18. Which of the following are possible causes of polyhydramnios?
    I. hydrocephalus
    II. esophageal atresia
    III. choanal atresia
    IV. Down syndrome
    V. cleft palate
        a. II, III, IV, V
        b. I, II, IV
        c. I, II, IV, V
        d. I, II, III, IV, V

REFERENCES

1. Liggins CG, Howie RN. A controlled trial of antepartum glucocorticoid treatment for prevention of the respiratory distress syndrome in premature infants. *Pediatrics.* 50, 1972.
2. Avery GB, Fletcher MA, MacDonald MG. *Pathophysiology and Management of the Newborn.* 6th ed. Philadelphia, PA: JB Lippincott Co., 2005.

BIBLIOGRAPHY AND SUGGESTED READINGS

Assali NS. *Biology of Gestation.* Vol 1, II. New York, NY: Academic Press, 1968.
American Thoracic Society. Mechanisms and limits of postnatal lung growth. *American journal of respiratory and critical care medicine.* 170:319–343, 2004.

Bayer-Zwirello LA, et al. Amniotic fluid surfactant-albumin ration as a screening test for fetal lung maturity. Two years of clinical experience. *J Perinatol.* 13, 1993.

Beachey W. *Respiratory Care Anatomy and Physiology, Foundations for Clinical Practice.* 3rd ed. St. Louis: Mosby, Inc., 2013.

Blackburn J, Loper D. *Maternal, Fetal, and Neonatal Physiology, a Clinical Perspective.* 4th ed. Philadelphia: Saunders, 2012.

Burton G, Hodgkin J, Ward J. *Respiratory Care: A Guide to Clinical Practice.* 4th ed. Philadelphia: Lippincott-Raven Publishers, 1997.

Chen C, et al. Clinical evaluations of the NBD-PC fluorescence polarization assay for prediction of fetal lung maturity. *Obstet Gynecol.* 80, 1992.

Comroe JH. *Physiology of Respiration.* Chicago, IL: Year Book Medical Publishers Inc.,1965.

Cottrell GP. *Cardiopulmonary Anatomy and Physiology for Respiratory Care Practitioners.* Philadelphia, PA: FA Davis, 2002.

Des Jardins T. *Cardiopulmonary Anatomy and Physiology.* 6th ed. Clifton Park, NY: Cengage Learning, 2012.

Fakhoury G, et al. Lamellar body concentrations and the prediction of fetal pulmonary maturity. *Am J Obstet Gynecol.* 170: 1(pt 1), 1994.

Hagen E, et al. A comparison of the accuracy of the TDx-FLM assay, lecithin-sphingomyelin ratio, and phosphatidylglycerol in the prediction of neonatal respiratory distress syndrome. *Obstet Gynecol.* 82, 1993.

Harker LC, et al. Improving the prediction of surfactant deficiency in very low-birth-weight infants with respiratory distress. *J Perinatol.* 12, 1992.

Herbert WN, et al. Role of the TDx-FLM assay in fetal lung maturity. *J AM Obstet Gynecol.* 168: 3(pt 1), 1993.

Klaus MH, Fanaroff AA. *Care of the High Risk Neonate.* 5th ed. Philadelphia, PA: WB Saunders, 2001.

Larsen WJ. *Essentials of Human Embryology.* Philadelphia, PA: Churchill Livingstone, 1998.

Lozon MM. *Emergency Pediatric Management.* Philadelphia, PA: WB Saunders, 2000.

Lowdermilk DL, Perry SE, Cashion, MC. *Maternity Nursing.* 8th ed. St. Louis: Mosby, Inc., 2011.

Schiff E, et al. Fetal lung maturity is not accelerated in preeclamptic pregnancies. *Am J Obstet Gynecol.* 169, 1993.

West J. *The Essentials of Respiratory Physiology.* 9th ed. Philadelphia, PA: Lippincott, Williams & Wilkins, 2011.

CHAPTER 2

Assessment of Fetal Growth and Development

OBJECTIVES

Upon completion of this chapter, the reader should be able to:

1. Describe at least three ways ultrasonography is used to assess fetal age.
2. Define amniocentesis and describe the role of each of the following:
   a. L/S ratio
   b. Determination of alpha-fetoprotein
   c. Bilirubin level
   d. Creatinine level
   e. Identification of meconium staining
   f. Cytologic examination of cells
3. Describe three different methods of measuring fetal heart rate (FHR).
4. Describe the cause and/or characteristics of the following:
   a. Baseline heart rate
   b. Beat-to-beat variability
   c. Bradycardia
   d. Tachycardia
   e. Accelerations
   f. Decelerations
5. Explain how fetal scalp pH is used to assess fetal asphyxia.
6. List and describe the five methods used to estimate the date of delivery.
7. Compare and contrast the contraction stress test (CST) and the nonstress test (NST). Describe how each test is performed, as well as their advantages and disadvantages.
8. Describe the use of vibroacoustic stimulation, fetal movements, and amniotic fluid volume as methods of assessing fetal well-being.
9. Describe the five tests used in the biophysical profile and how each is scored.
10. Explain the implications of meconium-stained amniotic fluid in assessing fetal status.
11. Describe chorionic villus sampling, cordocentesis, and magnetic resonance imaging in assessing fetal status.
12. Compare and contrast material estriol determination and human placental lactogen (HPL) levels as to their roles in determining fetal status.
13. Identify and list at least five factors that indicate a high-risk pregnancy.

KEY TERMS

alpha-fetoprotein (AFP)	fundus	meconium
amniocentesis	human placental	meningomyelocele
anencephaly	lactogen (HPL)	tocodynamometer
estriol		

INTRODUCTION

Prior to the late 1960s and early 1970s, the attitudes of medical professionals in terms of neonatal medicine was one of "live and let die." If an infant developed health issues in utero or after birth, there was generally little that could be done except take a wait and see approach for health care. The fetus was clearly an unknown and/or uninspected entity inside the mother's abdomen with little attention paid to its well-being other than the obvious physical notations of external growth and development.

As medicine advanced with new technologies and improved understanding of the unborn fetus, we entered a new era in neonatal medicine. The fetus is now treated like a patient, and concern for its well-being begins from the time of conception.

Modern technology has made it possible to monitor many aspects of the fetus. In this chapter, we will look at some of the technology now available to assess fetal development and well-being.

MODALITIES TO ASSESS FETAL STATUS

Fetal assessments are important for respiratory therapists so that they can gather and evaluate pertinent information and to make appropriate decisions about the care of the infant after delivery. Frequent assessments may be necessary to trend changes or evaluate the development of fetal abnormalities in utero. Clearly, every respiratory therapist must evaluate the reliability of and make judgments regarding the information assessed and make use of critical assessments necessary for treatment. Therapist-driven protocols may assist in making such judgments; however, the respiratory therapist needs to evaluate data based on all available information about the developing fetus. Knowledge of the technology and examinations that lend themselves to familiarizing respiratory therapists with information about the fetus can help to implement treatment plans upon delivery of the neonate.

Ultrasonography

Ultrasonography has proven to be one of the most important advances in neonatal medicine. Compared to radiography, ultrasound is a relatively safe procedure, and it has essentially replaced radiography as a mode of fetal assessment.

The modern ultrasound machine uses high-frequency sound waves to locate and visualize organs and tissues. These waves are well below the level of intensity that could potentially damage tissues. They are transmitted from a hand-held transducer and placed directly against the mother's abdomen or intravaginally through a transvaginal transducer. As the sound waves come in contact with different-density tissues, some are absorbed and others are reflected to the transducer. The reflected waves are converted into a screen image, visually duplicating the targeted organ (Figure 2–1).

New high-resolution, dynamic ultrasound equipment can give the caregiver dramatic insight into fetal structures, activities, and the intrauterine environment. Modern ultrasound can also give cross-sectional views of fetal organs, allowing for a detailed look at possible anomalies. The development of transvaginal ultrasound has enhanced the ability to assess the fetus during the first trimester, when its position in the maternal pelvis makes the transabdominal approach more difficult.

Ultrasound has evolved from crude static displays to high-resolution, real-time, B-mode displays that can illustrate two-dimensional, and more recently 3D and 4D

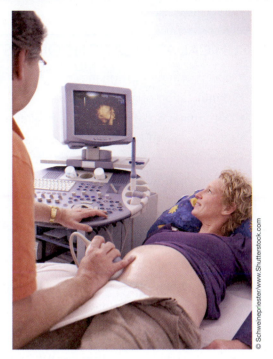

FIGURE 2–1. Ultrasonography is one of the most common methods used for fetal assessment.

images of fetal/organ movement or development. To clarify the definitions, 3D imaging sends the waves in multiple directions, rather than simply straight like in 2D. The result is the ability to see the height, width and depth of the fetal image. 4D technology adds the further dimension of motion to the image, allowing the fetus to be examined in real time. The improved applications of ultrasound have greatly enhanced the ability to identify at-risk fetuses.

Ultrasound is used during pregnancy for a variety of purposes usually beginning around 12–20 weeks gestation to evaluate fetal growth and development. Common usages are listed in Table 2–1.

The accurate determination of fetal age is vital in perinatal medicine in order to make appropriate clinical management decisions. This is one area in which ultrasound has influenced fetal assessment. Specific methods used to determine fetal age include crown-rump measurement (only accurate to 12 weeks gestation), biparietal diameter (the diameter of the fetal head), abdominal circumference, and femur length. The combination of head size, abdominal circumference, and femur length can be used to estimate fetal weight. Once gestational age and weight are determined, intrauterine growth retardation (IUGR) and excessive growth (macrosomia) can be determined.

Modern ultrasound has made fetal anomalies more recognizable for evaluation and management after delivery. Ideally, any anomaly in which there is an anatomic

Table 2–1

CLINICAL APPLICATIONS OF OBSTETRIC ULTRASOUND

- Identification of pregnancy
- Identification of multiple fetuses
- Determination of appropriate fetal age, growth, and maturity
- Observance of polyhydramnios and oligohydramnios
- Detection of fetal anomalies
- Determination of placenta previa
- Identification of placental abnormalities
- Location of the placenta and fetus for amniocentesis
- Determination of fetal position
- Determination of fetal death
- Examination of fetal heart rate and respiratory effort
- Detection of incomplete miscarriages and ectopic pregnancies

change in structure, or that results in a functional change in the organ or system is detectable in utero with ultrasound. The diagnostic accuracy of ultrasound in detecting anomalies increases with gestational age.[1]

Doppler Assessment of Blood Velocities

Doppler velocimetry is used to measure relative blood flow through the umbilical, placental, and fetal vessels in the umbilical cord of term infants. While it was hoped that monitoring umbilical artery blood flow would help estimate fetal compromise, thus far it has not proven to be effective. However, the benefits of Doppler may be evident in predicting some perinatal problems in high-risk pregnancies.[2] It is also suggested that Doppler velocimetry can decrease the number of cesarean sections, neonatal complications, and length of stay in the neonatal intensive care unit (NICU).

Amniocentesis

By obtaining of a sample of amniotic fluid, amniocentesis is divided into early (done before 15 weeks following the last menstrual period) and midtrimester amniocentesis (done during the second and third trimesters). Midtrimester amniocentesis is the most commonly performed and considered to be a primary examination or assessment for prenatal diagnosis. It is thought to be the "gold standard" to which other procedures are compared.[3]

Amniocentesis is performed by inserting a 3.5 to 4 inch, 20 to 22 gauge needle attached to a syringe into a pocket of amniotic fluid (Figure 2–2). The position for

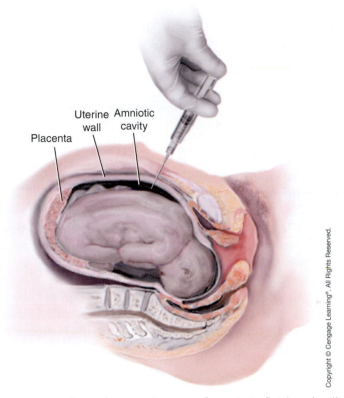

Placenta — Uterine wall — Amniotic cavity

FIGURE 2–2. Amniocentesis allows for examination of amniotic fluid and cellular elements.

insertion of the needle is guided by ultrasound. Once the needle is inserted, 20 to 30 mL of amniotic fluid are aspirated and placed in sterile tubes. Both the amniotic fluid and the cellular elements in the fluid are then examined and evaluated.

Complications of amniocentesis include fetal trauma, infection, and intrauterine hemorrhage. Accidental puncturing of the fetus, umbilical cord, and placenta may be minor, or may lead to intrauterine hemorrhage and death. However, amniocentesis is a relatively safe procedure with complication rates usually less than 1%.

Once amniotic fluid has been obtained, there are several tests for fetal development and well-being that can be performed on the amniotic fluid.

L/S Ratio Amniocentesis is used to determine lung maturity by determining the lecithin to sphingomyelin (L/S) ratio and the presence of phosphatidylglycerol (PG). This concept has been discussed in detail in Chapter 1.

Determination of Alpha-Fetoprotein Another test is the determination of **alpha-fetoprotein (AFP)** levels in the amniotic fluid. AFP is the main serum in the developing fetus. It normally peaks near the 12th week of gestation and then gradually decreases. Whenever there is a break in the fetal skin, as in **anencephaly**

(absence of the brain or brain tissues) or **meningomyelocele** (spina bifida), AFP leaks from the exposed tissues into the amniotic fluids. A high level of AFP, therefore, is an objective sign to some degree of neural tube defect. Acetylcholinesterase is also found in abnormally high concentrations when neural tube defects are present. Conversely, a low measurement of AFP has been useful in detecting the presence of Down syndrome in the fetus. Despite the success of AFP monitoring, Sepulveda and associates have found that high-resolution ultrasonography is more accurate in the detection of anomalies associated with elevated AFP levels.[4]

Bilirubin Level The level of bilirubin in amniotic fluid is an aid in detecting hemolytic diseases such as Rh incompatibility. Increases in amniotic bilirubin levels are proportional to the degree of hemolysis (blood loss).

Creatinine Levels Creatinine levels increase in the amniotic fluid as pregnancy progresses. In the presence of normal maternal levels, amniotic creatinine levels are used to help determine fetal kidney maturity.

Identification of Meconium Staining Amniocentesis can also be helpful to detect the presence of meconium in the amniotic fluid. Normally clear, amniotic fluid becomes greenish-black when meconium is present. This is discussed in more detail later in this chapter.

Cytologic Examination of Cells The cellular elements found in amniotic fluid include cells from the skin, amnion, and the tracheobronchial tree. These cells can be used to diagnose a variety of genetic and chromosomal disorders. Karyotyping of cells can be used to detect Down syndrome and other trisomy disorders.

A wide variety of disorders caused by errors in metabolism such as protein metabolism, carbohydrate intolerance, or glycogen storage can be screened or detected by performing biochemical and enzymatic assays on these cells.

Fetal Heart Rate Monitoring

The average heart rate in early gestation is 140/min, dropping to an average of 120/min near term. One important factor in the management of the fetus is that the fetal heart rate (FHR) and variability (discussed later in this chapter) correlate with fetal well-being. Fetal cardiac status is measured by simple auscultation with a stethoscope, or by sophisticated electronics that are relatively simple to use.

Monitoring the heart rate of the fetus has become so common that almost every labor room has a fetal heart monitor. The major reason for this popularity is that adverse results of delivery have diminished since its advent through continued use in the delivery room.

FHR monitoring can identify fetal distress that may be difficult to perceive otherwise. It is well established that labor and delivery are very stressful on the infant. For this reason, FHR is usually monitored along with uterine contractions so the correlation between the two can be evaluated.

Because the FHR monitor shows the response of the heart to asphyxia by fetal decelerations, it is an excellent way to identify those infants who are being asphyxiated in utero such that expedient treatment can be rapidly initiated after delivery.

Methods of Monitoring FHR FHR can be monitored in one of three ways. An external abdominal transducer can sense the movement of the fetal heart and its valves and can then determine heart rate (Figure 2–3). A second method is to place electrodes on the abdomen to pick up the electrical activity of the maternal and the fetal heart. The monitor can electronically pick out the fetal rate and display it. By far, the most accurate method is the placement of a small spiral electrode into the fetal scalp (Figure 2–4). This requires that the amniotic membranes be ruptured, with a small risk of infection, but the accuracy and dependability provided are unsurpassed through continuous monitoring.

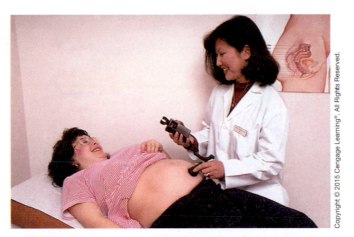

FIGURE 2–3. Monitoring fetal heart rate using an external abdominal transducer.

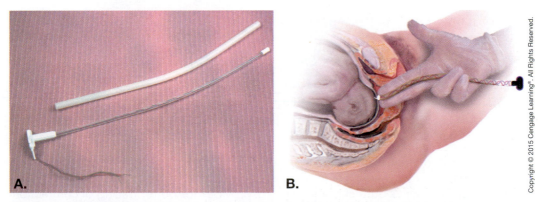

A.   **B.**

FIGURE 2–4. A. Fetal scalp electrode. B. Placing the electrode in the fetal scalp.

Monitoring Uterine Contractions Uterine contractions can be monitored by one of two devices. The most commonly used device is known as a **tocodynamometer**. The tocodynamometer is strapped to the mother's abdomen at the level of the uterine fundus (Figure 2–5). As the uterus contracts, the gauge is depressed. It then transforms the degree to which it is depressed into an estimate of intensity, timing, and duration of contractions. The main drawback is its susceptibility to artifact from a variety of sources. It is also, at best, a crude estimation of contractile intensity and does not measure actual intrauterine pressure.

A second device is the intrauterine pressure catheter. This instrument is inserted into the uterus through the cervix following rupture of the amniotic membranes. It can measure actual pressures in the uterus that are generated during each contraction. This device is mainly used during prolonged, difficult labors.

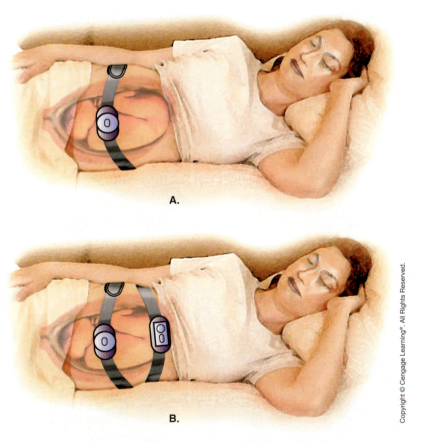

A.

B.

FIGURE 2–5. External fetal heart rate monitoring. A. Ultrasound transducer in place near the fetal heart. B. Tocotransducer in place over the uterine fundus. A tocotransducer placed over the infant's buttocks or lower back provides for better tracing of contraction pattern.

Determining Fetal Heart Patterns There are some basic patterns that are monitored with the FHR monitor. Each pattern is correlated with uterine contractions to help assess and identify possible problems.

Baseline Heart Rate The first pattern is the baseline heart rate, determined by watching the rate tracing for at least 10 minutes. The normal baseline heart rate will range between 120 and 160 beats per minute (bpm). Normal FHR will vary between the high and low end, but smaller gestation fetuses will usually be closer to the high end. Although rates of 120 to 160 bpm are considered normal, each fetus must be assessed carefully. An increase or decrease in baseline heart rate of 20 to 30 bpm may be abnormal even though still within normal limits.

Variability When first examining the fetal heart pattern, inspect the variability of the heartbeat. A healthy, awake fetus has a constantly changing heart rate, usually between 5 and 10 bpm. The beat-to-beat variability will be reduced in the presence of CNS depression secondary to hypoxia, immaturity of the fetus, fetal sleep, or narcotic and sedative use by the mother. Samueloff *et al.* have indicated that variability alone cannot be used as the sole indicator of fetal well-being but should be used in conjunction with other measures of assessment.[5]

Bradycardia A baseline heart rate of less than 100 bpm or a maintained drop of 20 bpm from the previous baseline rate is considered bradycardia. The most dangerous cause of fetal bradycardia is asphyxia. Oxygen administration to the mother may help reduce the severity of asphyxia to the fetus. Other causes of bradycardia include congenital heart block secondary to a congenital malformation, maternal systemic lupus erythematosus, administration of paracervical blocks, beta blockers to the mother, and fetal hypothermia.

Whenever fetal bradycardia is present, the primary concern should be to rule out fetal asphyxia as the cause. Fetal asphyxia can be diagnosed by the use of scalp blood pH determination, discussed later in this chapter.

Bradycardia seen during the second stage of labor (after the cervix is dilated to 10 cm through the delivery of the infant) is divided into end-stage and terminal bradycardia. End-stage bradycardia is accompanied by standard variability and a prior normal tracing. Normal vaginal delivery can be expected in the presence of end-stage bradycardia. In contrast, terminal bradycardia is accompanied by no variability, and delivery is performed in the quickest possible manner because it indicates fetal distress.

Tachycardia Tachycardia is present when the baseline is consistently above 180 bpm. The most common cause is maternal fever. Tachycardia can also be caused by fetal or maternal infection, fetal dysrhythmia, maternal dehydration, maternal anxiety, stimulation of the fetus, and asphyxia. Sympathomimetic drugs used to stop contractions, such as ritodrine, salbutamol, and terbutaline, and parasympatholytics, such as atropine, may cause fetal tachycardia when administered to the mother.

Accelerations If FHR exceeds 160 bpm for less than 2 minutes, it is called an acceleration. Accelerations during labor are a good sign that the fetus is reacting to the contraction in a positive way.

Decelerations When the FHR drops below 120 bpm for less than 2 minutes, it is called a deceleration. Decelerations, in contrast to accelerations, may either be threatening or harmless, depending on their characteristics and timing during the contraction. Categorizing decelerations can help predict fetal compromise or the severity of post-natal complications. The three types of deceleration are shown in Figure 2–6 A through C.

Early, or Type I, decelerations closely follow uterine contractions in onset and duration. The heart rate may drop to 60 to 80 bpm during the contraction, rapidly returning to baseline following the contraction. Type I decelerations are caused by compression of the fetal head against the cervix and are generally benign. Bradycardia due to a parasympathetic response is not indicative of hypoxia.

Late or Type II decelerations do not follow uterine contractions. They occur 10 to 30 seconds following the onset of the contraction, and heart rate does not return to baseline until after the contraction is over. Even a small decrease of 10 to 20 bpm from baseline can be suggestive of fetal problems. Type II decelerations are secondary to uteroplacental insufficiency during contractions, leading to fetal asphyxia.

During the contraction, the vessels of the uterus and placenta are compressed, leading to diminished transfer of oxygen from the maternal blood to the fetal blood. As the hypoxia worsens, the decelerations last longer and the beat-to-beat variability is lost. Progression of the hypoxia causes the decelerations to begin sooner and last longer with the heart rate dipping lower with each contraction.

Variable or Type III decelerations are independent of uterine contractions. They are random in their onset, duration, and severity. Type III decelerations are usually secondary to compression of the umbilical cord leading to hypoxia. The cord may either be wrapped around the infant's neck (nucal cord) or be pinched between the pelvis and the presenting body part. Type III decelerations may or may not be dangerous, depending on the frequency and severity of each occurrence. Alleviation of cord compression is accomplished by turning the mother from side to side or by assuming a knee-chest position. In emergency situations, the presenting body part may be elevated to try to prevent further cord compression.

Fetal Scalp pH Assessment

The assessment of fetal scalp pH is used as a secondary tool, following FHR monitoring, in the determination of fetal well-being. It is indicated in the absence of baseline variability, late decelerations with decreasing variability, and abnormal tracings.

The acid–base balance of the fetus is determined by the viability of the placenta and its ability to exchange oxygen and carbon dioxide between maternal and fetal blood through the circulatory system. If that exchange is disrupted, whether at the placenta or in the cord, the resultant drop in pH (acidosis) can be measured. The reason for the drop is twofold. First, as blood gas exchange decreases, fetal $PaCO_2$ increases, decreasing the pH. Second, in the face of hypoxia, the fetus begins to

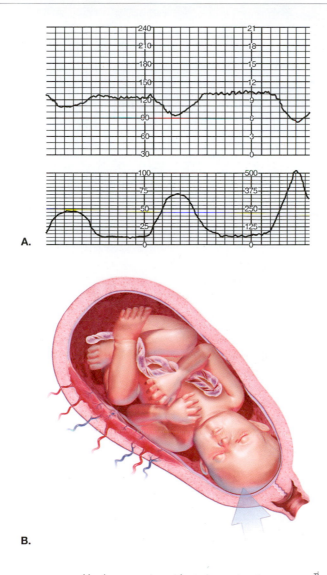

A.

B.

Head compression with uterine contraction

↓

Redistribution of cerebral blood flow

↓

Vagal response in triggered

↓

FHR slows gradually

↓

Early deceleration

C.   This process subsides when the head compression is relieved.

FIGURE 2–6A. A. Early decelerations. B. Fetal head compression. C. Physiology of early decelerations.

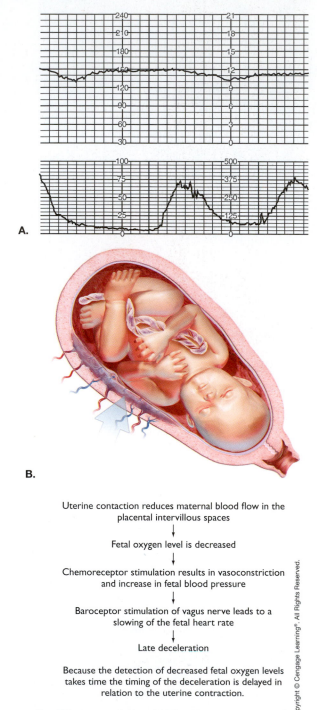

A. Late decelerations.

B.

Uterine contraction reduces maternal blood flow in the placental intervillous spaces

↓

Fetal oxygen level is decreased

↓

Chemoreceptor stimulation results in vasoconstriction and increase in fetal blood pressure

↓

Baroceptor stimulation of vagus nerve leads to a slowing of the fetal heart rate

↓

Late deceleration

Because the detection of decreased fetal oxygen levels takes time the timing of the deceleration is delayed in relation to the uterine contraction.

C. This process subsides when the uterine contraction ends.

FIGURE 2–6B. A. Late decelerations. B. Decreased flow of blood to the placenta. C. Physiology of late decelerations.

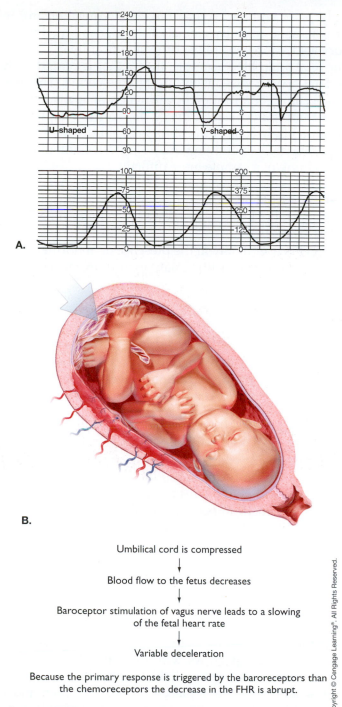

A. Variable decelerations.

B. Cord compression.

Umbilical cord is compressed

↓

Blood flow to the fetus decreases

↓

Baroceptor stimulation of vagus nerve leads to a slowing
of the fetal heart rate

↓

Variable deceleration

Because the primary response is triggered by the baroreceptors than
the chemoreceptors the decrease in the FHR is abrupt.

C.   The process subsides when the umbilical cord pressure is relieved.

FIGURE 2–6C. A. Variable decelerations. B. Cord compression. C. Physiology of variable decelerations.

metabolize glycogen without oxygen (anaerobic metabolism), resulting in a dramatic increase in lactic acid. This metabolic acid, combined with increased $PaCO_2$, the respiratory acid, causes the pH to drop significantly.

To get the fetal scalp blood sample, the mother is placed in the lithotomy position and the fetal head is visualized through the cervix. This is done with a long, cone-shaped speculum or an endoscope. An incision is made with 2×1.5 mm blade and the blood sample is collected into a heparinized capillary tube. The sample should be obtained between contractions to avoid decelerations, which may cause low values. Additionally, blood flow may slow substantially during a contraction, making the obtaining of a sample more difficult.

Fetal blood pH is considered to be normal above 7.25. A pH of 7.2 to 7.24 shows slight asphyxia, and a pH of less than 7.2 signifies severe asphyxia. Because maternal pH can influence fetal pH, it may be necessary to determine the acid–base status of the mother concurrently.

Fetal scalp pH is useful only in the presence of abnormal FHR tracings, because a normal tracing indicates a healthy infant in most instances.

ESTIMATING THE DELIVERY DATE

The delivery date is called the estimated date of confinement (EDC) and can be calculated by a variety of methods. Although none of the methods is exact, each will help determine the time when gestation will reach 40 weeks.

Nägele's Rule

Nägele's rule is the most common method of determining EDC. To determine the EDC, 3 months are subtracted from the first day of the last menstrual period. Seven days are then added to the result to determine the EDC. For example, if the first day of the last menstrual period was March 25, subtracting 3 months would arrive at December 25. Adding 7 days gives us an EDC of January 1.

The accuracy of Nägele's rule depends on a regular period of 28 days and the woman remembering her last menstrual period. The use of oral contraceptives or an irregular menstrual cycle reduces the accuracy of this method.

Fundal Height

The **fundus** of the uterus, which is the end opposite the cervix, can be measured on the abdominal wall as it grows with the fetus. It is fairly reliable during the first and second trimesters, but unreliable during the last trimester. To determine fundal height, a tape measure is placed on the abdomen and the distance from the symphysis pubis to the top of the fundus is measured (Figure 2–7). During the first two trimesters, gestational age correlates to this measurement in centimeters. Therefore, at 20 weeks, the fundus is roughly 20 cm above the symphysis pubis, and so forth.

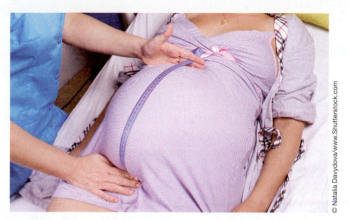

FIGURE 2–7. Measurement of fundal height.

Quickening

Quickening is the first sensation of fetal movement experienced by the mother. It generally occurs between 16 and 22 weeks, but on average occurs near week 20. Because of the large variations, quickening is at best only a very rough estimate of gestational age.

Determination of Fetal Heartbeat

The fetal heartbeat can be heard as early as week 16, but is nearly always heard no later than week 20. With the use of Doppler devices, the heartbeat can be detected much earlier, possibly as early as week 8. Again, the determination of fetal heartbeat is only a rough estimation of gestational age.

BIOPHYSICAL TESTS OF FETAL WELL-BEING

With the increase in knowledge and interest in the fetus, researchers increasingly became interested in the role of the heart rate and its relationship to fetal well-being. Researchers began looking at the response of the heart to uterine contractions as a method of fetal evaluation.

The Contraction Stress Test

The first test using this technique was called the contraction stress test (CST). The CST is used to determine the presence of uteroplacental insufficiency. One of the original forms of measuring fetal compromise, CST detects the uteroplacental insufficiency by subjecting the fetus to stress. The stress comes from an interruption of maternal blood to the intervillous spaces during contraction. A positive

CST is defined as more than 50% of contractions having late FHR decelerations. With a negative CST, no decelerations are seen after any contraction. In reality, most CST tests do not clearly fall into one of these categories. For this reason, there are several other classifications that the skilled respiratory therapist uses to interpret results, such as reactive, nonreactive, minimally reactive, and equivocal.[6]

Contraindications to the performance of the CST include placenta previa, previous vertical cesarean section, previous uterine rupture, premature labor, premature rupture of the membranes, and incompetent cervix.

A variation of the CST is the oxytocin contraction test (OCT). If spontaneous contractions are inadequate when the CST is done, the drug oxytocin at a dose of 0.5 to 1.0 mU/min increasing every 15 to 20 minutes is given through an intravenous line to start contractions (usually 3 contractions every 40 seconds within a 10 minute period). Additionally, it has been noted that self-stimulation of one nipple through the clothing may initiate uterine contractions. The procedure can be repeated every 5 minutes until an adequate pattern of contraction is initiated.

The Nonstress Test

In a healthy fetus, the heart rate increases in association with fetal body movement. Therefore, a second test was developed in which the response of FHR to fetal movements is observed. This test is called the nonstress test (NST). To classify NST results, a qualifying heart rate acceleration increases at least 15/min over baseline and lasts at least 15 seconds. A normal, reactive pattern shows at least two accelerations in conjunction with fetal movement, over a 20-minute window. A nonreactive NST occurs when the FHR does not accelerate during fetal body movement over two 20-minute periods. Some have extended the time period up to 120 minutes before declaring a nonreactive test.[7] A negative NST is often followed by a CST to evaluate the cause of the inactivity. A fetus suffering from prolonged hypoxia will have a positive CST with a negative NST. Negative CST results in the presence of a negative NST indicate the problem is one of fetal sleep or maternal narcotic or sedative ingestion.

The NST is popular mainly because it is simple to perform, is less time consuming than the CST, the patient has little discomfort, and there is little risk from induced contractions.

Vibroacoustic Stimulation

Another method of soliciting a fetal response, in addition to the NST, is by the use of vibroacoustic stimulation. In this test, a buzzer is held against the maternal abdomen. The FHR is then monitored and evaluated for accelerations. The healthy fetus responds to the acoustic stimulation with an acceleration of heart rate. Failure of the heart rate to increase may indicate a compromised fetus and further evaluation should be considered.

Monitoring Fetal Movement

Monitoring of fetal movement is probably the easiest means of fetal assessment. It serves as an indirect measurement of CNS integrity and function.[8] Movement can be monitored as simply as having the mother note movement, or as complex as observation with ultrasound over an extended time period. Jerky movement of the fetus has been detected as early as 7 weeks, and reaches its greatest activity between 28 and 34 weeks. Movements decrease toward term possibly due to increasing fetal size and decreasing amniotic fluid volume.

The mother first senses fetal movement sometime between 16 and 20 weeks. The test is simple in that it only requires the mother to note the number of fetal movements detected during a certain period (usually a 1-hour period). Less than 10 movements over an hour require further testing due to the fact that fetal inactivity is associated with fetal distress and/or stillbirth.

Assessment of Amniotic Fluid Volume

It has long been appreciated that there is a link between the volume of amniotic fluid and fetal well-being. This has been demonstrated by Hadi and colleagues who indicate that adequate amniotic fluid volume relates to longer pregnancies and higher neonatal survival.[9] Amniotic fluid volume measurement may offer clues to the presence of certain anomalies such as esophageal atresia, diaphragmatic hernia, cardiac, intracranial, spinal and ventral wall defects, and urinary trace abnormalities.

The Biophysical Profile

The biophysical profile (BPP), first proposed in 1980, uses information gained from five separate tests (Table 2–2). Those tests are: fetal breathing, fetal movement, fetal limb tone, the NST, and amniotic fluid volume. Each area is scored 0 or 1 depending on the finding. The BPP is typically done during the third trimester; however, it can be done in earlier trimesters in the event of a high-risk pregnancy. Vintzileos and colleagues modified the original BPP by adding placental grade to the evaluation and scoring each area 0, 1, or 2 based on the finding. The BPP is possibly the best overall method of fetal risk determination. The same group found that the biophysical profile is superior to the 1- and 5-minute Apgar scores for determining fetal acidosis.[10]

Meconium Presence in Amniotic Fluid

Meconium is the thick (tar-like), dark greenish stool found in the fetal intestine. The passage of meconium into the amniotic fluid occurs about 40% of the time in post-term fetuses of greater than 42 weeks gestation. The frequency drops to about 10% in the term infant and 3% to 5% in the preterm fetus.[11]

Table 2–2

THE BIOPHYSICAL PROFILE

Biophysical Variable	Normal (2)	Abnormal (0)
• **Fetal breathing**—at least one episode of at least 30 seconds during 30-minute observation	Present	Absent
• **Gross body movement**—at least three body/limb movements during 30-minute observation	3 or more	2 or less
• **Fetal tone**—one episode of extension/ flexion of limbs or trunk during 30-minute observation	Present	Absent
• **Reactive NST**—at least two episodes of 15 beats/min fetal heart rate accelerations during 30-minute observation	Yes	No
• **Amniotic fluid volume**—at least one pocket of at least 1 × 1 cm in two directions	Present	Absent

Normal Score: 8–10

Meconium staining of the amniotic fluid may result from a fetal asphyxia episode, but its reliability as evidence of fetal distress is debatable. This unreliability is based on the fact that low 5-minute Apgar scores are found in only 10% of meconium-stained neonates.

The presence of meconium in the amniotic fluid is determined by amniocentesis or amnioscopy, or is visualized when the amniotic sac ruptures. One theory of asphyxia-induced meconium passage is that fetal asphyxia causes relaxation of the fetal anal sphincter and increased peristalsis of the intestine.

The most severe result of meconium release is meconium aspiration syndrome (MAS), in which meconium is aspirated into the trachea and airways. MAS and its treatment are detailed in Chapter 7.

Chorionic Villus Sampling

As the name implies, chorionic villus sampling is the process of removing a small sample from the chorionic villus of the placenta, which contains fetal blood and tissue. The sample is then examined for the presence of chromosomal abnormalities. Sampling can be done transcervically, transvaginally, or transabdominally, depending on the location of the placenta. Most chorionic villus samplings are done between 9 and 12 weeks of gestation.[3] Indications for the procedure include advanced maternal age, previous child with chromosomal anomalies, or a parent carrier. It is particularly suited for DNA analysis because the amount of DNA obtained is significantly larger than that typically obtained with amniocentesis.

With the advent of high-resolution, real-time ultrasound and flexible catheters, the procedure carries a fetal complication rate of less than 1%, which is similar to that seen in amniocentesis.

Cordocentesis

Cordocentesis is the in utero sampling of fetal umbilical cord blood. The base of the umbilical cord is located with ultrasound and a 22-gauge needle is inserted through the maternal abdomen into the uterus. The umbilical cord is punctured and blood samples are drawn into tuberculin syringes.

The fetal blood samples are then checked for several fetal problems, including hemoglobinopathies (e.g., sickle cell), coagulopathies (e.g., hemophilia), specific IgM antibodies to fetal infections, metabolic disorders, suspected congenital anomalies, oxygenation, and acid–base status.

This technique has evolved to be an important part of the evaluation of fetal well-being. When properly done, both fetal and maternal risk is 1% or less.[3]

Biochemical Methods of Assessment

In addition to the previously discussed methods of fetal assessment, there have been other methods that were developed to help predict high-risk pregnancies, and hopefully adverse fetal outcomes.

Maternal Estriol Determination Estriol, a metabolite of estrogen, is secreted in high quantities by the placenta in the latter half of pregnancy. Adequate production of estriol depends on a properly functioning fetal liver and adrenal glands. Optimum levels of estriol in maternal urine require a healthy fetus, a properly functioning placenta, and a healthy mother.

With the growth and development of the fetus, the production of estriol increases. Growth retardation, fetal distress, and placental insufficiency all lead to decreased estriol production.

Estriol passes from the placenta into the maternal blood and is excreted in the mother's urine. Determinations of maternal estriol levels can be made using blood or urine samples. The mother's urine is collected over a 24-hour period and analyzed for the quantity of estriol present. Both blood and urine samples must be taken several times a week to be effective.

Fetal distress is indicated if there is a 50% to 60% decrease in results from the previous test, or if there is an ongoing decrease in serial values. This test is becoming unpopular owing to the high number of false-positive results, the inconvenience of 24-hour urine collection and/or weekly blood sampling, and the difficulty in outpatient management.

Recently, a review of a trial involving 622 women with high-risk pregnancies concluded that measuring estriol levels did not affect the outcome of the pregnancy.

Human Placental Lactogen Levels A second method of biochemical fetal evaluation is the determination of **human placental lactogen (HPL)** levels. Produced by the placenta and excreted into the maternal blood, HPL levels gradually increase until 37 weeks gestation, at which point the level remains the same or decreases slightly.

Maternal serum levels are evaluated on a weekly basis, with normal ranges near term of 5.4 to 7 µg/mL. Fetal compromise may be present if HPL levels fall below 4 µg/mL after 30 weeks gestation. As with estriol determination, HPL determination has become less popular in recent years.

Magnetic Resonance Imaging Magnetic resonance imaging (MRI) opened up new avenues not previously available to the assessment of the fetus. Unlike the CAT scan (computerized axial tomography), the MRI does not use radiation and, therefore, does not pose the risk of causing defects in the developing fetus.

MRI is especially suited for distinguishing between soft tissue structure and function. The MRI is capable of creating sagittal, axial, and coronal plane views of any part of the body. The sagittal view appears to be the most helpful in assessing fetal status in the prenatal period.

MRI imaging is indicated in those instances where ultrasonography is often insufficient, such as placental and fetal abnormalities and development of the fetal lungs and brain.

FACTORS IDENTIFYING A HIGH-RISK PREGNANCY

One of our greatest assets in caring for the sick neonate is the ability to predict those fetuses at high risk for anomalies or developing complications. Early in the development of perinatology it became clear that certain factors, both maternal and fetal, were present whenever a distressed infant was born. Some of these high-risk factors can be determined on the first office visit. Others appear as the pregnancy advances. Others still are only present during labor, delivery, and the postdelivery period.

Until these approaches are in common use, it is important that the neonatal respiratory therapist have an understanding of contributing high-risk factors. The ability to anticipate a distressed fetus will better prepare the respiratory therapist to care for the infant. These high-risk factors are outlined in Table 2–3.

Table 2–3

HIGH-RISK PREGNANCY INDICATING FACTORS

Socioeconomic Factors

1. Low income and poor housing
2. Severe social problems
3. Unwed status, especially adolescent
4. Minority status
5. Poor nutritional status

Demographic Factors

1. Maternal age under 16
2. Obese or underweight before pregnancy
3. Height less than 5 feet
4. Familial history of inherited disorders

Medical Factors

1. Obstetric history
    a. History of infertility
    b. History of ectopic pregnancy
    c. History of miscarriage
    d. Previous multiple gestations
    e. Previous stillbirth or neonatal death
    f. Uterine/cervical abnormality
    g. High parity (many pregnancies)
    h. History of premature labor/delivery
    i. History of prolonged labor
    j. Previous cesarean delivery
    k. History of low-birth-weight infant
    l. Previous delivery with midforceps
    m. History of infant with malformation, birth injury, or neurologic deficit
    n. History of hydatidiform mole or carcinoma
2. Maternal medical history
    a. Maternal cardiac disease
    b. Maternal pulmonary disease
    c. Maternal diabetes or thyroid disease
    d. History of chronic renal disease
    e. Maternal gastrointestinal disease
    f. Maternal endocrine disorders
    g. History of hypertension
    h. History of seizure disorder
    i. History of venereal and other infectious diseases
    j. Weight loss greater than 5 pounds
    k. Surgery during pregnancy
    l. Major anomalies of the reproductive tract
    m. History of mental retardation and emotional disorders

continued on the next page

Table 2–3

continued from the previous page

3. Current obstetric status
    a. Absence of prenatal care
    b. Rh sensitization
    c. Excessively large or small fetus
    d. Premature labor
    e. Preeclampsia
    f. Multiple gestations
    g. Polyhydramnios and oligohydramnios
    h. Premature rupture of the membranes
    i. Vaginal bleeding
    j. Placenta previa
    k. Abruptio placentae
    l. Abnormal presentation
    m. Postmaturity
    n. Abnormalities in tests for fetal well-being
    o. Maternal anemia
4. Habits
    a. Smoking
    b. Regular alcohol intake
    c. Drug use and abuse

SUMMARY

Modern perinatology has evolved over the past 40 years to a complex maze of tests and procedures used to evaluate, assess, and treat the fetal patient. While many old techniques are continually researched, updated, and improved, many new procedures and tests are being developed at a staggering pace.

Of all modes used to assess the fetus, none has had more of an impact than ultrasonography. With its ability to visualize the fetus and its organs, and its relative safety, it has become a mainstay in modern perinatal medicine. Once only a guessing game, ultrasound has made the determination of fetal gestational age a nearly exact science. It is also used to detect fetal anomalies, measure amniotic fluid volume, and safely guide the needles used for amniocentesis, chorionic villus sampling, and cordocentesis. Its counterpart, Doppler velocimetry, may also be helpful in predicting high-risk pregnancies.

One of the oldest methods of prenatal diagnosis is amniocentesis. Amniocentesis is useful in determining L/S ratio for lung maturity, alpha-fetoprotein levels to detect neural tube defects, bilirubin level to identify hemolytic disorders, to measure creatinine levels to determine kidney maturity, for identification of meconium staining, and for cell examination and karyotyping for genetic disorders.

Respiratory therapists' knowledge that FHR correlates well with underlying fetal distress has made monitoring of the FHR a common practice. When compared to uterine contractions, changes in rate and variability can be diagnostic of varying fetal distress. Bradycardia, tachycardia, and the accelerations and decelerations that occur during the contraction are useful diagnostic tools.

In the absence of baseline heart rate variability, late decelerations, or abnormal tracings during labor, scalp pH assessment is useful in determining the level of asphyxia present. Respiratory therapists must evaluate and use the gathered information as resources to make critical assessments about the newborn after delivery of the neonate.

Determination of the delivery date is accomplished by several methods. Nägele's rule utilizes the first day of the last menstrual period to calculate delivery date. The remaining methods—fundal height, quickening, detection of FHR, and ultrasonography—are used to assess approximate gestational age. Using a normal 40-week gestation period, the delivery date can be accurately calculated.

The CST and the NST continue to be useful in the detection of fetal compromise. Whether a test is reactive or nonreactive helps the respiratory therapist determine the amount of stress the fetus is undergoing and whether further investigation is required. Acoustic stimulation is used to stimulate the fetus to determine if it responds appropriately. Fetal movement is relatively easy to monitor and can yield important information to the respiratory therapist. Ordinarily, the mother is asked to monitor how long it takes her fetus to move 10 times. Times approaching an hour or longer require further follow-up. The amount of amniotic fluid present is diagnostic for fetal well-being. Normal amounts of fluid indicate less risk of early delivery and higher fetal survival.

The biophysical profile utilizes several tests in an effort to better analyze fetal well-being. The biophysical profile includes the NST, fetal movement, breathing movements, limb tone, amniotic fluid volume, and placental grade. Each area is given a numerical rating of 0, 1, or 2, depending on the test result. The higher the score, the fewer instances of fetal compromise.

The presence of meconium in the amniotic fluid may be indicative of fetal asphyxia and predisposes the fetus to possible aspiration of meconium into the trachea following delivery.

Chorionic villus sampling and cordocentesis are examples of the ability to work with the fetus while still in utero. Sampling of placental villus and fetal blood is used to detect possible genetic abnormalities, blood disorders, and acid–base imbalance.

The first step in treating a compromised fetus is predicting and anticipating those at high risk. Steps can then be taken to either prevent or minimize the effect of those risk factors. On the first visit, it is vital that a thorough history be taken to identify those patients at high risk.

It is hoped that with the basic understanding of techniques used to evaluate fetal wellness, the respiratory therapist can be better prepared to anticipate and care for these patients.

POSTTEST

1. Assessment of the fetus in the first trimester is facilitated by which technique?
   a. high-resolution ultrasound
   b. doppler velocimetry
   c. real-time displays
   d. transvaginal ultrasound
2. Which of the following cannot be detected by ultrasound?
   a. presence of infection
   b. position of the fetus
   c. position of the placenta
   d. volume of amniotic fluid
3. A high level of alpha-fetoprotein found during amniocentesis indicates which of the following?
   a. neural tube defect
   b. heart anomaly
   c. fetal infection
   d. Down syndrome
4. Which of the following tests done on amniotic fluid is used to help determine fetal kidney maturity?
   a. bilirubin level
   b. L/S ratio
   c. creatinine level
   d. cytologic cell examination
5. Monitoring of the fetal heart rate during labor and delivery is used to detect:
   I. uterine contractions
   II. placental insufficiency
   III. rupture of the amniotic sac
   IV. compression of the umbilical cord
   V. bradycardia secondary to a vagal stimulus
      a. I, II, III
      b. II, IV, V
      c. I, III, IV, V
      d. II, III, IV, V
6. The most accurate method of measuring fetal heart rate is:
   a. Doppler sensors
   b. stethoscope
   c. fetoscope
   d. fetal scalp electrode

7. A common cause of fetal bradycardia is:
   a. asphyxia
   b. congenital anomaly
   c. heart defect
   d. tocolytic drugs
8. Type III decelerations are caused by which of the following?
   a. uterine contractions
   b. placental insufficiency
   c. rupture of the amniotic sac
   d. compression of the umbilical cord
9. Which fetal scalp pH is the lower limit of normal?
   a. 7.30
   b. 7.25
   c. 7.20
   d. 7.15
10. A woman presents in her physician's office for an examination. The first day of her last menstrual period was October 21. Fundal height is 25 cm. Which of the following would be the estimated date of delivery?
    a. July 21
    b. July 28
    c. August 28
    d. June 21
11. What is the approximate gestational age of the fetus in question 10?
    a. 15 weeks
    b. 20 weeks
    c. 25 weeks
    d. 30 weeks
12. A fetus suffering prolonged hypoxia will demonstrate which of the following?
    a. a negative NST and positive CST
    b. a positive NST and negative CST
    c. a negative NST and negative CST
    d. a positive NST and positive CST
13. Which of the following statements are true regarding fetal movements?
    I. Fetal movements show the greatest activity between 28 and 34 weeks.
    II. Diminished fetal movements are normal early in gestation.
    III. Fetal distress and stillbirth are common findings when the fetus is inactive.
    IV. Movement has been detected as early as 7 weeks gestation.
    V. Fetal movements are very difficult to assess.
       a. I, III, V
       b. II, III,IV
       c. I, III, IV
       d. II, IV, V

14. Which of the following is not a part of the biophysical profile?
    a. nonstress test
    b. fetal movement
    c. fetal heart rate
    d. amniotic fluid volume
15. Which of the following involves removal of a fetal blood sample while still in utero?
    a. chorionic villus sampling
    b. cordocentesis
    c. amniocentesis
    d. transplacental aspiration
16. When measuring maternal estriol levels, fetal distress is indicated when:
    a. estriol is present in maternal urine
    b. estriol is absent from maternal urine
    c. levels exceed 5.4 to 7 mcg/mL
    d. estriol levels decrease 50 to 60% in maternal urine
17. Which of the following factors of maternal history places the fetus at high risk?
    I. maternal age of 37 years
    II. previous miscarriage
    III. previous premature delivery
    IV. asthma
    V. maternal obesity
        a. II, III, IV, V
        b. I, III, IV, V
        c. I, II, III, IV, V
        d. I, III, V

REFERENCES

1. Manning FA. Ultrasonography. In: Avery GB, Fletcher MA, MacDonald MG, eds. *Pathophysiology and Management of the Newborn.* 5th ed. Philadelphia, PA: JB Lippincott Co, 1999.
2. Maulik D. Doppler ultrasound velocimetry for fetal surveillance. *Clin Obstet Gynecol.* 38, 1995.
3. Drugan A, et al. Prenatal diagnosis: procedures and trends. In: Avery GB, Fletcher MA, MacDonald MG, eds. *Pathophysiology and Management of the Newborn.* 5th ed. Philadelphia, PA: JB Lippincott Co., 1999.
4. Sepulveda W, et al. Are routine alpha-fetoprotein and acetylcholinesterase determinations still necessary at second-trimester amniocentesis? Impact of high-resolution ultrasonography. *Obstet Gynecol.* 85, 1995.
5. Samueloff A, et al. Is fetal heart rate variability a good predictor of fetal outcome? *Acta Obstet Gynecol Scand.* 73, 1994.
6. Lagrew DC. The contraction stress test. *Clin Obstet Gynecol.* 38, 1995.

7. Paul RH, Miller A. Nonstress test. *Clin Obstet Gynecol.* 38, 1995.
8. Rayburn WF. Fetal movement monitoring. *Clin. Obstet Gynecol.* 38, 1995.
9. Hadi HA, et al. Premature rupture of the membranes between 20 and 25 weeks' gestation: role of the amniotic fluid in perinatal outcome. *Am J Obstet Gynecol.* 170, 1994.
10. Vintzileos AM, et al. The relationships among the fetal biophysical profile, umbilical cord pH, and Apgar scores. *Am J Obstet Gynecol.* 157, 1987.
11. Knuppel RA, Drukker JE. *High-Risk Pregnancy: A Team Approach.* 2nd ed. Philadelphia, PA: WB Saunders Co., 1992.

BIBLIOGRAPHY AND SUGGESTED READINGS

American Academy of Pediatrics. *Maternal and Fetal Evaluation and Immediate Newborn Care (2nd ed.),* Charlottesville, VA: University of Virginia Patent Foundation, 2012.

Avery GB, Fletcher MA, MacDonald MG. *Pathophysiology and Management of the Newborn.* 6th ed. Philadelphia, PA: JB Lippincott Co., 2005.

Cloherty JP, Stark AR, Eichenwald EC, Hansen AR, eds. *Manual of Neonatal Care.* 7th ed. Philadelphia, PA: Lippincott, 2012.

Cottrell GP. *Cardiopulmonary Anatomy and Physiology for Respiratory Care Practitioners.* Philadelphia: FA Davis, 2001.

Des Jardins T. *Cardiopulmonary Anatomy and Physiology.* 6th ed. Clifton Park, NY: Cengage Learning, 2013.

Merenstein GB, Gardner SL. *Handbook of Neonatal Intensive Care.* 7th ed. St. Louis, MO: CV Mosby Co., 2011.

Rhoades GG, et al. The safety and efficacy of chorionic villus sampling for early prenatal diagnosis of cytogenic abnormalities. *N Engl J Med.* 320, 1989.

Taussig LM, Landau LI. *Pediatric Respiratory Medicine.* 2nd ed. St. Louis, MO: Mosby, 2008.

Tucker SM. *Pocket Guide to Fetal Monitoring and Assessment.* 5th ed. St. Louis, MO: Mosby, 2004.

White L. *Foundations of Nursing: Caring for the Whole Person.* 3rd ed. Clifton Park, NY: Cengage Learning, 2011.

CHAPTER 3

Labor, Delivery, and Physiologic Changes after Birth

OBJECTIVES

Upon completion of this chapter, the reader should be able to:

1. List the five events that make up the birth process.
2. Compare and contrast cervical dilation and effacement.
3. Identify the most common presentation.
4. Define station and how it is expressed.
5. Describe the sequence of events that lead to the descent and delivery of the fetus.
6. Define tocolysis and describe the various methods used to achieve tocolysis.
7. Define dystocia and describe the three etiologic factors that cause it.
8. Describe each of the following:
   a. Complete breech
   b. Incomplete or footling breech
   c. Frank breech
   d. Face presentation
   e. Transverse lie
   f. Prolapse of umbilical cord and occult cord compression
9. Identify and describe the three types of placenta previa.
10. Describe the three categories of abruptio placentae.
11. List the indications for a cesarean birth.
12. Explain why multiple gestations create high-risk pregnancies.
13. List factors that are responsible for the first breath.
14. Describe the importance of overcoming surface forces in adapting to extrauterine life.

KEY TERMS

abruptio placentae	engagement	placenta previa
autosomal-recessive	gravida	preeclampsia
trait	multigravida	primigravida
breech	occult	prolapse
dilation	parity	stations
dystocia	parturition	tocolysis
effacement		

INTRODUCTION

The miracle of life follows a delicate balance of interaction between the mother and fetus we call pregnancy. Human pregnancy has been extensively studied, and yet we remain in awe of the process. This chapter will review the anatomy and physiology of pregnancy; however, it is important to not lose site of the emotional impact that pregnancy has on the mother and other family members. While it is mostly a happy adventure, it can also be devastating when things don't go right. As with all aspects of medicine, it is vitally important to remember the "art" as we help our patients through this process.

PREGNANCY

There are several medical terms used during pregnancy. **Gravida**, which comes from the Latin, gravidus meaning "heavy" is often the term used to describe the pregnant female. While rarely used in discussion, the term is often used in the literature and charting as well as defining the status of the patient. The term is combined with other prefixes to define the state of pregnancy in the patient. The female who is pregnant for the first time is called "**primigravida**" and subsequent pregnancies are termed "**multigravida**". A female who has never been pregnant is termed, "nulligravida". Another common term is **parity**, which is abbreviated as para. Parity describes the number of previous live births.

These terms are combined to describe the current status of the patient. For example, a patient in whom this is a first pregnancy would be termed gravida 1, para 0 (G_1P_0). The second pregnancy would then be termed gravida 2, para 1 (G_2P_1) and so forth. Gravida always includes the current pregnancy, while para only indicates previous successful viable births. Multiple gestations (twins, triplets) only count as 1 when describing para. Para is always lower than gravid due to the fact that it does not include the current pregnancy, and any miscarriages and abortions which are also not counted in para. Many hospitals and clinicians use the additional TPAL system to further delineate para. One easy mnemonic to remember TPAL is Texas Power And Light. The letters TPAL stand for Term births (>37 weeks gestation), Premature births (<37 weeks gestation), Abortions/miscarriages, and Living children.

Thus, a patient who is pregnant with her fourth child, who has two living term children and one miscarriage would be classified as G_4P_{2012} using the TPAL system.

PARTURITION

Parturition, the process of giving birth, is a complicated occurrence that is still not fully understood. Five distinct events make up the birth process: 1) Rupture of the membranes; 2) Dilation of the cervix; 3) Contraction of the uterus; 4) Separation of the placenta; and 5) Shrinking of the uterus.

The sequence of events that starts the birth process is complicated and also poorly understood. Three primary hypotheses, however, have emerged to help explain what starts labor: 1) the withdrawal of progesterone; 2) estrogen, causing uterine activation; and 3) stimulation of the uterus by factors such as oxytocin and prostaglandins.[1]

STAGES OF NORMAL LABOR AND DELIVERY

During the latter half of the third trimester, nature begins preparing the mother and the fetus for birth. The actual date of delivery may vary 2 weeks either way from the estimated date of delivery. As the gestation nears term, the placenta begins to slow its function down and the fetus becomes more and more self-reliant in preparation for birth. An understanding of normal labor and delivery is essential to understand what causes difficult deliveries that lead to fetal demise.

Labor and delivery are broken down into three major stages, as listed in Table 3–1. A fourth stage is often listed as a recovery stage, in which the uterus shrinks and homeostasis is reestablished. The duration of each stage of labor will vary based on whether the mother is in her first pregnancy (primigravida) or whether she has been pregnant before (multigravida).

Although every stage is distinct, labor and delivery are one continuous event. False labor may be present for some time during the pregnancy. These contractions, called Braxton-Hicks, are rhythmic and fairly mild compared to true contractions.

Stage I of Labor

The first stage of labor is called stage I. It begins with the onset of the first true contraction. Actual contractions are described as coming in waves, gradually increasing in strength. The first contractions usually are 10–15 minutes apart and last 30–90 seconds.

Effacement and Dilation of the Cervix With the onset of the first contraction, the cervix begins to stretch and widen. The stretching or thinning of the cervix is called **effacement**, and the widening is called **dilation**. Effacement of the cervix

Table 3–1			

STAGES OF LABOR AND DELIVERY

		Average Time	
Stage	**Occurences**	**Primigravida**	**Multigravida**
First	Onset of regular contractions to full dilation and effacement of the cervix	16–18 hr	7–12 hr
Second	Full dilation and effacement of the cervix to delivery of the fetus	1 hr (can last up to 2 hr)	20 min
Third	Delivery of the fetus to delivery of the placenta	3–4 min (can last up to 45 min)	4–5 min

is measured as a percentage. At 100% effacement, the cervix is imperceptible against the uterine wall. Dilation is measured in centimeters (cm) as the diameter of the cervical opening. The cervix is fully dilated at 10 cm. Effacement and dilation are a result of the continuous pushing of the amniotic fluid and the fetus against the cervix, resulting from uterine contractions. In normal labor, the cervix primarily effaces during the early portion of stage I. Dilation is minimal at first and then progresses rapidly toward the end of stage I, when effacement has almost completed. Effacement and dilation of the cervix are illustrated in Figure 3–1.

During the initial contractions, the uterus differentiates into a thick muscular upper portion and a thin lower section. This allows the contractions to push the fetus down the birth canal.

Stage I ends when the cervix is completely dilated and effaced. It averages between 7 and 12 hours in the multigravida, or 16 to 18 hours in the primigravida.

Stage II of Labor

The second stage of labor, stage II, is the actual delivery of the fetus. The descent of the fetus through the birth canal is aided by contraction of the abdominal muscles and diaphragm by the mother. This increases intra-abdominal pressure and, along with contractions, helps push the fetus out.

Position and Engagement of the Fetus Ninety-five percent of all births occur with the fetus in the head-down, or vertex, position. Figure 3–2 shows the possible presentations in the vertex position.

As the head advances down the birth canal, it reaches different degrees of engagement, or stations (Figure 3–3). The station is the location of the head as it relates to the level of the ischial spines on the maternal pelvis. Stations are expressed in cm above the ischial spines as negative numbers and below the spines as positive numbers. The head is said to be engaged in the birth canal when it reaches the spines, or a station of 0.

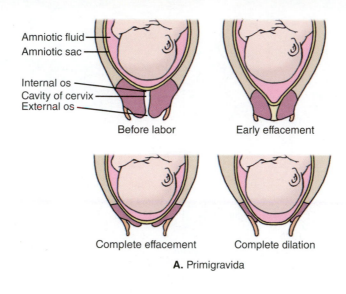

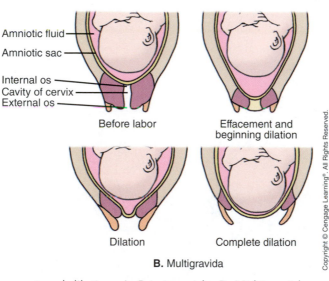

FIGURE 3–1. Effacement and dilation. A. Primigravida. B. Multigravida.

Delivery of the Fetus As the fetus begins its descent down the birth canal, the head turns to a face-down position to accommodate passage through the pelvis (Figure 3–4). Upon delivery of the head, the fetus rotates internally to ease the passage of the shoulders through the pelvis. The upper shoulder is delivered first, followed by the lower shoulder. The delivery to this point is the most time-consuming portion. Following delivery of the shoulders, the rest of the body exits quite rapidly. The umbilical cord is clamped following delivery, and the neonate begins to function outside the uterus for the first time.

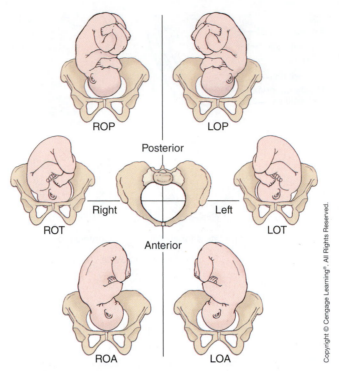

FIGURE 3–2. Positions of a vertex presentation.

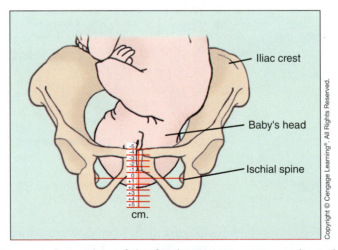

FIGURE 3–3. Station, or relationship of the fetal presenting part to the ischial spines. The station illustrated is +2.

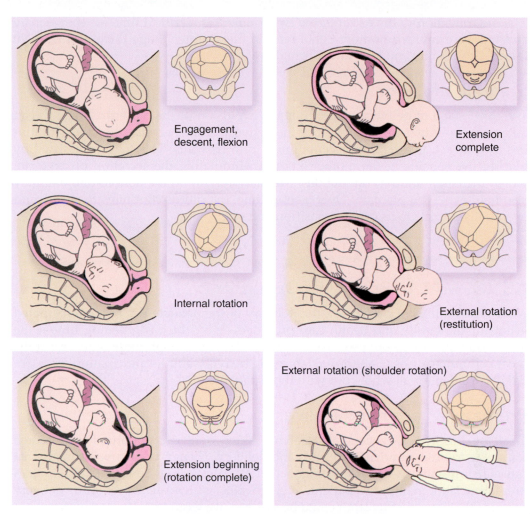

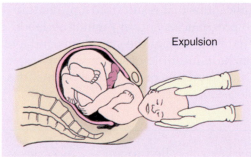

FIGURE 3–4. Mechanisms of labor.

The transition to the extrauterine environment is a critical time for the neonate and will be examined in more detail later in this chapter. Stage II can last from 20 minutes to 2 hours and be within normal range.

Stage III of Labor

The third stage of delivery, stage III, is the expulsion of the placenta. Stage III can take 5 to 45 minutes to achieve. After the delivery of the neonate, the uterus continues to contract, tearing the placenta loose from its walls. This may be assisted by placing the neonate at the mother's breast, stimulating the secretion of oxytocin, which increases uterine contractions. Manual pressure to the abdominal wall may also help expel the placenta. Over a short time, the uterus continues to shrink and eventually returns to its original position and size.

ABNORMAL LABOR AND DELIVERY

After nine months of pregnancy, the delivery of the neonate is a much anticipated event for the family and health care providers. It can be a frightening time if the labor and delivery do not progress as anticipated. A thorough understanding of the most common causes of abnormal labor and delivery and its anticipation, is essential knowledge for all who work with these patients.

Premature Labor and Delivery

Of all the directions that neonatal research is taking, none is as important as the search for a way to prevent premature labor and delivery. There is no incubator made that can match the uterus and no ventilator that can duplicate the placenta. The rate of premature labor in high-risk patients averages 40%, with a rate of premature delivery around 20%. If premature labor could be stopped, we would not have to worry about treating the many complications that result from a premature delivery.

Roughly 12% of all pregnancies end in premature labor. The chance of premature labor can be lowered by knowing the symptoms and avoiding the risk factors. Those at highest risk include multiple gestations, a history of previous premature births, and those with certain uterine or cervical abnormalities. Medical and lifestyle risks are shown in Table 3–2.

Tocolysis

The process of stopping labor is called **tocolysis**. Tocolysis is employed when premature labor threatens the premature delivery of the fetus.

Pharmacologic Tocolysis Many premature labors can be stopped, or at least slowed down, by the use of certain drugs. Tocolysis is often accomplished by the use of beta-sympathomimetic (adrenergic) drugs, which relax smooth muscle contractions. The common adrenergics used are terbutaline sulfate and ritodrine.

Table 3–2

RISK FACTORS FOR PREMATURE LABOR

Medical risk factors include:
- Recurring bladder and/or kidney infections
- Urinary tract infections, vaginal infections, and sexually transmitted infections
- Infection with fever (greater than 101 degrees F) during pregnancy
- Unexplained vaginal bleeding after 20 weeks of pregnancy
- Chronic illness such as high blood pressure, kidney disease, or diabetes
- Multiple first trimester abortions or one or more second trimester abortions
- Underweight or overweight before pregnancy
- Clotting Disorder (thrombophilia)
- Being pregnant with a single fetus after in vitro fertilization (IVF)
- Short time between pregnancies (less than 6–9 months between birth and beginning of the next pregnancy)

Lifestyle risks for premature labor include:
- Little or no prenatal care
- Smoking
- Drinking alcohol
- Using illegal drugs
- Domestic violence, including physical, sexual, or emotional abuse
- Lack of social support
- High levels of stress
- Low income
- Long working hours with long periods of standing

http://www.americanpregnancy.org/labornbirth/prematurelabor.html

Source: American Pregacy Association (http://americanpreganancy.org/labornbirth/prematurelabor.html)

Maternal side effects of the adrenergic drugs include tachycardia, hyperglycemia, hypokalemia, anxiety, nausea, and vomiting. Fetal effects include tachycardia and hyperglycemia. Neonates may develop a rebound hypoglycemia caused by an overproduction of insulin in response to intrauterine hyperglycemia.[2] Fetuses exposed to hyperglycemia in utero often are large for their gestational age; however, the hyperglycemia seen with terbutaline use does not appear to significantly affect birthweight.[3]

Another drug in widespread use, magnesium sulfate, is an anticonvulsant drug that is successful in stopping uterine contractions. It works by decreasing muscle contractility, inhibiting uterine contractions. Neonatal effects of maternal magnesium sulfate administration may include decreased muscle tone, drowsiness, and decreased serum calcium levels.[2] Nelson and Gretcher have conducted a study indicating that the use of magnesium sulfate may protect against cerebral palsy in very-low-birth-weight infants.[4]

With regard to their effectiveness as tocolytic agents, ritodrine and magnesium sulfate appear to be comparable according to one study by Wilkins and associates.[5] However, ritodrine seems to have more complications associated with its use. In addition to the shaking and nervousness accompanying the use of ritodrine, there is an increased incidence of maternal pulmonary edema. Blickstein and associates feel that the pulmonary edema may be secondary to an underlying cardiomyopathy and not the drug itself.[6] Pulmonary edema, which develops in patients receiving tocolytic therapy, also appears to be associated with the presence of maternal infection.

Drugs that inhibit prostaglandin synthetase, such as indomethacin, have been used experimentally to stop prostaglandin-induced labor. Adverse fetal effects seen with indomethacin use include constriction of the ductus arteriosus, pulmonary hypertension, reduced urine production, and rarely, small bowel perforation. A meta-analysis by University of Rochester Medical Center researchers concluded that there is an association between use of indomethacin and babies experiencing periventricular leukomalacia (white matter injury by decreasing blood flow in the brain, which may lead to cerebral palsy[7]).

Calcium channel blockers, such as nifedipine, have been shown to be effective in stopping labor. Side effects of this medication are principally seen in the mother and include nausea, flushing, headache, or dizziness. In the fetus, there is some concern that uterine and umbilical blood flow may be decreased.[8]

Indications for Tocolysis Tocolysis is indicated when stage I labor begins prior to 37 weeks gestation and when placenta previa is present. Preterm birth is a major cause of mortality and morbidity in the perinatal period. In one study, mortality of infants born before 37 weeks gestation was 83%, with 66% of deaths occurring in births less than 29 weeks. Tocolysis in the 20- to 29-week gestation group is aimed at increasing survival and reducing morbidity, whereas tocolysis between 30 and 36 weeks is aimed primarily at reducing morbidity. The prediction of perinatal morbidity and identification of neonates at risk for morbidity and mortality may be aided by measuring the amniotic fluid concentration of interleukin-6.[9]

Continued research is aimed at methods of identifying those mothers at high risk of preterm birth. One such method that showed some promise in early studies is the presence of prolactin in cervicovaginal washings. A more recent review has shown this procedure to not be clinically useful in predicting spontaneous preterm birth.

Tocolysis should only be done when certain factors are present. These factors, described by Knuppel and Drukker are: 1) true labor must be present with at least three contractions of moderate duration and intensity in a 20-minute period, 2) the cervix cannot be dilated more than 4 cm and effaced more than 50% with intact amniotic membranes, 3) the fetus must be between 20 and 36 weeks gestational age, 4) there should be no signs of fetal distress or disease, 5) there should be no medical or obstetric disorder that would contraindicate the continuation of labor, and 6) the mother must be willing and able to give her informed consent.[10]

Nonpharmacologic Strategies for Tocolysis Tocolytic drugs have not proven to be effective in stopping all premature labor. This has caused research to focus on other means of preventing premature labor. Bennett and associates present four nonpharmacologic strategies that do not use tocolytic drugs. They are: 1) comprehensive, accessible family planning; 2) risk assessment and counseling before conception;

3) risk assessment for prenatal patients; and 4) patient education to identify signs of premature labor and when to seek help.[11]

Dystocia (Prolonged Difficult Labor and Delivery)

Dystocia is a prolongation of labor secondary to uterine, pelvic, or fetal factors. Dystocia is present when the first and second stages of labor exceed 20 hours. Dystocia is also present when the second stage of labor exceeds 2 hours in primigravidas and 1 hour in multigravidas. Causes of dystocia are presented in Table 3–3.

As the length of labor increases, fetal morbidity and mortality increase for three main reasons. First, the likelihood of premature separation of the placenta from the uterus is increased, causing serious fetal asphyxia. Second, compression of the umbilical cord, with subsequent fetal asphyxia, is more likely, and third, the risk of premature rupture of the amniotic sac is increased. The danger of fetal infection rises significantly if the amniotic membranes have been ruptured for more than 24 hours. We will now examine the causes of dystocia.

Dysfunction of the Uterus A dysfunctioning uterus may contract excessively (hypertonic) or too mildly (hypotonic). When the uterus contracts hypertonically, the cervix does not dilate and efface as usual. The result may be hypoxia and asphyxia from compression of the placenta, and possibly the umbilical cord. Hypertonic contractions are the less frequent of the two varieties. Hypotonic contractions may be secondary to maternal overdosage of anesthetics or a failure of the fetus to descend normally. With hypotonic contractions, the cervix fails to dilate and efface normally, and contractions are not strong enough to expel the fetus.

Cephalopelvic Disproportion In this abnormality, the disproportion can either be too large a fetal head or too small a maternal pelvic opening. In either case, labor is delayed by the inability of the fetus to enter and then descend the birth canal. Possible causes of a large fetal head include hydrocephaly and a growth-accelerated fetus, which may occur in the presence of maternal diabetes.

Table 3–3

CAUSES OF DYSTOCIA

Uterine dysfunction (abnormal contractions of the uterus)
Abnormal fetal presentations
Excessive fetal size
Hydrocephalus
Abnormality in size or shape of birth canal

Contracture of the maternal pelvis is an infrequent occurrence. It is usually a congenital problem but may be secondary to malnutrition, neoplasms, pelvic fractures, and disorders of the spine or lower extremities. Small pelvic dimensions are also seen in Asian populations and in women younger than 20 years old.[12] The pelvic opening may be diminished in either the anterior/posterior or later dimensions. Both the upper portion of the pelvic opening, the inlet, and the lower portion, the outlet, are measured. The diameter of both pelvic openings is measured by estimating the distances anteroposteriorly and transversely. This is done by manually palpating and measuring the pelvis externally.

Abnormal Presentation Any fetal presentation other than vertex is considered abnormal. The **breech** presentation is the most common of all abnormal presentations, compromising about 3.5% of all births. Other abnormal presentations include face, brow, and shoulder or transverse lie of the fetus. Breech refers to the fetus being in a buttocks-down position.

The breech presentation is broken down into three varieties. When the feet, legs, and buttocks all present together, it is called a complete breech. An incomplete or footling breech occurs when one or both feet descend into the birth canal first. Frank breech occurs when the legs are flexed against the body, the feet being near the face, and the buttocks being the presenting part (Figure 3–5).

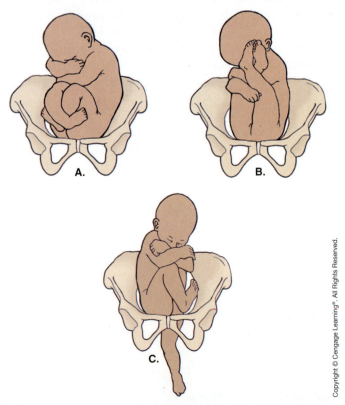

FIGURE 3–5. Breech presentations. A. Complete. B. Frank. C. Footling.

The primary complication of breech presentations occurs when there is a diminished pelvic size or enlarged fetal head. The problems arise after the body has been delivered and it is then discovered that the fetal head will not pass through the pelvis. At this point it is too late to perform a cesarean delivery and the head must be extracted from the pelvis. This is done by manipulation and pulling on the delivered fetal body by the obstetrician. The result is often spinal cord damage and hemorrhage in the brain. Placenta previa, discussed later in this chapter, is a common cause of the breech presentation.

The fetal skull (Figure 3–6) is not a solid structure as in the adult. It is made up of several bony plates separated by what are known as sutures. In normal presentations, as the head enters the birth canal, these sutures overlap, diminishing the diameter of the fetal skull and facilitating the birth of the fetus.

In face or brow presentation the head enters the birth canal in such a way that the sutures cannot override (Figure 3–7). The result is that the head must pass through the pelvis and the birth canal at its full size. This may or may not result in prolongation of labor, depending on the size of the maternal pelvic opening. The neonate may suffer from severe facial edema following this type of delivery. Fetal mortality is increased with this type of delivery, secondary to the asphyxia frequently seen with prolonged labor.

Shoulder presentation, or transverse lie, occurs when the fetus is lying perpendicular to the birth canal (Figure 3–8). Delivery of the fetus in this state is nearly impossible and requires a great deal of manipulation to straighten the fetus. If manipulation fails, a cesarean delivery is done.

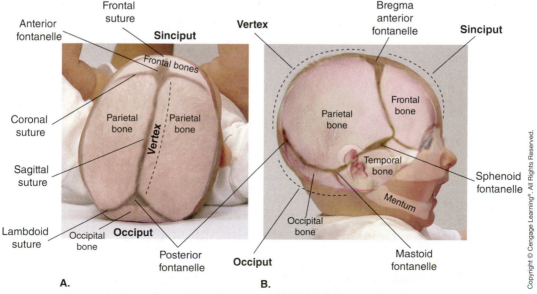

FIGURE 3–6. Fetal skull: sutures and fontanelles. A. Superior view. B. Lateral view.

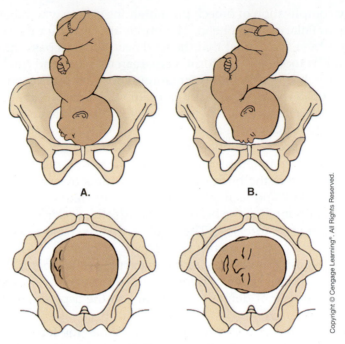

FIGURE 3–7. A. Brow presentation. B. Face presentation.

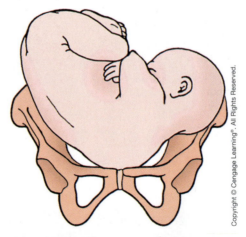

FIGURE 3–8. Shoulder presentation (transverse lie).

Problems Associated with the Umbilical Cord

Even though the Wharton's jelly, present in the umbilical cord, reduces the risk of the cord from bending to the point of occluding blood flow, it does not prevent the cord from being compressed between two body parts. This type of occlusion can occur in the uterus or in the birth canal.

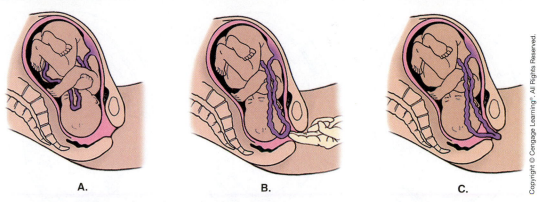

A.   **B.**   **C.**

FIGURE 3–9. Prolapsed cord. A. Occult (hidden, cannot be seen or felt). B. Complete (cannot be seen but may be felt). C. Visible (can be seen protruding from vagina).

Prolapse of the Umbilical Cord When the umbilical cord passes through the cervix into the birth canal ahead of the presenting part, it is called **prolapse** of the umbilical cord (Figure 3–9). This problem is common in breech presentations, especially footling and transverse lie, and in multiple gestations. As the fetus passes through the birth canal, the cord is easily compressed between the fetus and the maternal pelvis. Compression of the cord can also occur in the uterus and is called an **occult** prolapse.

Either of these occurrences can be dangerous to the fetus. Any interruption of blood flow through the umbilical cord leads to hypoxia, and eventual asphyxia to the fetus, and requires immediate intervention. This condition is monitored via the fetal heart monitor. Intrauterine cord compression can be reduced by artificially increasing the amniotic fluid volume through a process known as amnioinfusion.[13] By increasing the amniotic fluid volume, there is more room in the uterus and less chance of cord compression.

Placental Abnormalities

The placenta begins development at implantation and is finally delivered with the fetus at birth. The fetus relies on the placenta for all of the essentials needed for proper development and growth. With such an important role, it is vital that the placenta develop and function normally throughout pregnancy.

Placenta Previa In most pregnancies the blastocyst attaches itself somewhere near the upper portion of the uterine cavity. When the implantation occurs in the lower portion of the uterus, it is called **placenta previa**. Three varieties of placenta previa are recognized, according to their proximity to the cervix (Figure 3–10).

A low implantation occupies the lower portion of the uterus but does not cover the cervical opening. A partial placenta previa covers a portion of the cervical opening but does not cover it completely. Total placenta previa completely covers the opening of the cervix.

All types of placenta previa are readily diagnosed by ultrasound. It is obvious that with any type of previa, there will be varying degrees of obstruction to fetal

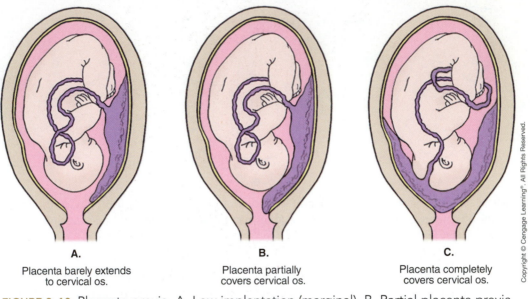

A.

Placenta barely extends
to cervical os.

B.

Placenta partially
covers cervical os.

C.

Placenta completely
covers cervical os.

FIGURE 3–10. Placenta previa. A. Low implantation (marginal). B. Partial placenta previa. C. Total placenta previa.

passage. A more serious complication is the early separation of the placenta from the uterus, abruptio placentae, discussed next.

Abruptio Placentae Any time a normally attached placenta separates prematurely from the uterine wall, it is called **abruptio placentae**. Separation of the placenta frequently causes labor to begin. Such a pregnancy is precarious at best and requires very close monitoring by the physician. Premature labor and delivery occur more commonly with abruptio placentae. This is due to the frequent commencement of labor when the placenta separates from the uterine wall. Maternal mortality ranges from 2% to 10% in severe cases ending in fetal death. Fetal mortality approaches 50% owing to the acuteness of blood loss.

The most common cause of abruption is maternal hypertension of any origin, which includes **preeclampsia**. Maternal preeclampsia is the development of hypertension with proteinuria, edema, or both. It is of unknown etiology and usually presents after week 20 of gestation.

Additionally, abruptio placentae may be present in someone with a history of abruption, a high number of previous pregnancies, trauma, short umbilical cord, sudden uterine decompression, uterine anomalies, and compression of the inferior vena cava.

Placental separation can be partial or complete. If bleeding from the vagina is present, it is called an apparent hemorrhage. If no bleeding is evident, it is called a concealed hemorrhage. Figure 3–11 shows the different combinations of abruptio placentae that are possible. A categorization of abruptio placentae is listed in Table 3–4.

The mother and the fetus are at risk in the presence of placental abruption. Severe abruptio placentae is clinically manifested by vaginal bleeding, tetany of the

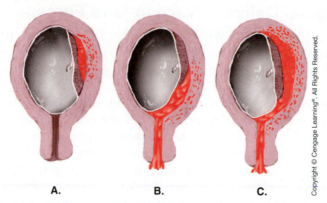

A. **B.** **C.**

FIGURE 3–11. Abruptio placentae. A. Central abruption, concealed hemorrhage. B. Marginal abruption, external hemorrhage. C. Complete abruption, external hemorrhage (could also be concealed).

uterus, tenderness of the uterus, absent fetal heart tones, and maternal hypovolemic shock. The risk to the fetus is the loss of placental surface area, resulting in severe fetal hypoxia and asphyxia. Premature separation of the placenta may also lead to fetal blood loss, with subsequent anemia and shock.

Treatment of abruptio placentae includes strict management of blood volume, maintaining a hematocrit volume of 30%. This is done by the intravenous administration of blood or crystalloid solutions. The mother is instructed to lie in the lateral position to allow maximal placental circulation. Intensive monitoring of both fetus and mother is essential, and those in charge of care should prepare for emergency delivery or cesarean delivery if the signs of maternal shock or fetal distress are seen.

Table 3–4

CLASSIFICATION OF ABRUPTIO PLACENTAE

Grade 0—Asymptomatic. Diagnosis is made after delivery when a small clot is found behind the placenta.

Grade 1—Vaginal bleeding. No signs of maternal shock or fetal distress. Tetany and tenderness of the uterus may be present.

Grade 2—External vaginal bleeding may or may not be present. No signs of maternal shock. Signs of fetal distress are present. Tetany and tenderness of the uterus are present.

Grade 3—External vaginal bleeding may or may not be present. Maternal shock and persistent abdominal pain are present. Fetal demise is present. Marked uterine tetany resulting in a very stiff, firm consistency. Thirty percent of cases show signs of coagulopathy.

Assisted Vaginal Delivery: Vacuum and Forceps

Assist devices are typically used when the second stage of labor stalls, or when fetal heart tones are atypical. Both the vacuum and forceps are capable of causing neonatal injury and should only be used when spontaneous vaginal delivery is not possible.

Vacuum Extraction Vacuum extractors are bell shaped and designed to fit over the fetal skull over the sagittal suture and in front of the posterior fontanelle. The most common extractors are made of a soft silicone and shaped like a funnel or bell.

Older extractors were made of metal and had a higher rate of trauma to the fetal scalp than the softer silicone. Complications to the fetus with the use of vacuum extraction most often involve a vascular rupture. The most common complication is subgaleal hemorrhage but also seen are cephalohematomas, and intercranial and retinal hemorrages. A nonbleeding complication is lateral rectus paralysis, however, it is almost always transient and not considered to be a clinically important occurrence.

Forceps Extraction Obstetrical forceps have been compared to long spoons or tongs (Figure 3–12). One blade of the forceps is placed individually on the side of the fetal head and then the second one is placed on the opposing side. They are then connected in order to articulate them, and they can additionally be locked with a wing nut to keep them from separating. Once in place, the forceps can be used to turn the fetus in utero and to assist delivery by applying traction to the fetal head. While they are less traumatic to the fetus, they are more likely to cause injury to the mother in the way of vaginal, perineal, or rectal tearing.

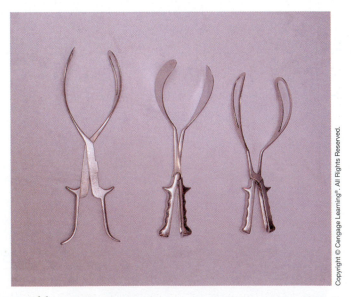

FIGURE 3–12. Types of forceps.

Cesarean Delivery

Some fetuses are delivered by way of a surgical incision through the maternal abdomen and uterus, called a cesarean delivery, or cesarean section. Cesarean deliveries are performed under anesthesia and should only be done in the presence of the following indications: prior cesarean delivery, dystocia, breech presentation, and fetal distress.[14]

Most cesarean deliveries result in a healthy neonate, but there are some possible complications. The most serious complications arise from accidental cutting of the placenta, umbilical cord, or fetus during the delivery. This can lead to serious hemorrhage and anemia. Another common complication is transient tachypnea of the newborn (TTN). This syndrome, discussed in Chapter 7 is thought to be caused by the retention of lung fluids, normally expelled as the fetus is squeezed through the birth canal.

Multiple Gestations

Multiple gestation is the presence of twins, triplets, quadruplets, or more fetuses during the same pregnancy. The incidence of mortality is higher in multiple than in single gestations.[15] This is due in part to the high incidence of premature labor and delivery in multiple gestations. There is also an increased incidence of congenital abnormalities, growth retardation, bacterial infection, and hypoglycemia.

Several factors increase the incidence of multiple gestations. Familial inheritance predisposes the carrier female to have fraternal twins. There is a high incidence of multiple gestation among blacks, and a very low incidence in the Asian population. Multiple gestations are also more common in the older female, ages 35 to 39. The administration of clomiphene citrate (Clomid®) to induce ovulation is associated with a high incidence of multiple gestations, as is the administration of gonadotropins. It is also speculated that there is an increase in twinning following discontinuation of oral contraceptives.

Twinning is the most common type of multiple gestation, occurring in about 1 out of 99 pregnancies. Two thirds of all twins are fraternal or dizygotic and arise from the fertilization of two separate ova. Fraternal twinning is an **autosomal-recessive trait** that is carried by the daughters of mothers of twins.

The remaining one third are identical twins, originating from one ova. They are of the same sex and have an identical appearance. In contrast to fraternal twins, identical twinning is a random occurrence. Identical twins have a higher mortality rate than do fraternal twins. Whenever there is a shared placenta or umbilicus between twins, there is an increase in risk factors. One twin may receive more nutrition, or actually deplete the other twin.

For some reason, the second twin is often more compromised than the first, and it appears that female twins are healthier than male twins.

ADAPTATION TO EXTRAUTERINE LIFE

Of all the adaptations that a human undergoes throughout life, none is quite so strenuous or important as the adaptation to extrauterine life. Within a short time following birth the neonate must undergo major changes that will allow it to survive outside the uterus. The neonate must begin spontaneous ventilation and respiration. The circulatory system must change to its adult pattern, and the neonate must now provide its own energy and rid itself of wastes. This chapter examines the establishment of breathing. Chapter addressed the changes in the cardiovascular system.

The First Breath

No single event is as thrilling as when a newborn takes its first breath. The breath is the sign of life, and the sound of the crying neonate is anxiously awaited by all in attendance at the delivery. What is unknown to many, however, is the magnitude of what must take place in order for the neonate to take that first breath.

Studies have shown that the fetus begins breathing movements while still in the uterus. Fetal respiratory movements have been detected as early as week 18, but most activity occurs during the last 10 weeks of gestation. These movements no doubt prepare the fetus for the time when it will be on its own.

The exact sequence of events that occur to stimulate the first breath is unknown; however, it is most likely the result of both physical and biochemical stimulations. Once the fetus has left the confines of the uterus, several events must occur to provide for an easy transition to extrauterine breathing. First, there must be something to stimulate the neonate to breathe. Biochemical and physical factors thought to be involved in the initiation of the first breath are listed in Table 3–5.

Biochemical and Physical Factors Thought to be Responsible for the First Breath Chemoreceptors found in the aorta and carotid arteries detect changes in PaO_2 and $PaCO_2$ levels in the blood. During the process of birth, the fetus is cut off from the placenta as it descends the birth canal. As a result, fetal PaO_2 falls and

Table 3–5

INITIATION OF THE FIRST BREATH

- BIOCHEMICAL:
  Asphyxia. Increased $PaCO_2$, decreased PaO_2, and pH stimulate the chemoreceptors, which then stimulate gasping.

- PHYSICAL:
  Recoil of the thorax. As the thorax passes through the birth canal during vaginal delivery, it is compressed. As the thorax exits the birth canal, the natural recoil of the thorax creates a negative pressure in the thoracic cavity, causing air to enter the lungs.

- Environmental changes. As the fetus passes from an environment of darkness and warmth into a bright, loud, cold environment, the abrupt change initiates a cry reflex. Additionally, tactile stimulus from handling further stimulates the cry reflex.

PaCO$_2$ rises. These two changes stimulate the chemoreceptors, which in turn stimulate the respiratory center in the brain. The brain signals the muscles of ventilation into action. This birth asphyxia is probably the most powerful influence on stimulating the initial breath.

A second contribution to the first breath occurs during vaginal delivery. The fetal thorax is compressed as it descends through the birth canal. As it exits, the chest expands to its original size and shape. A result of this expansion is the entry of air into the lungs. Additionally, during vaginal delivery the lung fluid is expelled, creating an "empty volume" in the lungs to be filled with air upon delivery.

A third influence is the abrupt change in environment from the dark and warm uterus to the bright, cold, and noisy delivery room. These changes, combined with the physical handling of the neonate, invoke the crying reflex, which also helps stimulate the first breath.

In order for the neonate to breathe successfully, surface forces in the lung must be overcome. In the term neonate this is aided immensely by the presence of pulmonary surfactant. Surfactant greatly reduces the surface tension of the alveoli and reduces the work required of the neonate to ventilate. Chapter 1 contains a detailed discussion of pulmonary surfactant.

The initial pressure needed to overcome the surface forces of the lung has been measured and found to be as high as −100 cm H$_2$O. Succeeding breaths require much less negative pressure due to the establishment of the functional residual capacity (FRC). This concept is illustrated in Figure 3–13. The FRC is simply air that remains in the lung following normal exhalation.

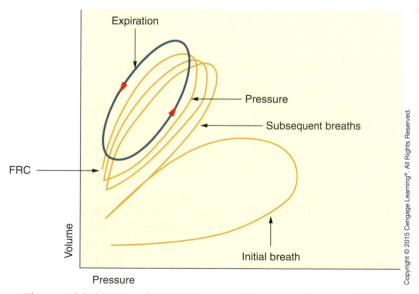

FIGURE 3–13. The establishment of FRC following delivery. With each ensuing breath, the FRC gradually increases, requiring less pressure to produce larger tidal volumes.

As the alveoli are deflated following the first breath, the presence of surfactant prevents them from collapsing completely, allowing them to remain partially filled with air. With each ensuing breath a little more air remains, causing the FRC to gradually expand in the first few hours of life. The result is that each successive breath becomes less difficult and requires less energy to accomplish. Thus, the healthy neonate quickly adapts to extrauterine breathing when the lungs are mature.

SUMMARY

The process of human birth is a complex event that is poorly understood. Normal birth starts with the first contraction, which signals the start of stage I of labor. During this stage, the cervix effaces and dilates to accommodate the passage of the fetus. Stage II is the actual delivery of the fetus, and stage III is the expulsion of the placenta.

Many factors can lead to an abnormal labor and delivery. Of all the causes of perinatal morbidity and mortality, none is as devastating as premature labor and birth. Preventing premature labor is a major focus of perinatal medicine and is accomplished with the use of tocolytic drugs, which help slow and hopefully stop uterine contractions. Another factor resulting in abnormal labor and delivery is dystocia caused by a dysfunctioning uterus, cephalopelvic disproportion, or an abnormal fetal presentation.

Labor and delivery can also be complicated by compression of the umbilical cord, either in utero (occult) or in the birth canal (prolapse). Complications are also seen with placental abnormalities such as placenta previa and abruptio placentae.

Approximately 25% of deliveries in the United States are done via cesarean section.[14] This mode of delivery can predispose the fetus to accidental trauma and blood loss, and TTN. Multiple gestations also have a higher incidence of mortality and can complicate the normal birthing process.

Once born, the fetus must adapt to the extrauterine environment. The stimulation of chemoreceptors, expansion of the fetal thorax, and stimulation are all factors that initiate extrauterine breathing. As the neonate continues to breathe, surface forces in the lungs are reduced by the presence of surfactant and FRC increases as compliance improves.

POSTTEST

1. A 32 year-old patient is admitted to the high-risk obstetric floor in premature labor. She is currently at 28 weeks gestation. She has three living children with one miscarriage and one previous premature delivery. Which of the following is her correct obstetrical history?
   a. G4 P2113
   b. G3 P1114
   c. G4 P3014
   d. G4 P2004

2. You are confronted by a worried parent in the waiting room who is concerned that her daughter seems to be taking too long to deliver her first grandchild. Her daughters first contractions started at 2:00 am, she was admitted at 4:00 am, and it is now 11:30 pm of the same day. You arrive at the nurses station and see that the patient is fully effaced and dilated to 8 cm. Which of the following is most likely?
   a. For a primigravida, this is still within the normal time variations.
   b. It is likely the daughter is preeclamptic.
   c. This is a classic case of cephalo-pelvic disproportion.
   d. The daughter has the signs of a dysfunctional uterus.

3. A 40-week gestation fetus is found to be in the breech position and is having severe heart rate decelerations. A vaginal examination is done, and it is found that the cervix is dilated to 10 cm with 100% effacement. The vaginal exam reveals no abnormalities and the amniotic sac ruptured nearly an hour previously. The most likely cause of the decelerations is:
   a. the breech presentation causing pressure on the head
   b. an occult prolapse of the umbilical cord
   c. hypoxia due to an extended stage I
   d. the loss of amniotic fluid

4. A 25-year-old female with a history of hypertension is admitted with a chief complaint of vaginal bleeding. She is 26 weeks gestation with her first pregnancy. On abdominal examination, her uterus is tender and feels contracted. Which of the following is most likely?
   a. Grade 0 abruption
   b. Grade I abruption
   c. Grade II abruption
   d. Grade III abruption

5. A G2P3 45 year old with a 20-pack/year smoking history is admitted to the hospital at 23 weeks gestation. Her blood pressure is measured at 160/98 and she has 2+ edema in both lower legs. You suspect preeclampsia; however, one additional test needs to be run to confirm the diagnosis. That test is:
   a. urinalysis
   b. blood culture
   c. fetal heart rate
   d. blood electrolytes

6. 5 hours postpartum following a forceps assisted vaginal delivery, a primigravida 29-year-old patient notices a small amount of frank blood on her pad. The nurse performs a vaginal examination and notices a small tear in the perineum. This is most likely caused by:
   a. the fact that she is primigravida
   b. the use of the forceps
   c. cepahalo-pelvic disproportion
   d. a weakened vaginal wall from an extended labor

7. During a routine prenatal class, a couple approaches you and reveals that they are expecting twins. They question whether the twins will be identical or fraternal. You discover that the mother of the pregnant woman was a twin. You tell them:
   a. that it is impossible to predict whether the twins will be fraternal or identical
   b. that there is an equal chance for fraternal or identical twins
   c. that they are more likely to be identical twins
   d. that they are more likely to be fraternal twins
8. Which of the following physical or biochemical factors initiating the first breath is a baby born via cesarean section likely to miss?
   a. chest recoil
   b. hypoxemia
   c. physical stimulation
   d. increased carbon dioxide level

REFERENCES

1. Roberts WE, et al. Risk of preterm delivery from preterm labor in high-risk patients. *J Reprod Med.* 40:95–100, 1995.
2. Merenstein GB, Gardner SL. *Handbook of Neonatal Intensive Care.* 7th ed. St. Louis: CV Mosby Co., 2011.
3. Robins GW, Blount BW, Airline A. Effective of terbutaline tocolysis on infant birthweight. *J Fam Pract.* 40:581–585, 1995.
4. Nelson KB, Grether JK. Can magnesium sulfate reduce the risk of cerebral palsy in very low birthweight infants? *Pediatrics.* 95:263–269, 1995.
5. Wilkins IA, et al. Efficacy and side effects of magnesium sulfate and ritodrine as tocolytic agents. *Am J Obstet Gynecol.* 159:685–689, 1988.
6. Blickstein I, et al. Ritodrine-induced pulmonary edema unmasking underlying peripartum cardiomyopathy. *Am J Obstet Gynecol.* 159:332–333, 1988.
7. University of Rochester Medical Center. Common drug for stopping preterm labor may be harmful for babies. *ScienceDaily*, Nov. 1, 2007.
8. Monga M, Creasy RK. Pharmacologic management of preterm labor. *Semin Perinatol.* 19:84–96, 1995.
9. Yoon BH, et al. Amniotic fluid interleukin-6: a sensitive test for antenatal diagnosis of acute inflammatory lesions of preterm placenta and prediction of perinatal morbidity. *Am J Obstet Gynecol.* 172:960–970, 1995.
10. Knuppel RA, Drukker JE. *High-Risk Pregnancy: A Team Approach.* 2nd ed. Philadelphia: WB Saunders Co., 1993.
11. Bennett NL, et al. New strategies for preterm labor. *Nurse Practitioner.* 14:27–28, 30, 33–34, 1989.
12. Lowdermilk DL, Perry SE, Bobak IM. *Maternity Nursing.* 5th ed. St. Louis: Mosby Inc., 1999.

13. Strong TH Jr. Amnioinfusion. *J. Reprod Med.* 40:108–114, 1995.
14. Paul RH, Miller DA. Cesarian birth: how to reduce the rate. *Am J Obstet Gynecol.* 172:1903–1907, 1995.
15. Gander MO, et al. The origin and outcomes of preterm twin pregnancies. *Obstet Gynecol.* 85:553–557, 1995.

BIBLIOGRAPHY AND SUGGESTED READINGS

Avery GB, Fletcher MA, MacDonald MG. *Pathophysiology and Management of the Newborn.* 6th ed. Philadelphia: JB Lippincott Co., 2005.

Des Jardins, T. *Cardiopulmonary Anatomy and Physiology, Essentials for Respiratory Care.* 6th ed. Clifton Park, NY: Cengage Learning, 2013.

Moore KL, Persaud TVN, Shiota K. *Color Atlas of Clinical Embryology.* 2nd ed. Philadelphia, PA : WB Saunders Co., 2001.

Olson DM, Mijovic JE, Sadowsky DW. Control of human parturition. *Semin Perinatol.* 19:52–63, 1995.

Tucker SM. *Pocket Guide to Fetal Monitoring and Assessment.* 5th ed. St. Louis: Mosby, 2004.

White L, Duncan G, Baumle W. *Foundations of Nursing: Caring for the Whole Person (3e).* Clifton Park, NY: Cengage Learning, 2011.

Techniques of Resuscitation and Stabilization of the Neonatal Patient

OBJECTIVES

Upon completion of this chapter, the reader should be able to:

1. List the four factors that can lead to fetal asphyxia.
2. Compare and contrast primary to secondary apnea.
3. Describe the cardiovascular events that occur during periods of intrauterine asphyxia.
4. Discuss the effects of asphyxia on the lungs.
5. List and describe the three factors that provide proper preparation for neonatal resuscitation.
6. Describe and discuss each step in the neonatal resuscitation process.
7. Describe each of the following skills as it relates to neonatal resuscitation:
   a. Thermoregulation
   b. Opening the airway
   c. Evaluation of respirations
   d. Evaluation of heart rate
   e. Evaluate color
   f. Positive pressure ventilation (PPV)
   g. Reevaluation
   h. Chest compressions
   i. Intubation
   j. Delivery of medications
8. List the drugs used during neonatal resuscitation. Include correct concentrations used, dosages, and routes of administration.
9. Assign an appropriate Apgar score when provided with patient data.
10. Describe the sources of fetal and neonatal glucose.
11. List the serum glucose values that indicate hypoglycemia. Include a description of the clinical signs.
12. List and describe the cause of hypoglycemia, techniques used to measure glucose, and the treatment for hypoglycemia.
13. Describe the procedure for obtaining arterial blood from the umbilical stump.

14. Discuss the indications, procedure for placement, and complications of an umbilical artery catheter (UAC).
15. Define the mnemonic S.T.A.B.L.E, and describe the purpose and function of the training.

KEY TERMS

acrocyanosis	flow-inflating bag	secondary apnea
asphyxia	glucagon	self-inflating bag
brown fat	necrotizing enterocolitis	supine
conductive	persistent fetal	thumb technique
convective	circulation (PFC)	T-piece resuscitator
erythroblastosis fetalis	primary apnea	two-finger technique
evaporative	radiant	vigorous

INTRODUCTION

For those who work with newborns, the skills and knowledge required for proper resuscitation are possibly the most important skills to possess. According to the American Academy of Pediatrics approximately 10% of newborns require some sort of resuscitative support and only 1% require extensive intervention to survive. In our society, it should be expected that each newborn receive appropriate skilled care provided by individuals who are properly trained and who have the necessary experience to perform a well-organized resuscitation that will result in the best possible outcome. It is anticipated that most respiratory therapists in a hospital setting will eventually be involved in a newborn resuscitation. For this reason, it is strongly recommended that each provider complete the Neonatal Resuscitation Program (NRP) offered jointly by the American Academy of Pediatrics and the American Heart Association. Although much of the information for this chapter was obtained from that program, this chapter is not a substitution for obtaining the NRP certification.[1]

WHEN TO RESUSCITATE

Asphyxia can cause severely damaging results to the fetus and the neonate. A successful intervention requires that the respiratory therapist know stages of primary and secondary apnea and the causes of fetal and neonatal asphyxia injuries. Understanding this information will better prepare the respiratory therapist to know when to resuscitate.

Primary and Secondary Apnea

The necessity to resuscitate a neonate is related to asphyxia, which can occur in utero during or after delivery. **Asphyxia**, which is a combination of hypoxia, hypercapnia, and acidosis, may lead to irreversible damage to the brain and other vital organs. Fetal asphyxia may be caused by any of the factors listed in Table 4–1.

Table 4–1

CAUSES OF FETAL ASPHYXIA

1. Maternal hypoxia
   a. Low environmental oxygen
   b. Apnea associated with seizures or eclampsia
   c. Acute asthma attack
   d. Pneumonia
   e. Hypoventilation from over sedation
   f. Carbon monoxide poisoning or anemia

2. Insufficient placental blood flow
   a. Diminished blood flow to the placenta secondary to congestive heart failure
   b. Hypotension and shock
   c. Vasoconstrictive states secondary to toxemia and essential hypertension
   d. Placenta previa
   e. Abruptio placentae

3. Blockage of umbilical blood flow
   a. Prolapse of the umbilical cord
   b. Occult prolapse of the umbilical cord
   c. Nuchal cord (wrapping of the cord around the fetal neck or body)

4. Fetal disorders
   a. Hydrops fetalis (fetal cardiac failure in utero)
   b. Fetal hypotension from hemorrhage or drugs
   c. Fetal hemolytic anemia

First, any disorder that leads to maternal hypoxia or asphyxia will in turn lead to asphyxia in the fetus. Second, insufficient placental blood flow or a reduction in the diffusion of oxygen and carbon dioxide will lead to decreased gas transfer from maternal blood to fetal blood and vice versa. Third, occlusion or blockage of blood flow through the umbilical cord stops blood flow to and from the placenta, which may lead to asphyxia. Finally, certain fetal factors such as anemia and drug toxicity can cause fetal asphyxia.

When any of these factors are present, the fetus initially becomes hypoxic. Because of the early development of chemoreceptors and baroreceptors in the fetal vasculature, the fetus can react to changes in blood gases while still in utero. The fetus attempts to reverse the hypoxia by beginning rapid respiratory effort. If the hypoxia is not corrected, the ventilatory effort ceases and the fetus enters a period of apnea called **primary apnea**. At this point, the heart rate and blood pressure begin to drop.

With continued hypoxia, $PaCO_2$ rises and the pH drops, leading to asphyxia. Continuation of the asphyxia leads to a second attempt by the fetus to ventilate.

This time, however, the respirations are weak, gasping, and ineffective. Again, this stage of attempting to regain ventilation may occur in utero or during the birthing process. The efforts weaken and cease, and the fetus enters another stage of apnea, known as **secondary apnea**. During secondary apnea, there will be no attempt to breathe again unless positive pressure ventilation (PPV) is initiated. When untreated, the heart rate and blood pressure drop until death occurs.

The return of spontaneous ventilation is a result of rapid initiation of PPV with supplemental oxygen adequate to stabilize pulse oximetry values within a normal range. The longer the patient has been in secondary apnea, the longer the PPV required until spontaneous breathing returns and the greater the chance of brain damage. As previously mentioned, a fetus may go through all of these stages in utero and be born in secondary apnea of unknown duration. One must, therefore, always assume that an apneic infant is in secondary apnea and begin resuscitative efforts immediately. Time wasted in trying to stimulate the infant only places it at a higher risk of developing brain damage.

Effect of Asphyxia on the Lungs

As discussed in Chapter 3, the initial adaptation of the fetal lungs to the extrauterine environment requires two steps. First, the lung must rid itself of the lung fluid and become filled with air. This requires the fetus to create significant negative pressures in the thorax to overcome the initial resistance and low compliance in the lungs. The second important step is the decrease in pulmonary vascular resistance secondary to the increasing levels of oxygen in the blood and ensuing vascular dilation.

As blood flow increases past the ventilated alveoli, PaO_2 further increases and $PaCO_2$ decreases, resulting in the eventual establishment of an adult pattern of circulation. When asphyxiation occurs, there is a disruption of one or both of these two vital steps, with the result being that the neonate does not adapt to the extrauterine environment.

A neonate who is born apneic or with shallow, ineffective respirations, may not be able to create the necessary negative force to open the alveoli and aid in lung fluid removal. The presence of hypoxia, hypercarbia, and acidosis causes significant pulmonary vasoconstriction to persist in the lungs, leading to a continuation of pulmonary hypertension. Blood flow continues to be shunted through the foramen ovale and the ductus arteriosus, completely bypassing the lungs as it did during fetal circulation. This occurrence is called **persistent fetal circulation (PFC)**, and it leads to further asphyxia, because little blood is coming in contact with the ventilated alveoli.

In severe cases of asphyxia, ventilation alone may not alter blood gases because of the significance of the shunt. $PaCO_2$ remains high in the face of adequate ventilation because of the blood bypassing the lungs. In these severe cases further intervention may be necessary. If pulmonary vascular resistance remains high, preventing adequate pulmonary circulation and impeding necessary gas exchange, the use of inhaled nitric oxide (iNO) may be used once the neonate is stabilized in order to achieve necessary pulmonary vasodilation.

PREPARATION FOR RESUSCITATION

An important determinant of a successful resuscitation is the amount of preparation that takes place before the delivery of a high-risk neonate (Table 4–2).

Anticipation of a High-Risk Delivery

The first step in preparing for neonatal resuscitation is anticipation of the depressed neonate. Anticipation involves a basic knowledge of the maternal history, the history of the pregnancy, and continuous monitoring of the mother and fetus during labor and delivery. Maternal history and history of the pregnancy should be examined with the high-risk factors discussed in Chapter 3 in mind.

Monitoring of the mother and fetus during labor and delivery includes maternal cardiovascular and pulmonary status and ongoing evaluation of the fetal heart rate. Proper identification and anticipation of a depressed neonate allows the team to be ready for the delivery and prepared to deal with potential problems. In some cases, this information is simply not available. If possible, the most basic information can be helpful. At a minimum determine the gestation of the neonate (term or preterm), if there are multiple neonates, and if there is meconium present. These three pieces of information provide the resuscitation team valuable information that will prepare them to respond, even in emergent cases where there is little time to prepare.

Equipment

The second important part of the preparation is the presence of properly functioning equipment at every delivery. Equipment and supplies that should be present at each

---

Table 4–2

PREPARATION FOR RESUSCITATION

1. Anticipation of a high-risk delivery requires:
   a. Maternal history
   b. History of the pregnancy
   c. Continuous monitoring during labor and delivery

2. Equipment
   a. Proper equipment
   b. Variety of sizes to suit various gestational ages
   c. Checked for proper function each shift

3. Trained personnel
   a. At least one person trained in all necessary skills
   b. Must be present in the hospital to respond to unexpected high-risk deliveries

resuscitation are listed in Table 4–3. The time to discover that a resuscitation bag is not working is not after the neonate is delivered. Equipment must be checked each shift, not only for its presence, but also for proper function. Equipment is checked again at the time of delivery in preparation for the resuscitation. When turning on all equipment and gathering supplies, each item should be checked for proper function. It is also wise to have back up supplies in case of equipment failure. This may include additional laryngoscope blades, endotracheal tubes, resuscitation bag and mask, suction supplies, etc.

Table 4–3

NEONATAL RESUSCITATION SUPPLIES AND EQUIPMENT

Suction Equipment
- Bulb syringe
- Mechanical suction and tubing
- Suction catheters, 5F or 6F, 8F, 10F
- 8F feeding tube and 20-mL syringe
- Meconium aspirator

Bag-and-Mask Equipment
- Neonatal resuscitation bag with a pressure-release valve or pressure gauge—the bag must be capable of delivering 90% to 100% oxygen
- Face masks, newborn and premature sizes (cushioned rim masks preferred)
- Oxygen with flow meter and tubing
- Oxygen blender to mix oxygen and compressed air to achieve desired oxygen percentage
- Pulse oximeter and oximeter probe

Intubation Equipment
- Laryngoscope with straight blades, No. 0 (preterm) and No. 1 (term)
- Extra bulbs and batteries for laryngoscope
- Endotracheal tubes, 2.5, 3.0, 3.5, 4.0 mm
- Stylet (optional)
- Scissors
- Tape or securing device for endotracheal tube
- CO_2 detector or capnograph
- Laryngeal mask airway (LMA)

Medications
- Epinephrine 1:10,000—3-mL or 10-mL ampules
- Isotonic crystalloid (normal saline or Ringer's lactate) for volume expansion 100–250 mL

- Dextrose 10%, 250 mL
- Normal saline for flushes

Umbilical vessel catheterization supplies
- Sterile gloves
- Scalpel or scissors
- Antiseptic prep solution
- Umbilical tape
- Umbilical catheters, 3.5F, 5F
- Three-way stopcock
- Syringes 1, 3, 5, 10, 20, 50 mL
- Needles, 25, 21, 18 gauge, or puncture device for needleless system

Miscellaneous
- Gloves and appropriate personal protection
- Radiant warmer or other heat source
- Firm, padded resuscitation surface
- Clock with second hand (timer optional)
- Warm linens
- Stethoscope (with neonatal head)
- Cardiac monitor and electrodes or pulse oximeter and probe (optional for delivery room)
- Adhesive tape, 1/2 or 3/4 inch

Trained Personnel

The third part of proper preparation is the presence of trained personnel who can direct the resuscitation and perform the necessary procedures. At a minimum, there should be two skilled persons present whose sole focus is the resuscitation of the neonate. If multiple births are expected, two additional personnel should be on hand to provide resuscitation for each additional neonate. Because many asphyxiated fetuses are born with no prior warning, it is of utmost importance that these skilled personnel be available to assist at all deliveries.

STANDARD PRECAUTIONS

Whenever there is a potential for exposure to any bodily fluids or blood, a high probability during a resuscitation, the respiratory therapist must follow standard or universal precautions. It is probable that, unless one is simply observing, the neonate will be handled, and the potential for a droplet of blood or fluid to hit those partici-pating is high. Therefore, gloves, masks, and protective eye wear should be worn by all present. Additionally, a gown or apron should be worn if the possibility of blood or body fluid splashing is present.

DETERMINE IF THE NEONATE REQUIRES RESUSCITATION

According to NRP guidelines there are three questions that should be asked upon the delivery of the neonate:

1. Is the neonate term?
2. Is the neonate crying or breathing?
3. Is there good muscle tone?

If the answer to one or more of these questions is 'no' then that is a good indication that the neonate will require some level of assistance through resuscitative efforts. If the answer is "yes" to all three questions, and the neonate has been assessed to have stable vital signs, then the neonate can be returned to the mother within minutes of delivery.

STEPS IN NEONATAL RESUSCITATION

After determining that the neonate needs resuscitation by answering the above questions, it is necessary to begin immediately. The steps in a neonatal resuscitation are outlined in Figure 4–1. The first steps include providing warmth, opening the airway, and clearing the airway. These first steps will decrease potential cold stress that can halt or significantly decrease the neonate's response to resuscitation efforts and provide the neonate with a clear, patent airway that will allow spontaneous respiration to resume or will provide a means for the respiratory therapist to provide assisted ventilation if necessary.

Thermoregulation

The first step in resuscitating the neonate is to provide some degree of thermoregula-tion. The importance of this cannot be overstated. A cold neonate will not respond to resuscitative efforts as well as one whose temperature is maintained. Even though it is impractical to attempt total thermoregulation, the neonate must be protected from the most probable causes of heat loss following delivery.

Radiant heat loss, which is the transfer of heat from one object to another with-out their coming in contact, is minimized by immediately placing the neonate under a radiant warmer. **Conductive** heat loss, which is the loss of heat through direct

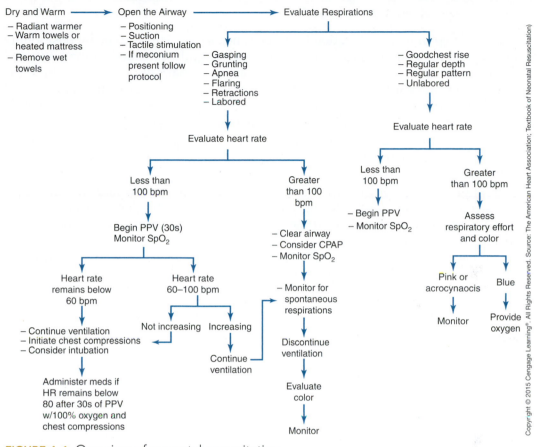

FIGURE 4–1. Overview of neonatal resuscitation.

contact of one object with a cooler surface, is minimized by placing the neonate on warmed blankets, towels, or heated mattresses. Because the neonate is wet when born, it is at a high risk of **evaporative** heat loss, which is the loss of heat through the evaporation of liquids from a surface. This is minimized by thoroughly drying the neonate with a warmed towel as quickly as possible. **Convective** heat loss, which is the loss of heat due to the movement of air past the skin and carrying away heat, is a strong possibility due to the nature of the open warmer and the necessity of keeping the neonate uncovered and accessible. Convective losses can be minimized, however, by the prevention of cold drafts over the bed and keeping movement to a minimum. Once the neonate is dried, the wet towel must be removed and placed in an appropriate receptacle.

Low-birth-weight, preterm neonates are at a higher risk of heat loss. For these very small preterm neonates it may be necessary to raise the temperature of the resuscitation room before delivery. Covering the neonate's trunk and legs with a clear plastic sheet has also been suggested as a possibility.

Opening of the Airway

The next step in the resuscitation is to open the airway. This is done by positioning the neonate in a supine position with the neck slightly extended to the "sniffing" position. Over or under extension of the neck may partially or fully occlude the airway and prevent free airflow during spontaneous respiratory efforts or manual ventilation. If no air movement is noted, the airway should be repositioned before further steps are taken, to ensure that the lack of air movement isn't simply due to poor head positioning. Elevating the shoulders ¾ inch to 1 inch with a rolled blanket or towel, as shown in Figure 4–2, helps in maintaining proper extension.

Once the proper position is achieved, the mouth is suctioned, followed by suctioning of the nose. Suctioning the mouth first removes debris that could be aspirated if the neonate gasps during nasal suctioning. Suctioning should be gentle and limited because stimulation of the vagal nerve in the oropharynx may induce a severe bradycardia.

If meconium is present in the amniotic fluid, further measures may be needed. Thin, watery discolored amniotic fluid requires no further measures; however, if

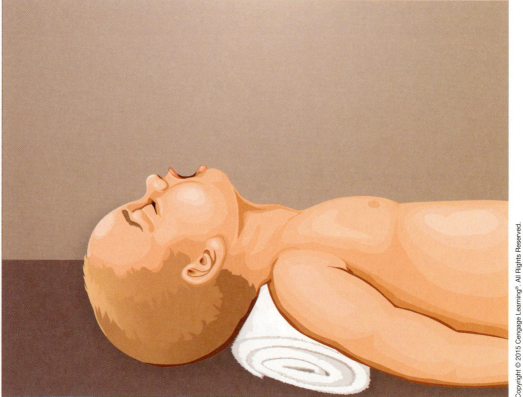

FIGURE 4–2. Elevation of the shoulders to extend and open the airway.

there is a presence of thick particulate meconium in the amniotic fluid AND if the neonate is not vigorous, further intervention is required at this time. A **vigorous** neonate is defined as one with strong respiratory effort, good muscle tone, and a heart rate that is greater than 100 beats per minute (bpm).

During a meconium delivery before the thorax is delivered, the mouth, oropharynx, and laryngopharynx should be thoroughly suctioned to remove any meconium that is present. Upon complete delivery of the neonate, it must be determined if the neonate is not vigorous. If there is meconium present and the infant is not vigorous, suction the trachea. This procedure is done by intubating the neonate with an appropriate endotracheal tube for the gestational age and size, then attaching a meconium aspiration device along with suction tubing to the end of the endotracheal tube (Figure 4–3). Suction is then applied for up to 3 seconds, then continued as the

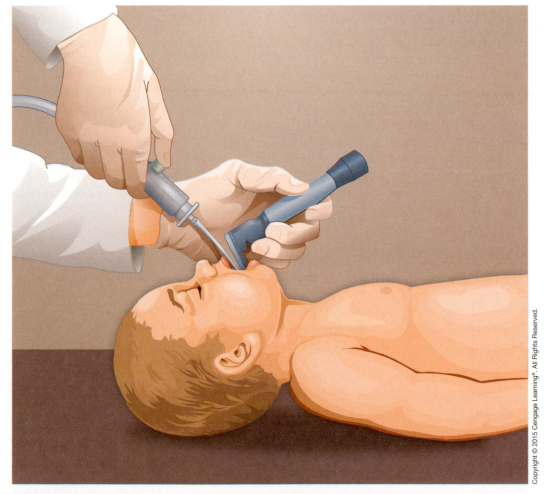

FIGURE 4–3. Suctioning meconium through the endotracheal tube.

endotracheal tube is slowly removed from the trachea. If a large amount of meconium is removed and the neonate remains unresponsive, reintubation with a new endotracheal tube may be necessary to clear excessive meconium. It is important to be mindful of how long this process takes since the neonate is not being ventilated or oxygenated during this process. It may be necessary to stop suctioning and proceed to PPV despite the possibility that some meconium may remain in the airways. Suction pressure should be set at 100 mmHg and suction applied no more than 3 to 5 seconds.

If no meconium is present or if there is meconium present and the neonate is vigorous, clear the mouth and nose of secretions with a bulb syringe or suction catheter. The mouth is always suctioned before the nose.

Other means of stimulation of the neonate include flicking the bottoms of the feet and gently rubbing the back, trunk, or limbs. Use caution to avoid overly aggressive stimulation, as it may cause injury to the neonate.

Evaluation of Respirations

Now that the neonate is warmed, dried, and the airway is open, it is necessary to assess the condition and determine if further resuscitation steps are required. An evaluation of respirations should take place. Respirations should produce good chest rise that is regular in depth and pattern and is unlabored and free of grunting, flaring, or retracting.

The neonate should have strong respiratory effort that increases in rate and depth after a brief period of tactile stimulation. If the neonate presents with any gasping, apnea, or a heart rate less than 100 bpm, PPV should be initiated. If the neonate presents with a heart rate greater than 100 bpm and labored breathing, grunting, flaring, or retractions, ensure the airway is clear and consider initiating continuous positive airway pressure (CPAP) to assist in decreasing the work of breathing. In both instances, oxygen saturation (SpO_2) should be monitored.

Evaluation of the Heart Rate

The heart rate should be greater than 100 bpm. Assess the heart rate by grasping the base of the umbilical stump between the middle finger and the thumb. Once the heart rate is easily palpated, the person assessing it should tap out the heart rate on the bed so all other care providers can visually observe the heart rate. Unlike adult patients, the heart rate is measured for six seconds and is multiplied by 10 to determine the bpm. Since the steps in a resuscitation of infant neonate happen so quickly, it is necessary to calculate the heart rate in this manner.

The evaluation of heart rate is based on the simple determination of whether it is above or below 100 bpm. If below 100 bpm, PPV is initiated. If above 100 bpm, the neonate's respiratory effort and color are evaluated.

Evaluate Color

The evaluation of the neonate's color consists of determining whether the skin is blue (cyanotic) or pink. It is best to evaluate the color of the neonate by directly observing the central portion or trunk of the body. It is not uncommon for neonates to have acrocyanosis, which is blueness of the hands and feet, for up to several hours after delivery. Acrocyanosis does not require intervention. On neonates with dark complexions, color assessment may need to be done on the mucous membranes. If the neonate is cyanotic oxygen should be provided.

Evaluate Oxygen Saturation

Since neonates take several minutes to transition to adult circulation, it is possible for oxygen saturation to be as low as 60% at the time of delivery. In a normal, uncomplicated delivery, it may take up to 10 minutes for a neonate to obtain an oxygenation saturation of >85%. The use of a pulse oximeter is necessary to confirm the presence of cyanosis and the need for supplemental oxygen. The proper placement of a pulse oximeter during resuscitation is on the right hand, wrist, or forearm. This will allow assessment of preductal oxygen saturation. If the probe is placed in another location on the neonate, the assessment may include blood flow through the ductus arteriosus, which has not participated in gas exchange, resulting in decreased oxygen saturation.

Supplemental Oxygen According to NRP guidelines, supplemental oxygen should only be given in instances where the neonate appears cyanotic or pulse oximetry monitoring has confirmed saturations lower than expected for the neonate according to the length of time since delivery. Although the use of supplemental oxygen can rapidly increase neonatal oxygen saturation, it must be used with extreme caution since oxygen toxicity can occur after only a few short minutes of administration of high levels of oxygen. Preterm neonates are even more susceptible to oxygen toxicity than term neonates. Because of the risk of toxicity, an oxygen blender is recommended, which allows the provider the ability to use a range of oxygen between 21% and 100% during the course of the resuscitation. Supplemental oxygen can be administered via several different devices. If the neonate is spontaneously breathing, the use of an oxygen mask or a flow-inflating bag and mask, T-piece resuscitator or oxygen tubing held near the neonate's mouth with your hand in the cupping position is appropriate. It is important to note that self-inflating resuscitation bags are NOT able to provide free flow oxygen due to the one-way valve they contain. Wean supplemental oxygen as tolerated by the neonate, always using the least amount of oxygen necessary to maintain an appropriate saturation as indicated by pulse oximetry monitoring. Saturations of 85% to 90% on room air are acceptable for a neonate breathing room air. If saturations remain below 85% despite administration of supplemental oxygen, the initiation of PPV may be indicated.

Positive-Pressure Ventilation (PPV) If PPV is indicated it must be started quickly and efficiently. PPV is indicated when the neonate is apneic, gasping, or when spontaneous breathing cannot maintain the heart rate above 100 bpm.

It is important to understand terms used in providing PPV including: peak inspiratory pressure (PIP), positive end-expiratory pressure (PEEP), continuous positive airway pressure (CPAP), and rate. PIP is the amount of pressure delivered to the lungs at the end of inspiration via PPV. PEEP is the amount of pressure that remains in the lungs after the end of expiration while administering PPV. CPAP is similar to PEEP, but is a continuous pressure administered to a spontaneously breathing patient.

Before beginning PPV, an appropriate delivery device should be selected. This may also be determined by the facility in which you work. Not all facilities have all available resuscitation devices on hand. It is important that you be familiar with the devices available in your facility, including their limitations. The most common resuscitation devices available to provide PPV include: flow-inflating bag, self-inflating bag, and a T-piece resuscitator.

A **flow-inflating bag** can deliver up to 100% oxygen. It requires a gas source to inflate the reservoir used to deliver positive pressure breaths. It is easy to determine if a leak is present because the bag will not inflate or maintain pressure. Without flow, this bag is unable to ventilate the patient therefore a gas source is necessary. This bag is capable of delivering free-flow, or blow-by, oxygen. Flow-inflating bags also have a flow-control valve that is used to titrate desired PEEP. This device should be used in conjunction with a pressure manometer if one isn't already built into the device to prevent lung over inflation.

A **self-inflating bag** is commonly found in delivery rooms and is thought to be easy to use by less skilled providers. It does not require a gas source to inflate the bag used to deliver positive pressure breaths. Because of this, it is possible for the gas source to become disconnected or for a leak to exist between the mask and the neonate's face, and the provider may be unaware of this. This device requires an attached reservoir in order to deliver the predetermined percent of oxygen. Additionally, the self-inflating bag is unable to deliver free-flow, or blow-by, oxygen to the neonate. This device contains a pressure-release or pop-off valve set at 30–40 cm H_2O that prevents over inflation.

A **T-piece resuscitator** requires a gas supply and is able to deliver precise and consistent pressures. A provider can deliver positive pressure breaths at a set PIP by occluding the tip of the T-piece. Exhalation occurs once the tip of the T-piece is no longer occluded, allowing the neonate to exhale to the preset PEEP. This device is also able to provide free-flow, or blow-by, oxygen and CPAP to spontaneously breathing neonates. If a leak is present, the T-piece resuscitator will not achieve the set pressures. This device has a built in pressure manometer for continuous pressure monitoring, however the pop-off is adjustable and must be manually set by the provider prior to use.

The resuscitation device should be checked when stocking the resuscitation room and prior to each resuscitation for proper function and to determine if there any cracks, leaks, or inoperable valves. This is generally accomplished by turning on the appropriate gas flow to the device, setting the necessary pressures if using a T-piece resuscitator, and occluding the patient interface. Squeezing the bag or occluding the T-piece opening should generate 30 to 40 cm H_2O or should open the pop-off valve, if a self-inflating bag is being used.

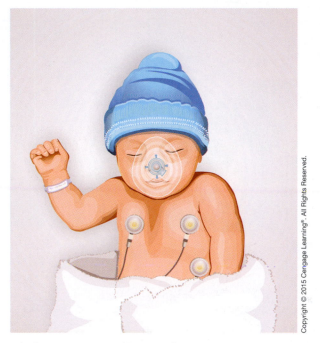

FIGURE 4–4. A properly fitting resuscitation mask.

The mask used to cover the mouth and nose should fit the neonate comfortably, as shown in Figure 4–4, without extending over the eyes or the chin. A mask that is too big or too small will make it difficult to maintain an adequate seal.

The neonate is now prepared by slightly extending the neck into the "sniffing" position, as described earlier in the chapter, being careful to avoid hyperextension, which may close off the trachea. The mask is positioned on the neonate's face and held in place by the fingers and thumb (Figure 4–5). Caution should be used when placing the fingers, which should be only on the mandible while creating a seal around the neonate's mouth. Any pressure beneath the mandible may occlude the neonate's airway. The bag is squeezed with the fingertips until chest expansion is observed, which may require higher than normal pressures. Start with pressures around 20 cm H_2O and gradually increase if necessary to achieve increased heart rate. Be careful to avoid excessive pressures and lung volumes, as they may result in lung injury. Once the lungs have been initially inflated, subsequent breaths will usually require 15 to 20 cm H_2O to maintain adequate chest expansion. Although breath sounds are a good indication of ventilation, chest rise is a better indication, especially in preterm neonates. The initial rate of ventilation should be 40 to 60 breaths per minute (BPM).

Reevaluation

To this point the neonate has been warmed, dried, and positioned. The respiratory therapist determined the neonate is in need of resuscitation due to prematurity, lack

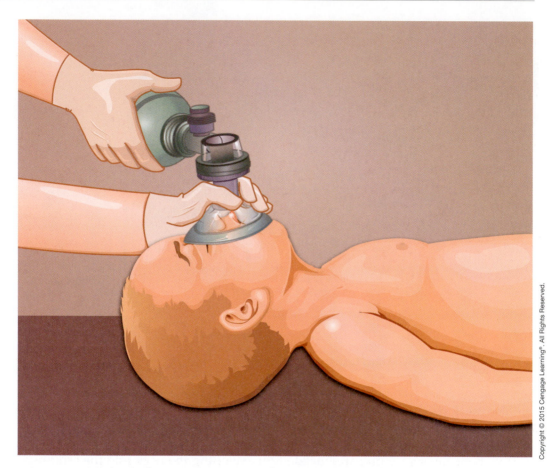

FIGURE 4–5. Method of securing a resucitation mask to fit the face of a neonate.

of respiratory effort or cry, or poor muscle tone. The airway is positioned in the sniffing position. The neonate didn't respond to tactile stimulus and presented with difficulty breathing or apnea. Thirty seconds of PPV via one of the devices discussed in this chapter was used. It is now time to reevaluate the neonate's condition. Despite all efforts, the neonate has not improved or has deteriorated.

During this evaluation, if the HR is more than 60 but less than 100, continue providing PPV and monitor oxygen saturation. Evaluate chest rise to verify adequate ventilation. Because positive pressure has been administered for some time, it is possible that air has entered the stomach. Consider decompressing the stomach by inserting an orogastric tube. Abdominal distension may impede ventilation efforts and may result in vomiting and aspiration of stomach contents. At this time the respiratory therapist should also troubleshoot equipment and consider any possible physiologic or pathologic reasons for lack of improvement.

If the HR is gradually increasing, the oxygen saturation should also be improving. Continue monitoring and supporting ventilation until spontaneous respirations return at a rate of 40–60 bpm and HR stabilizes at a rate greater than 100 bpm. Following discontinuation of the PPV, the neonate should be closely monitored.

Chest Compressions

A persistent HR of less than 60 bpm, despite tactile stimulation and 30 seconds of adequate PPV, does not provide adequate cardiac output to meet the needs of the neonate; therefore, chest compressions should be initiated. Properly performed chest compressions allow for increased blood circulation by increasing intrathoracic pressure and by compressing the heart against the spine. It is necessary to have at least two providers present; one to perform adequate compressions and one to continue providing PPV. Chest compressions can be administered by the thumb technique or the two-finger technique.

The **thumb technique** is performed by encircling the hands around the thoracic cage with both thumbs being placed on the sternum of the neonate. The thumbs are then used to compress the sternum, resulting in cardiac compression and improved circulation. This is the preferred method because it is easier to provide consistent depth and pressure with it.

The **two-finger technique** is performed by placing the fingertips over the lower third of the sternum, above the xiphoid process and below the nipple line (Figure 4–6). The two fingers used are the index and middle fingers, or the middle and ring fingers. If it becomes necessary to place an umbilical catheter for the administration of medications, the two-finger technique allows greater access to the umbilical stump for this procedure. If the provider is using the thumb technique, it is suggested he or she shift to the two-finger technique in this instance.

The sternum is compressed one-third of the anterior-posterior diameter at a rate of 90/min. Proper performance of chest compressions requires that the fingers or thumbs do not come off the thorax between compressions, although it is necessary to allow the chest to recoil fully after each compression. This ensures that the heart is able to fully

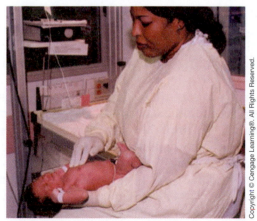

FIGURE 4–6. Demonstration of finger positioning for chest thrusts on a neonate.

refill before the next compression. It also provides for better chest expansion during the ventilation phases. Correct performance will reduce the chance of internal injuries to the infant, reduce time wasted in repositioning the hands, and allow control of the compression depth to be maintained. The proper rate of compressions and ventilations is 3 to 1. In order to maintain a compression rate of 90/min, the three compressions and one ventilation must be given in a 2-second time period. This breaks down to 1 compression every 0.5 second with a 0.5-second pause for the ventilation. In order to coordinate such a rapid sequence, it is necessary for both providers to communicate with each other effectively, each counting out loud their portion of the sequence. "One and two and three and breathe and…" and so on.

Although evaluations of HR have been outlined in this chapter as every 30 seconds, it is recommended in the current AAP/NRP guidelines that initial compressions continue for upwards of 45–60 seconds after well-established circulation before the first evaluation of HR. After the initial compressions are performed for 45–60 seconds, pause compressions only in order to assess HR. Ventilations should continue at one breath every 3 seconds. Measure HR as described previously for 6 seconds and times by 10 to calculate HR per minute. Compressions should be discontinued when the HR rises above 60 bpm and PPV continues until HR rises above 100 bpm.

If the neonate does not improve despite assisted ventilation and chest compressions, consider the underlying causes, possible equipment failure, or ineffective resuscitation techniques.

Intubation

Intubation is indicated during a resuscitation: 1) when thick meconium is present in a nonvigorous infant, 2) if bag and mask ventilation is difficult or ineffective, 3) if prolonged PPV is required due to lung disease, 4) if chest compressions have become necessary, and 5) in cases of extreme prematurity and need for surfactant administration. Intubation is also performed when a neonate is suspected of having a diaphragmatic hernia to prevent abdominal distension.

Intubation should only be attempted by someone who is proficient in the procedure. This procedure should be performed with a minimum of two people. The most skilled provider should perform the intubation and the other person should assist by handing the person intubating equipment, monitoring the infant's heart rate and oxygen saturation during the attempt, helping secure the endotracheal tube, and listening for breath sounds to confirm placement of the endotracheal tube following intubation. The intubation should be stopped if severe bradycardia and/or desaturations occur, allowing time to provide ventilation and oxygenation to return heart rate and oxygen saturation to normal limits.

The equipment needed for an intubation are a laryngoscope and blade with a functioning light, several endotracheal tubes of various sizes, a stylet (optional), laryngeal mask airway, end tidal carbon dioxide monitor or detector, equipment to suction the airway, adhesive tape or other securing device, scissors, oral airway, meconium aspirator, neonatal stethoscope, a resuscitation bag and mask or T-piece resuscitator, oxygen blender, and pulse oximeter with neonatal probe. All items necessary for resuscitation should be within comfortable reach of team members performing the resuscitation. Appropriately sized endotracheal tubes are outlined in Table 4–4.

Intubation of a term neonate will require a size 1 blade, and a size 0 blade is needed for premature neonates. Only straight (Miller) laryngoscope blades should be used in neonates and young children up to approximately 6–8 years of age. This is because the larynx is more superior and the epiglottis more horizontal than in adults.[3] Additionally, only uniform diameter, cuffless endotracheal tubes should be used, most of which have a black line near the distal tip that acts as a vocal cord guide. During placement of the endotracheal tube, the black vocal cord guide should be visualized at the level of the vocal cords, ensuring proper placement.

Some providers may opt to use a stylet when performing endotracheal intubation because it adds extra rigidity and a fixed curvature to the endotracheal tube. When this is the case, the endotracheal tube is prepared by placing the stylet just short of the tip of the tube to prevent trauma to the airway and then secured to prevent inadvertent forward advancement of the stylet into the airway. Placement of the stylet into the endotracheal tube should be done with the endotracheal tube still in the protective wrapper with only the connecting adapter exposed, to maintain sterility.

Suction pressures should be adjusted between 80 and 100 mmHg to minimize complications. This is achieved by occluding the suction tubing while adjusting the suction pressure. Several sizes of suction catheters should be available ranging from 5F to 10F. A bulb syringe or bulb suction device should also be readily available during resuscitation.

The neonate is prepared for intubation by placing it in the **supine** position and slightly extending the neck as previously mentioned. A small roll may be placed under the shoulders of the neonate to assist in airway positioning. The laryngoscope is taken in the left hand and held by the thumb and first 2–3 fingers. Use the right hand to position the head. If necessary, you may need to manually open the neonate's mouth with the right hand. Slide the blade inserted into the right side of the mouth. The tongue is swept to the left toward midline in a smooth motion using the left side of the blade. The blade is then lifted up and away from the roof of the mouth to visualize the glottic opening, as shown in Figure 4–7. The upper gums are *never* used as a fulcrum to pry the blade upward. At this point, it may be necessary to suction the

Table 4–4

SELECTING APPROPRIATELY SIZED ENDOTRACHEAL TUBES

Tube Size (ID MM)	Weight	Gestational Age
2.5	<1000 g	<28 weeks
3.0	1000–2000 g	28–34 weeks
3.5	2000–3000 g	34–38 weeks
3.5–4.0	>3000 g	>38 weeks

laryngopharynx free of mucus and secretions. If the epiglottis is not visualized, withdraw the blade until the epiglottis is seen. The tip of the blade is now used to lift the epiglottis away from the glottic opening, allowing insertion of the endotracheal tube. A gentle external pressure on the trachea may help visualize the glottis.

The endotracheal tube is now inserted into the right side of the mouth and guided through the glottic opening and into the larynx. Advancement of the tube should stop when the tip is seen passing the vocal cords. If the vocal cords are not open, wait for them to open. Attempting to advance the endotracheal tube through closed vocal cords may cause vocal cord spasm or injury. Once the endotracheal tube is in place, stabilize the tube against the hard palate by using the index finger of the right hand. Then remove the laryngoscope slowly. If a stylet was used during the procedure, it should be removed at this time as well.

Following intubation, the neonate should be clinically evaluated for proper tube placement. This includes auscultation of the right and left chest, and over the stomach. The neonate is also visually monitored for equal bilateral chest excursion when given a positive pressure breath. An end tidal carbon dioxide monitor or detector should be attached to the endotracheal tube to verify tube placement. If the endotracheal tube is in the trachea, you will also see mist in the tube on exhalation. When it is determined that the tube is properly positioned, it is secured with tape or another fastening device. A chest radiograph should be obtained as quickly as possible to verify proper position

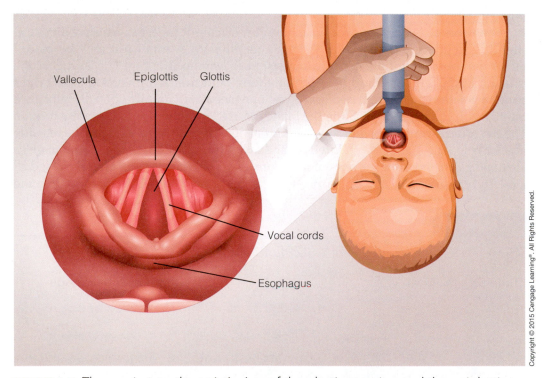

Vallecula   Epiglottis   Glottis

Vocal cords

Esophagus

FIGURE 4–7. The respiratory therapist's view of the glottic opening and the epiglottic area seen through a laryngoscope.

of the tip of the tube. The ideal placement of the tube will have its tip midway between the carina and the vocal cords, as determined on the chest radiograph.

Intubation attempts should be limited to 30 seconds to minimize hypoxia. Between attempts, the neonate is manually ventilated with sufficient oxygen to help stabilize the SpO_2. Following verification of tube position on the radiograph, the end of the tube is cut (between 13 and 15 cm), leaving only 4 cm outside the mouth. This helps reduce dead space and airway resistance. It also makes it easier to manage the tube.

If intubation was performed for the purpose of meconium removal, remember to minimize the length of time suction is applied to the airway and minimize the number of intubation attempts to remove meconium from the airway. If no meconium is removed on the first attempt, do not reintubate. Move directly to the next step of resuscitation.

Difficulties Intubating There are several problems that may occur during attempted intubation. It may be difficult to visualize the landmarks that are necessary for proper tube placement. The endotracheal tube may be accidently inserted in the esophagus rather than in the trachea. If the endotracheal tube is advanced too far down the trachea, the tip will slide into the right mainstem bronchus. Each of these difficulties can be eliminated or greatly reduced if the provider pays careful attention to detail and has taken the time to practice this skill and become proficient in performing endotracheal intubation.

If endotracheal tube placement is not possible by a skilled provider or if congenital anomalies, such as small mandible, large tongue, or abnormal upper airway anatomy exist, the use of a laryngeal mask airway (LMA) may be considered as an alternative means to oxygenate and ventilate the neonate.[2] An LMA can be inserted blindly by an unskilled provider. The recommended size 1 LMA is indicated for neonates over 2 kg. Once the LMA is slid into place with the tip of the cuff resting in the esophagus, the cuff is inflated with not more than 4 mL of air. Once inflated, this device is attached to a bag-mask or T-piece resuscitator. Assessment for equal breath sounds is necessary, then the LMA is secured with tape to prevent dislodging.

A number of complications can result from endotracheal intubation in neonates. An intubation procedure can produce or increase hypoxia, cause trauma to tissues, and introduce infection. However, when one is skilled in the procedure, the incidence of complications is minimized. Some of the common causes of complications of intubation are listed in Table 4–5.

Delivery of Medications

Although there are several medications that can be used to reverse narcotics (naloxone), treat metabolic acidosis (sodium bicarbonate), increase tissue perfusion and restore blood pressure (vasopressors such as dopamine), and treat special circumstances (atropine and calcium), these drugs are NOT recommended to be used during the acute stages of neonatal resuscitation. Epinephrine is the only medication indicated during this phase of resuscitation. In addition to epinephrine, volume expanders may be administered in cases of shock due to significant blood loss.

Epinephrine and volume expanders can be administered through a catheter inserted in the umbilical vein. Although epinephrine can be instilled directly into the

Table 4–5

COMPLICATIONS OF INTUBATION

Complication	Causes	Preventive or Corrective Actions
Hypoxia	Taking too long to intubate	Shorten intubation procedure to 30 seconds Bag-mask ventilation with appropriate oxygen concentration
	Incorrect placement of tube	Proper repositioning of ET tube
Bradycardia/Apnea	Hypoxia Vagal response due to the laryngoscope blade. ET tube, or suction catheter stimulating the posterior pharynx	Bag-mask ventilation Oxygenate after intubation Limit duration of intubation attempts and endotracheal suctioning
Pneumothorax	Over ventilation of one lung due to placement of tube in a main bronchus (usually the right)	Proper positioning of ET tube Appropriate ventilating pressures Consider transillumination and needle aspiration
Contusions or lacerations of tongue, gums, pharynx, epiglottis, trachea, vocal cords, or esophagus	Rough handling of laryngoscope or ET tube Laryngoscope blade too long or short	Additional practice/skill More appropriately sized equipment
Perforation of trachea or esophagus	Insertion of tube or stylet is too vigorous, or stylet protrudes beyond end of tube	Proper placement and curvature of stylet Gentler handling
Infection	Introduction of organisms via equipment or hands	More careful attention to clean/sterile technique

endotracheal tube, it is not recommended. The absorption of epinephrine through the lungs is unpredictable and it should only be used if venous access is not available or while venous access is being obtained in emergent situations. If the endotracheal administration route is selected, the dose of epinephrine should be increased to 0.5 to 1.0 mL/kg. After administering the medication via the endotracheal tube, manual positive pressure breaths should be delivered to assist in disbursement of the medication to the lung fields for absorption.

The umbilical vein is the most easily accessible route for direct administration of medication and fluids during an acute resuscitation. Placement of an umbilical venous catheter (UVC) is a sterile procedure that requires skill to perform. The provider will don sterile gloves and will create a sterile field prior to beginning the procedure (see *NRP 2011 guidelines for UVC placement instructions*). Placement of a UVC and administration of epinephrine and/or volume expanders is indicated when previous resuscitative efforts have not resulted in improvement of the infant.

Indications for the use of epinephrine during a resuscitation are: 1) the HR remains below 60 bpm despite 30 seconds of effective PPV and 30 seconds of chest compressions, or 2) the HR is zero.

Epinephrine is a powerful sympathomimetic drug that increases heart rate, improves the strength of heart contractions, and causes peripheral vasoconstriction. The net effect is to increase cardiac output and increase blood flow to vital organs. One mL of a 1:10,000 solution is drawn up and delivered at a dosage of 0.1 to 0.3 mL/kg of body weight. Epinephrine should be delivered rapidly regardless of the route of administration. When delivered via the endotracheal tube, the medication may be diluted with 1 to 2 mL of normal saline to aid delivery. Following delivery of the epinephrine, compressions should continue to ensure circulation of the medication. If the heart rate does not increase above 60 bpm in response to the medication, epinephrine can be readministered every 3 to 5 minutes. You may consider increasing the dose within the suggested range if no response is noted after the first dose.

The use of volume expanders is indicated in those infants showing signs of hypovolemic shock due to acute blood loss. Signs include low blood pressure, pallor in the face of adequate oxygenation, poor capillary refill, heart rate above 100 with weak pulses, and failure to respond to the resuscitation. Volume expanders used in neonatal resuscitation include normal saline and Ringer's lactate. O Rh-negative packed red blood cells may be considered in extreme cases of documented fetal anemia. The infant is then given 10 mL/kg intravenously over a 5 to 10 minute period. If the signs of hypovolemia persist, the dosage may be repeated. Table 4–6 summarizes the medications used in resuscitation of the neonate.

APGAR SCORE

The Apgar score was developed as an objective way to evaluate the condition of a neonate. The Apgar is an excellent method of assessing the effectiveness of neonatal resuscitation, but is not to be used as a basis for making resuscitative decisions. Resuscitation efforts should never be halted for the purpose of obtaining an Apgar score.

The five areas examined are respiratory effort, heart rate, muscle tone, reflex irritability, and color (Figure 4–8). Each area is given a score of 0, 1, or 2, depending on the response noted. The first score is assessed at 1 minute after delivery with a second evaluation performed at 5 minutes. Because the Apgar score is an objective

Table 4–6

MEDICATIONS FOR NEONATAL RESUSCITATION

Medication	Concentration To Administer	Preparation	Dosage Route*	Weight	Total Dose/Infant Total mL	Rate/ Precautions
Epinephrine	1:10,000	Calculated dose	0.1–0.3 mL/kg	1 kg	0.1–0.3 mL	Give rapidly
				2 kg	0.2–0.6 mL	
				3 kg	0.3–0.9 mL	
			IV	4 kg	0.4–1.2 mL	
				Weight	**Total mL**	
Volume	Normal saline	Calculated dose	10 mL/kg	1 kg	10 mL	Give over 5–10 minutes
Expanders	Ringer's lactate		IV	2 kg	20 mL	
	O Rh-neg packed red blood cells			3 kg	30 mL	
				4 kg	40 mL	

Apgar scoring system

	0	1	2	1 Minute	5 Minutes
Heart Rate	None detectable	Slow irregular	Over 100		
Respiratory Effort	Apnea	Irregular shallow, gasping	Yelling, crying		
Muscle Tone	Flaccid	Some flexion of extremities	Well flexed		
Reflex	None—no response to stimulus	Grimace (withdraws)	Crying		
Color	Pale blue (shock)	Blue hands and feed, body pink (Acrocyanois)	Pink all over		

FIGURE 4–8. The Apgar score.

assessment of neonatal status, a 5-minute score that is higher than the 1-minute score indicates the effectiveness of the resuscitation.

Apgars can be assessed every 5 minutes as needed up to 20 minutes, or when the resuscitation ends. Since the first Apgar is not given until 1 minute after birth, it cannot be used as a criterion to initiate resuscitation, but rather as an assessment of how well the neonate is responding to the resuscitation.

The 5-minute Apgar score is predictive of future impairment, with a low score being associated with a high risk of long-term damage.[4] The team can therefore use the Apgar score as an objective measurement of the response of the neonate to the resuscitation.

MANAGEMENT OF SERUM GLUCOSE

Glucose management is essential in neonates, especially those who have experienced prolonged resuscitation or who were born to diabetic mothers. This section covers signs and symptoms, causes, diagnosis and treatment of glucose abnormalities.

Sources of Fetal and Neonatal Glucose

During intrauterine life, the nutritional needs of the fetus are continuously supplied by the maternal circulation and regulated by the placenta. The fetus prepares for post-natal life by increasing energy stores and developing enzyme-dependent processes for rapid mobilization of stored energy. As carbohydrate stores become depleted postnatally, the neonate must develop the ability to produce hepatic glucose from alternate fuel sources. These sources, known as substrates, include ketones, glycerol, and lactate. This production is slight when compared to the major fuel sources derived from metabolism of glucose.

The rate of glucose uptake by the fetus through the placenta is directly related to the maternal blood glucose level. The glucose concentration in the fetal blood is approximately one third that in the maternal blood. Fetal stores of glycogen are present by the ninth week of gestation, and at term are approximately three times those of a healthy adult. Skeletal muscle glycogen is three to five times that of an adult, and glycogen in cardiac muscle ten times the adult.

Another energy source resides in fetal adipose tissue triglycerides that accumulate in the last trimester. These are known as **brown fat** stores. After glycogen stores are utilized, brown fat is metabolized for fuel. Brown fat is found in the scapulae, neck, axillary regions, mediastinum, and renal tissue (Figure 4–9). Due to the timing of accumulation of fat stores, neonates born prematurely are at a disadvantage, because they lack the adipose tissue stores that are used during stress.

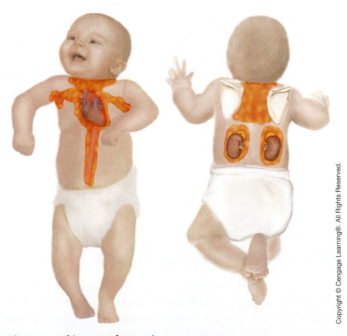

FIGURE 4–9. Distribution of brown fat in the neonate.

In the immediate postnatal period the concentration of glucose in the neonate declines to approximately 50 mg/dL by 2 hours of age, but equilibrates at approximately 70 mg/dL by 72 hours after birth. The concentration may be further influenced by disturbances in extrauterine adaptations, such as hypothermia, hypovolemia, and disruptions in acid-base balance.

Serum Values

Neonatal hypoglycemia is defined as a plasma glucose level of less than 30 mg/dL (1.65 mmol/L) in the first 24 hours of life and less than 45 mg/dL (2.5 mmol/L) thereafter[5] In most cases, concentrations below 50 mg/dL or greater than 125 mg/dL are abnormal after 3 days of age. Thus, any blood glucose level less than 50 mg/dL should be cause for concern and should be investigated more closely.[6]

The difficulty encountered in clinical diagnosis of hypoglycemia is the nonspecific nature of the symptoms. This is further complicated by the occurrence of symptoms at varying blood glucose levels in diverse patients.

Clinical Signs of Hypoglycemia

Clinical signs often associated with neonatal hypoglycemia are listed in Table 4–7.

Table 4–7
CLINICAL SIGNS OF HYPOGLYCEMIA
Tremors or jitteriness
Irritability
Exaggerated or decreased moro reflex
Apnea/tachypnea
Cyanosis
Seizures
Lethargy
Hypothermia
High-pitched or weak cry
Poor feeding
Vomiting
Cardiovascular failure and/or collapse

Causes of Hypoglycemia

Hypoglycemia can result from a wide variation of pathologic conditions. A common cause of hypoglycemia is hyperinsulinism. Several causes of hyperinsulinism will be discussed.

In utero, the fetus of a diabetic mother is subjected to high levels of maternal glucose, which freely crosses the placenta. In response, the fetal pancreas secretes high levels of insulin to counter the high glucose. Following delivery the continued increased production of insulin, coupled with the loss of the maternal glucose, results in neonatal hypoglycemia. Fetuses of diabetic mothers may also have problems with **glucagon** secretion, as well as utilization of substrates such as amino acids, for the production of glucose.

Neonates suffering from **erythroblastosis fetalis**, or Rh incompatibility, demonstrate hyperinsulinism due to pancreatic islet cell hyperplasia. Hyperinsulinism may also be a problem before and during exchange transfusion in these neonates.

Insulin-producing tumors of unknown etiology are another source of hyperinsulinism. Maternal tocolytic therapy with ritodrine or terbutaline, with resultant cessation of premature labor, can additionally lead to hyperinsulinism.

Several other causes of decreased glycogen stores are listed in Table 4–8.

Table 4–8
CAUSES OF DECREASED GLYCOGEN STORES
Prematurity
Intrauterine growth retardation (IUGR)
Starvation
Sepsis
Shock
Asphyxia
Hypothermia
Glycogen storage disease
Galactosemia
Adrenal insufficiency
Polycythemia
Congenital cardiac malformations
Iatrogenic causes (i.e., large volume and/or concentrations of glucose intravenously)

Measurement of Serum Glucose

Serum glucose levels should be routinely evaluated in neonates who demonstrate risk factors for hypoglycemia. High-risk factors include infants of diabetic mothers (IDMs), Rh incompatibility, prematurity, and neonates who are small for their gestational age (SGA).

Treatment of Hypoglycemia

Treatment should be instituted as soon as a neonate at risk for hypoglycemia is identified. Prophylactic care includes early oral or enteral feedings, if indicated, or parenteral administration of glucose. A glucose infusion of 10% dextrose and water intravenously will provide adequate glucose for most neonates.

Treatment is started with a 200 mg/kg bolus of $D_{10}W$ given over 1 to 3 minutes. This is followed by a continuous IV infusion of 4 to 8 mg/kg/min.[5] These requirements are increased as fluid and glucose requirements change over the first few days of life. Intravenous glucose should continue until enteral feelings can be instituted.

For acute symptomatic hypoglycemia, generally 1 to 2 mL/kg of $D_{10}W$, pushed through the IV, will render the neonate normoglycemic within 1 to 2 minutes. All neonates should be monitored at least hourly until stable.

Correction of acid–base disturbances, sepsis, maintenance of normal vital signs, and attention to thermoregulation should be instituted immediately to decrease physiologic stresses and energy requirements.

OBTAINING UMBILICAL VESSEL BLOOD SAMPLES DURING RESUSCITATION

In order to assess a neonate's ventilation and oxygenation status, it is necessary to gain access to an arterial site. The umbilical stump provides the most easily accessible route for arterial blood sampling.

Arterial Sampling through the Umbilical Stump

The umbilical vessels may be visualized through the Wharton's jelly of the umbilical cord. The umbilical vein is a single vessel of relatively large diameter that often appears filled with blood. The umbilical arteries are a pair of vessels of smaller diameter that usually are more opaque and whitish in appearance and appear to contain little blood.

After delivery, the umbilical arteries gradually spasm and close. Immediately after birth, however, they may be entered and an arterial sample obtained. This may be helpful in determining the neonate's status and the need for prolonged arterial access.

The cord stump should first be checked to ensure that the umbilical arteries are still pulsatile. To perform the procedure, the surface of the cord is cleaned with

Betadine® and then alcohol. The umbilical cord stump is punctured with either a scalp vein needle or other small-gauged needle attached to a syringe. The needle is directed toward one of the arteries in the direction of the umbilicus, as shown in Figure 4–10.

Upon entering the artery, connect a blood gas syringe and withdraw an appropriate amount for a blood gas sample. Remove the needle from the umbilicus and tamponade the artery proximal to the site of entry.

Although blood gas samples are obtained from the umbilical arteries, the umbilical vein may also be punctured and a sample obtained. The umbilical vein carries blood returning from the fetus to the placenta and, therefore, reflects fetal intrapartum metabolic status.

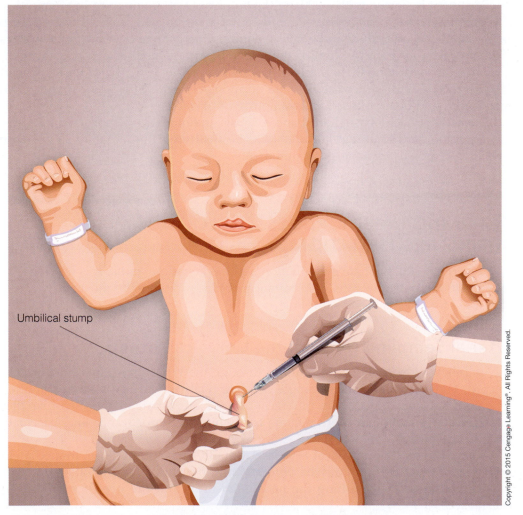

Umbilical stump

FIGURE 4–10. Obtaining a blood sample from the umbilical stump.

Placement of an Umbilical Artery Catheter (UAC)

The placement of an umbilical artery catheter (UAC) is an invasive procedure and should be performed by those skilled in the insertion of a UAC.

Indications An umbilical arterial catheter is indicated for use in a seriously ill neonate who may require frequent blood gas sampling, continuous arterial blood pressure monitoring, or less commonly, as a reliable route for parenteral infusions.

Procedure for Placement The usual site for insertion of a UAC is near the umbilicus. A 5 Fr. catheter is used for neonates weighing more than 1250 g, and a 3.5 Fr. is used on neonates of less than 1250 g.

The neonate is placed in a supine position and the arms and legs are restrained. Adequate control of thermoregulation, oxygenation, and ventilation must be maintained throughout the procedure.

Sterile gloves and a gown are put on following a thorough hand washing. The catheterization tray is then opened in a sterile manner.

The cord is prepared by cleaning with povidone-iodine and then alcohol. Any excess povidone should be cleaned up to avoid skin burns in neonates of less than 1000 g. The neonate is then draped in a sterile manner, with the umbilicus showing through the drape.

Umbilical tape is next tied around the base of the cord and is used for the control of bleeding. The umbilical cord is then cut 1 to 2 cm above the base. An umbilical artery is then isolated and dilated. Forceps are inserted into the artery and allowed to open, stretching the arterial wall until a catheter can be inserted.

A catheter, filled with sterile heparin flush solution, is introduced into the artery and advanced with slow, steady gentle pressure. A pulsatile blood return indicates that an umbilical artery has been cannulized. The catheter is then advanced until it is in the desired distance and an abdominal x-ray film obtained to confirm placement. Optimal placement for a low catheter is between L3–4 and at the level of T8 for a high catheter.

Complications Thrombus formation on the catheter tip is the most common complication and may lead to a decreased circulation to one of the legs. Additional thromboembolic complications include hypertension and **necrotizing enterocolitis**.

Perforation of the vessel wall is a direct complication of the procedure. Hemorrhage from inadvertent removal of the catheter or infusion system leaks or disconnects may also occur. Vasospasm of the arterial supply to a toe, foot, or leg is often predisposed by the presence of the UAC. If wrapping the opposite leg with a warm moist diaper does not quickly relieve the vasospasm, the catheter should be removed.

S.T.A.B.L.E[7] In 1998, a program was initiated to educate those who work with newborns to stabilize infants post-resuscitation. The S.T.A.B.L.E Program was developed to help train each member of the health care team who works with newborns in the specialized care needed to stabilize those who become ill. It utilizes a team approach to train each member his or her role in caring for the sick newborn in an efficient manner. The goal of the training is to affect not only the immediate health, but the infant's long-term outcome. The S.T.A.B.L.E. mnemonic stands for Sugar, Temperature, Airway, Blood pressure, Lab work, and Emotional support. A seventh module, Quality Improvement, teaches the need to evaluate and improve the care given. Each of these areas is taught as a module, and the course is designed to reduce infant morbidity and mortality and to improve the future health of children. A summary of the S.T.A.B.L.E. modules is shown in Table 4–9.

Table 4–9

S.T.A.B.L.E. PROGRAM MODULE OBJECTIVES

Module 1: Sugar and Safe Care

1. Issues of patient safety and error reduction in the delivery of nursing and medical care to neonates.
2. Infants at increased risk for becoming hypoglycemic and hyperglycemic.
3. Signs of hypoglycemia.
4. The initial, appropriate IV fluid therapy to provide for sick neonates.
5. The IV glucose treatment of hypoglycemia and when to reevaluate the blood glucose following treatment.
6. Candidates for placement of an umbilical catheter.
7. Principles for safe use of umbilical venous and arterial catheters.

Module 2: Temperature

1. Infants at increased risk for becoming hypothermic.
2. Ways infants lose body heat and protection from cooling.
3. Physiologic responses to hypothermia for premature and term infants.
4. Necessary precautions to observe when rewarming hypothermic infants.

Module 3: Airway

1. Evaluation of respiratory distress.
2. Indications for continuous positive airway pressure, positive pressure ventilation with bag and mask or endotracheal intubation.
3. How to provide assistance during endotracheal intubation.
4. How to secure an oral endotracheal tube and evaluation of ET tube depth on chest x-ray.
5. Blood gas interpretation and proper therapies to initiate in response to an abnormal result.
6. The initial ventilatory support for very-low-birth-weight, low-birth-weight and term infants.
7. The signs and symptoms of a pneumothorax, use of transillumination, and chest x-ray to evaluate for pneumothoraces and principles of emergent evacuation of a pneumothorax.

Module 4: Blood Pressure

1. The causes, presentation and initial treatment of hypovolemic, cardiogenic, and septic shock.
2. Physical exam for shock and laboratory tests that assist with recognition and evaluation of shock.
3. Indications for, and safe administration of, dopamine.

Module 5: Lab Work

1. Risk factors that predispose infants to infection and clinical signs of infection.
2. Laboratory tests indicated for evaluation of infection, including the complete blood count and blood culture.
3. Basic white blood cell development and calculation and interpretation of the absolute neutrophil count and immature to total ratio.
4. The relationship of thrombocytopenia to possible sepsis.
5. Initial antibiotic therapy with ampicillin and gentamicin and monitoring of gentamicin levels.

Module 6: Emotional Support

1. The crisis families experience when an infant requires care in a neonatal intensive care unit.
2. Ways healthcare providers can support parents of sick infants.

Module 7: Quality Improvement

1. Concerns regarding patient safety and methods to reduce medical errors and preventable adverse events.
2. The importance of self-assessment to evaluate care provided in the post-resuscitation/pre-transport stabilization period.
3. How to use the Pre-transport Stabilization Self-Assessment Tool (PSSAT).

Reprinted with permission from The S.T.A.B.L.E. Program, http://www.stableprogram.org/

SUMMARY

It is estimated that 80% of all babies born who weigh less than 1500 g will require resuscitation. Properly performed, resuscitation can make the difference between a healthy infant and a lifetime of neurologic and other problems. This chapter serves only as an overview of the steps involved in neonatal resuscitation and should not be used as a substitute for participation in an organized neonatal resuscitation program.

Typically, the neonate who requires resuscitation has undergone a certain degree of asphyxia in utero, which leads to primary and then secondary apnea. Any neonate born apneic must be assumed to be in secondary apnea and resuscitative efforts started immediately. The sooner efforts are started, the less chance of long-time sequelae from the asphyxia. The effects of asphyxia are many and include pulmonary hypertension, persistent fetal circulation, and acidosis.

A successful resuscitation begins with anticipation of the depressed neonate. This requires knowledge of the maternal history, and a history of the labor and delivery. Also required is the ready availability of proper, functioning equipment and the presence of personnel trained in its use.

Although the American Heart Association has updated CPR practices to focus on circulation, airway and breathing (CAB), neonatal resuscitation according to the American Academy of Pediatrics maintains initial assessment of breathing immediately after delivery with the clearing and positioning of the airway followed by an assessment of heart rate. Additional steps are added to meet the special needs of the newborn. Neonatal resuscitation follows a cycle in which the neonate is first evaluated regarding respirations, heart rate, and color. A decision is then made based on the evaluation, which leads to an action.

Before evaluation is performed, several steps are undertaken. These include thermoregulation, suctioning the trachea if thick meconium is present, positioning the neonate to open the airway, suctioning the mouth then nose, and providing tactile stimulus if needed. The neonate's respirations, heart rate, and color are then evaluated and the appropriate actions are taken as outlined on the resuscitation algorithm. The Apgar score is an excellent tool used to evaluate the overall condition of the neonate. It can also be used to assess the effectiveness of the resuscitation.

Once born, the neonate now has the responsibility to provide and maintain its own energy source—glucose. Initially, energy is derived from available glucose, stored glycogen, brown fat, and the production of glucose from ketones, glycerol, and lactate. These energy stores may be depleted more rapidly if the neonate is thermally stressed, and if the work of breathing is high owing to lung disease. Ideally, the blood glucose should be kept above 35 mg/dL to prevent problems associated with hypoglycemia.

Finally, obtaining blood from the neonate is often essential during and following resuscitation. In addition, the infusion of medications into the circulatory system is commonly necessary. Blood can be drawn immediately from an umbilical artery if done before the cord vessels ligate. A UAC provides not only access to the arterial system for obtaining blood samples, but also for the infusion of medications.

POSTTEST

1. Of the following, which does *not* cause fetal asphyxia?
   a. infection
   b. maternal asphyxia
   c. placental insufficiency
   d. occlusion of the umbilical cord

2. Which of the following is true of secondary apnea?
   a. the neonate begins gasping
   b. heart rate and blood pressure rise
   c. the neonate will not attempt to breathe
   d. stimulation will usually initiate breathing
3. The persistence of fetal circulation in the presence of asphyxia is secondary to:
   a. decreased cardiac output
   b. increased fluid volume
   c. arterial hypertension
   d. pulmonary hypertension
4. Equipment used for resuscitations should be checked at least:
   a. once a week
   b. every shift
   c. once a day
   d. just before use
5. During a resuscitation, which of the following are *first* evaluated?
   I. temperature
   II. color
   III. heart rate
   IV. respirations
   V. weight
       a. I, II, III
       b. II, III, IV, V
       c. II, III, IV
       d. I, II, III, IV, V
6. Assign an Apgar score to the following Caucasian neonate: 2150 grams, blue dusky color all over, flaccid, HR 90, weak gasping breaths, and a weak grimace when orally suctioned.
   a. 9
   b. 6
   c. 3
   d. 1
7. Following the positioning, suctioning, stimulation, and drying of a neonate, what is the next step in resuscitation?
   a. assess respirations
   b. assess heart rate
   c. assess color
   d. assess breath sounds
8. Which of the following would best minimize conductive heat loss in a neonate?
   a. place neonate under a radiant warmer
   b. place neonate on a warmed mattress
   c. dry the neonate immediately
   d. blow warm air over the neonate

9. During a resuscitation, positive-pressure ventilation is indicated when:
   I. breathing effort is absent
   II. PaO_2 is less than 60 mmHg
   III. $PaCO_2$ is greater than 50 mmHg
   IV. spontaneously breathing neonate's heart rate is below 100 bpm
   V. neonate is blue all over
      a. I, II
      b. I, II, IV
      c. I, IV
      d. I, III, V

10. Chest compressions are started when:
    a. the heart rate is below 100 bpm
    b. the heart rate is below 60 bpm
    c. spontaneous respirations are not present
    d. cardiac arrhythmias are present

11. Which of the following factors indicate the need to intubate?
    I. prolonged positive pressure ventilation is required
    II. bag and mask ventilation is ineffective
    III. thick meconium is present
    IV. chest excursion is poor
    V. breath sounds are absent
       a. I, III, V
       b. II, III, IV
       c. I, II, III
       d. I, II, IV

12. The correct concentration and dosage of epinephrine during a resuscitation is:
    a. 1:20,000 concentration given 0.1 to 0.3 mL/kg
    b. 1:10,000 concentration given 0.3 to 0.5 mL/kg
    c. 1:10,000 concentration given 0.1 to 0.3 mL/kg
    d. 1:20,000 concentration given 0.3 to 0.5 mL/kg

13. Which of the following are complications of umbilical artery catheters?
    I. thrombus formation
    II. perforation of the vessel wall
    III. hemorrhage
    IV. pneumothorax
    V. vasospasm
       a. II, III, IV
       b. I, II, III, V
       c. II, IV, V
       d. I, II, IV, V

14. Glucose concentration in the fetus is approximately what percent of the maternal concentration?
    a. 33%
    b. 50%
    c. 75%
    d. 90%

15. A serum glucose level in premature neonates below what level indicates hypoglycemia?
    a. 100 g/dL
    b. 80 mg/dL
    c. 35 mg/dL
    d. 20 mg/dL
16. Maternal tocolytic therapy with terbutaline may lead to:
    a. decrease of maternal glucose
    b. increased fetal glucose
    c. hyperinsulinemia
    d. hypoinsulinemia

REFERENCES

1. Bloom RS, Cropley C. *Textbook of Neonatal Resuscitation.* Evanston, Ill: American Heart Association/American Academy of Pediatrics, 2012.
2. Paterson SJ, et al. Neonatal resuscitation using the laryngeal mask airway. *Anesthesiology.* 80:1248–1253, 1994.
3. Finucane BT, Santora AH. *Principles of Airway Management.* 4th ed. New York, NY: Springer, 2011
4. Cloherty JP, Stark AR, eds. *Manual of Neonatal Care.* 7th ed. Philadelphia, PA: Lippincott, 2012.
5. Cranmer H. Neonatal Hypoglycemia, http://emedicine.medscape.com/article/802334-overview, 20123.
6. Halarnek LP, Stephenson T. Neonatal hypoglycemia, part II: pathophysiology and therapy. *Clin Pediatr.* 37:11–16, 1998.
7. The S.T.A.B.L.E. Program, http://www.stableprogram.org/index.php.

BIBLIOGRAPHY AND SUGGESTED READINGS

American Academy of Pediatrics and American Heart Association. *Neonatal Resuscitation Program.* 6th ed., 2011.

Avery GB, Fletcher MA, MacDonald MG. *Pathophysiology and Management of the Newborn.* 6th ed. Philadelphia, PA: JB Lippincott Co, 2005.

Fanaroff A, Martin R. *Neonatal Perinatal Medicine: Diseases of the Fetus and Infant.* 9th ed. St. Louis, MO: CV Mosby Co., 2011.

Goldsmith JP, Karotkin EH. *Assisted Ventilation of the Neonate.* 4th ed. Philadelphia, PA: WB Saunders, 2003.

Cairo JM. *Pilbeam's Mechanical Ventilation: Physiological and Clinical Applications.* 5th ed. St. Louis, MO: Mosby, 2012.

Taussig LM, Landau LI. *Pediatric Respiratory Medicine.* 2nd ed. St. Louis, MO: Mosby, 2008.

Tucker SM. *Pocket Guide to Fetal Monitoring and Assessment.* 5th ed. St. Louis, MO: Mosby, 2004.

CHAPTER 5

Assessment of the Neonatal and Infant Patient

OBJECTIVES

Upon completion of this chapter, the reader should be able to:

1. State at least 10 anatomic and physiologic differences between the infant and adult.
2. Given a patient's obstetrical history (PARA), identify the following: previous pregnancies, miscarriages, premature births, and living children.
3. Identify the physical and neurologic signs examined in the Dubowitz and the Ballard Gestational Age Assessments.
4. Compare and contrast the Dubowitz and Ballard Gestational Age Assessments.
5. Describe seven physical signs that are used to determine gestational age and relate findings of each to varying gestational ages.
6. List five purposes of the neonatal physical examination.
7. Describe each of the following as it pertains to the physical examination. Include a description of the unique aspects of each examination.
   a. Quiet examination
   b. Hands-on examination
   c. Neurologic examination
8. List four indications for performing pulmonary function tests on neonatal patients.
9. Describe two methods used to measure compliance and resistance, and two methods used to measure expiratory flows in the neonatal patient.
10. Briefly describe the use of helium dilution, nitrogen washout, and body plethysmography in assessing lung volumes.
11. When shown a volume-pressure loop, determine whether it is normal, or whether it demonstrates abnormal compliance or resistance.

KEY TERMS

acrocyanosis	lanugo	scaphoid
anencephaly	murmur	thoracic gas volume
caput succedaneum	paradoxical	(TGV)
Doppler	pinna	vernix
fontanelle	pneumotachograph	
hydrocephaly	rugae	

INTRODUCTION

Clinical correlation of the history and physical examination (signs/symptoms) is connected to a working diagnosis for evaluation and treatment of the problem. It is always associated with a thorough assessment of the infant patient, particularly because they often cannot communicate where it hurts or why. The information gathered in clinical observations can provide critical visual, auditory, or tactile clues (i.e., swelling, cyanosis, distension, chest abnormalities, breathing patterns, or wheezing and tactile fremitus) to evaluate and make sense of the underlying condition. These provide evidence by confirming suspicions that the assessment is targeted toward the working diagnosis. Therefore, the respiratory therapist must develop a working knowledge of the connectedness of particular assessments to pathology and to make recommendations for appropriate treatment of a specific disease process. The assessment of the neonate or infant patient is careful, systematic, and measured as each evaluation is considered as it compares or detracts from normal anatomy or physiologic function. Assessment begins with a thorough understanding of normal anatomy and how it compares to specific function in the human body.

ANATOMIC AND PHYSIOLOGIC CONSIDERATIONS

Before a successful physical assessment can be performed on a neonatal or infant patient, the respiratory therapist must have a clear understanding of the anatomic and physiologic differences between adults, infants, and children.

There is tremendous variation or difference in the anatomic structures and physiologic processes between various age group populations. In general, those differences are greatest during the neonatal period and become less apparent with increasing age.

Cardiopulmonary System

We will begin by contrasting the differences between the cardiopulmonary systems of adults and infants (recall that an infant is defined in age as between one month and one year old).

Beginning with the upper airways, in terms of area the infant tongue is proportionally larger than the adult tongue. Infants also have a large amount of lymphoid tissue in the area of the pharynx compared to the adult. These two factors greatly increase the risk of upper airway occlusion in infants.

The epiglottis of the infant is proportionally larger, less flexible, and omega-shaped (Ω), which makes it very susceptible to trauma. The infant epiglottis also lies more horizontally than the adult.

The infant larynx lies higher in the neck in relation to the cervical spine. Additionally, the narrowest segment of the larynx is at the level of the cricoid ring. In contrast, the narrowest portion of the adult larynx is at the glottis.

All of these factors make upper airway occlusion a greater risk in the infant than in the adult patient. Any swelling or inflammation of these structures greatly increases resistance and the patient's work when breathing.

The diameter of the trachea above the carina is roughly 4 mm at birth compared to 16 mm in the adult. The length of the trachea increases from 57 mm at birth to 120 mm in the adult.

The infant chest offers little stability because the ribs and sternum are mostly cartilage and offers little resistance to thoracic expansion. Adequate ventilation, therefore, requires the use of the diaphragm to determine tidal volume. Any increase in minute ventilation is accomplished by increasing the respiratory rate, not the tidal volume.

Three factors are responsible for the low pulmonary reserve in infants. First, the heart is large in proportion to thoracic diameter. Thus, it imposes on the lungs and reduces the volume of gas that an infant can inhale through diaphragmatic contraction. Second, as previously discussed, the thoracic cage offers little stability and makes it difficult for the patient to increase tidal volume by chest expansion. Third, proportionally large abdominal contents push up against the diaphragm, diminishing its ability to function properly.[1]

An additional difference in the pulmonary systems of adults and infants is the fact that infants are considered to be obligatory nose breathers. A study by Miller et al, however, has demonstrated that newborns are not totally dependent on nose breathing, but do in fact, mouth breathe for both spontaneous breathing and in response to nasal occlusion.[2] Although newborns breathe nasally under normal circumstances, it is important to understand the implications for alternative mechanisms in the airway operation of infants. Due to the small diameter of the nasal passages, any decrease in the caliber of the airway from secretions or inflammation can significantly increase resistance to airflow and increase the work of breathing for the infant.

Metabolism

The metabolic rate of neonates and infants is higher than in adults. The caloric requirement for neonates is approximately 100 cal/kg and decreases to 40 to 50 cal/kg in the adult.[3] The result of increased metabolism is that the neonate has a greater oxygen requirement proportional to body size than in the adult.

Due to the differences in metabolism, infants do not respond to medications and pharmacotherapy in any predictable manner. Similar patients may have dramatically different reactions to the same dosage of a particular drug. Because of this, there are recommended dosages but no definitive measures or frequencies of established medication administration. A respiratory therapist must assess and evaluate the risks and benefits of each prescribed medication. Each time a drug is given, the dosage must be adjusted for the individual patient.

Other Factors

Neonates have a large amount of skin surface area relative to their body weight proportional to size and weight. An adult male has a body surface area of about $0.02 \ m^2/kg$ of body weight. The term neonate has about $0.07 \ m^2/kg$, and a 28-week neonate has roughly $0.15 \ m^2/kg$.[4] This large surface area makes the neonate particularly prone to heat loss and often susceptible to cold stress.

Because 80% of the neonate's total body weight is water (as opposed to 50% to 60% in the average adult), and that water is mainly found in the extracellular spaces (as opposed to 2/3 total body water found in the cells of adults), fluid balance in neonates is precarious. Over hydration and dehydration can be very difficult to manage or avoid in the newborn.

PHYSICAL ASSESSMENT OF THE NEONATE

Following delivery and clamping of the umbilical cord, the neonate must undergo a transition from uterine life to survival outside the uterus. This initial transition is a critical time for the neonate. It is the responsibility of the respiratory therapist to assess, evaluate, and determine how well the neonate is adapting to its new environment.

It is crucial that the respiratory therapist be able to identify a neonate who is not adapting well. Clinical signs might include, tachypnea, tachycardia, grunting, retractions, inability to maintain body temperature, reduced vigor, or limp appearance. Recognition of these signs allows the respiratory therapist to react and treat the patient in a timely manner. The purpose of the physical assessment is just that—to determine how well the extra-uterine transition is taking place.

Another important aspect of the initial assessment of the neonate is understanding the patient's history. Of interest are those pertinent factors, which serve to focus the respiratory therapist's attention on possible risks or to consider potential complications or problems.

History

Before examining the neonatal patient, it is vital to know the important historical facts concerning the pregnancy, labor, and delivery. A basic history should also include the mother's obstetric past. The following offers a brief synopsis included in a minimal maternal history.

Obstetric History The respiratory therapist should know the pregnancy history (called PARA), which is typically recorded as four numbers representing the total prior term pregnancies, premature deliveries, abortions/miscarriages, and living children. For example, a woman for whom this is the fourth pregnancy and who has had one miscarriage, one premature delivery, and two living children, would be written as PARA 3-1-1-2. The PARA can be simplified by using the mnemonic for easier recall, *Texas Power And Light*, where the *T* stands for "term" pregnancies, *P* is for "premature" deliveries, *A* for "abortions/miscarriages," and *L* for "living" children.

Pregnancy History The information obtained in this history is directed toward those risk factors that may have jeopardized the growing fetus. These might include exposure to teratogenic drugs, maternal drug use, malnutrition, or if the infant is the product of a mother with diabetes (IDM).

Labor and Delivery History The history of a laboring mother can help identify a compromised fetus. It is important to obtain the following information: duration of the delivery stages I and II, presentation of the neonate, the use of birth assist devices, and fetal heart rate—including any changes that might indicate impending distress or further compromise the neonate.

Gestational Age Assessment

Until the late 1960s, the designations of prematurity, maturity, and post maturity were predominantly based on the birth weight of the neonate. A neonate of less than 2500 g was often characterized as premature. A neonate whose weight fell between 2500 and 3999 g was mature, and any weight above 4000 g was considered post mature or beyond term.

These weight designations assumed that all fetuses grow equally in utero. In reality, each fetus grows at its own rate, some reaching 2500 g well before 40 weeks, others never reaching 2500 g even at term.

The importance of determining the neonate's actual gestational age is to allow care that focuses on the special problems of premature gestations. Assessment of gestational age, compared to birth weight, allows the respiratory therapist to assess the neonate to be classified as growth retarded, growth accelerated, or of normal growth. This classification allows the respiratory therapist to generate a list of potential problems and take early steps to either avoid developmental complications or to manage and treat the parameters available to them.

Dubowitz Gestational Age Assessment Determination of gestational age was initially a guessing game, depending on the presence or absence of certain neonatal characteristics. In 1970, a group of investigators led by Lilly and Victor Dubowitz published several criteria to be used in assessing gestational age. The method they proposed was much more objective and reproducible than previous attempts at correlating characteristics. Using this method, the neonate's gestational age could be obtained during a routine physical examination. This scoring system is known as the Dubowitz Gestational Age Assessment and is shown in Figure 5–1A–C.

NEUROLOGICAL CRITERIA

Neurological Sign	Score						Record Score Here
	0	1	2	3	4	5	
Posture							
Square Window							
Ankle Dorsiflexion							
Arm Recoil							
Leg Recoil							
Popliteal Angle							
Heel To Ear							
Scarf Sign							
Head Lag							
Ventral Suspension							

Total Score	Gestational Age (weeks)	Total Score	Gestational Age (weeks)	Total Score	Gestational Age (weeks)
10	27.2	30	32.5	50	37.8
12	27.8	32	33.0	52	38.3
14	28.3	34	33.6	54	38.9
16	28.8	36	34.1	56	39.4
18	29.4	38	34.6	58	39.9
20	29.9	40	35.2	60	40.4
22	30.4	42	35.7	62	41.0
24	30.9	44	36.2	64	41.5
26	31.5	46	36.7	66	42.0
28	32.0	48	37.3	68	42.6

A.

FIGURE 5–1A. The Dubowitz Gestational Age Assessment.

Reprinted from The Journal of Pediatrics, Vol 77/1, Dubowitz, L.; Dubowitz, V.; Goldberg, C.; Clinical assessment of gestational age in the newborn infant, 1970with permission from Elsevier.

EXTERNAL (SUPERFICIAL) CRITERIA

EXTERNAL SIGN	SCORE					RECORD SCORE HERE
	0	1	2	3	4	
EDEMA	Obvious edema of hands and feet; pitting over tibia	No obvious edema of hands and feet; pitting over tibia	No edema			
SKIN TEXTURE	Very thin, gelatinous	Thin and smooth	Smooth, medium thickness. Rash or superficial peeling	Slight thickening. Superficial cracking and peeling, esp. hands, feet	Thick and parchment like; superficial or deep cracking	
SKIN COLOR (infant not crying)	Dark red	Uniformly pink	Pale pink; variable over body	Pale. Only pink over ears, lips, palms, or soles		
SKIN CAPACITY (Trunk)	Numerous veins and venules clearly seen, esp. over abdomen	Veins and tributaries seen	A few large vessels clearly seen over abdomen	A few large vessels seen indistinctly over abdomen	No blood vessels seen	
LANUGO (Over back)	No lanugo	Abundant; long and thick over whole back	Hair thinning, esp. over lower back	Small amount of lanugo and bald areas	At least half of back devoid of lanugo	
PLANTAR CREASES	No skin creases	Faint red marks over anterior half of sole	Definite red marks over more than anterior half; indentations over less than anterior third	Indentations over more than anterior third	Definite deep indentations over more than anterior third	

B.

FIGURE 5–1B. The Dubowitz Gestational Age Assessment.

(continues)

NIPPLE FORMATION	Nipple barely visible; no areola	Nipple well-defined; areola smooth and flat; diameter < 0.75 cm	Areola stippled, edge not raised; diameter < 0.75 cm	
BREAST SIZE	No breast tissue palpable	Breast tissue on one or both side < 0.5 cm diameter	Breast tissue both sides, one or both 0.5-1.0 cm	
EAR FORM	Pinna flat and shapeless, or no incurving of edge	Incurving of part of edge of pinna	Partial incurving of whole of upper pinna	
EAR FIRMNESS	Pinna soft, easily folded, no recoil	Pinna soft, easily folded, slow recoil	Cartilage to edge of pinna, but soft in places, ready recoil	Pinna firm, cartilage to edge, instant recoil
GENITALIA MALE/FEMALE (With hips half-abducted)	Neither testi in *scrotum* Labia majora widely separated, labia minora protruding	At least one testis high in scrotum Labia majora almost cover labia minora	At least one testis fully descended. Labia majora completely cover labia minora.	

FIGURE 5–1B. (continued)

GESTATIONAL AGE ASSESSMENT (Dubowitz)

Lily Dubowitz, M.D., D.C.H. and Victor Dubowitz, B.Sc., M.D., Ph.D., F.R.C.P., D.C.H.
Department of Paediatrics and Neonatal Medicine, University of London Royal Postgraduate Medical School, Hammersmith Hospital London W 12 OHS, England

NOTES ON ASSESSMENT TECHNIQUES FOR THE NEUROLOGICAL CRITERIA

POSTURE: Observed with infant quiet and in supine position. Score 0: Arms and legs extended. 1: Beginning of flexion of hips and knees, arms extended. 2: Stronger flexion of legs, arms extended. 3: Arms slightly flexed, legs flexed and abducted. 4: Arms and legs fully flexed and hips abducted.

SQUARE WINDOW: The hand is flexed on the forearm between the thumb and index finger of the examiner. Enough gentle pressure is applied to get as full flexion as possible, and the angle between the hypothenar eminence and the ventral aspect of the forearm is measured and graded according to the diagram. (Care is taken not to rotate the infant's wrist while doing this maneuver.)

ANKLE DORSIFLEXION: The foot is dorsiflexed onto the anterior aspect of the leg, with the examiner's thumb on the sole of the baby's foot and examiner's fingers behind the baby's leg. Enough pressure is applied to get as full flexion as possible, and the angle between the dorsum of the foot and the anterior aspect of the leg is measured.

ARM RECOIL: With the infant in the supine position, the forearms are first flexed for 5 seconds, then fully extended by pulling on the hands, and finally released. The sign is fully positive if the arms return briskly to full flexion (score 2). If the arms return to incomplete flexion or the response is sluggish, it is graded as score 1. If they remain extended or are only followed by random movements, the score is 0.

LEG RECOIL: With the infant supine, the hips and knees are fully flexed for 5 seconds, then extended by traction on the feet and released. A maximal response is one of full flexion of the hips and knees (score 2). A partial flexion scores, and minimal or no movement scores 0.

POPLITEAL ANGLE: With the infant supine and the pelvis flat on the examining couch, the thigh is held in the knee-chest position by the examiner's left index finger and thumb supporting the baby's knee. The leg is then extended by gentle pressure from the examiner's right index finger behind the baby's ankle, and the poplitcal angle is measured.

HEEL-TO-EAR MANEUVER: With the baby supine, draw the baby's foot as near to the head as it will go without forcing it. Observe the distance between the foot and the head as well as the degree of extension at the knee. Grade according to the diagram. Note that the knee is left free and may draw down alongside the abdomen.

SCARF SIGN: With the baby supine, take the infant's hand and try to put it around the opposite shoulder. Assist this maneuver by lifting the elbow across the body. See how far the elbow will go across and grade according to the illustrations. Score 0: Elbow reaches opposite axillary line; 1: Elbow between the midline and opposite axillary line; 2: Elbow reaches midline; 3: Elbow will not reach midline.

HEAD LAG: With the baby lying supine, grasp the hands (or the arms, if a very small infant) and pull the baby slowly toward the sitting position. Observe the position of the head in relation to the trunk and grade accordingly. In a small infant, the head may initially be supported by one hand. Score 0: Complete lag; 1: Partial head control; 2: Able to maintain head in line with body; 3: Brings head anterior to body.

VENTRAL SUSPENSION: The infant is suspended in the prone position with the examiner's hand under the infant's chest (one hand for a small infant, two for a large infant). Observe the degree of extension of the back and the amount of flexion of the arms and legs. Also note the relationship of the head to the trunk. Grade according to the diagrams.

Reprinted by permission of Dr. L.M.S. Dubowitz, Dr. V. Dubowitz and The Journal of Pediatrics.

References: Dubowitz, L.M.S., Dubowitz, V., Goldberg, C. Clinical assessment of gestational age in the newborn infant J Pediatr 77:1 10, 1970.

Dubowitz, L.M.S., Dubowitz, V.: Gestational Age of the Newborn, Reading, Mass.: Addison-Wesley Publishing Co., 1977.

C.

FIGURE 5–1C. The Dubowitz Gestational Age Assessment.

The Dubowitz examines 11 physical or "external" criteria and 10 neurologic signs evaluated in the newborn. These researchers found that the physical criteria are more accurate and reproducible for determining gestational age than the neurologic criteria. However, when both physical and neurologic criteria are evaluated together, the assessment of gestational age is more accurate than when either criteria are evaluated alone.

Each of the areas examined is assigned a point value from 1 to 5, depending on the physical characteristic or the neurologic response of the neonate. The points are added up from each category and the resulting number corresponds to the gestational age. The Dubowitz method is usually accurate to within 2 weeks and has consistent results when used in the first 5 days of life. The Dubowitz scoring system proved to be an important step forward in neonatology. However, the need for a more rapid method became clear.

Ballard Gestational Age Assessment In 1979, researchers presented a simplified method of assessing gestational age.[5] In their studies, they found that several of the criteria used in the Dubowitz assessment were not as good at indicating gestational age as others. Their studies resulted in an examination that scores six neurologic signs and six physical signs. This system is known as the Ballard score, shown in Figure 5–2. Using the Ballard score, gestational age can be assessed from 22 to 44 weeks.

The Ballard score is comparable to most assessments related in the Dubowitz scoring system in terms of reliability. The Ballard system is most reliable when the examination is done before 42 hours of life, with the ideal time being between 30 and 42 hours after delivery. With fewer categories to assess, the Ballard system takes less time to perform than the Dubowitz system. There is some question regarding the validity of shortening the Dubowitz system, because if one area is inaccurate, it has a heavier influence on the total score.

Physical Examination to Determine Gestational Age

Physical examinations are quick, easy, and fairly reliable for determining gestational age. There will be occasions when it will be necessary or prudent to do a quick assessment of gestational age to begin treatment without delay. One such time is during resuscitation.

A quick and fairly reliable assessment of gestational age can be made by inspecting the physical age signs, without taking the time for the neurologic examination. Using only physical signs, an assessment of gestational age can be determined in less than 1 minute by a skilled respiratory therapist. Rapid interpretation of the gestational age is important to determine what steps might be taken to reverse potential complications as a result of pre-term deliveries or reduced respiratory effort at birth. These signs will be examined individually.

Vernix One of the first criteria assessed on examination of a neonate is the presence of **vernix**. Vernix is a white, cream cheese-like material that covers the fetus in utero.

NEWBORN MATURITY RATING & CLASSIFICATION

ESTIMATION OF GESTATIONAL AGE BY MATURITY RATING
Symbols: X - 1st Exam   O - 2nd Exam

Side 1

Gestation by Dates _____ wks

Birth Date_____ Hour _____ am pm

APGAR _____ 1 min _____ 5 min

NEUROMUSCULAR MATURITY

	-1	0	1	2	3	4	5
Posture							
Square Window (wrist)	>90°	90°	60°	45°	30°	0°	
Arm Recoil		180°	140°-180°	110°-140°	90°-110°	<90°	
Popliteal Angle	180°	160°	140°	120°	100°	90°	<90°
Scarf Sign							
Heel to Ear							

MATURITY RATING

score	weeks
-10	20
-5	22
0	24
5	26
10	28
15	30
20	32
25	34
30	36
35	38
40	40
45	42
50	44

PHYSICAL MATURITY

Skin	sticky; friable; transparent	gelatinous; red; translucent	smooth; pink; visible veins	superficial peeling &/or rash; few veins	cracking; pale areas; rare veins	parchment; deep cracking; no vessels	leathery; cracked; wrinkled
Lanugo	none	sparse	abundant	thinning	bald areas	mostly bald	
Plantar Surface	heel-toe 40-50 mm: -1 <40 mm: -2	>50 mm; no crease	faint red marks	anterior transverse crease only	creases ant. 2/3	creases over entire sole	
Breast	imperceptible	barely perceptible	flat areola; no bud	stippled areola; 1-2 mm bud	raised areola; 3-4 mm bud	full areola; 5-10 mm bud	
Eye/Ear	lids fused loosely: -1 tightly: -2	lids open; pinna flat; stays folded	sl. curved pinna; soft; slow recoil	well-curved pinna; soft but ready recoil	formed & firm; instant recoil	thick cartilage; ear stiff	
Genitals male	scrotum flat; smooth	scrotum empty; faint rugae	testes in upper canal; rare rugae	testes descending; few rugae	testes down; good rugae	testes pendulous; deep rugae	
Genitals female	clitoris prominent; labia flat	prominent clitoris; small labia minora	prominent clitoris; enlarging minora	majora & minora equally prominent	majora large; minora small	majora cover clitoris & minora	

Scoring system: Ballard JL, Khoury JC, Wedig K, Wang L, Eilers-Walsman BL, Lipp R. New Ballard Score, expanded to include extremely premature infants. *J Pediatr.* 1991;119:417-423.

SCORING SECTION

	1st Exam=X	2nd Exam=O
Estimating Gest Age by Maturity Rating	_____Weeks	_____Weeks
Time of Exam	Date _____ am pm Hour _____	Date _____ am pm Hour _____
Age at Exam	_____Hours	_____Hours
Signature of Examiner	_____ M.D./R.N.	_____ M.D./R.N.

Provided Courtesy of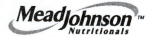

Reprinted from The Journal of Pediatrics, 119/3, Ballard, J. L., et al. New Ballard Score, 417-423, 1991, with permission from Elsevier.

FIGURE 5–2. Newborn Maturity Rating & Classification.

It appears around 20 to 24 weeks and remains thick on the fetus until week 36, at which point it begins to gradually disappear. It usually disappears by week 41 to 42.

Skin Maturity Next, the respiratory therapist examines the neonate's skin. The appearance of the skin is an excellent indicator of gestational age. At 25 to 26 weeks, the skin is gelatinous and transparent, the blood vessels readily visible. As gestation advances, the skin becomes pink and the vessels become less and less visible. The near-term neonate has adult-looking skin, with many cracks and wrinkles, and no visible vessels.

Lanugo While examining the skin, inspect the neonate for the presence of **lanugo**. Lanugo is the fine, downy hair that covers the fetal body (Figure 5–3). It appears around week 26 and quickly covers the thorax, head, and extremities. By 28 weeks, it begins to thin and then begins to disappear around week 32. The term neonate may have lanugo on the shoulders and forehead. This is more common in neonates with dark complexions. In general, though, the lanugo has disappeared by week 40.

Ear Recoil Examination of the **pinna**, or the external portion of the ear, is helpful in determining gestational age. The cartilage in the ear is not fully present until around

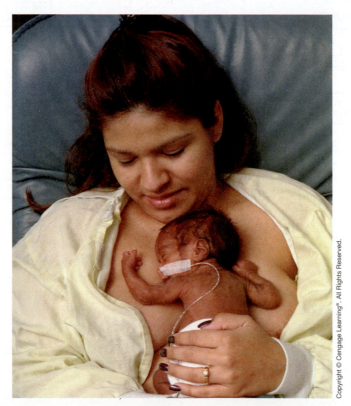

FIGURE 5–3. Lanugo is seen as the fine, downy hair on the arms and back"

34 weeks. At 25 to 26 weeks, the pinna is basically flat and will remain folded if doubled over. Cartilage first appears in the pinna around 27 to 28 weeks. At this point it has a slow recoil when folded. As each week of gestation proceeds, the pinna becomes more rigid and more adult looking, with a rapidly increasing recoil near term. At term the pinna recoils instantly, similar to that of an adult.

Breast Tissue The breast tissue is another physical sign used to determine gestational age. At 25 to 26 weeks, the breast is barely perceptible, if at all. At 27 weeks, the breast becomes a red circle, the areola, but there is no palpable tissue behind it. The breast bud forms around week 30 and is about 1 to 2 mm in diameter. The breast bud is a firm tissue that forms behind the areola that is easily felt when palpated between the fingers. The breast continues to develop until term, at which time the bud is 5 to 10 mm in diameter, raised, and the areola is fully developed.

Genitalia Examination of the genitalia is very useful in assessing gestational age. At 25 to 26 weeks, the male scrotum is hardly recognizable. It has no **rugae** (deep wrinkles in the mature scrotum), and the testicles have not descended. Rugae appear and the testes begin descending around weeks 30 to 32 and the scrotum continues its development until, near term, it is covered with deep rugae, and the testes have fully descended. The female genitalia undergoes very apparent changes from 24 weeks to term. At 25 to 26 weeks, the inner portion of the external genitalia, the labia minora and the clitoris, are very pronounced. As gestation advances, the outer portion, the labia majora, becomes equal in prominence. This occurs around weeks 30 to 32. The labia majora continue to grow until, at term, the clitoris and labia minora are completely covered.

Sole Creases Moving down to the neonate's feet, next examine the creases on the sole of the foot (Figure 5–4). Deep creases of wrinkles appear on the sole of the foot beginning at the anterior end near the toes and proceeding to the heel. The creases appear as faint red lines at roughly 26 weeks. At 30 weeks, the creases have covered

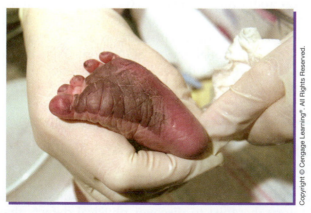

FIGURE 5–4. The plantar surface of the foot is assessed for creases as an indicator of gestational age.

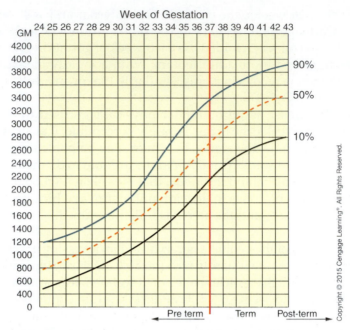

FIGURE 5–5. Intrauterine growth curve comparing weight and gestation.

the anterior portion of the foot. By 34 weeks, two thirds of the sole is covered with creases. By term, the entire sole is covered by continuous deep creases that are readily apparent.

Classification of the Neonate

After the gestational age of the neonate has been determined, and the weight measured, the patient can now be characterized by objective measures that inform the respiratory therapist about potential risks. At any given gestational age, 80% of all neonates will weigh within a normal range. These are classified as appropriate for gestational age, or AGA, while those with weights that fall below the 10th percentile are classified small for gestational age, or SGA. Conversely, those whose weight is above the 90th percentile are classified as large for gestational age, or LGA. A typical chart used for classifying infant weight is shown in Figure 5–5.

PURPOSE OF THE PHYSICAL EXAMINATION OF THE NEONATE

There are several purposes for the physical examination of the neonate. The exam allows the respiratory therapist to discover physical defects that may be present. These may be congenital or a result of a difficult labor and prolonged delivery. If defects are discovered, the respiratory therapist can then intervene and begin expedient treatment, if necessary.

The examination also helps to determine whether the neonate has made a successful transition to extra-uterine life and any adverse effect of labor and delivery on the neonate. This includes not only any physical effect, but also the consequence of anesthetics or analgesics on the neonate after delivery. This assessment usually includes a quick APGAR score evaluating heart rate, respiratory rate, muscle tone, reflex irritability, and skin color (See Chapter 4). The assessment is measured at 1 minute and at 5 minutes immediately after delivery and evaluates the adjustment to extra-uterine life. Scores of less than 6/10 at 1 minute and 7/10 at 5 minutes require immediate clinical intervention to restore postdelivery vigor. The gestational age of the neonate can be more thoroughly assessed after the neonate has been stabilized. By completely examining the neonate, the respiratory therapist can assess for signs of infection or verify metabolic disorders. Finally, the physical exam establishes a baseline for future comparisons.

The initial physical examination is usually done after the neonate has been stabilized and is somewhat adapted to its new environment. Of extreme importance is the maintenance of thermoregulation during the physical examination. Lacking the neurologic innervations to shiver, the neonate resorts to burning "brown fat" for producing heat in the transitional period. This process is an energy-requiring practice that increases oxygen consumption in the neonate. Therefore, the examination should be done in an incubator or under an open warmer to reduce heat loss.

The physical exam is usually done in two segments, a quiet observation exam followed by a hands-on exam. The quiet observation exam is necessary to observe the overall condition of the neonate in a nonstressed state, when it is not being handled or otherwise stimulated. It is difficult to assess the overall condition if the baby is upset and crying. Ideally, the neonate should be nude to observe all aspects of the body. Avoid the urge to touch the patient during this part of the exam.

Quiet Examination

The first part of the quiet exam is to observe various aspects of the neonate's color. A healthy neonate with a dark complexion may be difficult to assess for oxygenation via skin color. In these neonates, it may be possible to assess the color of the mucous membranes. These membranes should be pink in a well-oxygenated patient. Those neonates with light complexions are more readily assessed for oxygenation because they will have a pinkish hue to the skin. A blue (cyanotic) or pale color of the mucosa or skin may indicate hypoxemia (or tissue hypoxia), and treatment with oxygen should be started immediately, followed by further assessment of respiratory status. If the exam is done in the first few hours after birth, it is likely that the body will be pink, but the feet and hands will still be blue. This is known as **acrocyanosis** and is commonly present in the first 24 hours following birth.

A yellowish hue to the skin or the eyes is secondary to jaundice. If jaundice is present, further evaluation will be necessary to determine if the jaundice is pathologic or physiologic. The differentiation of jaundice is further explored in Chapter 6

The presence of greenish (tar-like), or dark green meconium on the skin may indicate distress or could alert the respiratory therapist that some degree of asphyxia was present in utero prior to delivery. Meconium staining that was acquired in utero may only be seen if the initial examination is done before the infant is cleaned and dried. Meconium seen on the skin following cleaning and drying may be secondary to normal bowel movements and not a sign of asphyxia.

While examining the skin, assess for the presence and amount of lanugo. This is followed by a determination of skin maturity. Both of these details are an important part of the gestational age assessment and their results should be noted accordingly.

Now focus your attention on a quick assessment the infant's condition and level of activity. Observe the infant for symmetry of movement, muscle tone, normal movements of the extremities, and respiratory effort. (It may be appropriate, in the absence of heart monitoring, to lightly palpate the umbilical cord for evidence of bradycardia to ensure the infant is responding suitably to treatment.) Any asymmetry or abnormal movements may indicate fractures, paralysis, or convulsive states. A lack of good muscle tone may signify a degree of neurologic impairment. The healthy neonate will move the extremities symmetrically. Asymmetry of arm or leg movements may mean a fracture or even paralysis. The movements may be jerky, but they are usually short in duration.

The arm and legs will be well flexed, showing good muscle tone. The healthy neonate will usually be in the fetal position, with the legs drawn to the abdomen and arms flexed and tight to the body.

Now inspect the overall look of the patient. Start at the head and visually inspect the entire patient, taking note of any malformations or apparent anomalies. A comparison of head size to body size may help diagnose **hydrocephaly** or **anencephaly**. Abnormal bulges or bumps may be cysts or tumors that require further examination. Many congenital defects or chromosomal disorders can readily be identified by simple observation.

The last part of the quiet examination involves a thorough examination of observing the infant's respiration. The respiratory rate is normally between 30 and 60 bpm. Neonates, especially those born prematurely, may have periods of apnea usually lasting 5 to 10 seconds but without cyanosis or bradycardia. This pause in breathing is called *periodic breathing* and is considered normal. True apnea, on the other hand, lasts longer than 15 to 20 seconds and is accompanied by cyanosis and/or bradycardia. The causes and treatments for apnea are covered in more detail in Chapter 7.

Tachypnea, or a respiratory rate above 60 bpm, could be a sign of respiratory distress and should be investigated further. Because of the relative noncompliance of the thoracic cage, newborns rely mainly on the diaphragm for their respirations. The neonate should be watched for good abdominal (paradoxical) movement during quiet breathing. This is a sign of an intact diaphragm. Chest movement should be symmetrical during inspiration and exhalation. There should also be noticeable chest excursion during inhalation, equal on both sides.

The three cardinal signs of respiratory distress are nasal flaring, grunting, and retractions. Nasal flaring is an attempt to get more gas volume into the lungs. It is identified by a widening of the nares during inspiration, returning to normal during expiration.

The term *grunting* may be misleading. The actual sound made is more of a high-pitched vocal tone rather than a low-pitched snore. The sound is made by closing the glottis over the trachea, causing an increased lung pressure during exhalation to allow for alveolar opening. The positive pressure created by grunting helps keep the alveoli from collapsing during exhalation. The effects and pathology of respiratory distress that are manifest by grunting are further elaborated in Chapter 7.

Retractions are the inward movement of the thoracic surface during inhalation (thoracic expansion). They may be mild, moderate, or severe and are found intercostally (between the ribs), above the clavicles, below the sternum, or may involve the entire sternum itself. As the lung becomes less complaint with advancing respiratory distress, greater subatmospheric pressures are required in the thorax to overcome the low lung compliance and alveolar collapse. As the subatmospheric pressures become greater, the external surface of the thorax is drawn inward, creating the characteristic retractions. One good method for evaluating the degree of respiratory distress is by the Silverman-Anderson Index, which examines the upper and lower chest and nares. To review the index visit http://pediatrics.aappublications.org and search for "Silverman and Anderson Index."

Hands-on Examination The next physical examination is the hands-on portion. The examiner should have warm hands and a warm stethoscope. Any touching should be done gently so as not to upset the patient. A pacifier may be used to help keep the neonate quiet. As with the quiet exam, the respiratory therapist starts at the head and works toward the extremities.

The head should be inspected for cuts or bruises secondary to the use of forceps or other intra-birthing process trauma. The head could be edematous from the pressure generated during labor. This produces what is called **caput succedaneum**. This is usually harmless and resolves in the first two days. The two soft spots, or **fontanelles**, should now be gently palpated. The anterior fontanelle is diamond-shaped and usually measures 1 to 4 cm. The posterior fontanelle is triangle-shaped and is smaller than the anterior one. Both fontanelles should be firm, but soft. A bulging, tense fontanelle may signify increased intracranial pressure. Shrunken or depressed fontanelles may be secondary to dehydration or volume depletion.

The mouth may now be examined for the presence of clefts (openings) in the palate and any other abnormality that may hinder breathing. The ears may now be examined to determine where they fall on the gestational age assessment scale. The neck should be palpated for the presence of any cysts or tumors.

Moving to the chest, the breast tissue may now be evaluated for the gestational age assessment (Figure 5–6).

With the stethoscope, the heart is now assessed by auscultation (Figure 5–7A). The normal heart rate is between 120 and 160 bpm. Heart rates below 100 bpm are considered bradycardia, and a heart rate above 160 bpm is considered tachycardia. The apical pulse, which is the point on the chest where the heart sounds are heard the loudest, is evaluated next. It is normally heard in the fifth intercostal space, mid-clavicularly on the left chest wall. This location, called the point of maximal impulse or intensity (PMI), is marked on the chest wall and used for future reference. Conditions that could cause the PMI to shift include pneumothorax, atelectasis, and an increase in heart size.

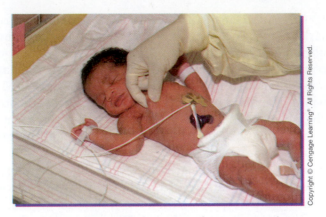

FIGURE 5–6. The breast tissue is examined to identify gestational age.

The heart normally has two distinct sounds, with the first sound being slightly louder and duller to auscultation than the second sound. Any sound that is heard besides the normal ones is considered to be a **murmur**. Murmurs are typically the result of turbulent blood flow in the heart. They can be caused by valvular defects, septal defects, increased blood flow, or a patent ductus arteriosus. Occasionally, a murmur of pulmonic or aortic stenosis is heard.

Systolic murmurs usually occur after the first heart sound and end before the onset of the second sound. Systolic murmurs make up most of the benign sounds, while diastolic murmurs are more indicative of heart disease. Murmurs are graded from I to IV, with I being soft and IV being loudest. Roughly 90% of murmurs in the neonatal period are benign; however, some severe heart defects may be present when no murmur is heard.

With the stethoscope on the chest, the lungs may now be evaluated (Figure 5–7). The healthy lungs will be well aerated in all segments and free of adventitious sounds. The presence of wheezes, crackles, or rhonchi should be examined further to determine their origin and to evaluate for the presence of any respiratory compromise.

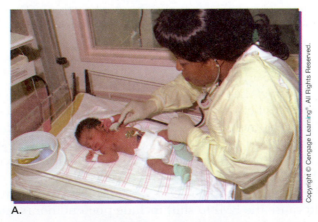

A.

FIGURE 5–7. A. Auscultation of the heart for rate and rhythm.

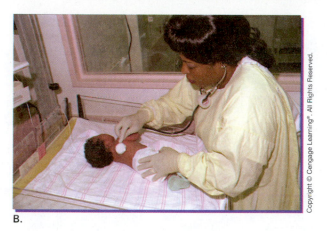

B.

FIGURE 5–7. B. Auscultation of the lungs for equal breath sounds and proper expansion.

Brachial pulses should now be evaluated and compared to femoral pulses (Figure 5–8A and B). Both pulses should be equal in intensity and strength and symmetrical in rhythm. Weak pulses may indicate hypotension, diminished cardiac output, or peripheral vasoconstriction. Decreased femoral pulses in the presence of normal brachial pulses may indicate a heart anomaly such as coarctation of the aorta or a patent ductus arteriosus and should be evaluated further. Conversely, bounding pulses may indicate a large right-to-left shunt through the ductus arteriosis.

Upon completion of the pulse evaluation, the blood pressure (BP) should be measured. Many factors cause neonatal BP to vary. Factors such as gestational age, weight, cuff size, and the neonate's state of alertness can all influence BP readings.[6] Neonatal BP is obtained by the use of a **Doppler** device and a cuff, an electronic BP cuff, or through the umbilical artery catheter. On the small neonate, BP is best taken from the femoral artery with the cuff around the thigh.

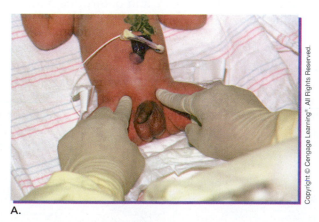

A.

FIGURE 5–8. A. Palpation of femoral pulses.

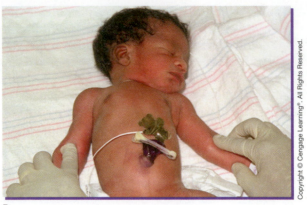

B.

FIGURE 5–8. B. Palpation of brachial pulses.

In many instances, diastolic pressure is difficult to assess. In such cases, systolic pressure is measured and documented. Neonatal BP begins low and increases with age and size. Normal neonatal blood pressures are listed in Table 5–1. BP continues to increase as the baby grows until it reaches its adult normal of 120/80 mmHg.

The abdomen should now be gently palpated to check for cysts or tumors. The liver may be palpated and measured in centimeters below the anterior, right lower chest margin. The liver can normally be palpated approximately 1.5 to 2 cm below the right costal border. In right-sided heart failure, the liver is engorged with blood and may be 5 to 6 cm below the costal border.

A normal neonate will have a protruding abdomen. However, if the abdomen is scaphoid (sunken or flat), the respiratory therapist should assess for presence of a diaphragmatic hernia.

If it is still possible, check the umbilical stump for the presence of three vessels. The presence of only two vessels is highly associated with urinary tract abnormalities.

The presence of bowel sounds should be documented with the stethoscope. The genitalia can now be examined to evaluate and determine maturity. Finally, the foot can be inspected for the presence of creases.

Table 5–1

NEONATAL BLOOD PRESSURE RANGE OF NORMALS

Weight	Systolic (mmHg)	Diastolic (mmHg)
750 g	34–54	14–34
1000 g	39–59	16–36
1500 g	40–61	19–39
3000 g	51–72	27–46

The neonate's temperature should now be measured to ensure proper thermoregulation. Temperature can be assessed rectally, aurally, or at the axilla, with the axilla being the preferred location. Axillary temperatures are reliable as indicators of thermoregulation and are within 0.10°C of rectal temperatures. Normal neonatal body temperature ranges from 36.2°C to 37.3°C.

Neurologic Examination The importance and necessity of the neurologic examination continues to be controversial. It is questionable whether the information obtained is useful for diagnosis of normal or abnormal neurologic status. Studies have shown that a fetus's neurologic system matures at a constant rate during gestation. The exam, therefore, is dependent on the degree of intrauterine development toward maturation.

Obviously, a 40-week neonate will respond differently to the neurologic exam than will a 32-week neonate. Apparent defects may be transient or permanent in nature. Until more studies are done to correlate gestational age with appropriate responses, the neurologic exam may be of limited use.

Much of the neurologic exam can be accomplished during the physical examination. The neonate's movements, crying, response to touch, and muscular tone are all signs that can be checked for neurologic development. All remaining information can be obtained by performing a series of reflex tests on the neonate to validate the assessment.

Neonatal Reflex Tests To elicit the rooting reflex, gently stroke the corner of the mouth, as shown in Figure 5–9. An appropriate response is for the baby to turn its head toward the side that was stroked. The suck reflex is determined by placing a pacifier or a clean finger into the mouth. The baby should begin sucking immediately; the strength of the suck depends on hunger and nursing instinct.

The grasp reflex is invoked by placing your index fingers into the patient's palm. The healthy neonate should immediately grasp your fingers. This is followed by

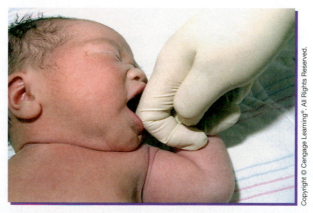

FIGURE 5–9. The rooting reflex is assessed by stimulation of the side of the neonate's mouth. The baby should turn its head toward the side that was stroked.

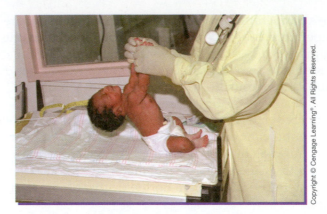

FIGURE 5–10. The grasp reflex is assessed by placing a finger in the neonates hand and gently pulling the neonate to an upright position.

placing your thumb over the fingers and gently pulling the patient to a sitting position (Figure 5–10). Be careful not to rely on the patient's grasp to be secure enough to pull him or her to an upright position. The degree of head control can be determined with the neonate in the upright position. A healthy patient should have enough control to keep the head upright and not limply hanging down. The Moro reflex can be tested by slowly lowering the neonate back to a lying position. Just before the head touches the bed, quickly remove your fingers, allowing the patient to fall to the bed. The normal response will be an upward and outward extension of the arms and rapid flexion of the hips and knees.

If desired, the neurologic evaluation portion of the gestational age assessment can now be performed following the guidelines of the Dubowitz or Ballard scoring systems. Findings of the neurologic examinations should be carefully evaluated in addition to physical characteristics because the incidence of false-positive and false-negative results is very high without their inclusion.

NEONATAL PULMONARY FUNCTION TESTING (PFT)

The purpose of testing pulmonary function in neonatal patients is to identify those patients at risk for pulmonary problems, diagnose the dysfunction, and aid in selection of treatments aimed at improving the dysfunction, and/or reducing acute and long-term complications.[7]

With the advent of computers, the performance of PFTs on neonates has become available to most NICUs. PFTs are used to reduce the risks associated with mechanical ventilation, while optimizing the patient/ventilator interaction synchrony). Technology has also produced airway connectors that have acceptable amounts of deadspace—a problem that severely limited PFTs on neonates prior to this development.

Pulmonary function values vary over a wide range of ages and sizes. Differences in anatomy and physiology between adults and infants must be considered when pulmonary tests are being performed. An additional concern that could potentially lead to inaccurate results is the lack of patient cooperation and inability to comprehend and follow commands, which is particularly seen in neonatal populations.

Indications for Pulmonary Function Tests

There are four main indications to the performance of PFTs on neonatal patients. They are: 1) diagnosis of lung disorders; 2) following the natural history of lung diseases and/or lung growth; 3) evaluation of therapeutic responses; and 4) prediction of subsequent dysfunction.[8]

Contraindications for Pulmonary Function Tests

The *AARC Clinical Practice Guideline* identifies nine absolute contraindications and seven relative contraindications that should be evaluated before performing PFTs on neonates. The absolute contraindications are: 1) active pulmonary bleeding; 2) open chest wound; 3) untreated pneumothorax; 4) past history of intolerance to sedation; 5) significant upper airway obstruction; 6) seizure disorder; 7) hemodynamically significant congenital heart disease; 8) recent intake of food or drink; and 9) naso-facial deformities. Relative contraindications include: 1) Medical conditions that could compromise patient's condition if ventilator support is temporarily interrupted; 2) central hypoventilation; 3) preexisting central nervous system depression or neurological impairment; 4) severe gastroesophageal reflux, esophagitis or gastritis; 5) uncooperative or combative patient; 6) patients with pacemakers; 7) febrile patients, or a recent history of URI, pneumonia or excessive coughing.[8]

Pulmonary Function Tests on Neonates

The ability to measure pulmonary compliance, resistance, and flow rates in the neonatal patient allows the respiratory therapist to maximize the benefit of therapeutic treatments. Following trends in compliance allows the respiratory therapist to optimize ventilator settings and avoid unnecessarily high pressures or respiratory rates.

Changes in resistance and flow can indicate bronchospasm or other obstructions that can then be further evaluated and treated. A gradual decreasing trend in values may help in the diagnosis and treatment of bronchopulmonary dysplasia.

The major disadvantage of performing pulmonary function tests on neonates is the inability of the patient to follow commands. The tests must be done using invasive measurements and often require sedating the patient, which may further compromise or invalidate the results. Either the "classic" method or occlusion method mentioned below can be performed on intubated or nonintubated patients.

The basic pulmonary function test requires the measurement of airflow rates and transpulmonary pressure (thoracic mechanics relating the difference between the alveolar pressure measured in the airway and pleural pressures. Several parameters can then be measured (frequency, tidal volume, and minute volume) by simple observation or calculated (compliance, resistance, and work of breathing) using measured parameters from the device in use. We will now examine how compliance, resistance, and work of breathing are determined.

Measurement of Compliance and Resistance The "classic method" is determined by gathering a few simple measurements. The first necessary measurement to calculate compliance (C_L) and resistance (R_{aw}) is airflow, obtained by placing a **pneumotachograph** in line with an endotracheal tube (ETT) or a face mask. The second measurement, transpulmonary pressure, is obtained by measuring the difference between airway and pleural pressures. Airway pressure is simply obtained by placing a pressure monitor inline to the ETT if intubated, or the pressure port on the face mask if the patient is not intubated. Pleural pressure is assessed by placing a catheter into the distal esophagus and measuring the pressure at the tip.[9]

A disadvantage with this testing is that accurate results are only obtained if the measured esophageal pressure actually represents an average pleural pressure. To measure lung compliance, three factors must be measured. The tidal volume is measured by the use of a pneumotachograph attached to a face mask. The proximal airway pressure is measured through a pressure port, while pleural pressure is estimated by the esophageal catheter. Measuring the proximal and pleural pressure at the same point during a breath allows for the determination of transpulmonary pressure. This is obtained by subtracting the pleural from the proximal pressure. Dividing the transpulmonary pressure into the patient's tidal volume results in the compliance (C_L) of the lung.

It is apparent that an inaccurate pleural pressure reading will result in an inaccurate compliance measurement. There are several factors that could result in the esophageal pressure differing from pleural pressure. One such factor is cardiac artifact from a misplaced catheter that could alter pressure readings. To avoid this problem, the catheter should be placed in the lower third of the esophagus. Additionally, **paradoxical** movement of the chest wall during ventilation causes different pleural pressures at any given tidal volume within the thorax. This paradoxical movement is caused by the horizontal position of the ribs and the lack of mineralization of the bony ribs, both giving rise to a very compliant chest wall. During REM sleep, the activity of the intercostal muscles changes, causing increased distortion of the rib cage and making the measurement of pleural pressures difficult.

In any of these situations, no clinically consistent pleural pressure exists and neither compliance nor resistance can be accurately measured.

Occlusion Techniques to Measure Compliance and Resistance Another method of determining lung compliance in the neonate is to measure alveolar pressure at a known lung volume. Alveolar pressure can be obtained by occluding the airway following an inspiration and measuring the pressure generated in the airway while the respiratory muscles are relaxed. This can be accomplished by the use of the face mask and pneumotachograph. A measured tidal volume is then delivered to the patient. Exhalation is prevented by occluding the expiratory valve on the mask.

The pressure is measured through the mask by a manometer once a plateau in pressure has been achieved. Exhalation is then allowed to occur and compliance is calculated by dividing the plateau pressure into the measured tidal volume. To be accurate, the occlusion time must be short enough so a spontaneous respiratory effort does not occur.

This technique is not without problems. First, a true pressure plateau must be reached at the mouth to ensure relaxation of the respiratory muscles. A struggling patient may not allow for accurate results. Second, in the diseased lung, diverse regional lung time constants may not allow for equilibration of pressures within the lung during the short time interval between occlusion of the airway and the onset of a spontaneous breath. This problem can be somewhat lessened by occluding the airway at several points before end inspiration, and averaging the compliances found at each point.

Measuring Work of Breathing Work of breathing reflects the amount of energy required by the lungs to overcome airway resistance. It is usually calculated by the area inside a pressure-volume loop created from modern pulmonary function technology. Pressure-volume loops are explained later in this chapter. As pulmonary mechanics worsen (resistance increases or compliance decreases), the amount of work increases and the neonate must expend more energy to maintain adequate ventilation.

Measurement of Expiratory Flows On the adult, forced expiratory flow rates are easily measured by instructing the patient to blow forcefully into the measuring device. It is obvious that this technique is not possible on the neonatal patient. Two methods are employed to measure forced expiratory flows. The first method is to physically squeeze the thorax to force exhalation.

Studies by England have shown that the external pressure needed to provide the desired results varies from patient to patient and is lower in patients with lung disease than in normal patients.[10] Thus, the use of a standard pressure to squeeze the chest of all patients will not result in accurate measurements.

The second method of measuring expiratory flows is to apply suction to the airway and measure the flows generated. With either described method, it is possible that the application of an external pressure, or the negative pressure applied to the airway, may alter the mechanical characteristics of the airway and give erroneous results.[10]

Measurement of Lung Volumes The measurement and evaluation of lung mechanics (tidal volume, dynamic compliance, and airway resistance) in the neonate is performed in healthy infants and those with respiratory disease. It requires specially trained respiratory therapists and specific equipment or facilities. Assessments are generally measured during sleep, in the supine position (often with light sedation), while breathing through a face mask or endotracheal tube (ETT). Volumes are compared to normal to evaluate the nature and severity of disease, airway reactivity, and responsiveness to therapeutic intervention.

Functional Residual Capacity (FRC) There are three basic methods used to measure the FRC of an infant or neonate: helium dilution, nitrogen washout, and body plethysmography. We will briefly examine each technique.

Helium dilution involves the closed-system rebreathing of a gas with a known helium volume and concentration. This technique, because of its effectiveness and simplicity, is probably the best method for use with neonates. Nitrogen washout is an open-system circuit in which the infant breathes 100% oxygen while the exhaled volume and concentration of nitrogen are analyzed. Both methods involve the placement of a mask over the mouth and nose, or attachment of the circuit to the endotracheal tube on intubated patients. Calculation of FRC is then done following prescribed equations. These techniques are most reliable in patients with good gas distribution and those with minimal small airway disease (manifest by reduced FEF_{25-75}).[11]

In contrast to the preceding techniques, body plethysmography is able to measure all of the thoracic gas volume, regardless of disease or distribution. To perform a measurement of **thoracic gas volume (TGV)** using plethysmography, the infant is placed in the body box and the airway is occluded at end expiration. As the infant attempts to inhale, the chest expands and produces an increase in volume in the plethysmograph. The change in volume is measured by a change in pressure in the plethysmograph. Mouth pressure is also measured with a differential pressure transducer. By applying Boyle's law, $P \times V - P' \times V'$, the TGV can then be calculated by the following equation[11]:

$$TGV = (\text{barometric pressure} - \text{water vapor pressure}) \times V/P - \text{deadspace}$$

where V/P = change in volume divided by the change in pressure. The amount of trapped gas in the thorax can be determined by subtracting the FRC from the TGV.

A relatively old technique, impedance plethysmography, is based on the concept that chest wall motion changes the impedance between two electrodes, which can then be converted to volume measurement. New research is using this concept and its possible use in neonates with a technique called respiratory inductive plethysmography.[12] As this procedure is perfected, it may prove to be an acceptable alternative to traditional methods of performing pulmonary functions.

Crying Vital Capacity The crying vital capacity has been advocated as an alternative to assess lung volume when FRC or TGV determinations are difficult to measure.[11] To assess the crying vital capacity, tidal volume is measured while the patient is crying. This may be useful in evaluating the course of RDS and other diseases that alter the FRC.

Pulmonary Function Profile

This data of lung volumes and pulmonary pressures provided by the PFT computer are used to create a profile of the patient's pulmonary function status using a volume-pressure and flow-volume loops. To obtain a volume-pressure loop, volume measurements are plotted on the vertical line and pressure on the horizontal. A normal

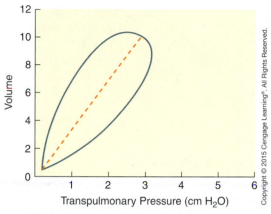

FIGURE 5–11. Normal volume-pressure loop.

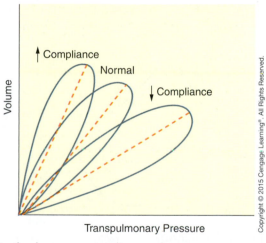

FIGURE 5–12. Change in the loop as compliance changes.

volume-pressure loop is shown in Figure 5–11. The compliance of the lung is indicated by connecting points of no airflow on the loop and examining the slope of the line, as shown in Figure 5–11. Changes in lung compliance are seen by a change in the slope of the line, as seen in Figure 5–12. Conversely, changes in airway resistance are seen as an increase or decrease in the area of the loop, as shown in Figure 5–13.

Another useful comparison is the relationship between tidal volume and airflow, called a flow-volume loop. The flow-volume loop, shown in Figure 5–14, detects abnormalities in the airways. In a patient with increased airway resistance, the loop narrows as shown in Figure 5–15.

To complete the profile, the calculated FRC is added to the preceding information. As an example, in the face of decreased compliance, knowing whether the FRC is normal or decreased can help the respiratory therapist narrow the possible causes between RDS (decreased FRC) and pneumonia (normal FRC).[13]

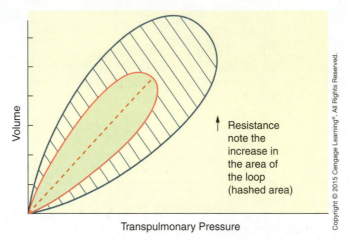

FIGURE 5–13. Change in the loop as resistance changes.

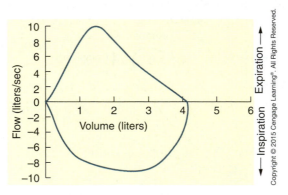

FIGURE 5–14. Typical flow-volume loop.

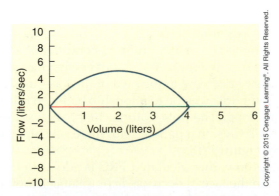

FIGURE 5–15. Narrowing of the loop as seen with increased airway resistance.

SUMMARY

Assessment of the neonatal patient requires the respiratory therapist to first understand the differences—both anatomic and physiologic—in comparison to the adult patient. Differences in the cardiopulmonary system make these patients more prone to airway occlusion, trauma, and afford them less pulmonary reserve. Understanding the difference in metabolism is vital before treating with medications and when considering caloric intake.

Assessment of the neonate is divided into history, physical examination, and neurologic examination, and serves several purposes. First, it allows the respiratory therapist to evaluate how well the patient is adapting to the extrauterine environment. Second, it allows for the identification of anomalies that may be present. Third, it allows for the determination of gestational age and establishing whether the neonate is appropriately grown for its gestational age.

The chapter also focuses on the assessment and evaluation of the cardiopulmonary system of the neonatal patient. A series of questions are presented, which will help the respiratory therapist focus attention on pertinent details that will aid in diagnosis and treatment. Physical examination of the same system allows the respiratory therapist to identify physical findings that support or rule out possible diagnoses determined from the history.

Pulmonary function testing, previously relegated to research laboratories, has become readily available for use in the neonatal populations with relative ease of use and safety, thanks to modern computer and microchip technology. Testing on neonates can identify and evaluate existing lung problems and monitor the efficacy of treatment. It can also be used to improve the patient/ventilator system by allowing the respiratory therapist to fine tune parameters to best meet the patient's needs. PFTs done in the pediatric population are usually well tolerated, but rely on patient cooperation to obtain accurate/reliable results.

POSTTEST

1. Which of the following are true regarding the anatomic and physiologic differences between adults and infants?
    I. Infants have a proportionally larger tongue.
    II. Infants have a proportionally larger epiglottis.
    III. Infants have a proportionally larger body surface area.
    IV. The infant's trachea is only a third the diameter of the adult's.
    V. Infants have a higher oxygen consumption.
        a. I, II, III, IV
        b. I, II,IV, V
        c. I, III, V
        d. I, II, III, IV, V

2. While reviewing a patient's chart before her delivery, you note the previous history shows PARA 3-1-0-2. Which of the following is TRUE?
   a. The patient has had 1 miscarriage.
   b. One previous birth is not living.
   c. This is her third pregnancy.
   d. There have been no premature deliveries.

3. Identify which of the following are included in the Ballard gestational age assessment.
   I. ear recoil
   II. presence of edema
   III. sole creases
   IV. skin appearance
   V. presence of lanugo
      a. I, III, IV, V
      b. I, II, III, IV
      c. II, III, IV
      d. I, III, V

4. Upon examination of a newborn, you find thick vernix covering the infant, gelatinous translucent skin, thick lanugo over the body, faint red lines on the soles of the feet, flat areola with no bud, slow ear recoil, male genitalia that shows no scrotal rugae or testicular descent. The proximate gestational age of this neonate is:
   a. 35–37 weeks
   b. 32–34 weeks
   c. 29–31 weeks
   d. 26–28 weeks

5. Which of the following are done during the quiet examination?
   I. assess skin color
   II. palpate the fontanelles
   III. assess patient movement
   IV. overall visual inspection
   V. auscultation of breath sounds
      a. II, II, V
      b. I, II,IV
      c. I, III, IV
      d. III, IV, V

6. Increased intracranial pressure is indicated when:
   a. The fontanelles are bulging or tense.
   b. The infant has an abnormal cry.
   c. The pulse is bounding and asynchronous.
   d. A caput succedaneum is present.

7. Which of the following is NOT an indication for performing PFTs on a neonatal patient?
   a. assess the extent of a pneumothorax
   b. diagnose lung disorders
   c. evaluate therapeutic response
   d. predict the risk of pulmonary dysfunction

8. Of the following, which may result in inaccurate pleural pressure readings when an esophageal balloon is used?

    I. increased airway resistance

    II. cardiac artifact

    III. paradoxical chest movement

    IV. REM sleep

    V. presence of infection

        a. I, II, III

        b. II, IV, V

        c. I, III, V

        d. II, III, IV

9. Body plethysmography uses which of the following gas laws to measure thoracic gas volume?

    a. $\dfrac{P}{T} = \dfrac{P'}{T'}$

    b. $\dfrac{V}{T} = \dfrac{V'}{T'}$

    c. $\dfrac{V \times P}{T} = \dfrac{V' \times P'}{T'}$

    d. $P \times V = P' \times V'$

10. This volume-pressure loop shows which of the following?

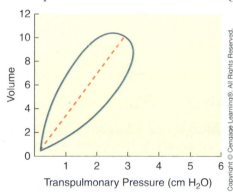

    a. decreased compliance

    b. increased airway resistance

    c. tracheal stenosis

    d. normal findings

REFERENCES

1. Shapiro BA, et al. *Clinical Application of Respiratory Care.* 4th ed. St. Louis, MO: Mosby-Year Book, 1991.

2. Miller MJ, et al. Oral breathing in newborn infants. *J Pediatr.* 107:465–469, 1985.

3. Whaley LF, Wong DL. *Essentials of Pediatric Nursing.* 5th ed. St. Louis, MO: CV Mosby Co., 1996.

4. Wilkins RL, et al. *Clinical Assessment in Respiratory Care.* 6th ed. St. Louis, MO: CV Mosby Co., 2010.

5. Ballard JL, et al. A simplified score for assessment of fetal maturation of newly born infants. *J Pediatr.* 95:769–774, 1979.

6. Merenstein GB, Gardner SL. *Handbook of Neonatal Care.* 4th ed. St. Louis, MO: Mosby Co., 1997.

7. Greenspan JS, Abbasi S, Bhutani V. Sequential changes in pulmonary mechanics in the very low birth weight (≤ 1000 grams) infant. *J Pediatr.* 113:732–737, 1988.

8. AARC Clinical Practice Guideline. Infant/toddler pulmonary function tests. *Resp Care.* 53:7, 2008.

9. Cullen JA, et al. Pulmonary function testing in the critically ill neonate, part II: methodology. *Neonatal Network.* 13:7–13, 1994.

10. England SJ. Current techniques for assessing pulmonary function in the newborn and infant: advantages and limitations. *Pediatr Pulmonol.* 4:48–53, 1988.

11. Thibeault DW, Gregory GA. *Neonatal Pulmonary Care.* Norwalk, CT: Appleton-Century-Crofts, 1986.

12. Alderson SH, Warren RH. Respiratory inductive plethysmography: application in infants. *Resp Care.* 40:114–120, 1995.

13. Greenspan JS, et al. Pulmonary function testing in the critically ill neonate, part I: an overview. *Neonatal Network.* 13:9–15, 1994.

BIBLIOGRAPHY AND SUGGESTED READINGS

Avery GB, Fletcher MA, MacDonald MG. *Pathophysiology and Management of the Newborn.* 6th ed. Philadelphia, PA: JB Lippincott Co., 2005.

Beachey W. *Respiratory Care Anatomy and Physiology.* 3rd ed. St. Louis, MO: Mosby, 2012. Walsh, BK, Czervinske MP, DiBlasi, RM, eds. *Perinatal and Pediatric Respiratory Care.* 3rd ed. Philadelphia, PA: WB Saunders Co., 2010.

Cloherty JP, Stark AR, Eichenwald, EC, Hansen AR, eds. *Manual of Neonatal Care.* 7th ed. Philadelphia, PA: Lippincott, 2011.

Des Jardins T. *Cardiopulmonary Anatomy and Physiology.* 6th ed. Clifton Park, NY: Cengage Learning, 2013.

Goldsmith JP, Karotkin EH. *Assisted Ventilation of the Neonate.* 4th ed. Philadelphia, PA: WB Saunders Co., 2003.

Harwood R. *Exam Reviews and Study Guide for Perinatal/Pediatric Respiratory Care.* Philadelphia, PA: FA Davis, 1999.

Hockenberry MJ, and Wilson D. *Wong's Nursing Care of Infants and Children.* 9th ed. St. Louis, MO: Mosby Co., 2010.

Lynam LE, Algren S. Pulmonary function testing: a tool for managing the mechanically ventilated patient. *Neonatal Network.* 12:61–64, 1993.

Pilbeam SP. *Mechanical Ventilation: Physiological and Clinical Applications.* 5th ed. St. Louis, MO: Mosby, 2012.

Taussig LM, Landau LI. *Pediatric Respiratory Medicine.* 2nd ed. St. Louis, MO: Mosby, 2008.

White L. *Foundations of Nursing: Caring for the Whole Person.* 3rd ed. Clifton Park, NY: Cengage Leaning, 2011.

Wilkins, RL, Sheldon, RL, Krider, SJ. *Clinical Assessment in Respiratory Care.* 6th ed. St. Louis, MO: Mosby Co., 2009.

Continuing Care of the Neonate

OBJECTIVES

Upon the completion of this chapter, the reader should be able to:

1. Explain the physiology of thermoregulation, including a description of the thermoneutral zone and nonshivering thermogenesis.
2. Define the internal thermal gradient (ITG) and describe the reasons why a preemie has a decreased ability to maintain its ITG.
3. Describe each of the following as it relates to the external thermal gradient (ETG). Include examples for each type of heat loss and a description of how each method of heat loss can be prevented or reduced in the nursery.
   a. Radiant
   b. Conductive
   c. Convective
   d. Evaporative
4. Describe how a neonate reacts to cold stress and to hyperthermia.
5. Discuss thermoregulation of the neonate in the delivery room and nursery, including methods of heat loss prevention.
6. Compare and contrast incubators and open warmers, focusing on the advantages, disadvantages, and thermoregulation in each.
7. Explain the physiologic effects of overstimulation of the premature neonate.
8. Identify and describe those factors involved in behavioral-based care.
9. Describe the use of environmental controls and parental involvement in reducing overstimulation and increasing more normal interactions and relationships.
10. Describe the physiologic factors that make the skin of the preemie more susceptible to trauma.
11. Discuss those factors that will reduce skin trauma on the neonate.
12. Describe the distribution of body water and its solutes. Compare and contrast the percentage of extracellular fluid (ECF) and intracellular fluid (ICF) between the preemie and the term neonate.

13. Describe the balance principle as it pertains to fluid and electrolyte balance. Identify the components of intake and output.
14. Identify and describe the three methods of determining fluid deficit. Estimate the degree of deficit when given patient clinical data.
15. Identify at least five factors that influence insensible water loss. Calculate the approximate insensible water loss when given the necessary information.
16. Describe the functions of sodium, potassium, calcium, magnesium, chloride, and phosphate in the neonate.
17. Relate the causes of hyponatremia, hypernatremia, hypokalemia, hyperkalemia, hypocalcemia, hypercalcemia, hypomagnesemia, and hypermagnesemia.
18. Describe how electrolytes are maintained and the importance of monitoring electrolytes.
19. With regard to jaundice, describe the following:
    a. Physiology
    b. Causes
    c. Pathologic jaundice
    d. Complications
    e. Treatment
20. Describe the clinical signs and treatment of necrotizing enterocolitis.

KEY TERMS

anaerobic	gastroschisis	myelomeningocele
brown fat	guaiac	omphalocele
conjugated	hydrops fetalis	parenteral
Crigler-Najjar syndrome	hyperosmolar	servo–controlled
encephalocele	hypotonia	sodium-potassium
enteral	internal thermal	exchange resin
excoriation	gradient (ITG)	stratum corneum
external thermal	kernicterus	thermoneutral zone
gradient (ETG)	Lucey-Driscoll	thermoregulation
galactosemia	syndrome	turgor

INTRODUCTION

Continuing care of the neonatal patient is a core component in the long-term outcome of these patients. A thorough understanding of thermoregulation techniques can aid tremendously in maintaining the growth and development of the newborn. Additionally, current research has shown the detrimental effect of overstimulation of these patients, making the use of behavioral-based care an essential skill. The delicate nature of the neonate, from the skin to the emotional aspects, demands effort from all those working with them to have the skills necessary to minimize those effects.

THERMOREGULATION

Homeostatic **thermoregulation** can best be defined as the maintenance of equality between heat dissipation and heat production by the body. Normal thermoregulatory mechanisms maintain a balance of heat production and heat loss to maintain a core temperature of 37°C (98.6°F). Thermoregulation is one of the most important aspects in the care of the neonatal patient. In particular, the human neonate is extremely vulnerable to cold stress and its complications at birth.

Heat balance must be considered in all aspects of the care of the neonate and must be constantly monitored and evaluated. Human infants have the ability to maintain fairly stable core temperatures when placed in a proper environmental temperature.

Neonatal Considerations

After delivery, an environmental temperature should be maintained that falls within the thermoneutral zone. The **thermoneutral zone** is that temperature range in which the metabolic rate is at a minimum and, thus, oxygen consumption is at its lowest. When this temperature is achieved, the neonate is thermally balanced with its environment, neither gaining nor losing heat. There is no exact environmental temperature at which all neonates will achieve thermoneutrality. This is the result of the diversity of metabolic rate, gestational age, and weight. Current recommendations are to maintain an environmental temperature that achieves a rectal temperature of 36.5°C to 37.5°C (98.6°F to 99.5°F) and an abdominal skin temperature of 36°C to 36.5°C (96.8°F to 97.7°F).

In the adult, heat can be produced by metabolic and physical activity (shivering). The newborn, however, has a diminished shivering response and relies entirely on the metabolism of brown fat for heat production. Around gestational weeks 26 to 30, the first **brown fat** cells appear. Brown fat, or brown adipose tissue, is abundant in the neonate and has a primary role of producing heat when shivering is not possible. The cells enlarge in size and number as the pregnancy advances. The fetus stores the brown fat around the great vessels, kidneys, scapulas, axilla, and the nape of the neck. Brown fat is highly vascularized and innervated by neurons from the sympathetic system.

In the presence of cold stress, the neonate responds by increasing stimulation of the sympathetic nervous system. Increased stimulation causes an increase in the amount of norepinephrine released. Norepinephrine is released from the nerve endings in the sympathetic system. Increased levels of norepinephrine activate lipase, which breaks the brown fat into free fatty acids. These acids are then hydrolyzed into glycerol and nonesterified fatty acids. The oxidation of the nonesterified fatty acids produces heat, which then increases the neonate's temperature. This breakdown of brown fat with the subsequent production of heat is called nonshivering thermogenesis.

THE PHYSIOLOGY OF HEAT LOSS

Heat loss from the core of the body in the environment follows two gradients: the internal thermal gradient (ITG) and the external thermal gradient (ETG) (Figure 6–1).

Internal Thermal Gradient

The **internal thermal gradient (ITG)** is the temperature difference between the warm body core and the cooler skin. The ITG is regulated by many factors. Among these are the metabolic rate, the amount of subcutaneous fat present, the amount of surface area available for dissipation of heat, and the distance from the body core to the skin surface.

A premature neonate has a diminished ability to maintain the ITG for several reasons. Neonates have a large amount of skin surface area in relation to body weight. This results in a large area for heat to dissipate from. The premature neonate has a relatively thin layer of skin and decreased amounts of subcutaneous and brown fat.

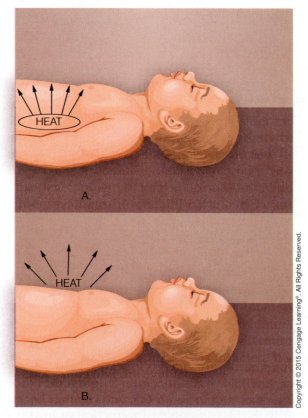

FIGURE 6–1. A. The internal thermal gradient. Heat travels from the warmer internal structures to the cooler skin. B. The external thermal gradient. Heat travels from the skin to the cooler environment.

Consequently, it has less insulation to prevent heat loss. Additionally, the brown fat stores deplete rapidly, resulting in a loss of the ability to generate heat through nonshivering thermogenesis.

Another factor is that the preemie is often unable to take in enough calories to maintain the level of nutrients for heat production. The metabolic response of the preemie to cold is impaired by hypoxemia. This presents a problem because most premature neonates suffer some degree of pulmonary problem, leading to hypoxemia. Frequent handling, which is often required in the care of the preemie, disposes the patient to the cold environment outside the incubator.

External Thermal Gradient

The temperature difference between the skin and the environment is called the **external thermal gradient (ETG)**. The ETG is determined by environmental factors that are controllable by the respiratory therapist. There are four factors that determine heat loss through the ETG, listed in Table 6–1 and described below.

Table 6–1

METHODS OF HEAT LOSS AND ITS PREVENTION

Type of heat loss	Definition	Prevention
Radiant	The dissipation of heat from the neonate to cooler objects surrounding but not touching the neonate	• At delivery, place a cap on the neonate and wrap it in a warmed blanket. • Use double-walled incubators. • Keep the incubator away from exterior walls and windows and drafts. • Line the inside of the incubator with reflective film.
Conductive	The transfer of heat from the neonate to a cooler surface in contact with the neonate	• Warm all items touching the neonate.
Convective	The loss of heat from the neonate to air current passing over the neonate	• Keep the neonate covered and out of areas with air movement. • Avoid the use of open warmers. • Warm any airflow passing over the neonate, including oxygen delivery.
Evaporative	The loss of heat that accompanies the evaporation of water from the surface of the neonate's skin	• Dry the neonate immediately upon delivery. • Keep the infant as dry as possible.

Radiant heat loss is the dissipation of heat from the neonate to cooler objects that surround the patient but are not in direct contact. The cooler objects are not limited to those within the incubator, but may be in the same room, or even outdoors if a window is nearby. The radiation of the sun's heat is an example of radiant heat. It is estimated that 55% to 65% of heat loss is through this mechanism.

Conduction is the transfer of heat from the body to a cooler surface on which the neonate is lying. The colder the surface, the more heat is lost. Conduction of heat can also occur in reverse if the surface is warmer than the skin.

Convection is the loss of heat from the skin to moving air. The velocity and the temperature of the air determine the amount of heat lost. Convection is the principle behind wind chill factors, which make temperatures colder in a wind. Combined, conduction and convection make up roughly 15% of heat loss.

As water changes states from a liquid to a gas, heat is released. This is called evaporation. Evaporative loss occurs as insensible (from the skin and respiratory tract), and sensible (sweating from the skin).

COLD STRESS: RESPONSE AND COMPLICATIONS

As previously mentioned, the thermoneutral zone is considered to be between 36.5°C and 37.5°C (97.7°F and 99.5°F). Once core temperature exceeds the thermoneutral zone, the body's responses are typically activated. Thermoreceptors located in the skin detect changes in environmental temperature. Receptors located in the face are the most sensitive and respond the quickest. A cold stress, or hypothermia, is any lowering of the thermoneutral temperature. It should be remembered that the adult thermoneutral zone is far below that of the newborn. A cold environmental temperature for the neonate may be uncomfortably warm or even hot to the adult.

Cold stress can be initiated by the opening of incubator doors or cold gas blowing onto the neonate from a resuscitation bag. It may also be triggered by placing the neonate on a cold scale or countertop.

The initial response to hypothermia is peripheral vasoconstriction. This results in a shunt of the blood away from the skin, helping to maintain the ITG. Peripheral vasoconstriction, however, leads to **anaerobic** metabolism and metabolic acidosis. The presence of acidosis may lead to pulmonary vasoconstriction with worsening hypoxemia and acidosis. Hypoxemia acts to further restrict the neonate's response to the cold stress and worsens the acidosis. Simultaneously, the hypothermia triggers nonshivering thermogenesis, which boosts heat output. With the increased metabolism of brown fat, glucose levels begin to fall, potentially leading to hypoglycemia.

The combination of peripheral vasoconstriction and brown fat metabolism causes the neonate's body temperature to remain homeostatic for a time. If the stress is corrected quickly, the patient may suffer no permanent effects. A continued cold stress, however, may lead to the deterioration of the patient condition and possibly death. A neonate who is being continually cold stressed may maintain normal body temperature, but at the expense of critical calories needed for growth.

As hypothermia progresses, all of the organ systems are affected, however the heart and CNS are the most noteworthy. As hypothermia worsens, the pacemaker cells of the heart are affected by a decrease in depolarization, leading to bradycardia. Accompanying the bradycardia is a decrease in arterial pressure and cardiac output. As core temperature continues falling, cardiac arrhythmias, including ventricular fibrillation and asystole, can occur.

In the CNS, hypothermia leads to decreasing metabolism and a subsequent drop in activity. The electrical activity of the brain becomes abnormal as core temperatures drop below 33°C (91.4°F) and at 20°C (68°F) the EEG mimics brain death.[1]

RESPONSE TO HYPERTHERMIA

Hyperthermia, as opposed to hypothermia, is temperature that is above normal. The effects of hyperthermia can be as severe as those associated with hypothermia. The initial response of the neonate is a vasodilation of the peripheral vessels to help dissipate heat. This is followed by an increase in metabolism and oxygen consumption. Additionally, cerebral blood flow diminishes. If hyperthermia continues, death can ensue from cardiac arrest and major organ failure.

Hyperthermia may result from infection, dehydration, improperly functioning incubators, radiant warmers, humidifiers, and phototherapy lights. Continuous monitoring of patient and environmental temperature is essential to avoid hyperthermia from malfunctioning equipment.

THERMOREGULATION IN THE DELIVERY ROOM

The goal of thermoregulation in the delivery room is to maintain an environmental temperature such that the neonate's core temperature remains in the normal range of 36.5°C to 37.5°C (97.7°F and 99.5°F). To achieve this goal, all avenues of heat loss must be minimized or eliminated.

Prevention of Evaporative Loss

The neonate is at the highest risk of heat loss shortly after delivery. Every newborn should immediately be completely dried with a prewarmed towel or blanket. The head and face are particularly important. This drying helps reduce evaporative heat losses.

Prevention of Radiant Loss

The neonate should then be wrapped in a warm blanket and immediately placed beneath a radiant heater for resuscitation or examinations. A cap or other covering should be placed on the head as shown in Figure 6–2. Due to a tremendous amount of heat loss from the head, placement of a cap greatly reduces heat loss.

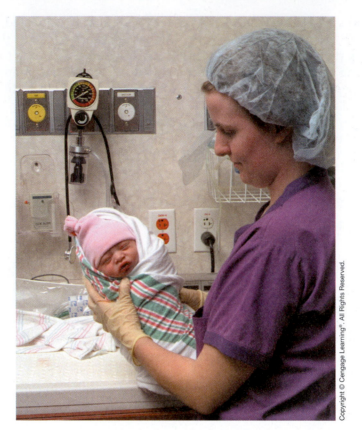

FIGURE 6–2. Knit caps and swaddling in a blanket help newborns maintain body heat.

PREVENTION OF CONVECTIVE AND CONDUCTIVE LOSS

The small preemie is more easily thermoregulated if placed on a warming mattress. The neonate should be kept covered as much as possible while on the open warmer to avoid convective losses (Figure 6–3). As quickly as possible, the neonate should be placed in a prewarmed incubator. The longer the patient is left out in the open, the greater the chance of hypothermia.

Skin-to-Skin Care

A relatively recent addition to the thermoregulation of the newborn is skin-to-skin care (SSC) or "Kangaroo Care." SSC is done by placing the newborn's bare chest against the bare chest of the mother (Figure 6–4). A warmed blanket is then used to cover the babies back. SSC has been shown to be effective in reducing the risk of hypothermia when compared to conventional incubator care[2]. Kangaroo care is also discussed later in this chapter as it pertains to parental involvement.

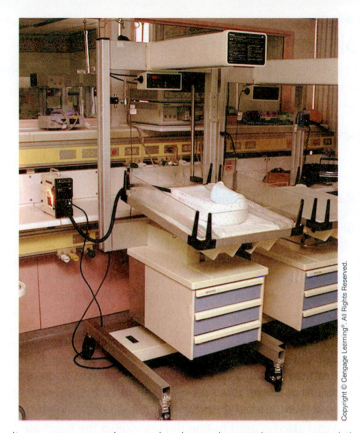

FIGURE 6–3. A radiant warmer can be used to keep the newborn warm while in an open warmer.

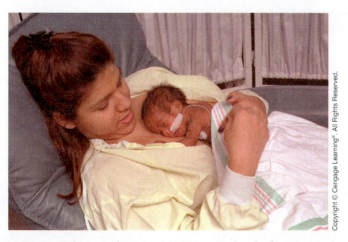

FIGURE 6–4. Kangaroo care (skin-to-skin contact) is a method of maintaining thermoregulation of the neonate.

THERMOREGULATION IN THE NURSERY

Management of thermoregulation in the neonate must also be maintained while the neonate is in the nursery. This is a critical part of the care provided to the neonate.

Incubators and Thermoregulation

Once in the incubator, several precautions can be taken to avoid unnecessary heat loss. Skin temperature should be maintained at 36.5°C (97.7°F) by a **servo-controlled** incubator. As previously discussed, at a skin temperature of 36°C to 36.5°C (96.8°F to 97.7°F), metabolism is at its lowest point. The servo-control uses the skin temperature to increase or decrease the heat output of the incubator into the environment. The operator designates a set point for skin temperature. If skin temperature falls below the set point, the incubator warms the environmental temperature until skin temperature rises above the set point. At that point, the heater returns to its normal output.

Modern incubators also monitor the environmental temperature and maintain it at neutrothermal ranges. When using a servo-control, it is vital that the skin probe be securely attached to the neonate. Hyperthermia could occur if the skin probe becomes loose.

Radiant heat losses can be lessened by several methods. Modern incubators incorporate an inner plastic wall on the interior of the incubator. This inner wall is warmed to the incubator's environmental temperature and, thus, reduces the amount of heat that is radiated by the baby to the external wall of the incubator. Aluminum foil can also be used to line the interior of the incubator to reflect radiant heat back toward the patient. Radiant losses can also be lessened if the incubator is kept away from air conditioner ducts and windows, which cool the external wall.

Conductive losses can be minimized by using warming mattresses or other warming devices under the patient.

A common cause of convective heat loss in the incubator is a resuscitation bag that is left on, blowing cold gas over the patient's head. If the resuscitation bag is to be left on, it should be positioned so it does not blow on the patient.

Evaporative heat loss can be controlled by creating a "swamp" environment around the patient. This is done by directing warmed and humidified gas into the incubator.

Thermoregulation in Open Warmers

Radiant heat loss is difficult to manage in the open warmer. Placing a shield over the neonate reduces the amount of radiant loss, but it also reduces access to the infant. Reduction of patient access takes away a major advantage of using an open warmer.

Evaporative heat loss in the open warmer can be minimized by providing a closed environment around the patient and creating a "swamp" as described above.

Convective heat loss is lessened by keeping the neonate out of areas of air movement. Convective losses are most profound in open warmers, where it may be necessary to cover the patient with plastic or a shield to protect it from air currents.

Shields and plastic sheets can also be used in the incubator to protect the small preemie from convective and radiant losses.

Conductive heat loss can be lessened by not placing the neonate on cold surfaces or allowing cold items to come in contact with the skin. In the open warmer, the patient should be placed on blankets that insulate the neonate from the cold mattress. A common source of conductive heat loss is weighing the neonate. The procedure of weighing requires that the patient be placed directly on the scale with only a paper covering. Weights should be done as quickly as possible to reduce conductive losses. An alternative method is to keep the patient covered while weighing, removing the coverings after the patient is returned to the incubator, and weighing the coverings alone. The weight of the coverings is then subtracted to arrive at the weight of the patient.

INCUBATORS VERSUS OPEN WARMERS

The perfect device to maintain thermoregulation in the neonate has yet to be developed. Modern incubators and open warmers each serve a distinct purpose.

Open Warmers

The primary advantage of the open warmer is access to the patient (Figure 6–5). This is critical during times of resuscitation or other emergencies where several people

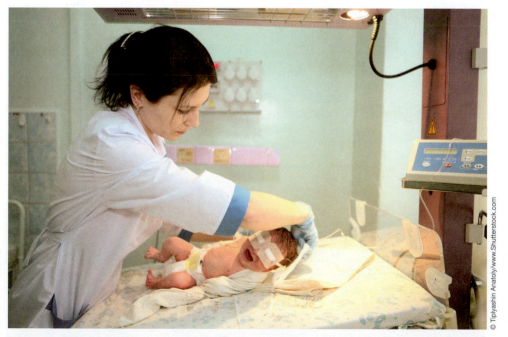

FIGURE 6–5. It is more challenging to maintain thermoregulation when an open warmer is in use.

must have access to the patient. Disadvantages include difficulty in thermal management and the inability to control the environment.

Incubators

One advantage to the use of an incubator is that it provides a controlled environment that allows for better thermal management (Figure 6–6). The closed environment may also serve as a barrier to excessive handling of the patient by nursery personnel. In addition, the incubator provides a somewhat quieter environment than the open warmer. The major disadvantage to an incubator is in patient access. During an emergency, it may be necessary to remove the neonate from the incubator to allow adequate access for procedures.

DEVELOPMENTAL NEEDS OF THE HIGH-RISK NEONATE

Much discussion and research has occurred over the past decade surrounding the developmental needs of high-risk neonates. Before the 1980s, the NICU was viewed as a sensory deficient environment. Many believed that hospitalized neonates needed considerable stimulation to overcome their functional disabilities. It was also believed that normal functioning would occur more quickly if aggressive development therapies were used.

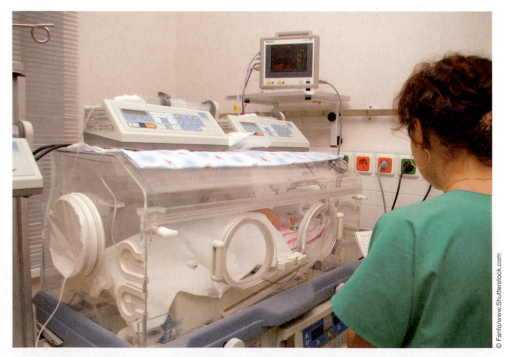

© Fanfo/www.Shutterstock.com

FIGURE 6–6. An incubator works well in maintaining thermoregulation.

More recently, concerns have centered on the impact of the environment on the developing nervous system of the neonate. There exists significant clinical evidence that the environment, as well as treatment protocols, affect the systemic and cerebral circulation, as well as oxygenation. These studies have revealed a possible causal relation between NICU caregiving protocols and physiologic stress. More recent studies have demonstrated that care must be individualized to the patient, because no two neonates respond to environmental stimulation the same way. It has been recommended that each infant be individually assessed and a specific care plan started.[3]

To this end, the Newborn Individualized Developmental Care and Assessment Program (NIDCAP) was developed to educate and offer support to NICU personnel to provide neurodevelopmentally supportive care. Through the foundation NIDCAP Federation International (NFI), this training and assistance is offered both domestically and internationally. A recent review of developmental care trials showed that, while these interventions may have outcome benefits, there continues to be conflicting evidence to support any one intervention.[4]

Physiologic Considerations

The nervous system of a neonate is anatomically immature. The chemical and physiologic function of the nervous system is primitive when compared to the adult. Additionally, the cerebral hemispheres show poor distinction between gray and white matter. Most neuronal cells, which conduct nerve impulses, are present at birth but are immature in their function. In the premature neonate, there is little nerve myelination and the synaptic junctions are at an early stage of formation. It appears that neurologic function in a neonate is largely controlled at the brain stem and spinal cord level, and that existing brain functions are hyperreactive.

The Effects of Overstimulation

Immature or stressed neonates have limited energy and can be exhausted by excessive stimulation. With the increased survival rate of premature neonates, the risk for developmental handicaps and morbidity in the presence of overstimulation is increased. Studies have shown that the preterm neonate finds itself in a "mismatch" between brain expectancy and environmental input leading to a form of self-analgesia.[3] It has been theorized that the NICU environment may interfere with both the maturation and the organization of the neonate's central nervous system. Furthermore, it is felt that another imbalance exists in that hearing and vision receive overwhelming overload, while tactile and vestibular needs are not met. A study by Zahr and Balian demonstrated significant changes in both behavioral and physiologic responses to typical nursing interventions and NICU noises.[5]

The importance for the respiratory therapist then is to reduce the amount of visual and acoustic stimulation in the NICU. Early intervention can reduce long-term disability in this patient group.

Behavioral-Based Care

Behavioral-based care is founded on the concept that care is provided to the neonate based on observed behaviors that indicate times of nonstress. The positive effects of intervention may be diminished if stimuli is offered at inappropriate times. It is, therefore, important to correlate interventions with times of nonstress. The approach then is to develop a plan of behaviorally supported care for each at-risk neonate. The timing of patient stimulation should be based on several factors, which are listed in Table 6–2.

Neonates should not be stimulated while they are asleep. Sleeping patients should not be disturbed, to allow a conservation of energy and to prevent a negative response by the neonate. Stimulation should be avoided when behavioral stress cues (such as gaze aversion, facial grimaces, hiccoughs, and irritability) and physiologic cues (cyanosis, hypoxemia) are present.

Neonates should be handled only when behavioral and physiologic signs dictate (Figure 6–7). The timing of interventions is an important key to an effective,

Table 6–2
THE TIMING OF PATIENT STIMULATION
Sleep/wake state
Activity level
Approachability
Oxygenation status

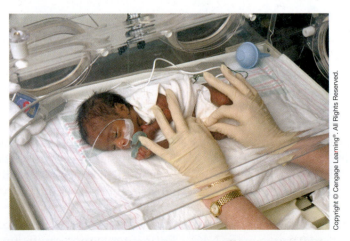

FIGURE 6–7. While this infant is awake, the nurse offers him a pacifier and schedules routine activities such as diaper change.

safe interaction. Clustering of caregiving and procedures should be minimized to allow adequate recovery time between treatments and to decrease the chance of overstimulation. Nonemergency procedures should be postponed or delayed if possible.

The respiratory therapist should ensure that oxygenation is adequate before and during interventions. If oxygen saturations decrease during intervention, it should be stopped and then restarted when saturation is acceptable. The neonate should be turned and positioned only as necessary. The neonate's response to procedures, especially if stressful, should be monitored for a minimum of 5 minutes following completion. One method that has shown promise in reducing the stress of minor pain and stress-inducing procedures is facilitated tucking. This is done by holding the patient's extremities flexed and close to the body.

Environmental Controls

Environmental controls to decrease excess stimulation should be instituted in the NICU whenever possible. These include scheduled periods without intervention or "quiet time." The patient should not be disturbed during this time, except in an emergency. Care should be taken to avoid loud noises and bright lighting. The importance of reduced lighting is detailed in a study that showed a significance in oxygen saturation in neonates who were subjected to increasing light brightness.[6] Both workers and parents should avoid loud laughing and talking at the bedside. Attention to details such as the quiet closing of garbage can lids and incubator portholes makes a tremendous difference. Critically ill neonates should be placed in a bedspace where traffic and noise level are minimal.

One method that has been shown to decrease the noise level in the incubator is to cover it with a custom-made blanket.[7] This method is not without its critics, however. They point out that covering the incubator does not allow for visualization of the patient. Thus, serious problems such as extubation, kinking of the endotracheal tube, IV problems, or loss of an umbilical artery catheter (UAC) may go unnoticed until serious complications have occurred.

Parental Involvement

Efforts to involve the parents in the care of their neonate should begin as soon as possible. Parents should be taught ways in which they can help in the care of their newborn. Being a part of the team not only helps the parents overcome feelings of helplessness, but also helps bond the infant-parent relationship. A strong relationship between the neonate and the parents is an accurate predictor of good future cognitive function in the neonate.

One previously described tool, kangaroo care, is beneficial for both the infant and parent. Kangaroo care has been shown to help parents overcome the feelings of separation with their infant. For the infant, it has been shown to reduce the amount of time in active states and to promote deep sleep.[8]

SKIN CARE OF THE PREMATURE NEONATE

Of special concern when working with premature neonates is the care and protection of the skin. Understanding several factors relative to fetal skin development will aid in good skin care.

Physiologic Factors

The skin of the premature neonate is very permeable to anything placed on it. Toxic substances used on adult skin for protection or to remove adhesive tape are absorbed very readily into the preemie's skin, creating the potential for systemic effects.

Another factor is a diminished cohesion between the surface epidermis and the underlying dermis. The bond between an adhesive tape and the epidermis may be stronger than the epidermal/dermal bond. The result is potential epidermal stripping when removing the tape.

The skin of the preemie is additionally sensitive because the **stratum corneum** layer is extremely thin. This is the top layer of the epidermis, which serves as the main barrier against microorganisms. Tape removal could very easily result in the removal of the stratum corneum.

Intensive care medicine requires that many monitors and other devices be taped to the skin of the neonate. These include temperature probes, umbilical artery catheters, endotracheal tubes, transcutaneous monitors, and pulse oximeters. Conventional medical tapes are traditionally used to secure these devices. Many times, barriers such as tincture of benzoin are sprayed or painted onto the skin to enhance adhesion of the tape. Because of the above-mentioned problems with the skin of these patients, severe damage may occur to the skin when these tapes are removed.

Skin Care Recommendations

With the above information in mind, some practical applications can be implemented to reduce damage to the skin of the preemie. Only mild soaps should be used when cleaning the skin. These soaps are best applied with a cotton ball to avoid abrading the skin.

Many spray-on skin barriers are plastic polymers, which may be absorbed into the skin and lead to systemic toxicity. Traditional adhesive removal swabs are saturated with a solvent that is readily absorbed through the premature patient's skin. There are adhesive removal swabs currently available that use citrus oils that are nontoxic to dissolve the adhesive barrier. These would be the preferred adhesive removers to use on the preemie.

One recent study examined the use of pectin-based adhesives. Pectin-based adhesives are used to secure ostomy bags to the abdomen. The study looked at the use of the barrier between the skin and the tape to lessen epidermal damage and at the same time allow adequate adhesion of the device to the skin. The results of this study show that pectin-based adhesive should be used between the skin and tape whenever the taping of equipment to the skin is necessary.[9]

Monitors such as transcutaneous monitors (TCMs) or pulse oximeters must be next to the skin to perform functionally. On the premature patient, both devices may be held in place with Coban-type wraps or fabric straps using a Velcro closure. Coban is a stretchable bandage material that sticks to itself but does not stick to skin.

A final recommendation is the use of transparent IV site dressing covers to protect areas of skin exhibiting **excoriation** or breakdown. This will protect the injured area from further damage and allow the skin to heal.

FLUID AND ELECTROLYTE BALANCE

Water is the major component of both the fetus and the newborn. Other compounds are dissociated, transported, dissolved, or transported in water. These compounds may also undergo chemical reactions within water and contribute to cellular and body functions. Compounds that dissolve in water and separate into charged particles (ions) capable of conducting an electric current are called electrolytes. Electrolytes are essential for cellular and organ functions and to maintain fluid and acid–base balance.

Fetal fluid and electrolyte status is regulated by both maternal and fetal mechanisms. Maternal disorders of fluid and electrolyte balance, diseases that affect uterine perfusion, and maternal IV therapy during labor may create a fluid and electrolyte imbalance in the neonate at birth. Most fetuses, however, are born in reasonable fluid balance for their gestation.

After birth, changes in fluid and electrolyte balance must occur, which are dependent on gestational age. The neonate's own regulatory mechanisms, combined with the interventions of the caretakers, unite to achieve fluid and electrolyte balance. Abnormalities in fluid and electrolyte balance occur with certain disease states. These diseases include respiratory disorders, asphyxia, congenital heart disease, **hydrops fetalis** (an accumulation of fluid in at least two fetal compartments), sepsis, renal disorders, urinary tract anomalies, endocrine disorders, and decreased skin integrity.

Distribution of Body Water

Total body water (TBW) decreases from a high of 95% of body weight at 13 to 14 weeks to approximately 78% of body weight at term. TBW is the total of extracellular fluid (ECF) and intracellular fluid (ICF). ECF is further divided into two compartments: interstitial fluid (ISF), which bathes many of the cells of the body, and intravascular fluid, which is the plasma volume (PV).

As gestation increases, and continuing postnatally, ECF decreases while ICF increases. ECF is greater in volume than ICF prenatally, but at about 3 months of age ICF volume passes and exceeds ECF. At term, ECF is roughly 45% of body weight, whereas ICF is 33% of body weight. This progression is shown in Figure 6–8. Postnatal changes in ECF are the most dramatic occurrence in the fluid and electrolyte adaptation of the neonate.

During the first days after birth most neonates experience a decrease in TBW caused by a reduction in ECF. The ECF volume shrinks secondary to a loss of water

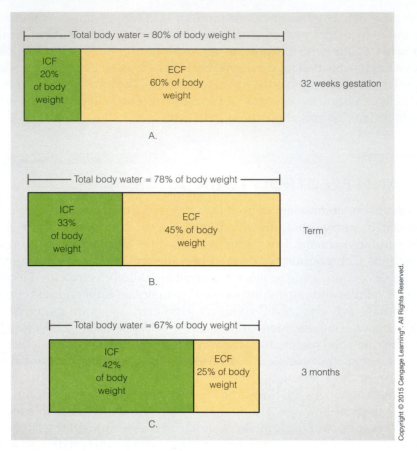

A.

B.

C.

FIGURE 6–8. The comparison of ECF to ICF: A. a 32-week preemie; B. A term neonate. C. A 3-month old infant.

and ECF electrolytes. This results in a 5% to 15% decrease in weight from birth weight. During these first few days, several periods of diuresis may occur, resulting in full-term neonates losing about 5% to 10% of their birth weight in water, and premature neonates about 5% to 15% of their birth weight.

The timing of this reduction in ECF is altered in certain disease states, most notably in those associated with respiratory distress. An improvement in the respiratory status often follows the onset of diuresis. An exception to this is respiratory distress syndrome (RDS), where induced diuresis is not followed by the same degree of improvement. Excess fluid and/or water intake during the first few days expands the ECF and may delay patient improvement or cause deterioration in cardiopulmonary status.

Distribution of Solutes

The total body solute composition changes as gestational age advances. The total amount of sodium and chloride per kg/weight decreases with increasing gestational age. These changes are a result of the decrease in ECF. Total body potassium content per kg/weight remains relatively constant throughout gestation.

The main electrolytes of the ECF are sodium and chloride. The minor electrolytes are potassium, calcium, magnesium, bicarbonate, and protein. Plasma and ISF are similar in composition, with the exception that plasma has a higher amount of protein.

The major electrolytes of ICF are potassium, magnesium, and phosphate, with sodium and bicarbonate being present in much smaller quantities than in ECF. Postnatally, the distribution of the electrolytes reflects the changes in body fluid distribution. For example, as ECF volume decreases with increasing postnatal age, total body sodium and chloride content per kg/weight continue to decrease. During the first weeks after birth, ICF electrolyte content per kg/weight remains relatively unchanged.

Postnatally, the intake of the neonate will influence the establishing of electrolyte homeostasis. Most important in this regard is sodium intake. Excess sodium intake delays contraction of the ECF in the early neonatal period. This is particularly true when combined with excess water intake.

Because sodium is mainly found in the ECF and water remains with the sodium, excess sodium prevents the reduction of the ECF and may even cause it to increase. The excess volume in the ECF may worsen and/or delay improvement in cardiorespiratory disorders. The premature neonate is especially vulnerable to this because of renal immaturity.

Balance Principle

Like other organisms, the neonate's body water composition is determined by input minus output. When the input equals the patient's output, it is said to meet the neonates' maintenance requirements. In this situation, the fluid, electrolyte, and nutritional requirements are the same as the losses. There will therefore be no weight gain or loss when input and output are balanced.

When intake and output are not equal, this balance is upset. When the intake of a given component exceeds its output, the neonate is said to be in positive balance with regard to that component. Conversely, when output is more than intake, there is a negative balance for that component.

Adequate growth requires that intake exceed output in the proper proportions. Weight gain is not synonymous with growth. As discussed previously excess water and/or sodium intake, or the inability to excrete water and/or sodium, may result in overexpansion of the ECF. Under these circumstances there is a weight gain but no growth of new tissues. Similarly, weight loss may reflect water or sodium losses in excess of intake, rather than inadequate nutrition.

In the first few days of life, there normally exists a negative balance for most components. The negative balance of sodium and water during this period results in the reduction of the ECF. With growth, there is a positive sodium and water balance, although the increase in ECF is proportionately less than the increase in the rest of the body.

Components of Intake and Output

Water and electrolyte intake for the newborn consists of that contained in feedings, IV fluid, medications, and transfusions. Patients on mechanical ventilators may even absorb water through the lungs from the humidity provided. The normal newborn regulates the intake of these, along with other nutrients.

In the case of the sick newborn, intake is generally controlled by the physician in amount and composition. Output of fluid and electrolytes occurs chiefly through the urine. Additional output occurs with stool, skin, and respiratory losses. Abnormal losses of fluid and electrolytes occur with diarrhea, emesis, nasogastric tube drainage, thoracotomy tube losses, damaged skin, and other factors that increase insensible water loss.

Urine losses primarily affect sodium and water balance. With diarrhea, bicarbonate loss may become significant. Gastric secretions contain considerable amounts of hydrogen, chloride, potassium, and sodium ions. Emesis and nasogastric tube drainage may, therefore, lead to a negative balance for these electrolytes in addition to the water loss. Thoracotomy tube drainage is similar to plasma in composition and results in a loss of ECF, including proteins.

Estimating Fluid Deficit

Fluid deficits may vary from minimal, with no apparent clinical consequences, to profound, with the clinical picture of hypovolemic shock. Assessing the patient for fluid deficit and estimating the amount requires looking at three categories of data: 1) history, 2) physical exam, and 3) laboratory values.

Historical information that is useful in assessing hydration is available from the nursing flow sheets and nurses' notes. A review of intake versus output may show whether intake and output have been deficient or excessive in relation to each other. Urine output may be diminished in the presence of advanced fluid deficit. Recent weight changes should be reviewed and the current percent of birth weight noted, because these can provide an estimate of the volume of fluid deficit.

A comparison of the weight change to the difference in intake and output will help determine if the weight change is expected. In addition, the patient must be assessed as to whether the weight change was beneficial. For example, in the first days of life when the ECF is reduced, a weight loss is expected and may bring about a clinical improvement. However, if the patient has lost more than expected and shows signs of hypovolemia or dehydration, a fluid deficit may exist. Vital signs may reveal a low or decreasing blood pressure, tachycardia, or increasing baseline heart rate.

Reviewing the amount of blood that has been withdrawn may indicate a compromise of the vascular volume. This occurs when about 10% of the baby's blood volume has been withdrawn over a short period.

Signs of dehydration or hypovolemia may be present on physical exam. Examination of the skin and head is most helpful when assessing for fluid deficit. The perfusion of the skin is decreased with larger fluid deficits, and decreased skin **turgor** may be present. Decreased turgor is manifested by skin that, when grasped and raised between two fingers, slowly returns to its previous position. Decreased turgor is difficult to assess in the premature neonate because of less subcutaneous fat.

The presence of edema may indicate that total body weight is adequate but does not rule out hypovolemia. In the presence of edema, the fluid deficit may be a deficit in vascular fluid. Examination of the head can show a sunken anterior fontanelle with increased overlapping of sutures in the presence of fluid deficit. Overlapping of sutures is not abnormal in newborns; therefore, changes from previous examinations are important.

Mucous membranes may also be noted to be dry. With increasing fluid deficits, the hematocrit, serum sodium, blood urea nitrogen (BUN), and serum protein tend to increase. Without these data, fluid deficits may be roughly approximated in the manner described in Table 6–3, providing the neonate has normal serum sodium values. Serial weights and observation of vital signs should follow efforts to replace fluid deficits. Reassessment of the deficit can then determine the adequacy of therapy and if modifications need to be made.

Insensible Water Loss (IWL)

Insensible water loss is water lost by evaporation from the skin and respiratory tract. This evaporative loss is proportional to the surface area of the skin and mucosa and is greatly influenced by the type of environment the patient is in—in particular, the relative humidity of that environment.[10] Other factors that influence IWL include temperature and skin integrity. Table 6–4 lists those factors that increase IWL.

IWL may be estimated by subtracting the patient's output from the input, and then subtracting the change in weight from the result [IWL = Intake − Output − (change in weight)]. This method is helpful in estimating IWL over several days, which is then used to estimate the patient's fluid needs. The instruments used to measure intake, output, and weight present enough inaccuracy to make this only an approximation. Also, the output includes measurable fluid losses only and, therefore, does not include water lost in stools. There are several clinical factors that influence IWL.

Table 6–3

ESTIMATION OF FLUID DEFICIT IN THE PATIENT WITH NORMAL SODIUM LEVELS

- 5% Dehydration—oliguria, dry mucous membranes, slightly sunken anterior fontanelle

- 10% Dehydration—signs of 5% dehydration plus: decreased skin turgor, decreased perfusion, sunken eyes, definite sunken anterior fontanelle

- 15% Dehydration—signs of 10% dehydration plus: signs of shock (tachycardia, hypotension, decreased pulses, poor perfusion), altered sensorium

Table 6–4

FACTORS THAT INCREASE INSENSIBLE WATER LOSS

Early gestational age
Respiratory distress
Environmental temperature above the neutrothermal zone
Elevated body temperature
Skin breakdown and excoriations
Congenital skin defects (neural tube disorders)
Radiant warmer
Phototherapy
Increased motor activity and crying

Level of Maturity Mature babies have increased skin thickness and, therefore, less evaporative loss per equivalent surface area. In contrast, premature neonates have greater evaporative losses due to decreased skin thickness.

Size Larger babies will have a greater surface area from which to have evaporative loss, resulting in a higher absolute IWL. Smaller babies, particularly those who are small for gestational age, will have higher surface area-to-body weight ratios. They will, therefore, have higher per kilogram IWL.

Respiratory Distress Increased gas movement through the respiratory tract will increase the amount of IWL from the airways.

Humidity Increased ambient or inspired humidity will decrease IWL from the skin and respiratory tracts, respectively. This is most important in very small babies with decreased skin thickness.

Temperature Increased environmental or body temperature increases IWL.

Skin Breakdown or Injury Even the skin of premature baby prevents some evaporative loss, and any break in skin integrity increases IWL. Similarly, lesions such as omphalocele, gastroschisis, myelomeningocele, or encephalocele, which are not covered with skin lead to increased evaporative loss (Figure 6–9). This is not only

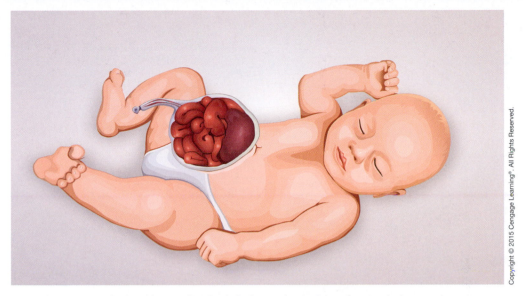

FIGURE 6–9A. Omphalocele is a birth defect in which the infant's abdominal organs protrude outside the belly through the umbilicus and are covered by a sac.

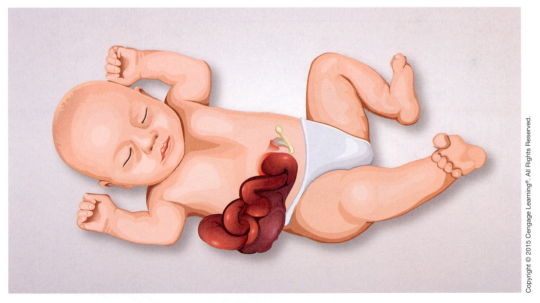

FIGURE 6–9B. Gastroschisis is a birth defect in which the infant's intestines protrude outside the abdominal wall near the umbilicus without an overlying sac.

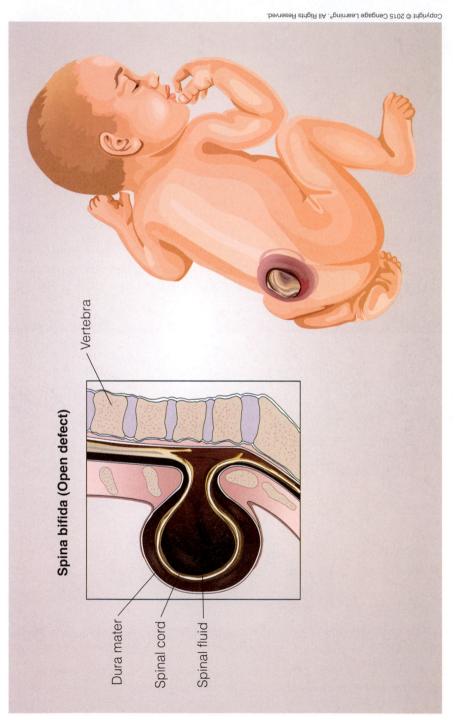

Spina bifida (Open defect)

Vertebra

Dura mater

Spinal cord

Spinal fluid

FIGURE 6–9C. Myelomeningocele is a birth defect in which the spinal cord protrudes through the spinal column.

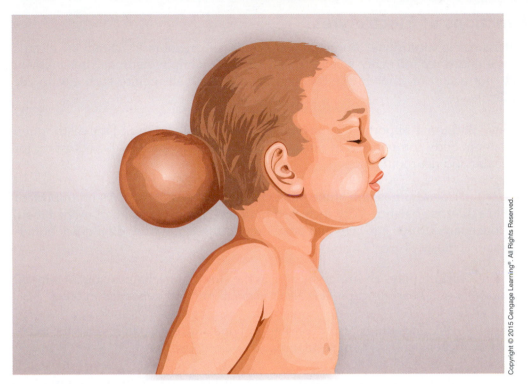

FIGURE 6–9D. Encephalocele is a birth defect in which the brain and membranes protrude through an opening in the skull.

because of a poorer barrier to evaporation, but also due to the increased surface area from which evaporation can occur. Occlusive dressings decrease this source of evaporative loss.

Radiant Warmers and Phototherapy Lights

Radiant heat increases evaporative losses and air currents that are common in open warmers which further increase IWL. Humidity under an open warmer depends on room humidity, unless a heat shield is used over the baby and humidity is added under the heat shield. Radiant heat from phototherapy lights increases evaporative water loss.

Heat Shields

Heat shields made of plastic may be placed over the baby to decrease radiant heat loss from the baby. This decreases the evaporative loss.

Motor Activity

Very active babies will have an increased IWL, whereas inactive babies will tend to have a lower IWL.

Functions of Electrolytes

Differences in electrolyte concentrations across cell membranes create an electric charge necessary for many cellular functions. For example, neuronal transmission and contraction of smooth, skeletal, and heart muscle all require such electrolytic gradients.

Sodium Sodium is important in the regulation of water balance and the distribution of water in body components by virtue of its osmotic activity. It is also necessary for muscular and neuronal function.

Potassium Potassium is one of the main constituents of ICF. It plays an important role in acid–base balance. With increased hydrogen ion concentration in the blood, hydrogen ion diffuses into cells and potassium diffuses out, providing quick buffering of an acidosis.

Calcium Calcium plays an important role in the clotting mechanism and is integral in muscular and heart function. It is also the major mineral deposited in bone.

Magnesium Magnesium is also deposited in bone and is also necessary for many enzyme functions and calcium regulation.

Chloride Chloride is a major anion providing electrical neutrality and is important in acid–base balance.

Phosphate Phosphate is an essential component in energy metabolism and bone deposition.

Electrolyte Disorders

Table 6–5 summarizes the types and causes of electrolyte disorders that can occur in the neonate.

Hyponatremia Hyponatremia, a decrease in body sodium, may be caused by inadequate sodium intake, excess sodium loss due to renal immaturity or diuretics, or dilutional from excess body water. In the first two instances, total body sodium content is decreased and treatment is directed toward increasing sodium intake. With dilutional hyponatremeia, the total body sodium content may actually be increased. Its treatment consists of eliminating the excess total body weight and with it the excess sodium.

Hypernatremia Hypernatremia, an excess of body sodium, is generally due to a loss of body water in excess of sodium. It is usually due to insensible water losses not replaced adequately with IV fluids or feedings. Treatment involves replacing the water deficit. Caution is required when replacing the water, because with severe degrees of hypernatremia, the baby may become **hyperosmolar** (excessive

Table 6–5

TYPES AND CAUSES OF ELECTROLYTE DISORDERS IN THE NEONATE

Disorder	Definition	Causes
Hyponatremia	Decrease in body sodium	Inadequate sodium intake, excess loss secondary to diuretics or renal immaturity, excess body water
Hypernatremia	Excessive body sodium	Loss of body water in excess of sodium
Hypokalemia	Deficit in body potassium	Inadequate potassium administration, diuretic therapy, gastric losses, high-output renal failure
Hyperkalemia	Excessive body potassium	Excessive administration of potassium, acute renal failure
Hypocalcemia	Decreased body calcium	Early onset: maternal factors— hyperparathyroidism, pregnancy-induced hypertension, diabetes mellitus
		Neonatal factors: asphyxia, cesarean delivery, prematurity
		Late onset: phototherapy, furosemide therapy, renal disease, intravenous lipid infusions, ingestion of formula with suboptimal calcium to phosphorus ratio
Hypercalcemia	Excessive body calcium	Excess IV calcium administration, maternal and neonatal factors
Hypomagnesemia	Deficit of body magnesium	Associated with hypocalcemia
Hypermagnesemia	Excessive body magnesium	Maternal magnesium sulfate therapy during labor, administration of magnesium containing antacid to the neonate

concentrations of solutes). Replacement of the water deficit will lead to water entering all cells. Seizures may result if water enters brain cells too rapidly.

Hypokalemia Hypokalemia, an inadequate amount of potassium, may be caused by several factors. Those factors include inadequate potassium administration, diuretic therapy, and gastric losses. Hypokalemia may also occur during the high-output phase of acute renal failure. Treatment consists of increasing the potassium supplement to the patient.

Hyperkalemia Hyperkalemia, an excess of body potassium, is caused by either excess potassium administration or acute renal failure. Treatment for mild-degree hyperkalemia involves restricting the patient's potassium intake. For severe hyperkalemia, treatment with sodium bicarbonate, calcium, insulin–glucose infusions, sodium–potassium exchange resin, or dialysis may be necessary. Sodium–potassium exchange resin (Kayexalate®) is administered orally or in an enema. In the gastric tract, and in particular the large intestine, the solution releases sodium ions which are then replaced by potassium ions excreted by the intestines. The solution is then evacuated, taking with it the excess potassium.

Hypocalcemia Hypocalcemia, a deficit of body calcium, is classified according to the timing of its onset. Early onset hypocalcemia begins in the first 3 days of life. It may be caused by maternal factors such as hyperparathyroidism, pregnancy-induced hypertension, or diabetes mellitus. It may also be caused by certain neonatal conditions such as asphyxia, cesarean delivery, or prematurity and its complications. Late onset hypocalcemia begins after 3 days of age. Causes include phototherapy, furosemide therapy, renal disease, intravenous lipid infusions, and ingestion of a formula with a suboptimal calcium-to-phosphorus ratio.

The clinical presentation of both forms can include jitteriness, irritability, apnea, and seizures. Treatment is the administration of calcium.

Hypercalcemia Hypercalcemia, an excess of body calcium, is much less common than hypocalcemia. It is frequently caused by excess IV calcium administration but may also be caused by maternal hypoparathyroidism or neonatal diseases beyond the scope of this text.

Hypomagnesemia Hypomagnesemia, an insufficient amount of magnesium, is most frequently associated with hypocalcemia and may present with the same clinical signs.

Hypermagnesemia Hypermagnesemia, or excess amounts of magnesium, is usually secondary to maternal magnesium sulfate therapy during labor, but it may also occur after administration of an antacid containing magnesium to the neonate. The patient presents with hypotonia, which is low muscle tone and lethargy, and may be apneic. Treatment includes ventilatory support and correction of acid–base and other electrolyte abnormalities.

Maintenance of Electrolytes

The ingredients of intravenous fluids may be adjusted in response to the needs of the patient. Parenteral or intravenous fluids may be used as a supplement to enteral feedings through a nasogastric tube, or may be the total nutrition. Enteral feedings of standard formulas or human milk meet the electrolyte requirements of most full-term newborns. For those babies with other requirements, there are special formulas designed to provide more or less sodium, or more calcium and phosphorus.

Monitoring of Fluid and Electrolytes

When total parenteral nutrition is being provided to the neonate, frequent monitoring of electrolytes is required. Sodium, potassium, chloride, calcium, and possibly phosphate are particularly important and must be monitored until a stable growth rate has been achieved. As feedings are started, continued monitoring is necessary to ensure that the neonate can meet electrolyte requirements as the intravenous portion is tapered. Once full feedings have been achieved, monitoring is not necessary unless there has been a persistent abnormality or signs of possible electrolyte disturbance.

Patients on diuretic therapy, particularly furosemide, need routine monitoring of electrolytes and acid–base status. Replacement therapy to correct chloride and phosphate deficiency is important in these patients and will help diagnose and treat metabolic alkalosis.

NEONATAL JAUNDICE

Jaundice is the yellowish-orange skin color that accompanies increased levels of bilirubin in the blood, called hyperbilirubinemia. Most bilirubin comes from the breakdown of old erythrocytes into its constituent parts. The globin portion is reused as a protein elsewhere in the body. The heme, which is the iron portion of the red blood cell, is the source of the bilirubin. Bilirubin is a waste product that is normally eliminated from the body through the intestinal tract or the kidneys.

Jaundice is common in neonates, occurring in 25% to 50% of all term neonates, with a higher percentage in preemies. It is important to distinguish between physiologic jaundice, which is normal, and pathologic jaundice, which is abnormal.

Typically, bilirubin is measured by taking a blood sample from the neonate and determining the plasma concentration. A noninvasive jaundice meter that can detect plasma bilirubin transcutaneously has recently been produced. One drawback is the influence of skin color on the readings. To offset this, a standardization curve was developed, which improves the predictive value of the readings.[11]

Physiology

Bilirubin is normally handled by the body in the following manner. Upon the destruction of the red blood cell, enzymes reduce the hemoglobin and produce bilirubin and carbon monoxide. The bilirubin at this point is called unconjugated, or indirect-reacting. It is released into the plasma, where it is bound to the protein albumin, which carries it in the blood to the liver. In this form, the unconjugated bilirubin is not water soluble, but is very soluble in fatty tissues, especially brain tissue. In the liver, the bilirubin is released from the albumin. The bilirubin then undergoes a series of reactions with a glucuronide radical, glucuronyl transferase, and the resultant bilirubin combines with the glucuronide and now is water soluble. This combining of glucuronide and the bilirubin is also called **conjugated**, or direct, bilirubin.

The conjugated bilirubin is passed into the intestine through the biliary tree. Direct bilirubin that enters the bloodstream may also be excreted by the kidneys. Of interest to note is that the process of conjugation requires oxygen and glucose to be present. Therefore, lack of either may contribute to hyperbilirubinemia.

Although hyperbilirubinemia is present to some degree in all neonates, jaundice does not appear until bilirubin levels exceed 4 to 6 mg/dL.

Causes of Jaundice

Most neonatal jaundice falls into the category of physiologic jaundice. There are several causes of neonatal jaundice.

Neonates have a large amount of bilirubin production in the first days of life. This is due in part to a higher percentage of erythrocytes in the neonate, and the fact that the erythrocytes have a shorter life span (70 to 90 days) than in adults. Therefore, as these cells break down, they release large amounts of bilirubin into the system. There is also a significant amount of reabsorption of bilirubin from the intestine.

These two factors greatly increase the amount of bilirubin present in the neonatal blood. The neonatal liver is unable to conjugate all the excess bilirubin, which further increases the amount of serum bilirubin.

Certain blood disorders cause jaundice in newborns. Maternofetal blood incompatibility, either Rh or ABO, is a frequent cause of jaundice. Premature black neonates are especially prone to a deficiency of the enzyme G-6-PD, which disrupts erythrocyte metabolism and leads to hemolysis. Abnormal erythrocyte contours also make them vulnerable to hemolysis. Hemolysis may occur when excess doses of vitamin K_3 are given, especially in the presence of G-6-PD deficiency.

Jaundice may result from hemorrhages in the fetal body. The hemorrhage may be in the skin, brain, or may be internal. A lack of the enzyme glucuronyl transferase, a major enzyme in the conjugation of bilirubin, has been linked to neonatal jaundice. Two syndromes, **Crigler–Najjar** and **Lucey–Driscoll**, are both disorders that affect the metabolism of bilirubin through a deficit of this enzyme. Bacterial and viral infections may impair liver function and lead to hyperbilirubinemia. Septic infections may also cause hemolysis of erythrocytes.

Several other factors are associated with jaundice. Infants of diabetic mothers have a high incidence of jaundice. The exact mechanism is unknown; however, it is believed that the frequency of prematurity and RDS in these patients are factors. Jaundice is often seen in breast-fed neonates. It is thought that substances in breast milk inhibit the activity of glucuronyl transferase in the liver. Interestingly, inadequacy of breastfeeding may lead to lowered caloric intake and dehydration, which are both associated with hyperbilirubinemia.

Jaundice is also seen in the presence of **galactosemia** and hypothyroidism. Galactosemia is a rare disorder in which the body is unable to metabolize the sugar galactose. The resultant toxins lead to liver injury and subsequent hyperbilirubinemia.

The administration of maternal drugs, especially oxytocin to induce labor, has been shown to increase neonatal bilirubin levels. Jaundice is often seen in neonates who are fed soon after delivery, possibly caused by immaturity of the hepatic system.

An uncommon but very serious disorder causing jaundice is biliary atresia. Although the exact cause is unknown, it has been seen with congenital rubella infections. Atresia of the biliary tree obstructs the outflow of bile, which is a major vehicle for ridding the body of bilirubin. It is seen mostly in term neonates and in females twice as often as in males.

Pathologic Jaundice

Pathologic jaundice can be determined by using the following criteria: 1) Jaundice appears within the first 24 hours following birth, 2) serum unconjugated (indirect) bilirubin levels exceed 13 mg/dL in term neonates and 15 mg/dL in premature neonates, 3) indirect levels rise more than 5mg/dL in a 24-hour period, 4) direct (conjugated) bilirubin levels exceed 1.5 mg/dL, and 5) the jaundice persists beyond 7 days in term neonates and beyond 14 days in the preemie.[10]

Complications and Treatment

The most serious complication of hyperbilirubinemia is **kernicterus** (bilirubin encephalopathy). Because of the high affinity for fat that unconjugated bilirubin possesses, in high levels it crosses the blood–brain barrier and attaches itself to the brain cells. This leads to neurologic deficits, including locomotor dysfunction, cerebral palsy, and hearing impairment.

The exact level of bilirubin that will produce kernicterus is unknown. Levels as low as 3.3 mg/dL have been reported to have caused kernicterus. Levels of 20 mg/dL for term neonates and 15 mg/dL for preemies are often listed as upper limits, with treatment beginning at levels of 10 mg/dL. It is important to treat hyperbilirubinemia quickly and efficiently because of this unknown association between bilirubin levels and kernicterus.

Treatment must begin with the determination of whether the jaundice is physiologic or pathologic. Pathologic symptoms must be further investigated as to their cause. The most common method of treatment for moderate levels of hyperbilirubin is the use of phototherapy lights. The most effective light is in the blue spectrum. The blue light causes the bilirubin to decompose by photooxidation forming water-soluble bilirubin products that are then excreted by the kidneys and through the bile. Phototherapy lights increase insensible water loss, so care must be taken to counteract the loss.

New methods of phototherapy involve the use of fiberoptics. The infant is covered in a blanket in which fiberoptic fibers have been placed. The light is then able to reach a larger area of the patient's skin while reducing the effects of IWL. These devices have been shown to be superior to traditional phototherapy in recent studies.[12, 13]

High levels of hyperbilirubinemia are treated by exchange transfusion in an attempt to rid the neonatal body of factors causing hemolysis. The indications for exchange transfusion are listed in Table 6–6. Exchange transfusions usually involve

Table 6–6

INDICATIONS FOR EXCHANGE TRANSFUSION

- Correction of severe anemia

- Treatment of hemolytic disease by removing antibody-coated red blood cells

- Removal of excessive amounts of unconjugated bilirubin

a two-volume exchange. The patient's blood volume is estimated by weight, which approximates 80 mL/kg. The procedure is performed by withdrawing 5 to 20 mL of blood, depending on the weight of the patient, from the catheter. The same amount of fresh blood is then replaced to the patient. This is done until all of the fresh blood is gone. Two-volume exchange transfusions remove and replace about 87% of the patient's blood volume.

Other treatments include the administration of phenobarbital and albumin. Phenobarbital induces microsomal enzymes and increases bilirubin conjugation and excretion. It has numerous side effects, however, and so must be used cautiously. The administration of albumin increases the capacity of the blood to transport unconjugated bilirubin to the liver.

NECROTIZING ENTEROCOLITIS (NEC)

NEC is an idiopathic disorder characterized by ischemia and necrosis of the intestine. In its mildest form, abdominal distention is present. At its worst, perforation of the intestine occurs, leading to sepsis and eventually death. Risk factors include prematurity, asphyxia, and formula feeding.[14]

Etiology

The cause of NEC is known to be multifactorial, but three main factors are seen as key etiological factors: 1) mucosal wall injury, 2) bacterial invasion into the damaged intestinal wall, and 3) formula in the intestine.[15] Injury to the intestinal mucosa may be secondary to ischemia and/or decreased blood flow to the gut. Maternal cocaine abuse has also been implicated. Factors leading to ischemia and decreased blood flow are listed in Table 6–7.

The next step in the onset of NEC is the invasion of bacteria into the damaged intestinal tissue. Following mucosal wall injury, the intestine loses its defense against bacterial invasion. Once the bacteria have invaded the intestinal tissue, necrosis and the formation of gas in the intestinal wall, called pneumatosis intestinalis, occurs. Pneumatosis intestinalis is visible on x-ray, as shown in Figure 6–10. In some cases, the bacterial invasion is unrelenting and leads to the passage of bacteria into the

Table 6–7	
FACTORS LEADING TO ISCHEMIA AND DECREASED BLOOD FLOW	
Injury	**Possible Causes**
Ischemia	RDS
	Apgar scores <5
	Abruptio placentae
	Apnea
	Hypertonic oral medicines
	Bowel obstruction
Decreased blood flow	PDA with left to right shunting
	Exchange transfusion
	Umbilical artery catheter
	Polycythemia
	Shock

circulation, causing sepsis, or perforation of the intestine, allowing bacteria into the abdominal cavity, causing profuse peritonitis, organ failure, and death.

The final factor, formula feeding, is seen in 95% of infants with NEC.[15] It is theorized that formula may interfere with intestinal blood flow, contribute to mucosal damage, and provide the substrate for the intestinal bacteria. In contrast to formula, human breast milk may enhance gastrointestinal function and has been shown to be protective against NEC.[16]

Clinical Signs and Treatment

The first confirmatory sign that will be seen in the presence of NEC is guaiac-positive stools, which is the presence of blood in the stools. The invasion of the bacteria results in bleeding, which may not be visible in the stool. It is, therefore, important to perform a **guaiac** check on each stool to determine if blood is present. Abdominal distention becomes apparent as the disease advances by increasing abdominal girth measurements. The patient may have bile residuals and bile-tainted emesis. Feedings may be poorly tolerated, demonstrated by increased residuals and frequent emesis. Lastly, the patient may show general signs of sepsis, which are lethargy and increased F_iO_2 requirements.

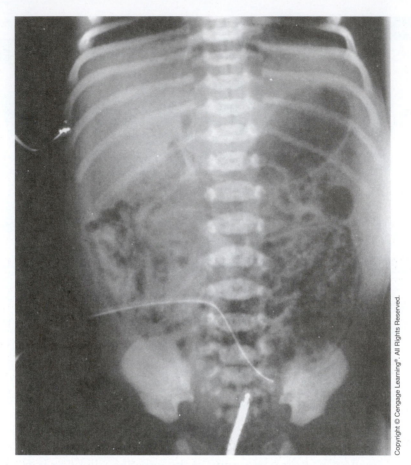

FIGURE 6–10. Gas bubbles seen in the intestinal wall with necrotizing enterocolitis (NEC).

The best treatment of NEC is avoidance of factors that lead to its presence. Good hand washing is mandatory when treating all neonates, especially those with suspected NEC. Oral feedings are stopped immediately and nasogastric suctioning started to empty the stomach of bile residuals. Feeding is started via hyperalimentation through an IV, and antibiotics, such as ampicillin and gentamicin, are administered. Abdominal x-rays are done frequently for follow-up and to rule out intestinal perforation. The F_iO_2 is also increased to raise arterial PaO_2 levels and aid in mucosal regeneration. Studies have indicated that nitric oxide maintains the integrity of gastric mucosa. Because of this, it has been suggested that a potential treatment for NEC is L-arginine, a nitric oxide substrate. In a piglet study, a continuous infusion of L-arginine was shown to markedly reduce intestinal injury.[17]

The presence of gastrointestinal perforation or full-thickness necrosis requires surgical resection of the affected area.

SUMMARY

This chapter focuses on several aspects of continuing care that are important for the respiratory therapist to have an understanding. Thermoregulation is of utmost importance in the ongoing care of a neonate. A patient who is not thermoregulated will waste energy and reserves in an attempt to stay warm. Ideally, the thermoneutral temperature should be maintained as much of the time as possible. The thermoneutral temperature varies from patient to patient. It is the environmental temperature that maintains a rectal temperature of 36.5°C to 37.5°C (97.7°F to 99.5°F), or an abdominal skin temperature of 36.0°C to 36.5°C (96.8°F to 97.7°F).

Heat loss occurs by one of four mechanisms: 1) radiant—the dissipation of heat from the patient to cooler surroundings not in direct contact, 2) conduction—the transfer of heat to cooler surfaces in contact with the patient, 3) convection—the loss of heat from the body to air moving across the skin, and 4) evaporation—the heat lost when water is changed to a gas. An understanding of these four mechanisms allows the respiratory therapist to take precautions in preventing unnecessary heat loss.

Another very important consideration in the care of the premature infant is control of the NICU environment in order to meet the developmental needs of the patient. The premature infant is developmentally immature, both physiologically and neurologically, and excessive stimulation in either area can have serious consequences. Interventions such as planning procedures during times of nonstress, keeping the lights and sound levels low, facilitated tucking, and kangaroo care have all been shown to reduce the amount of stimulation the infant receives.

As an organ system, the skin of a preemie is also immature and very susceptible to injury. Additionally, absorption through the skin is enhanced, and use of solvents or polymers on the skin may lead to toxicity. Skin injury can be reduced by using a pectin-based adhesive between the skin and tape. The pectin-based adhesive allows the skin to grow and develop while protecting it from the trauma associated with tape removal. Monitors can be applied using Velcro closures, or Coban tape, which do not stick to the skin.

One of the most difficult components in the care of a premature neonate is fluid and electrolyte balance. Because a preemie's body weight is mostly water, and a majority of the body water is extracellular, fluid balance can be difficult to achieve. Because of their effect on the lungs and compliance, a basic understanding of fluid balance and the major ions and their function helps the respiratory therapist. Additionally, an understanding of insensible water loss and those mechanisms that increase it, aids the respiratory therapist in helping control fluid balance.

Jaundice is a common occurrence in newborns. While it is common, it is important to distinguish normal physiologic jaundice from pathologic jaundice. Hyperbilirubinemia can lead to severe neurologic complications, called kernicterus. Knowing the normal mechanisms of bilirubin production as well as when and how to treat, can prevent kernicterus from occurring.

Finally, necrotizing enterocolitis is a serious gastrointestinal disorder that every respiratory therapist working with neonates needs to be aware of. The importance of good hand washing cannot be emphasized enough in helping prevent this disease. Rapid and effective identification of the disease may prevent serious complications such as sepsis and peritonitis. Assurance of adequate oxygenation may also help prevent the disease, or slow its progression.

POSTTEST

1. While performing an aerosol treatment on a 30-week gestation neonate, you have the incubator open for access and notice the skin temperature is 36°C. To maintain the neonates oxygen consumption at its lowest this temperature:
   a. The neonate needs to be warmed by at least 1°C.
   b. The neonate should be protected to avoid any lowering of the skin temperature.
   c. The neonate is well within the range of acceptable skin temperature and no additional protection is needed.
2. In which of the following situations would non-shivering thermogenesis be triggered?
   a. fever
   b. infection
   c. increased convective heat loss
   d. aspiration
3. During a resuscitation of a 28 week neonate, the baby is placed on an open warmer and dried vigorously. A radiant warmer is turned on above the infant. Following drying, the neonate is wrapped in a warmed blanket. Ten minutes later, the blanket is removed in order to place an umbilical artery catheter (UAC) but the neonate is left on a warmed pad. During the placement of the UAC the neonate is susceptible to what type of heat loss?
   a. conductive
   b. radiant
   c. evaporative
   d. convective
4. A 33-week neonate, 1 week old, is noted on a blood gas to have a metabolic acidosis. Which of the following could be a contributor to the acidosis?
   a. too many calories in the feedings
   b. oxygen from the resuscitation bag blowing on the neonates face
   c. the temperature inside the incubator is too warm
   d. the neonate is being overstimulated
5. While performing a ventilator check on a 32-week neonate, you note that the legs and arms are mildly cyanotic and pale, while the trunk is pink. You should:
   a. obtain an arterial blood gas
   b. increase the F_iO_2 on the ventilator
   c. check the baby's temperature
   d. check the IV to make sure it is patent

6. During chest physiotherapy on a 29-week-gestation neonate, you note that the baby is hiccoughing. This could be a sign of:
   a. hyperkalemia
   b. cold stress
   c. hypoxemia
   d. overstimulation

7. A neonate is due for suctioning, which has been ordered q4h. As you observe the neonate, you note that the oxygen saturation is 97% and the baby is sleeping quietly. Following the guidelines of environmental control, you should:
   a. not disturb the neonate
   b. proceed with the suctioning, but limit it to 5 seconds or less
   c. hyperoxygenate the neonate prior to suctioning and perform the suction as ordered
   d. only perform oral suctioning and postpone nasal suctioning

8. A 32-week neonate weighed 2500 gm at birth and 2 days later weighs 2175 gm. You would:
   a. increase the IV fluids
   b. increase the caloric intake
   c. do nothing as that amount of weight loss is within normal range
   d. add humidity to the incubator to reduce water loss

9. While assessing a 3-day-old neonate, 30 weeks gestation, you note decreased skin turgor and a mildly sunken fontanelle. This neonate shows signs of:
   a. hypotension
   b. weight loss
   c. fluid deficit
   d. low hematocrit

10. A full-term infant is admitted to the PICU for dehydration following a week-long bout of vomiting. Three days later, it is noted that the baby has developed edema in the legs and arms. Which of the following scenarios is most likely the cause of the edema?
    a. hyperkalemia
    b. hypernatremia
    c. hypocalcemia
    d. hypomagnesemia

11. Three days postdelivery, a 38-week neonate is being evaluated following a seizure. On review of the nursing notes, it is noted that the infant has been showing increased irritability and apnea for the previous 8 hours. What is the most likely cause of these symptoms?
    a. hypermagnesemia
    b. hyponatremia
    c. hyperkalemia
    d. hypocalcemia

12. You are called to the pediatric unit to assess a 5-day-old infant with jaundice. Which of the following would lead you to believe this is a pathologic condition?
    a. The conjugated bilirubin is 2mg/dL.
    b. The jaundice appeared 30 hours after delivery.
    c. The indirect bilirubin is 12mg/dL.
    d. The indirect bilirubin was 9mg/dL 24 hours ago.
13. Of the following, which is NOT a risk factor for NEC?
    a. shock
    b. hyperthermia
    c. maternal cocaine use
    d. formula feedings

REFERENCES

1. Elelstein JA. et al. Hypothermia. http://emedicine.medscape.com/article/770542-overview.
2. McCall EM, et al. Interventions to prevent hypothermia at birth in preterm and/or low birthweight infants. *Cochrane Database of Systematic Reviews* 2010, Issue 3. Art. No.: CD004210. DOI: 10.1002/14651858.CD004210.pub4.
3. Gorski PA, et al. Handling preterm infants in hospitals: stimulating controversy about timing stimulation. In: *Infant Stimulation.* Skillman, NJ: Johnson and Johnson; 1987.
4. Pinelli A. Developmental care for promoting development and preventing morbidity in preterm infants Symington, http://www.nichd.nih.gov/cochrane/symington/symington.htm
5. Zahr LK, Balian S. Responses of premature infants to routine nursing interventions and noise in the NICU. *Nurs Res.* 44:179–185, 1995.
6. Shogan MG, Schumann LL. The effect of environmental lighting on the oxygen saturation of preterm infants in the NICU. Neonatal Network. 12:7–13, 1993.
7. Treas LS. Incubator covers: Health or hazard? *Neonatal Network.* 12:50–51, 1993.
8. Ludington-Hoe SM, et al. Kangaroo care: research results, and practice implications and guidelines. *Neonatal Network.* 13:19–27, 1994.
9. Dollison EJ, Beckstrand J. Adhesive tape vs. pectin-based barrier use in preterm infants. *Neonatal Network.* 14:35–39, 1995.
10. Horns KM. Physiologic and methodologic issues: neonatal insensible water loss. *Neonatal Network.* 13:83–86, 1994.
11. Linder N. Noninvasive determination of neonatal hyperbilirubinemia: standardization for variation in skin color. *Am J Perinatol.* 11:223–225, 1994.
12. Garg AK, et al. A controlled trial of high-intensity double-surface phototherapy on a fluid bed versus conventional phototherapy in neonatal jaundice. *Pediatrics.* 95:914–916, 1995.
13. Tan KL. Comparison of the efficacy of fiberoptic and conventional phototherapy for neonatal hyperbilirubinemia. *J Pediatr.* 125:607–612, 1994.

14. Caplan MS, et al. Role of asphyxia and feeding in a neonatal rat model of necrotizing enterocolitis. *Pediatr Pathol.* 14:1017–1028, 1994.
15. Parker LA. Necrotizing enterocolitis. *Neonatal Network.* 14:17–26, 1995.
16. Schanler RJ. Suitability of human milk for the low-birthweight infant. *Clin Perinat.* 22:207–222, 1995.
17. Di-Lorenzo M, et al. Use of L-arginine in the treatment of experimental necrotizing enterocolitis. *J Pediatr Surg.* 30:235–240, 1995.

BIBLIOGRAPHY AND SUGGESTED READINGS

Bernardo LM, Henker R. Thermoregulation in pediatric trauma: an overview. *Int. Trauma Nurs.* 5:3, 101–105, 1999.

Cloherty JP, Star, AR, eds. *Manual of Neonatal Care.* 7th ed. Philadelphia, PA: Lippincott, 2011.

Corff KE. An effective comfort measure for minor pain and stress in preterm infants: facilitated tucking [abstract]. *Neonatal Network.* 12:74, 1993.

D'Apolito K. Hats used to maintain body temperature. *Neonatal Network.* 13:93–94, 1994.

Hockenberry MJ, Wilson D. *Wong's Nursing Care of Infants and Children.* 9th ed. St. Louis, MO: Mosby, 2011.

Klaus MH, Fanaroff MB. *Care of the High-Risk Neonate.* 6th ed. Philadelphia, PA: WB Saunders Co., 2013.

Merenstein GB, Gardner SL. *Handbook of Neonatal Intensive Care.* 7th ed. St. Louis, MO: CV Mosby Co., 2011.

Patten BM. *Human Embryology.* 2nd ed. New York, NY: The Blakiston Co. Inc., 1953.

Thomas K. Thermoregulation in neonates. *Neonatal Network.* 13:15–22, 1994.

White-Traut RC, et al. Environmental influences on the developing premature infant: theroretical issues and applications to practice. *J Obstet Gynecol Neonatal Nurs.* 23:393–401, 1994.

Perinatal Lung Disease and Other Problems of Prematurity

OBJECTIVES

Upon completion of this chapter, the reader should be able to:

1. Describe each of the following as it relates to respiratory distress syndrome (RDS):
   a. Etiology
   b. Pathophysiology
   c. Clinical signs
   d. Treatment
   e. Complications
2. Describe the pathophysiology, diagnosis, and treatment of bronchopulmonary dysplasia.
3. Discuss the pathophysiology, clinical signs, and treatment of pulmonary dysmaturity (Wilson–Mikity syndrome).
4. Summarize the stages of eye development in the fetus.
5. Identify and describe the factors that lead to retinopathy of prematurity (ROP), how diagnosis is made, and a treatment rationale to prevent damage to the developing ocular membranes in the newborn.
6. Compare and contrast the pathophysiology and complications of intracranial and intraventricular hemorrhages.
7. Identify and describe the four stages of intraventricular hemorrhage.
8. Define asphyxia and identify its incidence in neonates.
9. Describe the pathophysiologic changes that occur with asphyxia, its consequences, and treatment.
10. Identify the cause of meconium release in utero and describe the diagnosis, pathophysiology, and treatment of meconium aspiration.
11. Relate the diagnosis and treatment of a pneumothorax in contrast to a pneumomediastinum and pneumopericardium.
12. Describe the pathophysiology and treatment of pulmonary interstitial emphysema.
13. Identify the factors that lead to pulmonary air embolism and subcutaneous air leaks.

14. Describe the etiology, diagnosis, and treatment of persistent pulmonary hypertension of the newborn (PPHN).
15. Identify and discuss several factors responsible for the onset of transient tachypnea of the newborn (TTN).
16. Compare and contrast central and obstructive apnea with regard to causes and treatments.

KEY TERMS

amblyopia	micrognathia	titration
amnioinfusion	myopia	tonic posturing
choroid plexus	ora serrata	transillumination
cryotherapy	periventricular	vaso-obliteration
disseminated	leukomalacia	ventricular-peritoneal
intravascular	posthemorrhagic	shunt
coagulation (DIC)	hydrocephalus	ventriculostomy
germinal matrix	(PHH)	vernix
hypoxic-ischemic	strabismus	
encephalopathy	systolic ejection click	

INTRODUCTION

Fetal growth during the 40 weeks of gestation is a complex interaction within the fetus and between the fetus and the mother. Most of the time, these interactions occur with seeming flawlessness; however, an interruption of the process frequently results in the underdevelopment of organ systems and all the subsequent sequelae. This chapter will discuss those interruptions as they pertain to the pulmonary system and the brain.

CONSEQUENCES OF PREMATURE BIRTH

The major factor of morbidity and co-mortality in the premature neonate is the degree to which the organ systems are under developed. Clearly, the earlier in gestation that birth occurs, the higher the degree of morbidity and co-mortality. Although the fetus can be maintained outside the uterus as early as 23 to 24 weeks of gestation, it cannot survive without some degree of therapeutic intervention to assist the under developed organ systems. Of all the organ systems of the developing fetus, the pulmonary system is most vulnerable to premature delivery and subsequent complications arising from mechanical ventilation.

Respiratory Distress Syndrome

Respiratory distress syndrome (RDS), also called hyaline membrane disease (HMD), is the primary cause of respiratory disorders in the neonate. According to Avery, RDS is estimated to be the cause of 30% of neonatal deaths.[1] As many as 70% of all preterm deaths are also attributed to RDS. RDS was first reported in 1903 by the German physician Hochheim. Since its first report up to the present time, several names have been added to RDS. Older terms include IRDS, for infant RDS, or idiopathic RDS. More current terminology is to simply use RDS, or NRDS for neonatal RDS.

Etiology The name hyaline membrane disease arises from the change in the alveolar membrane (tissue metaplasia) that occurs with the progression of the disease. The scar-like tissue that replaces the normal alveolar tissue is called *hyaline membrane*, thus the name.

The etiology of RDS is well understood. It is known that the underlying etiology of RDS in the neonate results from a deficiency of surfactant production by alveolar type II cells. Although many factors contribute to this deficiency, the main contributor is prematurity of the pulmonary system. It can also be the result of genetic problems with lung development.[2] Although surfactant is produced near gestational week 22, it is easily disrupted by hypoxemia, hypothermia, and acidosis, all of which plague the premature neonate. It is not until the mature surfactant is produced near week 35 that the above stressors do not disrupt or influence its production and the fetal lungs are considered mature.

Several risk factors have been recognized to help identify those neonates at risk for developing RDS (Table 7–1). At greatest risk are neonates born before 35 weeks and particularly those born before 28 weeks. The shorter the gestational period, the higher the risk involved from premature delivery. The presence of maternal diabetes is another risk factor, presumably because of the effect of diabetes on lung maturation and the high incidence of premature labor and delivery with diabetic mothers. A history of RDS in siblings also places the neonate at high risk. Statistically, males have a higher incidence of RDS, as does the second-born twin and infants born by cesarean delivery without labor. Neonates with poor Apgar scores are also predisposed to RDS, possibly due to complications associated with asphyxia.

Pathophysiology Continuing research on RDS has demonstrated that deficiency in surfactant production is not the only cause of the disease. Overall immaturity of other organ systems contributes to its development. The immaturity of the terminal air sacs and associated vasculature result in poor gas exchange across the alveolar-capillary membrane. Additionally, the immaturity of the chest wall from non-ossified bones allows very little stability during inspiration. As a negative pressure is created for inspiration, the chest retracts inward, reducing the effectiveness of the inspiratory effort. Immaturity of the diaphragm and other muscles of respiration may cause further inspiratory difficulty and/or insufficiency.

Apnea is also common in the premature neonate due to the immaturity of the central nervous system. Add to these the effects of hypothermia, tissue hypoxia, and acidosis on surfactant production, and RDS becomes a multifactorial pathologic process of newborn dysfunction. The role of surfactant in the lung is previously discussed in Chapter 1.

Table 7–1

FACTORS THAT INCREASE THE INCIDENCE OF RDS

1. Prematurity—incidence of RDS is inversely proportional to gestational age

2. Birth weight—incidence of RDS is greater in preemies weighing less than 1200 g

3. Gender—premature males outnumber females 2:1 in acquiring RDS

4. Persistence of fetal circulation

5. Atelectasis

6. Multiple gestations—higher incidence in the second and subsequent siblings

7. Prenatal maternal or delivery complications
   a. Hypoxia
   b. Hemorrhage
   c. Shock
   d. Hypotension
   e. Hypertension
   f. Anemia

8. Maternal diabetes

9. Abnormal placental conditions
   a. Placental previa
   b. Abruptio placentae

10. Umbilical cord disorders
    a. Cord compression
    b. Cord prolapse

Focusing on the effects of a decreased surfactant activity, we will examine the pathogenesis of RDS (Figure 7–1).

With diminished or absent surfactant in the alveoli, alveolar surface tension increases resulting in widespread collapse. As surface tension increases, the compliance of the lung decreases, and the lung becomes stiff. The neonate now must generate tremendous negative intrathoracic pressures to inflate the lung. With each successive breath, the infant weakens and uses up vital energy stores.

The diminished surfactant supply eventually leads to widespread atelectasis in the lungs, which in turn leads to a worsening of ventilation perfusion (V/Q) ratios and tissue hypoxia. Atelectasis also contributes to a decreasing functional residual capacity (FRC) in the lungs. FRC is the amount of gas left in the lungs following a normal expiration. It is made up of the residual volume (RV) and the expiratory reserve volume (ERV). A reduction in the FRC is mainly due to a decrease in the RV.

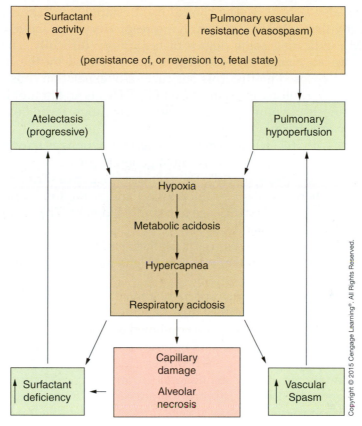

FIGURE 7–1. The pathogenesis of RDS.

As FRC decreases, the patient must work ever harder to create the negative pressures necessary to open the shrinking alveoli.

Along with hypoxia, hypercapnia develops due to the increased work of breathing and often leads to respiratory acidosis. The lack of oxygen at the cellular level leads to anaerobic metabolism with resultant metabolic acidosis. The net effect of the hypoxia and combined acidosis results in damage to the capillaries and alveolar tissues. The condition is now worsened as the damaged alveoli and capillaries result in surfactant deficiency.

The combined acidosis also leads to increasing pulmonary vasospasm. Pulmonary vasospasm is further enhanced by the hypoxemia, which contributes to pulmonary hypoperfusion. Hypoperfusion leads to a further worsening of the V/Q ratio and extenuates hypoxemia from inadequate gas exchange.

The neonate is now caught in a vicious circle that begins again with worsening atelectasis, leading to more profound hypoxia and acidosis, increased pulmonary vascular spasm, and further hypoperfusion. If it continues unchecked, the cycle continues until the patient fatigues and can no longer overcome the effects of the disease.

Clinical Signs and Diagnosis The clinical manifestations of RDS usually begin at birth, or shortly thereafter. The patient has a respiratory rate above 60 breaths per minute (BPM), indicating some degree of respiratory difficulty. The patient then begins grunting, so named because of the sound created by the infant exhaling against a partially closed glottis. This obstruction of exhalation causes a back pressure in the alveoli, resulting in an increased FRC. This is an attempt by the neonate to combat the effects of volume loss in the stiffening lungs. It can be thought of as a natural PEEP in the airways.

The neonate with RDS will also manifest chest retractions as the disease worsens. With ever-stiffening lungs, the patient must generate greater and greater negative pressures to open collapsing alveoli. The increased negative intrathoracic pressure causes the spaces between the ribs (intracostal) and at the top (supra-sternal) and bottom (substernal) of the thoracic cage to be pulled inward. This inward movement of the skin is called a *retraction*.

Another sign of worsening distress is the flaring of the external nares of the nose. This is an attempt by the neonate to get more gas into the lungs by widening the airway passage.

Cyanosis may also be present, especially if the patient is breathing room air. The blood gases are typical of respiratory distress with worsening or refractory PaO_2 to oxygen therapy, increasing $PaCO_2$, and combined acidosis.

The chest x-ray helps establish a diagnosis with the lungs appearing underaerated bilaterally. Their appearance has been described on x-rays as clouded, opaque, reticulogranular, and frosted or as bilateral ground glass opacities. As atelectasis worsens throughout the lungs, air-bronchograms appear in the lung periphery.

Other nonrespiratory signs may also be present in the patient with RDS. Hypothermia is a common problem in the RDS patient. Observation of the skin may reveal pallor and/or severe edema. The muscle tone may be flaccid, with a general muscular hypoactivity. An historical method of determining the presence of pulmonary surfactant, the "shake" test, has been touted as a tool to rapidly diagnose RDS.[3]

In most cases, the symptoms of RDS gradually worsen for the first 48 to 72 hours which may be followed by stabilization and a slow recovery period. Stabilization of the disease is often associated with the onset of diuresis. The highest incidence of mortality from RDS occurs within the first 72 hours. If death occurs following 72 hours, it is usually secondary to complications such as barotraumatic air leaks, intracranial hemorrhages, or infections and not due to the lung disease.

Treatment The ideal treatment for RDS would be to prevent the pathology from occurring. The administration of glucocorticoids to the mother, if done at least two days before delivery, has been shown to promote fetal lung and surfactant development. It is of interest to note the use of antenatal steroids for reducing the need for blood pressure support in premature infants, in addition to promoting lung maturation.[4] No discussion of treating RDS would be complete without examining the use of artificial surfactant replacement. This subject is covered in detail in Chapter 20. A policy statement by the American Academy of Pediatrics was updated in 2008 regarding the use of surfactant in the treatment of RDS.[5] As beneficial as surfactant replacement is, it is apparent that it does not work on all patients equally. Many still require ventilatory support and others appear to get no benefit from the surfactant treatment. Therefore, we will examine conventional treatment of the RDS patient at this point.

The difficulty in treating RDS is in maintaining adequate alveolar ventilation without inflicting damage on the lungs. This then becomes the goal of treatment: to support the patient's respiratory system adequately while minimizing complications. This is easy to envision, but difficult to accomplish clinically. The nature of the disease, and the means we have to treat it, often combine to create other problems that lengthen the recovery of the neonate. The overriding rule to follow when treating the patient with RDS is to treat the symptoms quickly, using inspiratory pressures or CPAP and F_iO_2's as low as possible. However, never compromise the patient's status by using parameters that are too low. Use pressures and F_iO_2's that restore blood gas values to acceptable ranges, whatever those pressures and percents may be. PaO_2 should be maintained at a minimum between 50 and 80 mmHg, with the $PaCO_2$ maintained below 60 mmHg. The pH should be greater than 7.25, as a more acidotic pH leads to decreased surfactant production, organ dysfunction, and an increased risk of intraventricular hemorrhage.

Depending on the severity of the disease, the neonate may require positive pressure ventilation immediately or later in the course of the disease. Some institutions intubate and begin mechanical ventilation when it is apparent the patient's condition begins to deteriorate, indicated by a $PaCO_2$ greater than 60 mmHg and pH less than 7.25, or a worsening of clinical signs, such as grunting, flaring, and retracting. Others advocate the use of nasal CPAP before intubating the patient. Heated and humidified high-flow nasal cannulas have also shown promise in the delivery of nasal CPAP.[6]

Regardless of the technique used, one must intervene before the onset of fatigue or impending respiratory failure. By waiting too long to begin advanced support, the respiratory therapist faces an uphill battle of trying to get ahead of the patient. Early intervention allows supportive steps to be taken that may reduce the amount of total support needed in the care of the patient. Dexamethasone, administered early in the course of RDS has been shown in a study to improve pulmonary compliance and tidal volume, reducing the requirements for F_iO_2 and mean airway pressure. Additionally, its use is associated with reduced time on the ventilator and a decreased incidence of chronic lung disease.[7] Short-term improvements in the respiratory mechanics of ventilated neonates are also seen with the use of salbutamol and ipratropium bromide given via MDI and spacer to ventilated neonates in a study by Lee and associates.[8]

Treatment of RDS also requires adequate hydration, including electrolyte balance. Diuretics are used widely in the management of fluid balance in the neonate. Furosemide (Lasix) is often used because of its excellence in unloading water off the patient. Ironically, researchers have demonstrated that furosemide appears to increase the incidence of patent ductus arteriosus (PDA) threefold.[9] However, it works so well as a diuretic that the benefit outweighs the risk of a greater incidence of PDA.

Of vital importance in the treatment of RDS is the maintenance of thermoregulation. A neonate who is not thermoregulated will not respond as well to treatment as a temperature regulated neonate.

The use of a pulse oximeter and transcutaneous monitor, along with supportive blood gases, allows for the gradual adjustment of ventilatory support to optimize the patient's needs (**titration**). Their use should be considered mandatory equipment for treating RDS.

Complications Most complications of RDS are secondary to the use of positive pressure ventilation. Successful management of the patient requires close monitoring and anticipation of potential complications. Such close scrutiny can aid in the prevention of some complications and assist in the rapid treatment of complications in others.

Intracranial hemorrhage occurs in more than 40% of infants weighing less than 1500 g.[10] The risk increases significantly as positive pressure is initiated to assist ventilation. The positive pressure inside the thorax is transmitted to the cranial cavity, where the immature vasculature of the developing brain may rupture, leading to intraventricular hemorrhage.

Barotraumatic injury that leads to pulmonary air leaks is a common complication in RDS. As the lung compliance drops, higher ventilator pressures are needed to maintain adequate ventilation and oxygenation. This can lead to rupture of the lung and the development of pneumothoraces and other barotraumatic diseases.

Disseminated intravascular coagulation (DIC) is an insidious disease caused by a disruption of coagulation factors, leading to profuse bleeding throughout the body. It has been shown that neonates with RDS have an increased incidence of DIC.

Infection is also a common complication resulting from the institution of positive pressure ventilation, often due to the presence of an endotracheal tube in the trachea. Gram-negative organisms often infect the lung, causing low-grade, chronic pneumonias, which can be very difficult to eradicate. The pneumonia further injures the lung tissue and makes additional ventilatory support necessary. Use of sterile technique when intubating and suctioning, along with sterile humidifiers and disposable tubing, reduce the incidence of a pulmonary infection.

A patent ductus arteriosus (PDA) is another common complication of RDS. A PDA can lead to severe right-to-left shunting of blood, with accompanying hypoxemia, tissue hypoxia, hypercapnia, and acidosis. During the healing stages of RDS, a PDA can cause left-to-right shunting and subsequent right-sided heart failure. PDA is covered in detail in Chapter 8.

Bronchopulmonary Dysplasia

Bronchopulmonary dysplasia (BPD) was first described in 1967 by Northway and associates, who found secondary lung injuries following prolonged exposure to oxygen and high ventilatory pressures required during invasive forms of mechanical ventilation.[11] Most incidences of BPD occur following the treatment of RDS. Ironically, the treatment for RDS is considered to be the prime cause of BPD, that is, high pressures and high F_iO_2 over a period of time predisposes very-low-birth-weight infants (<1500 g) to require respiratory intervention to preserve life. Symptoms of BPD present in a patient without the concurrent radiologic signs is termed *neonatal chronic lung disease (NCLD)* yet specific signs of the disease remain difficult to define due to variations and subtle definition differences.

Pathophysiology The pathophysiology of BPD appears to be linked to four factors: 1) oxygen toxicity; 2) barotrauma; 3) presence of a PDA; and 4) fluid overload. Exposure to high concentrations of oxygen leads to local inflammation, edema, and thickening of the alveolar membrane. As the exposure is prolonged, the alveolar tissues hemorrhage and become necrotic. The interstitial spaces become fibrotic as the disease progresses. As the lung attempts to heal itself, the new cells are damaged by the same factors, and the disease is perpetuated.

A study by Strayer and associates showed a strong link between the development of BPD and the presence of antisurfactant protein A antibodies in the neonate.[12] They found that levels of these immune complexes correlated well with the development of BPD, more strongly than gestational age and birth weight. Another study showed that preemies that went on to develop BPD had a diminished ability to secrete cortisol due to adrenal fatigue. It is speculated that this inability leaves the preemie vulnerable to continued lung injury.[13] The effect of positive airway pressure on the development of BPD is well documented.[14] The incidence of BPD increases with higher peak airway pressures and declines as lower pressures and long inspiratory times are used.[15] The incidence of BPD has found to be higher also in those patients with PDA who subsequently develop congestive heart failure.[1,16] Patients with left-to-right shunting through the PDA develop pulmonary congestion with worsening lung compliance. The result is higher ventilatory pressures and oxygen percents needed to ventilate and oxygenate the patient. This may partly explain the higher incidence of BPD in these patients.

Neonates who have developed symptoms of fluid overload in the first few days of life are also inclined to have a higher incidence of BPD. This is especially common in very small preemies, in which water balance is often difficult to manage. The predisposing factor may be an exacerbation of pulmonary edema caused by increased intervascular pressure changes in these patients. Additionally, a study by Nickerson and Taussig linked a family history of asthma to an increased incidence of BPD.[17]

Despite rapid advances in scientific study regarding BPD, its exact etiology remains misunderstood although concomitant connections are evident. The key to understanding the development of BPD lies in the ability to understand the interrelationship between all of the mentioned factors, their occurrence in underdeveloped organ systems and their role in its development and progression towards illness.

Diagnosis The diagnosis of BPD is elusive even with the advancing technology and trends for less invasive treatment of the disease but is generally made from the chronic need for oxygen therapy and ventilator support and is verified by serial chest radiographs and laboratory studies. The CXR characteristics in BPD were first described by Northway and coworkers as falling into four stages.[11]

In stage I, usually the first 3 days of life, the CXR is typical of RDS, with a bilateral frosted or ground glass appearance. In stage II (days 3 to 10 of the disease), the lungs become opaque with granular infiltrates that obscure the cardiac markings. Stage III occurs during the first 10 to 20 days of life and begins showing multiple small cyst formations within the lung fields with a visible cardiac silhouette. Stage IV occurs following day 28 of life and is manifest by an increased lung density and the formation of larger, irregular cysts. Weinstein, et al, had previously described a scoring system to standardize the reading of chest x-rays in determining the severity of BPD.[18] It is generally categorized as mild, moderate or severe disease in signs present with patients requiring supplemental oxygen and/or continued mechanical ventilation after 28 days. Treatments that minimize exposure to high F_iO_2's and high-pressure mechanical ventilation have been shown to decrease the incidence of BPD. A nationwide inpatient sample between 1993 and 2006 was analyzed in a study by Stroustrup & Trasande that suggests a decrease in incidence of 4.3% annually for the years reported. The study suggests that very-low-birth-weight (VLBW) infants benefit from less invasive forms of mechanical ventilation with improved respiratory outcomes noted.[19]

Laboratory studies include arterial blood gas analysis, which shows evidence of chronic lung disease, that is, hypoxemia with or without tissue hypoxia, hypercarbia, and increased bicarbonate levels. As the patient progresses through the disease, the ECG will show a right axis deviation of the heart and possible hypertrophy of the right ventricle.

Pulmonary function studies will show an increased respiratory rate, decreased tidal volumes, and normal minute ventilation. Airway resistance, especially in the lower airways, is increased and lung compliance is typically decreased as a result of airway and lung parenchymal damage.

Prevention and Treatment The incidence of BPD is reported to be about 25% to 35% of discharged neonatal intensive care unit (NICU) graduates (<1500 g) based on multicenter studies at large academic institutions.[20] Radiologic evidence can be observed as early as two weeks and as late as three months. The goal in treating BPD is to avoid or reduce those factors that lead to its development and perpetuation. Using the lowest possible airway pressures to achieve sufficient gas exchange is the goal of mechanical ventilation. One recommendation is to use pressures, rates, and F_iO_2 that maintain the PaO_2 at 50–70 mmHg and the $PaCO_2$ at 45–55 mmHg.[21] Transcutaneous monitors and pulse oximeters are used to maintain these parameters and avoid the need for numerous arterial blood gases.

Mechanical Ventilation The endotracheal tube should be small enough to allow a small leak during the mechanical breath. This helps reduce the chance of subglottic stenosis in the long-term ventilated patient. If the patient requires mechanical ventilation for longer than 1 to 2 months, a tracheostomy may be more appropriate than endotracheal intubation.[22] Ideally, the patient should be extubated as quickly as can be tolerated: however, weaning should be done slowly and cautiously so as not to compromise the patient's status. The use of nasal CPAP may be of help in the transition from mechanical ventilation.

High-frequency oscillatory ventilation (HFOV) and volume guaranteed (VG) ventilation has shown some evidence of successful treatment of pulmonary interstitial emphysema seen in RDS associated with the development of BPD.[23]

Adequate humidification of inspired gases must be monitored closely. Patients with BPD requiring long periods of intubation must have the artificial airway sufficiently humidified to avoid mucus plugging from thickened secretions.

Respiratory Therapy Procedures Chest physical therapy is done as needed to prevent the accumulation of secretions and to maintain good bronchial hygiene. The frequency of treatment should be dictated by the amount and viscosity of the patient's secretions, not simply on a routine basis. Suctioning of the airway must be done aseptically to prevent the possibility of infection which may potentially complicate the clinical course. Aerosolized bronchodilators may be used to improve airway bronchospasm. However, they have not been shown to reduce airway resistance in the small BPD patient.[24] This is possibly due to the immaturity of the bronchial smooth muscle in the preemie. Historically, there were some who advocated for the use of theophylline to aid in the weaning from mechanical ventilation; however, more recently theophylline has been replaced by caffeine as the drug of choice due to its reduced toxicity and longer half life.[25, 26]

Fluid Therapy Fluid therapy is aimed at maintaining adequate hydration and urination. Diuretics such as furosemide are often needed in addition to fluid restriction to reduce pulmonary edema and help in maintaining fluid balance. Patients receiving diuretic therapy may rapidly lose excess water in the body. In these instances, lung compliance may quickly improve, subjecting these patients to possible pneumothoraces if pressures and rates are not weaned quickly. Close observation of urine output, breath sounds, and chest excursion will help the respiratory therapist identify an improvement in compliance. Patients receiving long-term diuretics must also have calcium and phosphorus levels monitored and maintained to avoid the weakening of developing bones.

Right Heart Failure Symptomatic right-sided heart failure may be treated with diuretics. The effect of closure of the PDA, either chemically or surgically, on the development of BPD is unknown, but it may reduce the degree of severity by improving heart function. Digoxin may also be used to improve the effects of right-sided heart failure in the BPD patient. A patient with BPD must have frequent blood work, which depletes the blood volume to various degrees. In such instances, blood transfusions are given as needed to maintain a hematocrit above 40%.[10]

Nutrition BPD patients must have adequate nutrition to meet increased metabolic requirements. The patient with BPD may require 120–150 cal/kg/day to achieve growth and meet the needs of lung tissue repair.

Patients with inadequate nutrition may suffer a delay in the growth and development of new alveoli. Additionally, they may be very difficult to wean from the ventilator and are more prone to infection.[22]

Two precautions must be observed when administering a high number of calories to BPD patients. First, oxygen consumption increases in newborns as their caloric intake increases. The BPD patient has a limited ability to oxygenate and, therefore, may become hypoxic as more oxygen is used to metabolize the added calories. Second, the metabolism of glucose results in increased CO_2 production. The BPD patient may be unable to remove the excess CO_2, resulting in hypercapnia and a worsening acidosis.

Vitamin E Administration A deficiency of vitamin E has been shown to increase the incidence of oxygen toxicity. Additionally, the administration of vitamin E reduces lung injury caused by the administration of excessive oxygen. Subsequent tests in BPD patients did not demonstrate conclusive evidence that vitamin E reduced the incidence of BPD.[1]

Future Outlook Because of the advent and rapid technical progression of mechanical ventilation strategies for neonates, and by demonstrating that strategies that improve ventilation with limited pressures can prevent the development of BPD, few studies are available to examine the long-term effects of BPD in later life. An investigation into early management practices demonstrated a decrease in BPD in extremely preterm infants following surfactant administration and CPAP at delivery, decreasing O_2 saturation goals, and early amino acid supplementation.[27] Some have suggested that there is an increased risk of developing asthma and even chronic obstructive pulmonary disease (COPD) later in life. These suggestions, however, have not been scientifically analyzed and documented. Early reports that BPD patients suffer from poor growth throughout childhood have recently been downplayed.[28]

Pulmonary Dysmaturity (Wilson–Mikity Syndrome)

Wilson–Mikity syndrome is a rare disease of functional and structural pulmonary changes seen in premature neonates with no apparent underlying lung disease.

Pathophysiology The underlying pathophysiology of Wilson–Mikity syndrome remains unknown. The only common finding is prematurity, with a majority of afflicted neonates weighing less than 1500 g at birth.[1] One etiologic theory is that lung immaturity leads to emphysematous changes in the lungs due to treatments required to sustain life. There may also be an association between maternal bleeding and asphyxia and the development of the syndrome.

The radiographic picture of the lungs is very similar to stage III and IV BPD, with the exception that the neonate with Wilson–Mikity has not been ventilated. Lung biopsies done on patients early in the course of the disease show little if any structural change in the pulmonary tissue. Later biopsies show immaturity of the alveolar septa, causing overexpansion and atelectasis of the lungs.[1]

Clinical Signs The initial symptoms usually appear near the end of the first week or later and are usually mildly evident. Early symptoms include hyperpnea, transient cyanosis, and retractions. Lower levels of arterial PO_2 along with progressive hypercarbia and respiratory acidosis is apparent as symptoms persist. The symptoms gradually worsen over the following 2 to 6 weeks, leading to the acute phase of the disease. The acute phase may last from days to weeks and presents as severe respiratory distress, poor feeding, and vomiting.

Two thirds of infants survive this acute phase and begin a gradual recovery with clearing of the disease by age 2.

Treatment Treatment of Wilson–Mikity syndrome is supportive. The patient is routinely placed on mechanical ventilation to treat apnea and progressive hypercarbia. Oxygen is titrated to treat hypoxemia. Once the patient is ventilated, the disease becomes impossible to differentiate from BPD and is, therefore, treated as BPD would be treated.

Retinopathy of Prematurity

Retinopathy of prematurity, formally called retrolental fibroplasia (RLF), was initially described by Terry in 1942.[29] The term RLF literally means the formation of a scar behind the lens, which is the culmination of the disease. The term retinopathy of prematurity (ROP) was introduced by Heath in 1951.[30]

ROP is a more descriptive term of the actual events that the neonate passes through, leading to scar formation. The term ROP has now been expanded to include all stages of the disease, so that the term RLF is no longer used.

Following an epidemic of ROP that occurred in the 1940s and 1950s, a reduction in the use of supplemental oxygen led to a decline in the incidence of the disease. The reduction in oxygen use, however, led to an increase in mortality and cerebral palsy.[1]

More recent studies have identified a definite link between the development of ROP and oxygen use, but have also identified various other factors that contribute to its development. These include retinovascular immaturity, and circulatory and respiratory instability.[31]

Typically, ROP affects infants born before 31 weeks of gestation that weigh 1250 gms or less. There seems to be a direct relationship between size and the probability of developing ROP with smaller preemies being more likely to develop it.[32] The disorder, which usually develops in both eyes, occurs in 25% to 35% of preemies up to 35 weeks, gestation, with 5% to 10% having stage 3 or more and 3% to 5% resulting in blindness.[31] Another study showed an ROP incidence of 26.5%, with 40% of those resulting in blindness or severely impaired vision.[33] In a study performed in 10 schools for the blind, 17.6% of all children with severe visual loss were found to have a history of ROP.[33] In recent years, while survival of the extremely low birth weight patient has increased, the rate of ROP has not been shown to increase proportionally.[34] It is estimated that 14,000–16,000 infants born yearly are affected by some degree of ROP with 90% of them having a mild form not requiring treatment.[32] Infants with ROP are at a higher risk of developing other eye problems later in life such as retinal detachment, **myopia**, **strabismus** (misalignment of the eyes), **amblyopia** (impaired vision in one eye), and glaucoma.[32]

Physiology of the Developing Eye An understanding of retinal development is basic to the understanding of ROP. The capillaries of the retina begin branching out at approximately 16 weeks. Capillaries begin from the optic nerve and grow toward the **ora serrata**, the retina's anterior end. The capillaries do not completely reach the entire ora serrata until 40 weeks. As the capillary network expands, arteries and veins form in its path. The capillaries of a prematurely born neonate have not had time to reach the ora serrata. Depending on several factors, the network can either develop normally or cease to grow and cause ROP.[35]

Pathophysiology of ROP In the presence of high PaO_2, the retinal vessels constrict. If not relieved, the constriction leads to a necrosis of the vessels, called **vaso-obliteration**. In an attempt to reestablish a blood supply to the retina, those vessels that have not necrosed begin to proliferate. The proliferation may extend into the liquid portion of the eye, the vitreous, where the vessels hemorrhage, depicted in Figure 7–2. The result is the formation of a scar behind the retina with later traction,

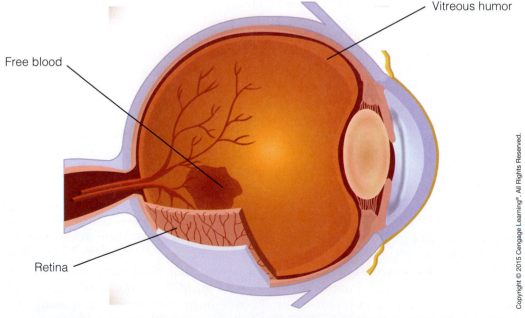

Vitreous humor

Free blood

Retina

FIGURE 7–2. Hemorrhage of blood into the vitreous humor, resulting in scar formation behind the retina.

detachment, and blindness. It is important to note that at any time the process may stop, with no further damage occurring.

Although oxygen has long been implicated in the development of ROP, many downplay its role.[36, 37] Studies of several risk factors led Lucey and Dangman to identify several factors that may contribute to the development of ROP.[38] Those factors include immaturity, hyperoxia, hypoxia, blood transfusions, intraventricular hemorrhage, apnea, infection, hypercarbia, PDA, prostaglandin synthetase inhibitors, vitamin E deficiency, lactic acidosis, prenatal complications, and genetic factors. Bright lighting in the nursery may also contribute to the development of ROP.[35] Additional factors related to the occurrence of ROP are early intubation, hypotension, and necrotizing enterocolitis.[32] A study by Wright and Wright showed that birth weight and duration of supplemental oxygen were significant predictors of stage 2 or higher ROP.[39] These data show the multifactorial processes involved in the development of ROP and help to illustrate why its development is difficult to prevent. However, it is clear that close monitoring of the infant and maintenance of physiologic conditions in the NICU may forestall its development.

Diagnosis ROP is classified into five stages, listed in Table 7–2. ROP is diagnosed by ophthalmologic examination of the internal eye anatomy. Capillary damage occurs in one of three zones shown in Figure 7–3. The extent of the disease is described by using the hours of a clock superimposed over the three zones. The disease is described by the stage number and the clock hours it is located in, for example, 3 clock hours of stage 2 ROP in zone 3. It appears that the most unfavorable outcomes are associated with injury involving zone 1 at a stage 3 or better.[40]

ROP appears between 35 and 45 weeks' gestational age and may progress from stage 1 to stage 5 in the next several weeks.

Table 7–2

STAGES OF RETINOPATHY OF PREMATURITY

Stage Number	Classification
1	A thin white demarcation line is seen separating the avascular retina anteriorly from the vascularized retina posteriorly.
2	A ridge is now formed and rises up from the plane of the retina. New vessels may be seen posterior to the ridge.
3	In this stage, there is a proliferation of extraretinal fibrovascular tissue. It is often seen posterior to the ridge or connected to the posterior aspect of the ridge.
4	In stage 4, there is a subtotal detachment of the retina.
5	Continued traction and buildup of fluids; the retina becomes completely detached.

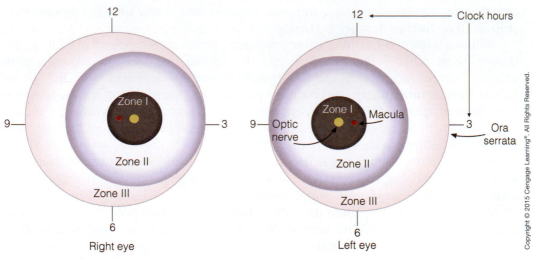

FIGURE 7–3. The three zones of the internal eye.

Treatment and Prevention The knowledge that vitamin E is a natural antioxidant led researchers to experiment with its use to prevent ROP. Studies concluded, however, that administration of vitamin E does not decrease the incidence or development of ROP.

The traditional treatment for stage 3 ROP is cryotherapy. **Cryotherapy** is performed by introducing a probe that has been cooled to −20°C with nitrous oxide behind the eye and freezing the avascular portion of the retina, preventing further abnormal vessel proliferation. Complications include retinal scarring, cell destruction, and possible retinal detachment.[41] Cryotherapy has also been linked to visual field changes later in life.[42]

Laser therapy is used as an alternative to cryotherapy. Either argon or diode lasers are used to photocoagulate the avascular portion of the peripheral retina. It is less invasive and less traumatic to the eye than cryotherapy. Complications include scarring, choroidal hemorrhage and, rarely, pain.[41]

Surgical interventions, such as vitrectomy and lensectomy are also being investigated as possible treatments for severe ROP. There is some evidence that in stage 5 ROP, vitrectomized eyes function better than nonvitrectomized eyes.[43] A sclera buckle technique involves placing a silicone band around the eye which is then tightened. The band prevents the vitreous from pulling on the scar tissue allowing the retina to flatten against the wall of the eye. This is the same treatment used for retinal detachment.[44]

Until more is known about the development of ROP, prevention is based on cautious use of oxygen delivery to the patient. TCMs, pulse oximeters, and blood gases are all used to maintain levels of oxygen between hypoxia and toxicity.

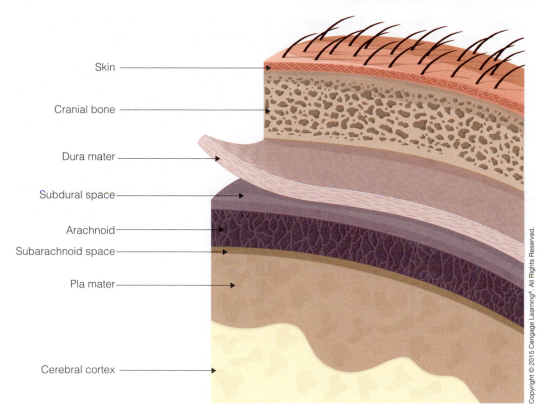

Skin

Cranial bone

Dura mater

Subdural space

Arachnoid

Subarachnoid space

Pla mater

Cerebral cortex

FIGURE 7–4. The location of subdural and subarachnoid bleeding.

Intracranial/Intraventricular Hemorrhage (ICH/IVH)

Bleeding in the cranium is a major source of morbidity in the premature population. It can occur in any one of several areas. Subdural or subarachnoid bleeding occur secondary to trauma or asphyxia, within the respective spaces of the cranial bone, shown in Figure 7–4. These bleeds are most commonly found in term neonates following birth trauma.

Bleeding can also occur within the cerebellar tissue itself. This type of bleed is usually found in preterm neonates and is associated with the periventricular-intraventricular hemorrhages. The majority of cranial hemorrhages in neonates are the periventricular-intraventricular hemorrhages, or IVH. These bleeds occur in preterm neonates of between 24 and 32 weeks' gestation. Neonates with birth weights of less than 1500 g are also at a high risk.

Pathophysiology In the developing fetus, the brain is perfused in highly vascular, extremely fragile tissues. In the term neonate, the area of most frequent bleeding is called the **choroid plexus** of the lateral ventricles, shown in Figure 7–5. In the premature neonate, the **germinal matrix**, located in the subependymal region (Figure 7–6), is the most common source of bleeding.

The inability of the cerebral vascular system to regulate blood flow, probably due to immaturity, is the underlying cause of hemorrhage at these areas. Small bleeds may be confined to the immediate area, with no residual effect. With severe hemorrhages, the blood enters the ventricles, enlarging their size and compressing the parenchyma of the brain. Hemorrhaging may also extend into the brain tissue, resulting in further damage to the patient.

The triggering factors that lead to a fluctuation in blood flow include shock, acidosis, hypernatremia, transfusion of blood, seizures, and rapid expansion of blood volume.[14] Increasing intracranial pressure by placing the neonate in the Trendelenburg position or by mechanical ventilation may also lead to IVH. It has also been reported that the premature infants of mothers who consume alcohol during pregnancy have a substantially increased risk of developing IVH.[45] Table 7–3 lists a few specific factors that may lead to IVH. It lists some additional patient historical factors often seen with IVH.

While most IVHs occur one to several days post-delivery, it is possible that up to one third are congenital or are of immediate postnatal onset.[46]

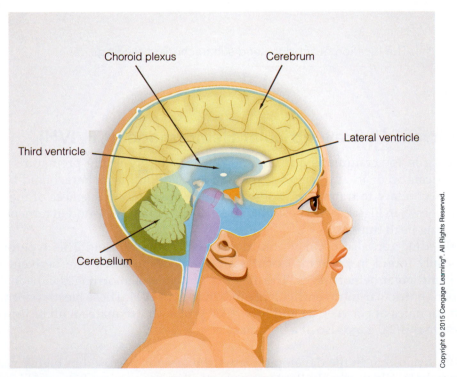

FIGURE 7–5. The choroid plexus, common site of bleeding in term neonates.

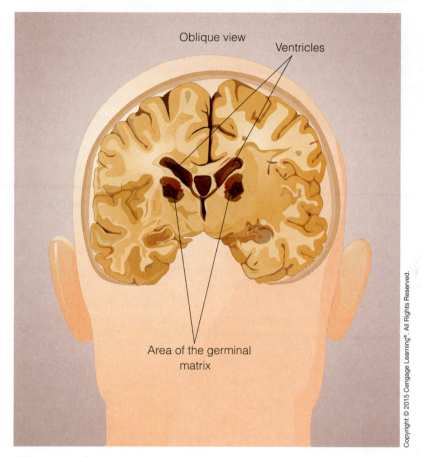

FIGURE 7–6. The area of the germinal matrix in the developing brain.

Table 7–3

ETIOLOGY AND HISTORY OF INTRAVENTRICULAR HEMORRHAGE

Etiologic Factors	Historical Factors
Hypernatremia	Less than 1500 g birth weight
Shock	Less than 34 weeks' gestation
Acidosis	Hyaline membrane disease
Blood transfusions	Coagulopathy
Seizures	Hyperviscocity
Rapid volume expansion	Hypoxia
Fluctuation in cerebral blood flow	Birth asphyxia

The physical signs the IVH patient demonstrates depend on the severity of the bleeding. They range from severe, rapid deterioration in patient condition to having no apparent side effects. Some common signs of bleeding in the germinal matrix include apnea, hypotension, reduced hematocrit, flaccidity, bulging fontanelles, and the flexion and extension of opposite arms (**tonic posturing**).[14]

IVH is classified into four grades diagnosed by CT scan or ultrasound. If no bleeding is present, it is categorized as Grade 0. Hemorrhage that is limited to the germinal matrix is grade I. A Grade II hemorrhage involves the germinal matrix with blood extending into the ventricles. With this degree of bleeding, there is no ventricular dilation. Grade III IVHs are comparable to Grade II, with the exception that the ventricles are dilated. The most severe hemorrhages are Grade IV. Grade IV hemorrhages dilate the ventricles and extend into the brain parenchyma. Grades I through IV are depicted in Figure 7–7.

Complications Implications of IVH are related to the severity of the bleeding and the underlying causes. In general, increased bleeding, results in severe complications and sequelae manifest in the patient.

The most serious complication of IVH is **posthemorrhagic hydrocephalus (PHH)**. PHH is caused by the obstruction of cerebrospinal fluid (CSF) outflow and impairment of CSF resorption in the brain. Treatment of PHH is initiated to maintain

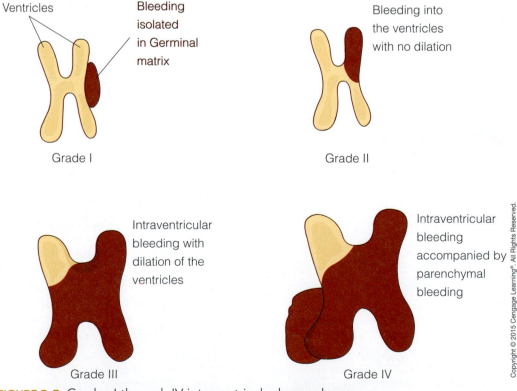

FIGURE 7–7. Grades I through IV intraventricular hemorrhages.

a normal cerebral perfusion pressure as intracranial pressure rises. This is initially done by removing CSF by lumbar puncture. If PHH persists with the use of lumbar punctures, surgical placement of a **ventricular-peritoneal shunt** or creating a surgical hole in the ventricles (**ventriculostomy**) with an external drain is indicated.

Complications seen as the child grows include cerebral palsy, vision loss, hearing loss, epilepsy, and intellectual disability.[47]

Treatment The best treatment of IVH is to avoid those factors that lead to its occurrence. Careful avoidance of those factors that cause fluctuations in cerebral blood flow will help in preventing IVH. Caregivers must avoid wide fluctuations in blood pressure, oxygenation, and pH. Low-dose indomethacin, given prophylactically, has been shown to significantly lower the incidence and severity of IVH.

Treatment following an IVH is mainly supportive. Clearly, little can be done to treat the IVH once it has occurred. Every precaution must be taken to prevent further hemorrhage and damage once a bleed has occurred.

Osmotic agents such as blood and plasma should be carefully and slowly administered. Caregivers should carefully monitor and treat the patient for hyperbilirubinemia, which is a common occurrence. Hypotension must be avoided in the presence of an elevated intracranial pressure to prevent a reduction in cerebral blood perfusion.

PROCESSES OF INTRAUTERINE ORIGIN

Adequate and proper growth and development of the fetus requires an intricate relationship between the fetus and the mother. That interaction requires an interface between the two, which is the placenta and umbilical cord. When there is a disruption of that interface, the fetus faces a range of possible complications, which will be discussed in this section.

Asphyxia

Asphyxia is a combination of hypoxia, hypercarbia, and acidosis in the fetus or neonate. It begins as either a lack of oxygen or a lack of perfusion to various tissues.

In utero, the placenta is the organ of respiration where the initial insult occurs, and in the neonate, it is the lung. Asphyxia is present in 1% to 1.5% of all births, increasing to 9% in neonates of less than 36 weeks' gestation.[10] Intrauterine growth retardation, breech delivery, and postmaturity also increase the risk of asphyxia.

Pathophysiology Asphyxia in utero is a result of placental insufficiency with an inability to exchange oxygen and remove carbon dioxide from the fetus. Asphyxia after delivery is caused by pulmonary or cardiac problems.

During normal labor, the blood flow to the placenta is diminished during contractions with resultant diminished gaseous exchange. Prolonged compression of the umbilical cord may further interrupt blood flow, with resulting hypoxia to the fetus.

Both the mother and fetus require significantly increased oxygen consumption secondary to the stress of the labor. Maternal hyperventilation may even further reduce placental blood flow. The net result of all these factors is reduced oxygen delivery to the fetus and ensuing decrease of oxygen reserve, even in the normal neonate.

Any maternal, placental, or cord problem that interferes with the exchange of gas in the placenta or fetus leads to asphyxia. These factors are listed in Table 7–4. In addition, impairment of maternal oxygenation will impair blood flow to the placenta and cause less oxygen to be available for the fetus, resulting in asphyxia. In the presence of asphyxia, blood is shunted away from the lungs, skeletal muscle, liver, kidneys, and gut. The blood flow is directed to the brain, heart, and adrenal glands.

Patient symptoms begin with a decreased heart rate and blood pressure. The fetus attempts to correct the asphyxia by starting a gasping reflex. If the asphyxia remains uncorrected, the fetus enters a period of apnea, known as primary apnea.

Table 7–4

FACTORS LEADING TO FETAL ASPHYXIA

1. Maternal hypoxia
   a. Maternal shock
   b. Acute asthma attack
   c. Carbon monoxide poisoning
   d. Anemia
   e. Oversedation
   f. Apnea from any cause
   g. Congestive heart failure
   h. Low ambient F_iO_2
   i. Severe pneumonia

2. Disruption of uteroplacental blood flow
   a. Maternal shock
   b. Maternal vasoconstrictive states
   c. Inferior vena cava syndrome

3. Dysfunction of the placenta
   a. Placenta previa
   b. Abruptio placentae

4. Impairment of blood flow through the umbilical cord
   a. Compression of the cord

5. Intrinsic fetal disorder
   a. Fetal cardiac failure (hydrops fetalis)
   b. Fetal hypotension secondary to hemorrhage or drugs

With continuation of the asphyxia, the heart rate and blood pressure continue to drop during primary apnea. The fetus then commences a series of deep, ineffective gasps, which gradually slow and, finally, cease. The fetus then enters a period of secondary apnea. If the asphyxia is untreated, the heart rate and blood pressure continue to fall, resulting in permanent damage or death.

Asphyxia in utero is detected by the fetal heart monitor and the presence of meconium in the amniotic fluid. The fetal heart monitor will show a loss of baseline variability, late decelerations, and prolonged periods of bradycardia.

Consequences and Treatment

The major complication of prolonged asphyxia is hypoxic-ischemic brain injury. In the term neonate, the resultant brain injury is called **hypoxic-ischemic encephalopathy**. It is the result of necrosis to the neurons of the cerebral cortex and basal ganglia. The injury in the preterm neonate is most often associated with hemorrhage into the ventricles of the brain. This condition is termed periventricular-intraventricular hemorrhage.

Another lesion that affects both term and preterm neonates is called **periventricular leukomalacia**, which is an area of infarct in the periventricular region. Victims of asphyxia may also suffer cardiac ischemia as a result of the insult. This is usually transient in nature with normal ECGs returning within 3 months.

The asphyxiated patient is also at risk of developing tubular necrosis of the kidneys and gastrointestinal effects such as bowel ischemia and necrotizing enterocolitis. Disseminated intravascular coagulation (DIC) may be present due to blood vessel damage. Severe asphyxia may also lead to liver damage, to the point that the liver may not provide its basic functions.

Asphyxic damage to the lung is manifest by increased pulmonary vascular resistance (pulmonary hypertension), hemorrhage, and possible damage to the production of surfactant with resultant RDS.

The treatment of asphyxia requires the immediate reversal of hypoxia and acidosis. Asphyxia that occurs in utero requires the rapid delivery of the fetus, possibly by cesarean delivery if normal labor is not rapidly progressing. Once delivered, the neonate is dried, warmed, and stimulated. The airway is then opened and maintained while breathing is assisted using 100% F_iO_2 and positive pressure. Circulation is assisted as needed with drugs and external massage. The neonate is then closely monitored and treated as needed for continuing hypoxia and hypercarbia. Prevention of asphyxia will prevent the need for treatment in the postdelivery patient. Clinical observation along with laboratory analysis of blood gases will help in avoiding and treating asphyxia.

Meconium Aspiration Syndrome

Meconium is the name given to the sterile contents of the fetal bowel. It is a thick, tar-like dark green material that consists of swallowed amniotic fluid, bile salts and acids, squamous cells, **vernix**, the thick white substance on fetal skin, and intestinal enzymes. It is the first stool of the newborn and typically passes within the first 48 hours postpartum. The name meconium is from the Greek word *mekonion*, which has an interesting origin. Near the ancient city of Corinth was a small city named Mekonê, which is translated as "poppy-town." It got its name from the extensive cultivation of poppies in the area.[48] The name *mekonion* came to mean "poppy-juice" or "opium." Aristotle used the term meconium either because of its thick tarry appearance, or because he thought it induced sleep in the fetus.[49]

Meconium Aspiration Syndrome (MAS) occurs when the fetus passes meconium while still in utero. Intrauterine passage of meconium has been associated with low Apgar scores, fetal hypoxia, acidosis, and abnormal fetal heart tracings.[50] It has also been linked to fetomaternal stress and infection.[51] MAS is predominantly a disease of the term or postterm neonate that has experienced some degree of asphyxia either before or after the onset of labor. Meconium passage into the amniotic fluid occurs in 9% to 20% of all births.[53] Actual aspiration of meconium into the trachea occurs in about half of the neonates born with meconium staining the amniotic fluid and can occur before or during delivery, or with the first breath. Postterm patients are at a high risk, possibly due to diminished amniotic fluid levels, which dilute the meconium; and diminishing placental function, leading to increased asphyxia. Several perinatal risk factors have been linked to MAS. These include placental insufficiency, maternal hypertension, maternal diabetes mellitus, preeclampsia, oligohydramnios, and maternal smoking.[52]

Pathophysiology The sequence of events that results in the aspiration of meconium into the trachea involves a complex series of asphyxia-induced occurrences. During an asphyxial episode in utero, there is an apparent shift in blood distribution to the vital organs. The response to the fetal bowel is increased peristalsis and relaxation of the anal sphincter, resulting in the passage of meconium into the amniotic fluid. Additionally, vagal stimulation from compression of the head or umbilical cord during labor may lead to increased peristalsis and relaxation of the rectal sphincter, allowing meconium to enter the amniotic fluid.[54]

In response to asphyxia and/or vagal stimulation, the fetus begins gasping, attempting to relieve the asphyxia. With severe asphyxia, deep gasping movements may allow the passage of meconium into the oropharynx and upper levels of the tracheobronchial tree.

Meconium that is aspirated into the tracheobronchial tree has two potentially devastating effects on the neonate. The physical presence of the meconium in the airways can lead to blockage of the airway and air trapping. This obstruction is enhanced by the ball-valve effect, illustrated in Figure 7–8, in which the airway dilates during inspiration owing to the negative pressures generated in the thorax. With the airway dilated, the meconium advances further into the airway. Upon exhalation, the airway constricts and traps the meconium in the lumen, trapping the gas behind the obstruction.

This leads to disruption of V/Q ratios and ensuing hypoxia and hypercarbia. Increasing obstruction leads to widespread atelectasis, which further impairs gas exchange, worsening the hypoxia, and hypercarbia. Air leaks, such as pneumothoraces, occur as the trapped gas increases in volume and eventually ruptures the lung.

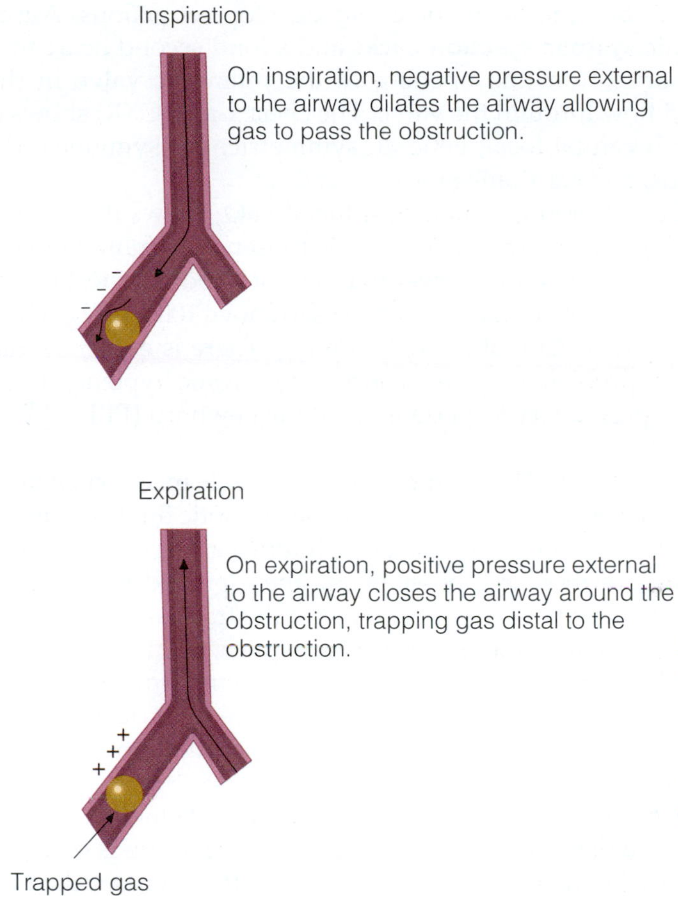

Inspiration

On inspiration, negative pressure external to the airway dilates the airway allowing gas to pass the obstruction.

Expiration

On expiration, positive pressure external to the airway closes the airway around the obstruction, trapping gas distal to the obstruction.

Trapped gas

FIGURE 7–8. The ball-valve effect: inspiration dilates the airway, allowing gas to pass the obstruction; on exhalation, the airway collapses, trapping air distal to the obstruction.

Another effect of meconium aspiration is an inflammatory response of the tracheobronchial epithelium to the presence of meconium. This is called a chemical pneumonitis and results from the irritating effect of the acidic meconium on the epithelium. The inflammation results in mucosal edema, decreasing lung compliance, and further impairment of gas exchange.

Vasospasm of the pulmonary vasculature occurs in many MAS patients in response to the effects of intrauterine asphyxia leading to persistent pulmonary hypertension (PPH). In these patients, blood flow follows fetal routes, bypassing the lungs and leading to an increased shunt and worsening arterial blood gases. It is important for the respiratory therapist to ascertain the degree of PPH in these patients.

Persistent fetal circulation (PFC) in these patients is detected by several factors. Worsening cyanosis that does not respond to increased F_iO_2 is a common sign.

The≈patient may become tachypneic and develop retractions. Auscultation often reveals pulmonic **systolic ejection clicks** and a loud second heart sound. Pulmonic ejection clicks arise from the opening of the pulmonic valve in the presence of increased blood flow through the valve. The chest x-ray (CXR) shows diffuse patchy infiltrates, which can be focal, general, symmetric, or asymmetric, hyperinflation, pleural effusions, and cardiomegaly.

A comparison of preductal and postductal PaO_2 shows the presence or absence of ductal shunting. One definitive test for the presence of pulmonary hypertension in the neonate is the hyperoxia-hyperventilation test. A positive test is when the patient has a PaO_2 of less than 50 mmHg, which rises to above 100 mmHg when the patient is hyperventilated to a $PaCO_2$ of 20 to 25 mmHg. There is evidence that the primary pathophysiologic problem may be secondary to chronic hypoxia in-utero and subsequent persistent pulmonary hypertension of the newborn (PPHN).[55]

Diagnosis and Treatment The diagnosis of MAS is only made when meconium is aspirated from the trachea. It is suspected when the amniotic fluid is stained with the dark green meconium. The neonate is called meconium stained until meconium aspiration into the trachea is verified. It is possible that the aspirated meconium has advanced to the point where it cannot be suctioned out of the trachea. These patients may show classic signs of respiratory distress such as tachypnea, tachycardia, and hypoxemia.

As the condition progresses, the severity of symptoms increases with ensuing hypercarbia and acidosis. The chest x-ray shows irregular densities throughout both lungs, similar in appearance to pneumonia. Hyperinflation may be present as the disease advances.

Prevention of meconium aspiration is the ideal. Fetal status must be continuously monitored to detect early signs of stress. If meconium is detected in the amniotic fluid, an infusion of sterile, warm saline into the uterus, called **amnioinfusion**, may help dilute the meconium and reduce the chance of problems with aspiration. However, two studies did not support the use of routine amnioinfusion to prevent MAS.[50,56]

Recommendations by the American Congress of Obstetricians and Gynecologists do not advise for the routine suctioning of infants with meconium staining.[57] Additionally, the consistency of the meconium does not justify routine suctioning.[58]

The American Academy of Pediatrics has developed guidelines to manage newborns exposed to meconium. They are available in the Academy's Neonatal Resuscitation Program and are summarized here.

Upon delivery of the head, before the delivery of the thorax, the mouth and oropharynx are thoroughly suctioned and cleared of any meconium that is present using at least a 10 Fr. oral suction catheter. Once delivered, the infant is placed under an open radiant warmer and dried by a team member. A newborn that has depression of respiratory effort, a heart rate below 100 beats/min and poor muscle tone, is described as "not vigorous" and should be intubated and suctioned immediately following delivery. Suctioning should be limited to 5 seconds.

The largest endotracheal tube possible is used to aspirate the meconium. Upon completion of the intubation, suction is applied to the end of the endotracheal tube

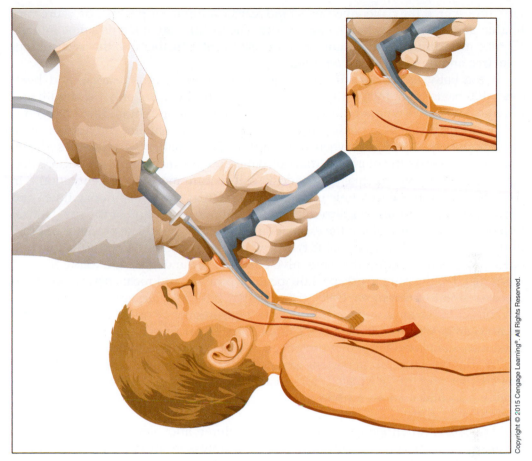

FIGURE 7–9. Applying suction to the endotracheal adapter to remove meconium from the trachea.

for no longer than 5 seconds, either by mouth or by suction tubing attached to wall suction, as illustrated in Figure 7–9.[59] The ET tube is withdrawn and examined for the presence of meconium. Attempts to suction meconium from the trachea by passing a suction catheter through the endotracheal tube should not be made. The small size of the catheter makes it ineffective to remove meconium.

If meconium is aspirated, and the baby is not bradycardic, the procedure is repeated, using a new endotracheal tube, until no meconium is aspirated from the trachea. The general condition of the neonate must be taken into account while performing the intubations. The repeated intubation and suctioning of the patient must be performed rapidly, to reduce the effects of possible bradycardia and hypoxia. Exhaustive attempts to remove meconium that is beyond the carina are inadvisable.

If no meconium is returned during the first suctioning attempt, no more attempts are made. Throughout the procedure, 100% oxygen should be blown by the patient's face, however, if the patient becomes bradycardic administer positive pressure ventilation and consider suctioning again later. The instillation of sterile saline into the ET tube may dilute the meconium and cause it to enter further into the tracheobronchial tree and therefore is not advised.

If the baby has a normal respiratory effort, normal muscle tone, and heart rate >100 beats/min, then intubation is not done. In this case, only the mouth and nose are suctioned with a bulb syringe or catheter. Warmed, humidified oxygen is used to treat persistent hypoxia. An optimal thermal environment and minimal handling both help to reduce oxygen consumption. If the patient is agitated, sedation may be necessary. In roughly a third of patients with meconium aspiration, persistent hypoxia, hypercarbia, and acidosis will require mechanical ventilation.[60] In these cases, the presence of air trapping requires that short inspiratory times and longer expiratory times be utilized to allow adequate expiration of the gas. Utilization of PEEP may also aid in the exhalation of trapped gases. The presence of PEEP in the airways mechanically holds the airway lumen open and does not allow it to collapse. This may reduce the ball-valve effects to some degree and allow trapped gases distal to the plug to escape. Low peak inspiratory and mean airway pressures are desirable to prevent air leaks. If traditional positive-pressure ventilation does not correct hypoxemia and/or hypercarbia, high-frequency oscillation and jet ventilation can be effective. In all cases, caution must be taken to not hyperventilate the patient as there is evidence that prolonged alkalosis may lead to neuronal injury.[61]

In the presence of persistent pulmonary hypertension, discussed later in this chapter, the use of inhaled nitric oxide (iNO) is the treatment of choice. NO inhibits vascular smooth muscle contraction, leading to a lowering of pulmonary hypertension.

Pay careful attention to systemic blood volume and blood pressure. Volume expansion, transfusion therapy, and systemic vasopressors are critical in maintaining systemic blood pressure greater than pulmonary blood pressure, thereby decreasing the right-to-left shunt through the patent ductus arteriosus.

Recently, the use of surfactant replacement therapy has been shown to reduce the severity of disease.[62] Surfactant is thought to both replace surfactant in the lungs as well as act as a detergent to remove any remaining meconium. The routine use of corticosteroids is not recommended. When all other options have been exhausted, ECMO may be considered, however, it is associated with poor neurologic outcomes.[63]

Because meconium promotes the growth of bacteria, broad-spectrum antibiotics should be administered to those patients who present with infiltrates on CXR. Tracheal cultures should then be obtained to identify specific pathogens.

BAROTRAUMATIC DISEASES: AIR LEAK SYNDROMES

Air leak syndromes appear with increased frequency in the newborn infant. The incidence is higher in patients with RDS, meconium aspiration, and transient tachypnea of the newborn. Most air leaks are caused by mechanical ventilation; however, some may occur spontaneously. Pulmonary air leak and its sequelae include pneumothorax, pneumomediastinum, pneumopericardium, pulmonary interstitial emphysema (PIE), subcutaneous emphysema, and air embolism.

All air leaks develop from a common event. The initial event is a rupture of the alveoli, usually secondary to uneven ventilation in alveoli exposed to pressure. Where the air goes after it leaks from the alveoli determines what kind of air leak will develop.

Pneumothorax

Pneumothorax is the most common of the air leaks, occurring in 1% to 2% of all newborns. A pneumothorax develops when the extraalveolar air ruptures to the external surface of the lung and into the pleural space.

Pneumothoraces are divided into two categories: spontaneous and tension. A spontaneous pneumothorax is an isolated pocket of free air in the pleural space that is not fed by a continuous inflow of gas from the point of the leak. Spontaneous pneumothoraces are the result of the rupture of a weak alveolar tissue and are often asymptomatic. It may resolve without complication and is frequently not detected.

A tension pneumothorax is so named because of the addition of new air through the rupture with each breath, creating a larger and larger air pocket that is under pressure. As the air accumulates in the pleural space, the lung collapses and is displaced under the added pressure. Additionally, the accumulated air causes the great vessels to shift toward the unaffected side and cardiac function becomes compromised.

Diagnosis Physical symptoms are usually the first signs of a pneumothorax. The onset may be gradual or very rapid, depending on the severity of the air leak. Physical signs begin with an increase in respiratory distress, with retractions and tachypnea. The patient then becomes bradycardic, cyanotic, and may have periods of apnea and hypotension. Examination of the chest reveals asymmetry in chest excursion, a movement of the maximal impulse point of the heart, and a change in breath sounds.

Any patient showing a sudden demise in status should be transilluminated with a fiber-optic light source. **Transillumination** involves the placement of a high-intensity light source, usually fiber optic, on the thoracic surface. When the light is placed against the thorax of a neonate with normal lungs, the light is reflected to the surface of the thorax by the lung tissue, forming a uniform circle around the light. In the presence of free air in the thorax, the light is reflected at odd angles due to the collapse of the lung. The result is an irregular-shaped reflection on the chest wall, with fingers of light possibly appearing away from the light source, as seen in Figure 7–10.

Transillumination is a quick method of diagnosing a pneumothorax. However, a negative transillumination does not rule out a pneumothorax. Chest x-rays taken during expiration will show severe pneumothoraces. Taken in both AP and lateral views, the pneumothorax appears as a dark bleb with no lung markings present. The lung is often seen collapsed and unaerated. The mediastinum may be shifted away from the air pocket.

Treatment Treatment of pneumothoraces depends on the severity of symptoms. Patients who are not on a ventilator, have small leaks, and are in no respiratory

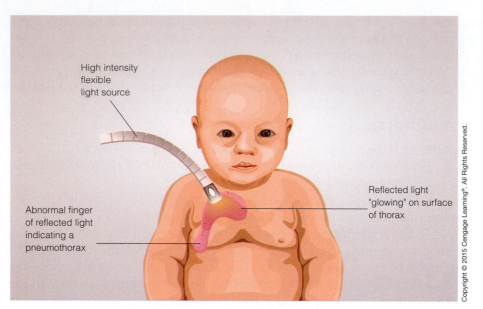

High intensity
flexible
light source

Reflected light
"glowing" on surface
of thorax

Abnormal finger
of reflected light
indicating a
pneumothorax

FIGURE 7–10. The appearance of a positive transillumination indicating a pneumothorax.

distress can usually be managed by close observation. The patient in severe distress should have the trapped air removed through needle aspiration. Needle aspiration is an emergency procedure to be used only in a life-threatening situation until a chest tube can be inserted.

The patient with a continuous air leak who is receiving continuous positive pressure ventilation should have a chest tube placed as quickly as possible. This is only to be done by experienced nursery personnel trained under the direction of a physician. The chest tube is then attached to a one-way valve, water seal, or suction. The level of suction should range from −15 cm H_2O for small leaks to −25 cm H_2O for large air leaks.[10]

The chest tube is removed when the patient's respiratory disease is resolved, there has been no leakage from the tube for 24 to 48 hours, and the extrapulmonary air has been resolved for 24 to 48 hours. Often, the tube is clamped for 24 hours before removal to ensure complete resolution of the air leak.

Pneumomediastinum

A pneumomediastinum occurs when extra-alveolar air dissects through the lung interstitium and ruptures into the mediastinum. Although rarely severe, it may compromise venous return and cause a tamponade on the heart in severe cases.

The symptoms depend on severity, with the most common sign being distant, crackly heart sounds. Diagnosis is made by chest x-ray, which shows free air in the mediastinal space. The air highlights the border of the heart, but does not surround the heart. Treatment involves close observation for other air leaks and, if possible, lower ventilatory pressures.

Pneumopericardium

Air that dissects through the perivascular sheaths to the great vessels may rupture into the pericardial sac, causing a pneumopericardium. Air may also rupture through mediastinal connective tissue, near the pleural-pericardial connection. As the air builds up in the pericardial sac, it compresses and tamponades the heart, impeding cardiac output and causing a severe, rapid demise in patient status. These patients may have severe bradycardia, with muffled or distant heart sounds. A chest x-ray shows the presence of air completely around the heart.

Treatment of symptomatic patients is by needle aspiration of the air in the pericardial sac. Because this is a dangerous procedure, it should only be performed by trained personnel.

Pulmonary Interstitial Emphysema (PIE)

PIE occurs when air dissects throughout the interstitial tissue of the lungs. It results from the chronic use of high PEEP, high peak inspiratory pressures, and prolonged inspiratory times.

PIE develops into one of two classifications. If the air remains in the lung tissue, it is called intrapulmonary interstitial pneumatosis. Intrapleural pneumatosis is the name given when the extra-alveolar air is confined by the visceral pleura, forming blebs. One or both forms may be present in the affected lung. PIE can lead to a pneumothorax, pneumomediastinum, and possibly pneumopericardium if the free air follows those routes.

Pathophysiology As the air dissects and collects in the interstitium, the small airways and vessels are compressed. Widespread ventilation to perfusion mismatches follow and lead to a deterioration of blood gases. A vicious circle begins as higher ventilator pressures are required to correct the worsening blood gases. Higher pressures may cause more air to leak into the interstitium and the mismatch of ventilation to perfusion worsens.

The chest x-ray of PIE resembles bubbly, cystic areas throughout the lung parenchyma.

Treatment PIE is best treated by prevention. Close attention to low ventilator pressures, while maintaining ventilation and oxygenation, may help avoid the onset of PIE. Mild cases may clear spontaneously with reabsorption beginning in 5 to 7 days.

The treatment of moderate and severe cases begins by lowering ventilator pressures while maintaining oxygenation and ventilation. Selective intubation of the unaffected or less affected lung may allow the injured lung time to heal. Several published studies report that high-frequency ventilation is successful in treating patients with pulmonary air leaks, including PIE.[64]

Survivors of PIE have a high incidence of BPD due to the necessity for vigorous mechanical ventilation.

Pulmonary Air Embolism

Air embolism is extremely rare but may occur when high pressures are being used to ventilate stiff lungs. It is thought that air enters the pulmonary vasculature through lacerations in the parenchyma. Infants suffering from air embolism have an extremely rapid deterioration of physical condition with eventual circulatory collapse. There is no effective treatment for air embolism.

Subcutaneous Emphysema

Subcutaneous air is usually secondary to other air leaks, with the air dissecting into the subcutaneous spaces between muscle tissues. Clinically, it has little importance other than that it indicates the presence of a pulmonary air leak. Subcutaneous emphysema resolves when the causative air leak is treated.

OTHER RESPIRATORY DISEASES OF THE NEONATE

Although uncommon, there are other maladies that can affect the pulmonary system of the neonate. It is important that the respiratory therapist be aware of these problems along with their evaluation, diagnosis and treatment.

Persistent Pulmonary Hypertension of the Neonate (PPHN)

PPHN is also known as persistent fetal circulation (PFC) for reasons that will become apparent. PPHN is most frequently seen in term or postterm infants and often in patients suffering from asphyxia, meconium aspiration, sepsis, congenital diaphragmatic hernia, pulmonary hypoplasia, congenital heart disease, and premature closure of the ductus arteriosus.[65] Additional clinical disorders associated with PPHN include HMD, bacterial pneumonia, myocardial dysfunction, and pulmonary hypoplasia.[10] PPHN also occurs more frequently in neonates with Down syndrome.[66]

Affected infants have severe, persistent pulmonary vasoconstriction, which causes increased blood pressure in the lungs and decreased pulmonary blood flow. Right-sided heart pressures may rise higher than arterial pressures. The result is a continuation of the factors that allow fetal circulation to occur, with blood shunting through the foramen ovale and ductus arteriosus and away from the lungs. This shunting is illustrated in Figure 7–11.

The profound mismatch in ventilation and perfusion that follows leads to metabolic and respiratory acidosis and hypoxia, which further worsen pulmonary vasoconstriction. There are three types of PPHN that have been categorized: PPHN that is secondary to pulmonary vascular constriction due to lung parenchymal diseases; PPHN that is characterized by hypoplastic pulmonary vasculature; and

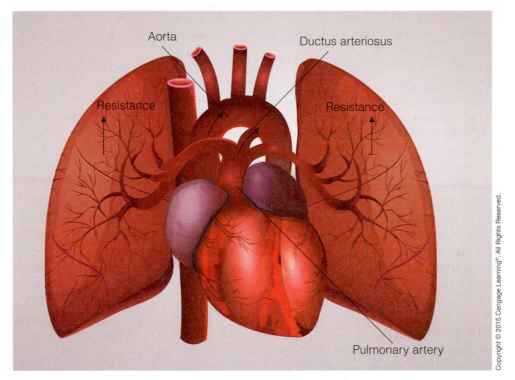

FIGURE 7–11. Right-to-left shunting through the ductus arteriosus resulting from an increase in pulmonary vascular resistance.

idiopathic PPHN in which there is normal lung parenchyma and remodeling of the vasculature.[67]

Etiology The underlying cause of the persistent vasoconstriction is unknown, but numerous factors that cause the initial constriction are involved to some degree. PPHN is primarily a disease of the term and postterm neonate. This is because the pulmonary arterial musculature does not develop until late gestation. The manifestations of PPHN suggest a dysfunction of pulmonary vasoregulation resulting in abnormally high pulmonary vascular resistance.[68] PPHN is also associated with chronic intrauterine events.[69] It is possible that genetic factors may play a role in increasing the susceptibility to develop pulmonary hypertension.[70]

The most common scenario in the development of PPHN is an acute vasoconstriction of the pulmonary vasculature. Conditions that lead to parenchymal lung injury, such as MAS, RDS, and pneumonia, can cause alveolar hypoxia and subsequent pulmonary vasoconstriction. Acute vasoconstriction can also follow hypothermia, hypoglycemia, or hypoventilation.[71] Hypoplasia of the pulmonary vasculature secondary to diaphragmatic hernia can lead to PPHN. Pulmonary hypoplasia can also develop in the presence of oligohydramnios. A third cause of PPHN is idiopathic in which the ductus arteriosus constricts in utero. This can happen with maternal ingestion of NSAIDS during the last part of pregnancy. There is current research examining the role of maternal SSRI ingestion as another link to idiopathic PPHN.[72]

Diagnosis and Evaluation The physical examination of the newborn with PPHN will typically show cyanosis with tachypnea and respiratory distress, usually occurring within a few hours after delivery. Additionally, the presence of tricuspid regurgitation can cause a loud single S2 or a harsh systolic murmur. In the presence of severe or worsening hypoxemia in a full-term neonate, one of three possible differential diagnoses should be considered: parenchymal lung disease, cyanotic congenital heart lesion, and PPHN. To help differentiate among the three disorders, a series of tests have been developed that can be done noninvasively at the patient's bedside.

The simplest test is the hyperoxia test. It is performed by administering an F_iO_2 of 1.0 to the patient for 5 to 10 minutes. An arterial sample is then obtained and the PaO_2 is measured. If the PaO_2 is below 100 mmHg, the diagnosis is a right-to-left shunt, found in both PPHN and cyanotic heart lesions. Because of the association between high PaO_2 and the development of ROP, the use of this test on premature neonates is questionable.

Right-to-left shunting is also detected by measuring preductal and postductal PaO_2 levels. In the presence of a significant right-to-left shunt, the preductal sample may be 15–20 mmHg higher that the postductal sample. The difference between the two is increased when the F_iO_2 is increased.

A third test, the hyperoxia-hyperventilation test, is the most accurate of the three to differentiate PPHN. The patient is hyperventilated to achieve a $PaCO_2$ of 20–25 mmHg and raise the pH to 7.50 or greater. The alkalosis reduces the pulmonary vasoconstriction, improving lung perfusion and oxygen content. If the PaO_2 is less than 50 mmHg before hyperventilation and rises to above 100 mmHg follow hyperventilation, it is regarded as an almost certain diagnosis of PPHN.

The use of echocardiograms in the NICU has advanced the diagnosis of PPHN. The presence of PPHN is documented by an echocardiogram showing increased pulmonary artery pressures, right-to-left shunting at the ductal or atrial level, regurgitation through the tricuspid valve, and dilation of the right ventricle.[65]

Once the diagnosis has been established, there are several lab studies that are indicated. First, arterial blood gases are evaluated regularly through an indwelling line. If the site of withdrawal is preductal, the PaO_2 could be elevated as blood shunts through the ductus arteriosus and dilutes the arterial blood. In cases where there is significant ductal shunting taking place, the Oxygen Index (OI) can be used to assess the adequacy of oxygenation. The OI is calculated by multiplying the mean airway pressure (MAP) by the F_iO_2 and multiplying the result by 100. The product is then divided by the post ductal PaO_2. The formula is

Oxygen Index

$$OI = (MAP \times F_iO_2 \times 100)/PaO_2$$

The blood should be monitored by checking the hematocrit. Polycythemia with hyperviscocity can exacerbate PPHN. The white blood count can also help identify an underlying sepsis or pneumonia. Serum glucose and electrolyte levels are also critical to monitor frequently. In particular, calcium should be maintained at a normal level as hypocalcemia as well as hypoglycemia can both worsen PPHN. A chest x-ray can help to rule out the presence of parenchymal lung disease. It can also determine the presence of a diaphragmatic hernia. The chest x-ray often appears with normal lung fields and decreased vascular markings in the presence of idiopathic PPHN. The heart shadow can appear normal or slightly enlarged.

As previously mentioned, an echocardiogram is vital in not only the diagnosis, but the identification of shunting through the ductus arteriosus and/or foramen ovale. Measuring the peak velocity of regurgitant blood flow across the tricuspid valve, right ventricular and right vascular pressures can be calculated. The echocardiogram is needed to rule out any obstructions to left-sided outflow before NO treatment can be started. Obstructions such as a hypoplastic left ventricle, interruptions in the aortic arch and severe aortic stenosis require right to left shunting through the ductus, negating treatment with NO.

Treatment The treatment of PPHN is a delicate balance requiring the maintaining of temperature, fluids and electrolytes, blood sugar, oxygenation, blood pressure and perfusion. Minimal stimulation protocol is used to minimize the handling of the patient. Oxygenation and ventilation issues can be addressed with several high-end therapies. In patients with concurrent lung parenchymal disease associated with MAS, the use of surfactant can help reduce the need for Extracorporeal membrane oxygenation (ECMO).[73] Traditional mechanical ventilation is almost always necessary in the presence of PPHN. The overall goal is to maintain as close to normal blood gases as possible, while minimizing mean airway pressures. The use of high F_iO_2's and pressures to keep the PaO_2 at normal levels, could lead to extended ventilator support and barotraumas. Additionally, the high oxygen levels could be toxic to the developing lung. A PaO_2 of 50 mmHg or higher typically provides for adequate oxygen delivery.[74] The use of sedatives may be necessary to keep the neonate from fighting the ventilator. When peak airway pressures exceed 30 cm H_2O and/or the mean airway pressure exceeds 15 cm H_2O, high frequency ventilation can be valuable to help keep the airway pressures low.

If the OI reaches 25 or more, iNO therapy is indicated. Typically, NO comes in an H-cylinder that contains 450–1000 parts per million (PPM) of NO mixed with nitrogen. When NO comes in contact with high concentrations of oxygen, it forms nitrogen dioxide (NO_2), which is very irritating to lung tissue. In order to minimize the production of NO_2, NO is usually delivered in very small quantities, 5 to 6 ppm. When delivered to a patient, NO is introduced to the inspiratory limb of the mechanical ventilator just proximal to the ETT. This further reduces the contact time between NO and O_2. In the bloodstream, excess NO is quickly absorbed by hemoglobin, forming methemoglobin.

When used in line with mechanical ventilation, the amount of NO introduced into the circuit is regulated by a flow controller. The concentrations of NO, NO_2, and F_iO_2 are all measured inline near the ETT. Protocols for administration of iNO vary among institutions. Ideally, the amount of inhaled NO and NO_2 are balanced to maximize the vasodilatory effects while minimizing methemoglobinemia and the toxic effects of NO_2. While it is generally thought that concentrations of 5 to 20 ppm of NO are considered usual, reports of concentrations up to 80 ppm with no side effects have been documented.[75, 76]

Transient Tachypnea of the Newborn

Transient tachypnea of the newborn (TTN) is also called RDS Type II because of the similarities in patient symptoms. Although the exact etiology is unclear, the retention of fetal lung fluid following birth is felt to play a major role in the development of TTN. It most commonly occurs in near-term or term infants with a history of cesarean or precipitous deliveries. In either of these types of deliveries, the gradual compression of the thorax that develops during a vaginal delivery does not occur, possibly leading to the retention of lung water.

Diagnosis Within the first few hours following delivery, the infant shows signs of respiratory distress including tachypnea, nasal flaring, retractions, and grunting. The patient may be cyanotic when breathing room air. Blood gases are usually normal but may show varying degrees of hypoxemia. Hypercapnia is a rare occurrence.

The chest x-ray may mimic early RDS, with streaky infiltrates that radiate from the hilum of the lung. Fluid in the interlobar fissures is commonly seen. The chest x-ray gradually clears within 24 to 48 hours following the onset of symptoms.

The diagnosis of TTN is only made after other potential problems have been ruled out. It is important to rule out pneumonia as the source of the symptoms. The presence of an elevated white blood count, hyperglycemia, persistent metabolic acidosis, and poor perfusion all indicate a possible pneumonia.

Treatment Treatment of TTN involves taking appropriate measures to treat the patient's clinical symptoms. Warmed, humidified oxygen is delivered via oxyhood to treat hypoxia. More severe symptoms may require the use of positive pressure to treat hypoxemia. Continuous positive airway pressure (CPAP) delivered via nasal prongs may be used to treat refractory hypoxemia. The use of mechanical ventilation may be necessary when nasal CPAP does not improve arterial oxygen.

Frequent turning of the infant with gentle chest physiotherapy may help in the absorption of lung fluids. Broad-spectrum antibiotics are given, as the symptoms of pneumonia are often mistaken for TTN.

Apnea

True apnea is defined as a cessation of breathing for a period sufficient to produce bradycardia and/or cyanosis. That period is usually 10 to 20 seconds or longer. Apnea is categorized into central or nonobstructive apnea, which is the absence of airflow and ventilatory effort, and obstructive apnea, which is the absence of airflow despite a ventilatory effort.

The mechanisms that provide for adequate ventilation and homeostasis are diverse. The respiratory centers in the medulla and pons receive information from numerous receptors and then send out impulses to the ventilatory muscles to maintain homeostasis. Apnea may be present when there is a dysfunction of any of the various mechanisms involved. We will briefly examine potential dysfunctions at each site. Causes of apnea are found in Table 7–5.

Table 7–5

CAUSES OF APNEA IN PREMATURE INFANTS

Respiratory
- RDS
- Congenital upper airway anomalies
- Airway obstruction
- Postextubation
- CPAP
- Pneumonia
- Hypoxia

Cardiovascular
- Congestive heart failure
- Patent ductus arteriosus
- Anemia
- Tachycardia and bradycardia
- Sepsis
- Polycythemia

Central Nervous System
- IVH
- Meningitis
- Seizures
- Pharmacologic sedation
- Kernicterus
- Immaturity of the respiratory centers
- Tumors

Gastrointestinal
- Necrotizing enterocolitis
- Gastroesophageal reflux

Metabolic
- Hypoglycemia
- Hypo- and hypernatremia
- Hypocalcemia
- Hypo- and hyperthermia

Environmental
- Increased environmental temperature
- Suctioning
- Feeding

Apnea of Prematurity A common type of central apnea is identified as apnea of prematurity. As the gestational age of the preemie decreases, the incidence of apnea of prematurity increases. Apnea of prematurity is a result of one or more of the following factors.

Chemoreceptor Sensitivity Evidence from apnea research has demonstrated that newborns, especially premature newborns, have a somewhat blunted response from peripheral chemoreceptors located in the aortic arch and the bifurcation of the carotid artery. These receptors sense changes in PaO_2, pH, and $PaCO_2$ and send impulses to the respiratory centers to either increase or decrease ventilation.

Although both premature and term infants show an initial response to blood gas changes, the response is transient. It is not until around day 18 that the infant shows a sustained response to changes. This blunting in chemoreceptor sensitivity can potentially initiate an apneic spell or can prolong an apneic spell that is started by other factors.

Arousal Response In the adult, periods of hypoxemia and/or hypercapnia during sleep cause arousal. There is some evidence that this response is not present in some infants who suffer apneic spells. The level of sleep also influences response to hypercapnia and hypoxemia. Nonrapid eye movement (NREM), or quiet sleep, has been shown to be controlled by metabolic and chemical factors, whereas REM, or active sleep, is controlled by behavioral and reflex mechanisms. Studies on infants suffering apneic spells have shown an apparent blunting of the sensitivity to CO_2 during NREM sleep.

Stimulation of Airway Reflexes One of the protective mechanisms of the airways is to induce coughing, constriction, and apnea when a foreign substance is aspirated. This mechanism serves to prevent the material from entering deeply into the tracheobronchial tree and occluding the airways. Apnea that is present in patients suffering from gastroesophageal reflux and infections such as RSV may be caused by an activation of this protective airway mechanism. Research indicates that as many as one third of patients diagnosed with apnea of prematurity in reality are suffering from apnea secondary to gastroesophageal reflux.[77] While the main response of the adult to airway stimulus is coughing, the response of the newborn is apnea.

Dysfunction of the Respiratory Centers Dysfunction of the centers in the brain responsible for maintaining ventilation can be caused by several factors. In the preterm infant, inadequate development of the brain centers themselves may be the cause of dysfunction. The respiratory centers may also be damaged by trauma or bleeding in the brain, leading to hypoperfusion and increased pressures that damage the brain tissue.

The presence of certain drugs in the maternal or fetal circulation depresses the respiratory centers and leads to apnea.

Dysfunction of the Ventilatory Muscles The muscles of ventilation, especially the diaphragm, may be dysfunctional and unable to increase ventilation in the face of hypercapnia and hypoxia, leading to apnea. At special risk are infants with chronic lung diseases that interfere with gas exchange. As $PaCO_2$ rises and PaO_2 falls, the muscles may not be able to respond by increasing ventilation due to chronic fatigue and underdevelopment. Studies have shown that fatigue of the ventilatory muscles leads to apnea in the newborn.

Dysfunction of the Peripheral Nervous System Apnea may occur when a disease that affects neurotransmission to the ventilatory muscles is present. Illnesses such as Guillain-Barré syndrome block transmission of the nervous system and may lead to apnea. The defect may be a maldevelopment of the motor neurons in the spinal cord as in Werdnig-Hoffmann disease. Toxins such as botulism and certain drugs disrupt and inhibit the neuromuscular junctions. Finally, trauma to the CNS leads to a loss of neurotransmission and subsequent apnea.

Other Factors That Cause Apnea Other factors that have been linked to apnea in newborns are thermal instability, metabolic disorders, PDA, shock, anemia, sepsis, and NEC.

Treatment Treatment of central apnea is accomplished by the administration of drugs that stimulate ventilatory mechanisms. The most commonly administered drugs are the methylxanthines, theophylline, and caffeine citrate, which stimulate the central respiratory chemoreceptors. Which drug is more effective is a matter of debate; however, caffeine citrate offers the advantages of once daily dosing and a wider therapeutic range, with a lower risk for toxicity [78].

The drug primidone, chemically related to phenobarbital, is a drug that traditionally has been used to treat neonatal seizures. It is now being investigated as a possible treatment option for apnea in those cases that are resistant to theophylline.

Mechanical ventilation may be necessary to support the patient whose apnea leads to acute respiratory failure. In these patients, inspiratory pressures and ventilator rates are kept as low as possible to avoid barotraumatic injuries.

While apnea of prematurity can present a difficult challenge and may have long-term consequences in the presence of other events, it appears as though the apnea in and of itself is not associated with any significant developmental problems later in life.

Obstructive Apnea In the adult, and in the healthy newborn, the upper airway is protected from obstruction by the presence of protective reflexes. During inspiration, negative intrapharyngeal pressures are countered by the presence of elastic fibers and smooth muscle in the pharyngeal wall to prevent collapse. Any time that negative intrapharyngeal pressures exceed the force of the fibers and muscle, the pharynx will collapse. The most common cause of airway obstruction is the tongue.

Many infants who suffer from obstructive apnea have anatomic abnormalities that cause obstruction. Prematurity or agenesis of the pharyngeal musculature may lead to pharyngeal collapse. Enlarged tonsils and adenoids, underdevelopment of the mandible, (**micrognathia** or Pierre–Robin syndrome), and facial anomalies lead to airway obstruction. The presence of choanal atresia, laryngeal webs, and vocal cord paralysis has also been shown to cause apnea.

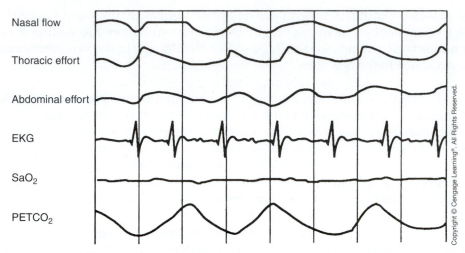

Nasal flow

Thoracic effort

Abdominal effort

EKG

SaO$_2$

PETCO$_2$

FIGURE 7–12. A polysomnographic tracing.

Obstructive apnea in suspect patients is documented by the use of the polysomnogram. The polysomnogram monitors chest wall and abdominal movement, oral and nasal airflow, heart rate and rhythm, arterial oxygen levels, and end-tidal CO$_2$ levels. The level of sleep is often determined by the use of electroencephalograms.

The pattern observed in obstructive apnea shows movement of the chest and abdomen, with no airflow at the nose or mouth. Significant apnea is present if the oxygen saturation drops 5% or more, the PaO$_2$ drops 8 mmHg or more, or end-tidal CO$_2$ increases 2% or more. A polysomnographic tracing is shown in Figure 7–12.

Treatment The treatment of obstructive apnea can range from pharmacologic agents to surgery. Antihistamines, decongestants, cromolyn sodium, and topical application of corticosteroids may help reduce the airway narrowing. Surgical correction normally involves the removal of the offending tissue or obstruction. Obstructive apnea may also be treated by the use of nasal CPAP during sleep periods to maintain a patent airway.

Nasal CPAP is used as an adjunct in the treatment of obstructive apnea, to stabilize and support the airway structures. The patients best suited for treatment with nasal CPAP are those suffering from obesity or those with enlarged or edematous tissues in the upper airways. CPAP mechanically holds the airway open during expiration, helping to prevent the airway collapse that leads to apnea.

SUMMARY

As is apparent from the length of this chapter, the consequences of premature birth are many and complex. Prematurity affects all organ systems, and the respiratory therapist must be aware that interaction between the systems is also diminished.

Of all the problems associated with prematurity, none is as significant in its implications as RDS. The premature respiratory system is often unable to adequately provide oxygenation and ventilation for the neonate. The main reason for this is underdevelopment resulting in a lack of surfactant, which makes the lungs very noncompliant. As compliance worsens, atelectasis ensues with widespread V/Q mismatching the blood gas instability. Work of breathing also increases significantly, wasting the valuable energy reserves of the patient. The resultant hypoxia causes damage to the capillaries and alveolar tissue. Soon, the neonate enters a cycle of hypoxemia, surfactant deficiency, atelectasis and tissue damage that, if not corrected, frequently leads to death.

A consequence of RDS is often BPD, also called neonatal chronic lung disease (CLD). The presence of BPD often requires the patient to remain on mechanical ventilation for long periods. Once off the ventilator, the patient often requires supplemental oxygen for long periods thereafter.

Pulmonary dysmaturity (Wilson–Mikity syndrome) is a disease similar to BPD; however, the patient often does not have RDS preceding its onset. Treatment of this, as well as the other pulmonary disorders, is mainly supportive with respiratory care procedures such as CPT and SVN used to aid lung recovery.

ROP is a disorder of the developing retina in which the retinal vasculature becomes constricted, leading to necrosis of the vessels. This is followed by a proliferation of new vessels in an attempt to reestablish the blood supply. This proliferation causes hemorrhage into the vitreous, scarring of the retina and possible detachment, and blindness. Treatment with laser is a promising technology.

Intraventricular bleeding is a major source of mortality and morbidity among the premature population. On the very tiniest of preemies, the simple act of raising the hips to place a diaper under may increase intracranial pressure enough to cause a bleed. Prevention is the key, because little can be done once the bleed has occurred. The bleeding is graded from I to IV, with grades III and IV resulting in the most sequelae.

Problems occurring in utero also cause some significant problems for the neonate. Fetal asphyxia can be secondary to maternal hypoxia, disruption of uteroplacental blood flow, dysfunction of the placenta, umbilical cord compression, or an intrinsic fetal disorder. Asphyxia leads to meconium release into the amniotic fluid, gasping, fetal heart decelerations, and if long enough, encephalopathy. The release of meconium predisposes the fetus to aspiration of the meconium. This can lead to serious pulmonary complications such as air trapping and V/Q imbalances.

The presence of RDS with resultant positive-pressure ventilation, combined with the fragility of the premature lung, often leads to air leak syndromes such as pneumothorax, pneumomediastinum, and pneumopericardium. An air leak that remains in the lung tissue is called pulmonary interstitial emphysema (PIE). Because the air dissects into the lung tissue, this type of air leak can be very difficult to treat and has serious consequences.

Persistent pulmonary hypertension of the neonate (PPHN) is often seen in term or postterm infants. Increased vascular resistance in the pulmonary vasculature causes blood to shunt away from the lungs and leads to profound mismatch between ventilation and perfusion. Traditionally, PPHN is treated with hyperventilation, which raises pH. The increasing pH causes some vasodilation of the pulmonary vessels and allows more blood to enter the lungs. A relatively new treatment involves the use of iNO, a powerful vasodilator. When inhaled in small quantities, nitric oxide has been shown to be successful in treating PPHN.

Transient tachypnea of the newborn, or RDS type II, is the result of retained lung water. It is often seen following cesarean delivery. Because it mimics RDS, the patient must be monitored closely and treated as needed. Most often, treatment involves only supplemental oxygen, but more aggressive treatments may be needed. CPT and postural drainage are often helpful in aiding the reabsorption of lung fluids.

Apnea in a newborn can either be the result of prematurity or obstruction. Either way, it can often avoid detection and is seen as frequent drops in the heart rate. Treatment involves the use of respiratory stimulants such as caffeine or theophylline, or correction of the obstruction. Polysomnography can be a useful adjunct in determining the cause and severity of apnea.

POSTTEST

1. You are working as a respiratory therapist on the night shift in the NICU. You are called to the delivery room and find a newborn infant with signs of distress, including expiratory grunting and nasal flaring. A pulse oximeter is placed and shows a saturation of 90% on room air. A chest x-ray is ordered. Which of the following would you expect to find on the x-ray?
   a. evidence of a pneumothorax
   b. a "ground glass" appearance to the lung fields
   c. hyperinflation of the lungs
   d. an enlarged cardiac silhouette

2. An urgent call comes from the emergency room notifying you of a 25-year-old woman, G2P1011 who has been admitted for premature labor at 28 weeks' gestation. One of the best options to help reduce the risk of RDS in the fetus if it delivers is:
   a. administer 100% oxygen to the mother
   b. administer terbutaline to the mother
   c. administer glucocorticoids to the mother
   d. place the mother in a Trendelenberg position

3. You are asked to assess, at 1 month postpartum, a 32-week baby with a history of PDA, and 3 weeks on a ventilator with high inspiratory pressures. The chances of the baby developing BPD is increased if which of the following is also present?
   a. history of fluid overload
   b. a forceps or vaccum assisted delivery
   c. a diagnosis of necrotizing enterocolitis
   d. a history of hypothermia

4. You are working with a 1-month-old neonate diagnosed with BPD. The neonatologist has ordered an increase in the caloric intake to the patient. Which of the following will need to be monitored closely?
   a. the possible need for increased oxygen demand
   b. the patient's abdominal girth
   c. the reaching of neurologic milestones
   d. any evidence of seizure activity
5. While examining the retina of an NICU patient, an ophthalmologist notes necrosis of the retinal vessels. This condition is called:
   a. strabismus
   b. glaucoma
   c. hereditary cataract
   d. vaso-obliteration
6. Of the following, which is linked to the most unfavorable outcomes with ROP?
   a. Stage 1 retinal injury in zone 3
   b. Stage 3 retinal injury in zone 1
   c. Stage 2 retinal injury in zone 2
   d. Any stage of retinal injury in zone 2
7. During an assessment, a 31-week-gestation neonate is found to have bulging fontanelles, hypotension, and a decreased hematocrit. A cranial ultrasound is ordered and shows bleeding into the germinal matrix extending into the ventricles. This represents what grade of IVH?
   a. Grade I
   b. Grade II
   c. Grade III
   d. Grade IV
8. You are called stat to the delivery room with a report of meconium stained amniotic fluid. The neonate is term. Upon delivery, you note that the infant has meconium on his skin. The recommended treatment is:
   a. immediate intubation and airway suctioning
   b. administer 100% oxygen via blowby
   c. chest physiotherapy with postural drainage for at least 20 minutes following delivery
   d. Observation is all that is needed.
9. You are called to the bedside of a 33-week-gestation neonate being mechanically ventilated. The peak pressures have gone up and the patient is cyanotic, bradycardic, and hypotensive. Auscultation of the lungs reveals diminished breath sounds. Your next step should be to:
   a. extubate the patient and begin bag/mask ventilation at 100% oxygen
   b. transilluminate the chest
   c. order a stat chest x-ray
   d. rapid IV infusion of sterile saline

10. A routine chest x-ray of a 30-week-gestation neonate being mechanically ventilated shows evidence of PIE. Which of the following strategies would best reduce harmful sequelae?
    a. start the patient on glucocorticoids
    b. reduce the delivered oxygen to keep the saturations between 85 and 90%
    c. maintain as low of ventilator pressures as possible without compromising oxygenation and ventilation
    d. start the patient on broad spectrum antibiotics

11. A newborn is suspected of having PPHN. Which of the following tests is the most accurate in helping to diagnose this disorder?
    a. chest x-ray with Doppler cardiac ultrasound
    b. VQ scan
    c. hyperoxia-hyperventilation test
    d. serial arterial blood gases every 30 minutes following an elevation in the inspired oxygen at 10% increments.

12. You are a respiratory therapist working in the NICU with a patient being treated with inhaled nitric oxide (iNO). The patient's oxygen saturation via pulse oximetry is 85% despite high levels of inspired oxygen. This could be a result of which of the following?
    a. methemoglobinemia
    b. the pulse oximeter is invalid in the presence of NO
    c. NO in the bloodstream causes a reduction in PaO_2
    d. iNO therapy frequently results in a re-opening of the ductus arteriosus

13. Which of the following is typically NOT seen in the presence of TTN?
    a. hypoxemia
    b. nasal flaring
    c. retractions
    d. hypercarbia

14. A patient with micrognathia is at risk for what type of apnea?
    a. apnea of prematurity
    b. obstructive apnea
    c. central apnea
    d. dysfunction of the respiratory centers

REFERENCES

1. Avery GB, Fletcher MA, MacDonald MG. *Pathophysiology and Management of the Newborn*. 5th ed. Philadelphia: JB Lippincott Co., 1999.
2. http://www.nlm.nih.gov/medlineplus/ency/article/001563.htm
3. Skelton R, Jeffery H. "Click test": rapid diagnosis of the respiratory distress syndrome. *Pediatr Pulmonol*. 17:383, 1994.
4. Moise AA, et al. Antenatal steroids are associated with less need for blood pressure supports in extremely premature infants. *Pediatrics*. 95:845–850, 1995.

5. Angle WA, et al. Surfactant-replacement therapy for respiratory distress in the preterm and term neonate. *Pediatrics*. 121(2): 419-432, Feb. 2008.

6. Zuzanna J, et al. Heated, humidified high-flow nasal cannula therapy: Yet another way to deliver continuous positive airway pressure? *Pediatrics*. 121:82, 2008.

7. Durand M, et al. Effects of early dexamethasone therapy on pulmonary mechanics and chronic lung disease in very low birthweight infants: a randomized, controlled trial. *Pediatrics*. 95:584, 1995.

8. Lee H, et al. Bronchodilator aerosol administered by metered dose inhaler and spacer in subacute neonatal respiratory distress syndrome. *Arch Dis Child*. 70: F218–F222, 1994.

9. Green TP, et al. Furosemide promotes patent ductus arteriosus in premature infants with respiratory distress syndrome. *N Engl J Med*. 308:743–748, 1983.

10. Cloherty JP, Stark AR, eds. *Manual of Neonatal Care*. 7th ed. Philadelphia, PA: Lippincott, 2012.

11. Northway WH, et al. Pulmonary disease following respiratory therapy for hyaline membrane disease. *N Engl J Med*. 276:357, 1967.

12. Strayer DS, et al. Levels of SP-A-Anti-SP-A immune complexes in neonatal respiratory distress syndrome correlates with subsequent development of bronchopulmonary dysplasia. *Acta Paediatr*. 84:128–131, 1995.

13. Watterberg IL, Scott SM. Evidence of early adrenal insufficiency in babies who develop bronchopulmonary dysplasia. *Pediatrics*. 95:120–125, 1995.

14. Merenstein GB, Gardner SL. *Handbook of Neonatal Intensive Care*. 7th ed. St. Louis, MO: CV Mosby Co., 2010.

15. Korones SB. *High-Risk Newborn Infants*. 4th ed. St. Louis, MO: CV Mosby Co., 1986.

16. Jacob J, et al. The contribution of PDA in the neonate with severe RDS. *J. Pediatr*. 96:79–87, 1979.

17. Nickerson B, Taussig L. Family history of asthma in infants with BPD. *Pediatrics*. 65:1140–1144, 1980.

18. Weinstein MR. A new radiographic scoring system for bronchopulmonary dysplasia. *Pediatr Pulmonol*. 18:284, 1994.

19. Stroustrup, Trasande. Epidemiological characteristics and resource use in neonates with bronchopulmonary dysplasia: 1993–2006 *Pediatrics* 126(2): 291–297, Aug. 2010.

20. Ibid, 292.

21. Hicks MA. A systemic approach to neonatal pathophysiology: understanding respiratory distress syndrome. *Neonatal Network*. 14:29–35, 1995.

22. Carlo WA, Chatburn RL. *Neonatal Respiratory Care*. 2nd ed. Chicago: Year-Book Medical Publishers Inc., 1988.

23. Lista G, et al. Volume guarantee versus high-frequency ventilation: lung inflammation in preterm infants Archives Of Disease In Childhood. *Fetal And Neonatal Edition*. 93(4):F252–F256, Jul. 2008.

24. Cabal L, et al. Effects of metaproterenol on pulmonary mechanics, oxygenation and ventilation in infants with chronic lung disease. *J. Pediatr*. 110:116, 1987.

25. Capers CC, et al. Use of theophylline in neonates as an aid to ventilator weaning. *Ther Drug Monit*. 14(6):471-4, Dec. 1992.

26. Larsen SC. Weaning neonates from mechanical ventilation: is there a right way? http://www.perspectivesinnursing.org/pdfs/Perspectives32.pdf.

27. Geary C, et al. Decreased incidence of bronchopulmonary dysplasia after early management changes, including surfactant and nasal continuous positive airway pressure treatment at delivery, lowered oxygen saturation goals, and early amino acid administration: a historical cohort study. *Pediatrics.* 121(1):89–96, Jan. 2008.

28. Vrlenich LA, et al. The effects of bronchopulmonary dysplasia on growth at school age. *Pediatrics.* 95:855, 1995.

29. Terry TL. Extreme prematurity and fibroblastic overgrowth of persistent vascular sheath behind each crystalline lens [preliminary report]. *Am J Ophthalmol.* 25:203, 1942.

30. Heath P. Pathology of the retinopathy of prematurity; retrolental fibroplasia. *Am J Ophthalmol.* 34:1249, 1951.

31. Bossi E, Koerner F. Retinopathy of prematurity. *Intensive Care Med.* 21:241–246, 1995.

32. Arroe M, Peitersen B. Retinopathy of prematurity: review of a seven-year period in a Danish neonatal intensive care unit. *Acta Paediatr.* 83:501–505, 1994.

33. National Eye Institute. Facts About Retinopathy of Prematurity. http://www.nei.nih.gov/health/rop/rop.asp#a.

33. Gilbert CE, et al. Causes of blindness and severe visual impairment in children in Chile. *Dev Med Child Neurol.* 36:326–333, 1994.

34. Keith CG, Doyle LW. Retinopathy of prematurity in extremely low birth weight infants. *Pediatrics.* 95:42–45, 1995.

35. George DS, et al. The latest on retinopathy of prematurity. *MCN.* 13:254–258, 1988.

36. Kushner BJ, Gloeckner E. Retrolental fibroplasia in full-term infants without exposure to supplemental oxygen. *Am J Ophthalmol.* 97:148–153, 1984.

37. Schulman J, et al. Peripheral proliferative retinopathy without oxygen therapy in a full-term infant. *Am J Ophthalmol.* 90:509–514, 1980.

38. Lucey JF, Dangman B. A reexamination of the role of oxygen in retrolental fibroplasia. *Pediatrics.* 73:82–96, 1984.

39. Wright K, Wright SP. Lack of association of glucocorticoid therapy and retinopathy of prematurity. *Arch Pediatr Adolesc Med.* 148:848–852, 1994.

40. Cryotherapy for Retinopathy of Prematurity Cooperative Group. The natural ocular outcome of premature birth and retinopathy. Status at one year. *Arch Ophthalmol.* 112:903–912, 1994.

41. Hunsucker K, et al. Laser surgery for retinopathy of prematurity. *Neonatal Network.* 14:21–26, 1995.

42. Kremer I, et al. Late visual field changes following cryotherapy for retinopathy of prematurity stage 3. *Br J Ophthalmol.* 79:267–269, 1995.

43. Seaber JH, et al. Long-term visual results of children after initially successful vitrectomy of stage V retinopathy of prematurity. *Ophthalmology.* 102:199–204, 1995.

44. VisionRX. Encyclopedia–Scleral Buckle http://www.visionrx.com/library/enc/enc_sbuckle.asp.

45. Holzman C, et al. Perinatal brain injury in premature infants born to mothers using alcohol in pregnancy. Neonatal brain hemorrhage study team. *Pediatrics.* 95:66–73, 1995.
46. Paneth N, et al. Incidence of timing of germinal matrix/intraventricular hemorrhage in low birth weight infants. *Am J Epidemiol.* 137:1167–1176, 1993.
47. Aziz K, et al. Province-based study of neurologic disability of children weighing 500 through 1249 grams at birth in relation to neonatal cerebral ultrasound. *Pediatrics.* 95:837–844, 1995.
48. Kritikos PG, Papadaki SP. The history of the poppy and of opium and their expansion in antiquity in the eastern Mediterranean area. http://www.unodc.org/unodc/en/data-and-analysis/bulletin/bulletin_1967-01-01_3_page004.html.
49. Sawyer TL, et al. Intubation and tracheal suctioning for meconium aspiration http://emedicine.medscape.com/article/1413467-overview.
50. Velaphi S, Vidyasagar D. Intrapartum and postdelivery management of infants born to mothers with meconium-stained amniotic fluid: evidence-based recommendations. *Clin Perinatol.* 33(1):29–42, Mar. 2006.
51. Ahanya SN, et al. Meconium passage in utero: mechanisms, consequences, and management. *Obstet Gynecol Surv.* 60(1):45–56, Jan. 2005.
52. Walsh MC, Fanaroff JM. Meconium stained fluid: approach to the mother and the baby. *Clin Perinatol.* 34(4):653–65, Dec. 2007.
53. Houlihan CM, Knuppel RA. Meconium-stained amniotic fluid. Current controversies. *J Reprod Med.* 39:888–898, 1994.
54. Clark MB, et al. Meconium aspiration syndrome http://emedicine.medscape.com/article/974110-overview#a0104.
55. Ghidini A, Spong CY. Severe meconium aspiration syndrome is not caused by aspiration of meconium. *Am J Obstet Gynecol.* 185(4):931–938, Oct. 2001.
56. ACOG Committee No. 346: Amnioinfusion does not prevent meconium aspiration syndrome. *Obstet & Gynecol.* 108(4):1053–1055, Oct. 2006.
57. ACOG Committee Opinion No. 379: Management of delivery of a newborn with meconium-stained amniotic fluid. *Obstet Gynecol.* 110(3):739, Sept. 2007
58. *Textbook of Neonatal Resuscitation.* 6th ed. Chicago: American Heart Association, American Academy of Pediatrics, 2011.
59. Sawyer TL, et al. Intubation and tracheal suctioning for meconium aspiration http://emedicine.medscape.com/article/1413467-overview.
60. Wiswell TE, Tuggle JM, Turner BS. Meconium aspiration syndrome: have we made a difference? *Pediatrics.* 85(5):715–729, May, 1990.
61. Collins MP, et al. Hypocapnia and other ventilation-related risk factors for cerebral palsy in low birth weight infants. *Pediatr Res.* 50(6):712–719, Dec. 2001.
62. El Shahed AI, et al. Surfactant for meconium aspiration syndrome in full term/near term infants. *Cochrane Database of Systematic Reviews* [serial online]. 2, 2007.
63. Clark MB, et al. Meconium aspiration syndrome treatment & management. http://emedicine.medscape.com/article/974110-treatment.
64. Goldsmith JP, Karotkin EH. *Assisted Ventilation of the Neonate.* 5th ed. Philadelphia, PA: WB Saunders Co., 2010.

65. Holowaty L. Nitric oxide. *Neonatal Network.* 14:83–86, 1995.

66. Sylvester, B. Down's syndrome newborns show higher incidence of idiopathic persistent pulmonary hypertension. http://www.docguide.com/downs -syndrome-newborns-show-higher-incidence-idiopathic-persistent-pulmonary -hypertension-presented.

67. http://emedicine.medscape.com/article/898437-overview#a1

68. Kinsella JP, Abman SH. Recent developments in the pathophysiology and treatment of persistent pulmonary hypertension of the newborn. *J Pediatr.* 126:853–864, 1995.

69. Fineman JR, et al. Chronic nitric oxide inhibition in utero produces persistent pulmonary hypertension in newborn lambs. *J Clin Invest.* 93:2675–2683, 1994.

70. Pearson DL, et al. Neonatal Pulmonary Hypertension—Urea-cycle intermediates, nitric oxide production, and carbamoyl-phosphate synthetase function. http://www.nejm.org/doi/full/10.1056/NEJM200106143442404.

71. Sallaam S, et al. Persistent newborn pulmonary hypertension. http://emedicine.medscape.com/article/898437-overview#aw2aab6b3.

72. Chambers CD, et al. Selective serotonin-reuptake inhibitors and risk of persistent pulmonary hypertension of the newborn. *N Engl J Med.* 354(6):579-87, Feb. 9, 2006.

73. El Shahed A, Surfactant for meconium aspiration syndrome in full term/near term infants. http://www.nichd.nih.gov/cochrane_data/shaheda_01/shaheda_01.html.

74. Sallaam S, et al. Persistent newborn pulmonary hypertension. http://emedicine.medscape.com/article/898437-overview#a11.

75. Finer NN, et al. Inhaled nitric oxide in infants referred for extracorporeal membrane oxygenation: dose response. *Pediatrics.* 124:302, 1994.

76. Roberts JD, et al. Inhaled nitric oxide in persistent pulmonary hypertension of the newborn. *Lancet.* 340:818–819, 1992.

77. Krishnamoorthy M, et al. Diagnosis and treatment of respiratory symptoms of initially unsuspected gastroesophageal reflux in infants. *Am Surg.* 60:783–785, 1994.

78. Buck ML, et al. Caffeine citrate for the treatment of apnea of prematurity. *Pediatr Pharm.* 14(6), 2008.

BIBLIOGRAPHY AND SUGGESTED READINGS

American Academy of Pediatrics Committee on Fetus and Newborn.Use of onhaled nitric oxide. *Pediatrics.* 106(2): 344–345, Aug. 1, 2000.

Chernick V, Boat TF. *Kendig's Disorders of the Respiratory Tract in Children.* 8th ed. Philadelphia, PA: WB Saunders Co., 2012.

DiBlasi RM, Myers TR, Hess DR. Evidence-based clinical practice guideline: inhaled nitric oxide for neonates with acute hypoxic respiratory failure. *Respir Care.* 55(12):1717–1745, 2010.

Medline Plus. Intraventricular hemorrhage of the newborn. Medline Plus. http://www.nlm.nih.gov/medlineplus/ency/article/007301.htm.

Medscape Reference. Persistent newborn pulmonary hypertension. http://emedicine.medscape.com/article/898437-overview.

Periventricular Hemorrhage-Intraventricular Hemorrhage. Medscape Reference. http://emedicine.medscape.com/article/976654-overview.

Soll RF. Inhaled nitric oxide in the neonate. *Journal of Perinatology* 29: S63–S67, May 2009.

Taussig LM, Landau LI. *Pediatric Respiratory Medicine.* 2nd ed. St. Louis, MO: Mosby, 2008.

UpToDate. Management and complications of intraventricular hemorrhage in the newborn. http://www.uptodate.com/contents/management-and-complications-of-intraventricular-hemorrhage-in-the-newborn.

CHAPTER 8

Causes of Persistent Perinatal Illness

OBJECTIVES

Upon completion of this chapter, the reader should be able to:

1. Explain how infections are acquired by the fetus and neonate.
2. Identify the organisms in the TORCH acronym.
3. Define chorioamnionitis and discuss the role of Group B strep in perinatal illness.
4. Describe the three stages of HIV and its pathophysiology.
5. Describe the following tests used to diagnose HIV: western blot, ELISA, PCR, P24 antigen, and HIV culture. For each list at least one advantage and disadvantage.
6. Briefly describe the following HIV medications and their mechanism of action in inhibiting HIV: Fusion inhibitors, integrase inhibitors, NNRTI's, NRTI's, and protease inhibitors.
7. Describe the postpartum care of the neonate exposed to HIV.
8. Identify the effects of cytomegalovirus, rubella, herpes simplex, and toxoplasmosis on the developing fetus.
9. Discuss each of the following as it relates to standard precautions and infection control:
   a. Hand hygiene
   b. Use of personal protective equipment
   c. Safe injection practices
   d. Safe handling of potentially contaminated equipment or surfaces in the patient environment
   e. Respiratory hygiene/cough etiquette
9. Describe the role of each of the following antibodies:
   a. IgA
   b. IgD
   c. IgE
   d. IgG
   e. IgM

10. Describe the pathophysiology, diagnosis, and treatment of the following:
    a. Tracheoesophageal anomalies
    b. Choanal atresia
    c. Micrognathia (Pierre-Robin sequence)
11. For each of the following cardiac anomalies, identify the defect from an artist's rendering and describe the diagnosis and treatment:
    a. Patent ductus arteriosus
    b. Atrial septal defect
    c. Ventricular septal defect
    d. Tetralogy of Fallot
    e. Complete transposition of the great vessels
    f. Subaortic stenosis
    g. Coarctation of the aorta
    h. Tricuspid atresia
    i. Anomalous venous return
    j. Truncus arteriosus
    k. Hypoplastic left heart syndrome
12. Describe the respiratory care of a neonatal patient with any of the above anomalies.

KEY TERMS

afterload	disseminated	hypoplastic
balloon septostomy	enzyme-linked	immunoglobulins (Ig)
choanal atresia	immunosorbent assay	petechiae
chorioamnionitis	(ELISA)	TORCH
color flow mapping	Fontan procedure	Western blot

INTRODUCTION

It's not unusual for children to have health problems during infancy. Most of the time the illness is short and doesn't interfere with their daily lives. This chapter will look at some of the conditions that have the possibility of affecting health on an ongoing basis in the neonate.

INFECTIONS

A neonate is susceptible to infection from several routes. Prenatal infection of the fetus always follows some degree of maternal involvement, which may be asymptomatic. An infection may be acquired prenatally either through the placenta, or an infection may ascend upward through the birth canal. During delivery, the fetus may become infected from direct contact with infected maternal tissue in the birth canal. Following delivery, the neonate is at risk of acquiring infection from NICU personnel, other patients, or the equipment being used for treatment.

As in most circumstances, the earlier the gestational age, the more vulnerable the neonate is to picking up an infection. Of interest is the emerging literature linking prenatal infections to the development of schizophrenia and autism.[1, 2, 3]

TORCH Complex

The acronym **TORCH** is used to identify those perinatal infections that are associated with severe fetal anomalies and even death. These infections include bacteria, viruses and protozoans. The most common use of the acronym is as follows:

T – Toxoplasmosis
O – Other
R – Rubella
C – Cytomegalovirus
H – Herpes simplex Type 2

The "other" infective agents are syphilis, HIV, coxsackie virus, varicella-zoster virus (chicken pox), and parvovirus B19.

In 2007, International Prenatal Infection Awareness Month was created to help educate pregnant women and prevent infection. In conjunction, the CDC has created a web page devoted to educating pregnant women in infection prevention.[4]

Implications for the Respiratory Therapist

Generally speaking, neonates and children with persistent illnesses require a team effort to deal with problems that often involve multiple organ systems. The respiratory therapist is an integral part of that team, providing support and care for all issues that involve the cardiopulmonary system. A thorough understanding of the pathophysiology of these chronic problems is necessary to anticipate problems that may arise early or late in the course of the disease.

BACTERIAL INFECTIONS

Bacterial infections in the neonate are often caused by organisms found in the maternal intestinal and genital tracts. Prenatally, although some organisms may enter the uterus through an intact amniotic membrane, most bacterial infections ascend the birth canal and enter the uterus through a rupture in the amniotic sac. Amniotic membranes ruptured for more than 24 hours before delivery greatly predispose the fetus to infection.

Once in the uterus, the organisms may enter the fetal mouth and infect the lungs, intestinal tract, and may even enter the bloodstream from one of these sites. The presence of bacteria in amniotic fluid begins an inflammatory response known as **chorioamnionitis**, characterized by an outpouring of leukocytes into the fluid from inflamed amniotic tissues. Chorioamnionitis does not always lead to fetal infection, it but greatly enhances the neonate's susceptibility. Chorioamnionitis is suspected when the neonate and birth fluids are malodorous, and it is diagnosed by culturing a tissue sample of the amniotic membrane.

Bacterial infections are also contracted from poor aseptic technique in the nursery or with equipment. One of the most common and challenging bacterial infections seen in neonatal care is pneumonia, covered in detail in Chapter 14.

Streptococcus agalactiae, or Group B strep (GBS), has arisen as a cause of serious illness and even death in the neonate. GBS is a normal flora of both the intestinal tract and the female genital tract and roughly 25% of females are colonized with the bacteria in the vagina. For this reason, the CDC recommends the universal prenatal screening for vaginal and rectal GBS colonization of all pregnant women at 35–37 weeks' gestation.[5] The various bacterial agents and their effects on the fetus are listed in Table 8–1.

Table 8–1

COMMON DISEASE-PRODUCING AGENTS IN THE FETUS AND NEWBORN

| Organism | Abortion | Intrauterine | | Congenital Disease | Neonatal Disease |
		Premature Birth	Growth Retardation		
VIRUS					
Hepatitis A	NE	SE	NE	NE	NE
Hepatitis B	NE	SE	NE	RA	SE
Herpes simplex (type I or II)	SE	SE	RA	RA	SE
Cytomegalovirus	QUA	SE	SE	SE	SE
Enterovirus (ECHO virus, poliomielitis, coxsackie virus A and B)	SE	QUA, RA	NE	RA	SE
Human immunodeficiency virus	QUA	QUA	QUA	SE	SE
Measles	SE	SE	NE	RA	RA
Respiratory syncytial virus	NE	NE	NE	NE	SE
Rubella	SE	SE	SE	SE	RA
Varicella	NE	NE	RA	RA	SE

BACTERIA

Group A streptococcus	SE	SE	NE	SE	SE
Group B streptococcus	SE	SE	NE	SE	SE
Group D streptococcus	NE	NE	NE	RA	SE
Anaerobic bacteria (*Bacteriodes, Clostridia, Peptostreptococcus, Veillonela*)	QUA	QUA	NE	RA	RA
Escherichia coli	QUA	QUA	NE	SE	SE
Hemophilus influenzae	NE	NE	NE	RA	SE
Staphylococcus aureus	NE	NE	NE	RA	SE
Staphylococcus epidermidis	NE	NE	NE	RA	RA
Klebsiella species	NE	NE	NE	RA	RA
Listeria monocytogenes	SE	SE	NE	SE	SE
Neisseria gonorrhoea	QUA	SE	NE	RA	SE
Neisseria meningitidis	NE	NE	NE	NE	SE
Proteus species (*Pseudomonas aeruginosa*)	NE	NE	NE	RA	RA
Salmonella species	NE	NE	NE	RA	SE
Shigella species	NE	NE	NE	RA	SE

SE = strong evidence for; NE = no evidence for; RA = rare association; QUA = questionable association.

Source: Bruhn FW, et al. Infection in the neonate. In Merenstein GB, Gardner SL, eds. *Handbook of Neonatal Intensive Care.* 7th ed. St. Louis: Elsevier, *2010.*

VIRAL INFECTIONS

Although viral infections are less common in the fetus and neonate, special attention is given them due to the serious effects that many of them have on the neonate. Refer to Table 8–1 for viral infections and their effect on the neonate.

Human Immunodeficiency Virus (HIV)

First identified in 1981, HIV is a retrovirus that infects humans by contact with mucous membranes and breaks in the skin. It has the unfortunate ability to mutate which enables it to become resistant to previously effective medications. In general, the virus is slowly progressive with infection being divided into three stages. The first stage is identified as the primary infection and usually occurs within several weeks of exposure to the virus. Primary infection often manifests with flu-like symptoms that resolve after several weeks. The second stage is a time of chronic infection in which the patient is asymptomatic. This stage can last up to 8 to 10 years. The final stage is symptomatic infection in which the immune system is suppressed and complications begin to develop. This stage is also called the acquired immunodeficiency syndrome or AIDS. At this stage, the HIV has severely damaged the immune system, putting these patients at risk for opportunistic infections.

The overriding goal of drug therapy is to stop the suppression of the immune system by the virus and delay the progression of the infection.

Risk Factors A vast majority (93%) of neonatal HIV infection is acquired from an infected mother during pregnancy, labor and delivery, or by breast feeding.[6] Therefore, the primary risk factors for prenatal infection involve high-risk parental (primarily maternal) activities, such as: IV drug use and exposure to infected bodily fluids. The remaining cases are acquired by exposure to infected blood products, exposure to infected breast milk, and a small percentage in which the cause is unknown.

Transmission With regard to prenatal HIV infection, the virus passes transplacentally from the infected mother to the fetus. It apparently crosses early, as antibodies specific to HIV have been found as early as 9 weeks' gestation.[7] Not all HIV-infected mothers pass the virus to the fetus. A study by Goedert and associates found that the presence of certain antibodies in the mother may prevent the transmission of the virus.[8] A reduction of nearly two thirds in the transmission rate was seen in a study where zidovudine was given before delivery to the mother and then for 6 weeks to the neonate.[9]

During delivery, the fetus may acquire the virus by contact with maternal blood.[10] Postdelivery, feeding with infected breast milk, and transfusion with infected blood products serve as other transmission mechanisms. Unfortunately, sexual abuse by an infected adult is another possible cause of transmission that must be considered in older pediatric patients.

AIDSinfo, a service of the U.S. Department of Health and Human Services (HHS), recommends combined antepartum, intrapartum, and infant antiretroviral prophylaxis to prevent perinatal transmission of HIV.[11]

Pathophysiology The causative organism of AIDS is the retrovirus HIV-1. Upon entering the body, it infects the T-helper lymphocytes (T4) by attaching to the CD4+ molecule. It also infects monocytes, macrophages, and cells of the central nervous system. Once the T4 cell is infected, it is destroyed by the virus. This results in abnormal humoral and cell-mediated immunity. This insidious destruction of the immune system makes the patient vulnerable to opportunistic infections that are usually kept in check by the immune system.

Diagnosis Current methods to diagnose AIDS infection are based on the presence of serum antibodies against the HIV. Current tests detect the presence of antibodies, antigens, or RNA of the HIV in the serum, saliva, or urine. In the serum, the **enzyme-linked immunosorbent assay (ELISA)** and **Western blot** tests, if positive, show the presence of antibodies against the HIV, not the actual presence of the HIV. Of the two, the Western blot is more specific and has a higher sensitivity. It is always run following a positive ELISA test. Both tests are nondiagnostic in patients under 14 months, because both tests may be positive from antibodies passed transplacentally from the mother, when in reality, the infant has not been exposed to the virus.

Several new techniques are being used to diagnose HIV infection. These include polymerase chain reaction (PCR), which detects HIV DNA or RNA sequence, P24 antigen, HIV cultures, enzyme-linked immunospot (ELISPOT) which is a modified version of the ELISA test, in vitro antibody production assay (IVAP), and IgA and IgM assays.

Of the new techniques, PCR detects the presence of the virus and not the antibodies, making it more promising for diagnosis in newborns. Both the P24 antigen and HIV cultures take 2 to 5 weeks to get results, which is a disadvantage to their use. ELISPOT detects antibody-secreting cells. HIV infection stimulates the infant's immune system to produce antibody-producing B lymphocytes, which can then be detected by IVAP. Because both IgA and IgM molecules do not pass through the placenta, their increasing level in the infant signals HIV infection. When HIV is perinatally acquired, the infection can be diagnosed by the time the child is 4 to 6 months of age with the use of current tests available. Rapid, point of care tests can be done in the office or at home and use blood, saliva, or urine to check for the presence of HIV antibodies. Any positive point of care test should be verified with a Western blot.

Treatment The treatment of HIV is complex and ever changing. Due to frequent resistance issues, HIV treatment is always done with combination therapy. Current treatment regimens include the following categories of medications: fusion inhibitors, integrase inhibitors, non-nucleoside reverse transcriptase inhibitor, nucleoside reverse transcriptase inhibitor, and protease inhibitor.[12]

Fusion Inhibitors Fusion inhibitors work by blocking HIV's ability to merge with and infect healthy cells. Examples of this type of medicine are enfuvirtide and maraviroc.

Integrase Inhibitors Integrase inhibitors work by blocking integrase, an HIV enzyme. Blocking integrase prevents the integration of HIV DNA into the host DNA. Raltegravir is this type of medicine.

Non-Nucleoside Reverse Transcriptase Inhibitor (NNRTI) NNRTIs work by binding to and blocking HIV reverse transcriptase, an HIV enzyme. This prevents HIV RNA from converting to DNA. NNRTIs are always used in combination with other anti-HIV medications. Current NNRTIs include delavirdine mesylate, efavirenz, etravirine, nevirapine, and rilpivirine hydrochloride.

Nucleoside Reverse Transcriptase Inhibitor (NRTI) NRTIs are similar to NNRTIs in that they also work by blocking HIV reverse transcriptase. NRTIs differ slightly in that they do not bind the virus structure in the way NNRTIs do. Two NRTIs are always given together as combination therapy and are the drug of choice over the NNRTIs. Examples of NRTIs include abacavir, zidovudine, didanosine, emtricitabine, lamivudine, stavudine, and tenofovir disoproxil fumerate.

Protease Inhibitor (PI) Protease inhibitors work by blocking the cleavage of viral DNA into mature virus particles that are then packaged and excreted from infected cells. PIs have a major interaction with the CYP450 enzyme system and must be used with caution. Like NRTIs, PIs are always used in combination with other HIV medications and are often combined with ritonavir for enhancement. Preferred combinations with ritonavir include atazanavir and darunavir. Other examples of PIs include fosamprenavir, indinavir, lopinavir, nelfinavir, saquinavir and tipranavir.

Postpartum Care of the Neonate Exposed to HIV Recommendations have been proposed for the follow-up care and treatment of neonates born to HIV infected mothers. These recommendations by the HHS sponsored AIDSinfo, include a complete blood count (CBC) and differential to be done soon after delivery and before the initiation of ARV therapy. The initial CBC serves as a baseline. All treatment decisions depend on the baseline hematologic values. Zidovudine, at gestational-age-appropriate doses, should be initiated as close to the time of birth as possible, preferably within 6 to 12 hours of delivery. In addition to the CBC, gestational age at birth, clinical condition of the infant, the dose of zidovudine being administered, the receipt of other ARV drugs and concomitant medications, and maternal antepartum ARV therapy should all be evaluated when making treatment decisions. Virologic tests are required to diagnose HIV infection in infants <18 months of age and should be performed within the first 14 to 21 days of life, at 1 to 2 months, and at 4 to 6 months of age. Infants born to HIV-infected women who have not received antepartum antiretroviral (ARV) drugs should receive prophylaxis with zidovudine given for 6 weeks, combined with three doses of nevirapine in the first week of life (at birth, 48 hours later, and 96 hours after the second dose), begun as soon after birth as possible. All infants born to women with HIV infection should begin PCP prophylaxis at ages 4 to 6 weeks, after completing their ARV prophylaxis regimen, unless there is adequate test information to presumptively exclude HIV infection.

Cytomegalovirus (CMV)

CMV is a member of the herpes virus family, designated as human herpesvirus 5, and is passed transplacentally from the asymptomatic mother, via aspiration of secretions in the birth canal and by breastfeeding. CMV is most devastating to the fetus early in gestation, while having few, if any, effects on the term neonate. Of all the human herpes viruses, CMV causes the most morbidity and mortality.[13] Patients with suspected CMV infections should not be treated by any pregnant personnel. The wearing of gloves when handling urine and secretions and good hand washing help prevent the spread of the virus.

Symptoms include intrauterine growth retardation, direct hyperbilirubinemia secondary to liver damage, hepatosplenomegaly, microcephaly, brain damage, and progressive sensorineural hearing loss. Treatment consists primarily of nutritional support and general supportive care.

Rubella

Rubella infections of the fetus in the first 5 months of gestation have a high incidence of congenital abnormalities. Rubella is preventable by appropriate vaccination of the mother before conception.

Symptoms of early gestation infection include cataracts, cardiac defects, hearing loss, intrauterine growth retardation, chronic encephalitis, direct hyperbilirubinemia, and microcephaly. The various organs of the growth-retarded fetus are underdeveloped (**hypoplastic**) as the rubella virus impairs the proliferation of cells, if acquired in early gestation. The combined presence of cataracts and congenital cardiac disease strongly suggests the diagnosis of congenital rubella infection.

Herpes Simplex Types I and II

Type I herpes is the common variety of the virus that causes recurrent lesions on the lips and on other parts of the skin, usually above the waist. Type II is the variety most commonly acquired by the neonate. Following infection, the viruses become latent in the sensory neural ganglia.

The fetus is infected by the ascent of the virus up the birth canal, from infected genitalia, or from the direct contact with infected tissues during delivery. There may also be a rare transplacental passage of the virus. The fetus of a mother with known Type II herpes is best delivered via cesarean delivery, although the possibility of infection still exists.

In the infected neonate, symptoms are both **disseminated**, or widespread, and nondisseminated. or localized. Neonates with disseminated symptoms have a 96% mortality rate, while those with nondisseminated symptoms have a 25% mortality rate. Disseminated symptoms include hepatosplenomegaly, hepatitis with jaundice, bleeding disorders, widespread skin lesions, and neurologic abnormalities. Convulsions, abnormal muscle tone, bulging fontanelle, lethargy, and coma are common neurologic abnormalities. The nondisseminated forms of the disease attack the eyes, central nervous system, and the skin.

Diagnosis is usually made from cultures of the virus from skin lesions. Some studies have shown a decreased mortality from herpes infections in the neonate with the use of adenine arabinoside (ara-A).

Several antiviral drugs are available for the treatment of herpes simplex and zoster. Acyclovir (Zovirax®) is indicated for the treatment of neonatal herpes simplex, varicella zoster with CNS and pulmonary involvement, and herpes simplex encephalitis.[14] Two newer antiviral drugs, famcyclovir (Famvir®) and valacyclovir (Valtrex®) have shown significant effectiveness in the treatment of herpes and may gain use in the neonatal and pediatric populations in the future.

PROTOZOAL AND FUNGAL INFECTIONS

Protozoa are single-celled parasites that can cause human infection. Like most parasites, they are opportunistic. These infections are rare in the United States, but more common in underdeveloped countries.

Toxoplasmosis

Toxoplasma gondii is the protozoa organism responsible for toxoplasmosis infections. It is contracted by the mother via contact with cat feces or from eating raw meat. The organism is transmitted from the mother to the fetus through the placenta. The infected mother may be asymptomatic or may show influenza-like signs.

Transmission of the disease occurs mainly during the third trimester for unknown reasons. In the neonate, symptoms may be present immediately or may be delayed for several weeks. Those symptoms include neurological abnormalities such as microcephaly, coma, convulsions, and hydrocephalus. Other symptoms are hepatosplenomegaly, jaundice with both direct and indirect hyperbilirubinemia, small skin hemorrhages (**petechiae**), and pallor secondary to anemia.

Diagnosis is verified by the presence of specific toxoplasma IgM antibodies in the blood serum.

Pneumocystis carinii

Pneumocystis carinii, recently renamed *Pneumocystis jiroveci*, is an inhaled yeast-like fungus that is seen primarily in immunocompromised patients, such as those with HIV/AIDS. It is the most common opportunistic infection in these patients, and even though it is classified as a fungus, it does not respond to antifungal medications.

The initial workup includes measuring the LDH (lactic dehydrogenase). LDH levels typically elevate in patients infected with HIV who also have pneumocystis. Another promising test is the β-D-glucan, which is found in the cell wall of the pneumocystis.[15]

The treatment of pneumocystis is dependent upon the degree of illness when the diagnosis is made. The degree of illness is determined by the alveolar-arterial gradient and is classified as mild (<35 mmHg), moderate/severe (35–45 mmHg) and severe (>45 mmHg). Treatment primarily consists of trimethoprim–sulfamethoxazole for 21 days.

DIAGNOSIS AND TREATMENT OF INFECTION

In most instances, diagnosis of infection is made by isolating and identifying the antigen from specimens taken from the neonate or by serologic diagnosis, which shows an antibody response to the specific agent.

Viral diseases are treated by proper prevention of the disease in the mother. Proper immunization against rubella in the mother will prevent fetal infection. Toxoplasmosis is best prevented by avoidance of cat litter boxes and raw meat by pregnant mothers and by those attempting to get pregnant.

Bacterial infections may be treated by administering broad-spectrum antibiotics to the neonate until the pathogen is identified. Upon identification of the causative organism and its sensitivities, a specific antibiotic is selected. The ideal antibiotic will be the least toxic to the patient and lethal to the organism. Many institutions will administer broad-spectrum antibiotics for 48 to 72 hours any time the amniotic membranes have been ruptured for more than 24 hours, due to the high risk of infection imposed upon the fetus.

It is often very difficult to differentiate between bacterial pneumonia and RDS. For this reason, the respiratory therapist must closely monitor the patient's ventilatory status and be prepared to ventilate the patient if the status worsens.

PREVENTION OF INFECTION

The Centers for Disease Control and Prevention (CDC) have developed protocols for minimum infection prevention practices that apply to all patient care, regardless of suspected or confirmed infection status of the patient, in any setting where health care is delivered. Key areas identified by the CDC as standard precautions include hand hygiene, use of personal protective equipment, safe injection practices, safe handling of potentially contaminated materials and equipment in the patient environment, and respiratory hygiene/cough etiquette. Each of these elements is summarized in Table 8–2.[16]

Table 8–2

STANDARD PRECAUTIONS

1. Hand hygiene: Use of alcohol-based hand rubs is the preferred method for hand hygiene with two exceptions: when hands are visibly soiled with dirt, blood, or body fluids and after caring for suspected infectious diarrhea. In both cases, soap and water should be used. Hand hygiene should be performed:
   - Before touching a patient, even if gloves are to be worn
   - Before exiting the patient's care area after touching the patient or the patient's immediate environment
   - After contact with blood, body fluids, excretions, or wound dressings
   - Prior to performing an aseptic task such as placing an IV or preparing an injection
   - If the hands will be moving from a contaminated body site to a clean body site during patient care
   - After glove removal

2. Personal protective equipment (PPE): PPE is wearable and intended to protect the health care provider from exposure to or contact with infectious agents. Items include gloves, gowns, face shields and masks, goggles, and respirators. Recommendations include:
   - Sufficient and appropriate PPE should always be available and readily accessible.
   - All health care providers should be educated on the proper selection and use of PPE.

continues on the next page

Table 8–2

continued from the previous page

- Remove and discard PPE before leaving the patient room or area.
- Wear gloves for potential contact with blood, body fluids, mucous membranes, non-intact skin, or contaminated equipment.
- Do not wear the same gloves for the care of more than one patient.
- Do not wash gloves for the purpose of reuse.
- Perform hand hygiene immediately after removing gloves.
- Wear a gown to protect skin and clothing during procedures or activities where contact with blood or body fluids is anticipated.
- Do not wear the same gown for the care of more than one patient.
- Wear mouth, nose, and eye protection during procedures that are likely to generate splashes or sprays of blood or other body fluids.
- Wear a surgical mask when placing a catheter or injecting material into the spinal canal or subdural space.

3. Injection Safety: Injection safety is intended to prevent the transmission of infectious diseases between one patient and another, or between a patient and health care provider during the preparation and administration of parenteral medications.
   - Use aseptic technique when preparing and administering medications.
   - Cleanse the access diaphragms of medication vials with 70% alcohol before inserting a device into the vial.
   - Never administer medications from the same syringe to multiple patients, even if the needle is changed or the injection is administered through an intervening length of intravenous tubing.
   - Do not reuse a syringe to enter a medication vial or solution.
   - Do not administer medications from single-dose or single-use vials, ampoules, or bags or bottles of intravenous solution to more than one patient.
   - Do not use fluid infusion or administration sets for more than one patient.
   - Dedicate multidose vials to a single patient where possible. If multidose vials will be used for more than one patient, they should be restricted to a centralized medication area and should not enter the immediate patient treatment area.
   - Dispose of used syringes and needles at the point of use in a sharps container that is closable, puncture-resistant, and leak-proof.
   - Adhere to federal and state requirements for protection of the health care provider from exposure to bloodborne pathogens.

4. Environmental cleaning: The cleaning and disinfection of environmental surfaces is an essential part of an infection prevention plan. Emphasis should be placed on surfaces that are most likely to become contaminated with pathogens, both those in close proximity to the patient and frequently touched surfaces in the patient care environment.

- Establish policies and procedures for routine cleaning and disinfection of environmental surfaces in ambulatory care settings.
- Focus on those surfaces in proximity to the patient and those that are frequently touched.
- Select EPA-registered disinfectants or detergents/disinfectants with label claims for use in health care.
- Follow manufacturer's recommendations for use of cleaners and EPA-registered disinfectants.

5. Medical equipment: Medical equipment is labeled by the manufacturer as either reusable or single-use. Reusable medical equipment should be accompanied by instructions for cleaning and disinfection or sterilization as appropriate. Single-use devices may not be reprocessed except by entities cleared by the FDA.
   - Facilities should ensure that reusable medical equipment is cleaned and reprocessed appropriately prior to use on another patient.
   - Reusable medical equipment must be cleaned and reprocessed and maintained according to the manufacturer's instructions. If the manufacturer does not provide such instructions, the device may not be suitable for multipatient use.
   - Assign responsibilities for reprocessing of medical equipment to health care providers with appropriate training.
   - Ensure health care providers have access to and wear appropriate PPE when handling and reprocessing contaminated patient equipment.

6. Respiratory hygiene/cough etiquette: This strategy is targeted primarily at patients and accompanying family members or friends with undiagnosed transmissible respiratory infections, and applies to any person with signs of illness including cough, congestion, rhinorrhea, or increased production of respiratory secretions when entering the facility.
   - Implement measures to contain respiratory secretions in patients and accompanying individuals who have signs and symptoms of a respiratory infection, beginning at point of entry to the facility and continuing throughout the duration of the visit.
   - Post signs at entrances with instructions to patients with symptoms of respiratory infection to:
     - Cover their mouths/noses when coughing or sneezing
     - Use and dispose of tissues
     - Perform hand hygiene after hands have been in contact with respiratory secretions
   - Provide tissues and no-touch receptacles for disposal of tissues.
   - Provide resources for performing hand hygiene in or near waiting areas.

continues on the next page

Table 8–2

continued from the previous page

- Offer masks to coughing patients and other symptomatic persons upon entry to the facility.
- Provide space and encourage persons with symptoms of respiratory infections to sit as far away from others as possible. If available, facilities may wish to place these patients in a separate area while waiting for care.
- Educate health care providers on the importance of infection prevention measures to contain respiratory secretions to prevent the spread of respiratory pathogens when examining and caring for patients with signs and symptoms of a respiratory infection.

Source: Centers for Disease Control and Prevention Guide to Infection Prevention for Outpatient Settings: Minimum Expectations for Safe Care. Atlanta: Centers for Disease Control and Prevention, 2011.

FETAL IMMUNITIES

The fetus is endowed with certain immunities from its mother and also produces immunities of its own. These immunities are in the form of antibodies. An antibody is a type of protein produced by plasma cells in response to the presence of an antigen. An antigen is defined as anything that stimulates the production of antibodies.

The immunities that will be examined circulate in the plasma and are called **immunoglobulins (Ig)**. Immunoglobulins are classified into five classes: IgA, IgD, IgE, IgG, and IgM. Of the five classes IgA, IgG, and IgM play major roles in the immunities of the neonate.

IgA Antibody

IgA is not transported transplacentally and is not produced by the neonate until approximately 1 month of age. The importance of the IgA antibody lies in a subclass of antibody called secretory IgA. Secretory IgA is found in tears, saliva, bronchial and intestinal secretions, and breast milk. Its presence enables the body to defend against antigens at the source of entry into the body. Breast-fed neonates gain immunity from the IgA in the milk while their own systems are maturing. Breast milk IgA protects the intestinal system from *Escherichia coli, Vibrio cholerae,* poliovirus, and rotovirus.[17] As the neonate grows, it begins producing and secreting its own IgA.

IgD Antibody

The IgD antibody is a specialized protein found in serum tissue. The exact role of IgD is not known, but it increases in quantity in the presence of allergic reactions to milk, penicillin, insulin, and various toxins.

IgE Antibody

IgE is concentrated in the lung, skin, and the cells of the mucous membranes. IgE is responsible for allergic reactions that cause the release of the allergic mediators from the mast cell. It provides the primary defense against environmental antigens.

IgG Antibody

The IgG antibody is the only immunoglobulin that is transported through the placenta from mother to fetus. It accumulates in the fetus during the third trimester, reaching its highest level at birth. Because the majority of antibodies in the maternal circulation are of the IgG fractions, the fetus receives a healthy portion of them.

The IgG antibody protects the neonate from infections to which the mother has acquired immunity. These infections include pneumococcus, streptococcus, meningococcus, *Hemophilus influenzae,* viruses, and the toxins of tetanus and diphtheria. The baby begins to synthesize its own IgG antibody as the maternal level falls to lower levels. This occurs around the third month following delivery.

IgM Antibody

The IgM antibody is produced by the fetus around the 30th week of gestation and does not cross the placenta from the mother. Any IgM present at birth represents the baby's own synthesis of the antibody. The measurement of IgM levels in the neonate is used to detect the presence of infection. IgM levels do not rise for a week to 10 days following the appearance of disease. This makes it unreliable for early detection of infection. IgM levels rapidly increase during the first month of life and then gradually slow.

IgM synthesis is stimulated by most infectious organisms and is the main fetally produced antibody present in the baby.

CONGENITAL ANOMALIES

Congenital anomalies are those birth defects that are present from the time of birth. They can be mild or severe enough to become life-threatening. Congenital anomalies have a variety of causes and can occur during pregnancy or at birth. Common causes are genetic malformations and in-utero viral infections but many times a cause cannot be found.

Pulmonary System Anomalies

Anomalies in the pulmonary system are often associated with gastric anomalies; however, the pulmonary system can also develop anatomic abnormalities that can greatly affect the health of the newborn.

Tracheoesophageal Anomalies Atresia of the upper esophagus, with an accompanying fistula between the lower esophageal tube and the trachea, shown in Figure 8–1A, accounts for 75% to 80% of all tracheoesophageal anomalies. Other combinations of atresias and fistulas occur in much less frequency.

The next most common problem, accounting for about 8% of esophageal anomalies, is atresia of the esophagus, without any fistula attachment to the trachea, shown in Figure 8–1B. Other possible combinations, occurring very infrequently, are the so-called H-type fistula, illustrated in Figure 8–1C; esophageal atresia with attachment of the upper esophagus to the trachea, depicted in Figure 8–1D; and attachment of the upper and lower portions of the esophagus to the trachea, represented in Figure 8–1E.

Diagnosis and Treatment Diagnosis of tracheoesophageal anomalies is usually based on the presence of three distinct clinical symptoms: 1) accumulation of secretions in the mouth, 2) sporadic or continuous respiratory distress, especially during feedings, and 3) repeated regurgitation of feelings.

In the presence of these signs, insertion of a nasogastric tube (NG) is attempted. Air is then injected into the catheter while listening with a stethoscope over the stomach. Absence of any sounds in the stomach requires the obtaining of a CXR. The air-filled pouch of the esophageal atresia can often be visualized on the x-ray.

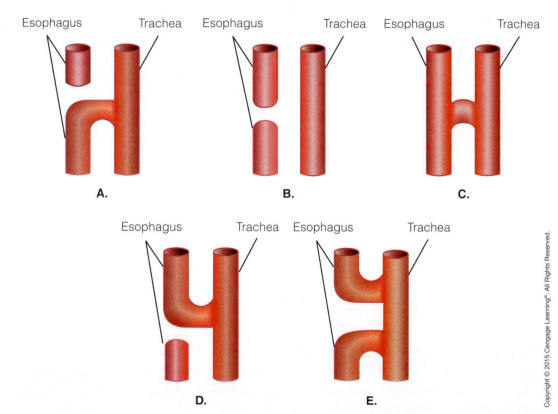

FIGURE 8–1. A. The most common variety of tracheoesophageal anomaly. B. Esophageal atresia without a fistula to the trachea. C. The "H" type of tracheoesophageal anomaly. D. A lower esophageal atresia with upper attachment to the trachea. E. Upper and lower attachment of the esophagus to the trachea.

Upon diagnosis of this disorder, the patient should be kept in a 30° upright position to help prevent aspiration. Treatment is always surgical repair of the defect. Although not an emergency procedure, the surgical repair of the defect should be done as quickly as possible. Surgical correction is done through an incision in the right retropleural area. The distal esophagus is divided from the trachea, and the ends of the esophagus are sutured together.

Caregivers should observe the patient for signs of worsening ventilatory status that may follow aspiration pneumonitis.

Choanal Atresia The portion of the nasal cavity that opens into the nasopharynx is called the choana. **Choanal atresia**, illustrated in Figure 8–2, occurs when the membrane that separates the nasal cavity from the nasopharynx during embryologic development fails to disintegrate and blocks the passage of air.

This defect is apparent almost immediately in the neonate, as severe respiratory distress is usually present. The neonate's reliance on nasal breathing as its prime

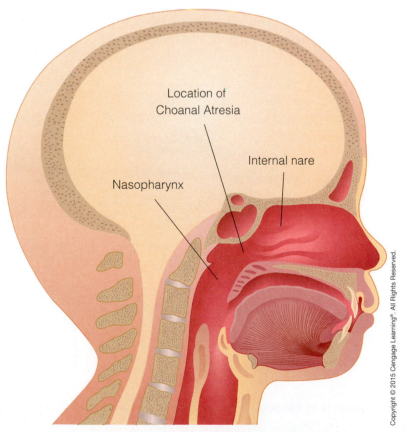

Location of
Choanal Atresia

Internal nare

Nasopharynx

FIGURE 8–2. Choanal atresia located at the opening to the nasopharynx.

method of ventilation accounts for the severity of the distress. Choanal atresia is suspected as respiratory distress improves when the neonate cries. Diagnosis is verified by the inability to pass an NG tube past the obstruction.

Immediate treatment requires the use of an oral airway. Some neonates may require intubation to relieve the distress. Long-term treatment involves surgical removal of the membranes covering the choanae.

Pierre-Robin Sequence (Micrognathia) Pierre-Robin sequence has in the past been referred to as a "syndrome"; however, it is the result of several events that occur early in development and is more appropriately referred to as a "condition." It can occur alone or as part of another disorder. More than 30 syndromes have been identified that include Pierre-Robin sequence within their symptoms.[18] Essentially, it is hypoplasia of the mandible, which forces the tongue to be positioned posteriorly in the pharynx, creating an obstruction to breathing. Estimates of its frequency vary between 1 out of 8000 births and 1 in 30,000 births. As many as 50% to 70% have a concurrent cleft palate. The diagnosis is made by observation of a short jaw or receding chin during examination (Figure 8–3).

The treatment is to maintain the patient's airway patency until the mandible grows to its appropriate size, usually by 6 months to a year of age. This may require procedures such as facial slings, metal appliances passed through the lips to support the tongue, suturing the tongue to traction, and tracheostomy.

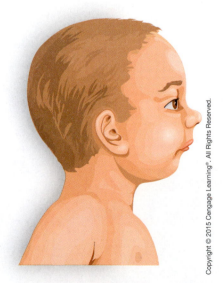

FIGURE 8–3. Physical features seen upon assessment of a child with Pierre-Robin Sequence.

Care should be taken during feedings to prevent choking on formula. Special feeders (Breck) are used to prevent aspiration. Often the patient's airway patency is maintained by having the neonate in a face-down position while sleeping.

Cardiac System

Congenital cardiac defects occur in approximately 1 out of 100 deliveries. Depending on the type and degree of defect, the patient may have mild signs that require no intervention or may have life-threatening symptoms that require immediate intervention. This section will look at the different types of cardiac defects, their signs, diagnosis, and treatment.

Patent Ductus Arteriosus (PDA) Anatomically, the ductus arteriosus connects the pulmonary artery to the aorta, shunting blood away from the lungs in the fetus. The smooth musculature that surrounds the ductus arteriosus develops toward the end of gestation. The vessel is maintained patent in the fetus by the presence of prostaglandins, which causes the smooth muscle to remain in a dilated state.

Closure of the ductus arteriosus following delivery is caused by several factors, including blood oxygen tension, levels of circulating prostaglandins, and the muscle mass present in the vessel. Studies have additionally connected the constrictive effects of acetylcholine, low pH, bradykinin, and catecholamines to ductal closure.[17] Closure of the ductus arteriosus usually occurs a few hours to a few days following delivery.

Pathophysiology As the pressure in the pulmonary vasculature drops below arterial pressure, blood is shunted from the aorta through the ductus arteriosus into the pulmonary system, creating a left-to-right shunt, as shown in Figure 8–4A. The blood shunted into the pulmonary artery greatly increases intrapulmonary vascular and right-heart pressures. The result is a hyperperfusion and engorgement of the pulmonary vessels with resulting pulmonary edema. When large amounts of blood are shunted through the ductus, hypoperfusion occurs to all postductal organs and tissues, leading to necrotizing enterocolitis and other disorders. Right-sided heart failure may follow long bouts with a PDA. If pulmonary vascular pressures exceed aortic pressures, blood is shunted from the pulmonary artery to the aorta, creating a right-to-left shunt, depicted in Figure 8–4B.

A PDA is not always undesirable. In the presence of certain heart defects, such as transposition of the great vessels, a PDA may be the only life-sustaining connection between pulmonary and systemic circulation. In this instance, it is desirable for the ductus arteriosus to remain open. This can be accomplished by the administration of prostaglandin E_1 (PGE_1), which can reopen a constricted ductus arteriosus and prevent the ductus from closing.

PGE_1 is indicated for any defect in which the left heart is obstructed or pulmonary perfusion is decreased. Following the administration of the drug, arterial

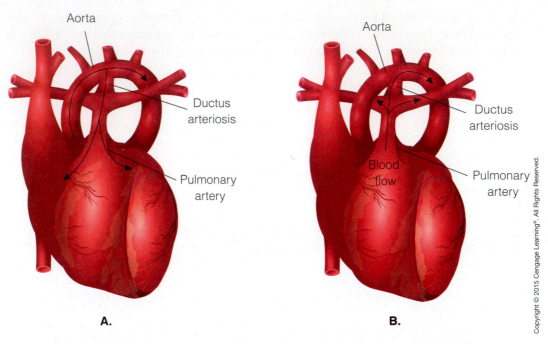

FIGURE 8–4. A. Left-to-right shunt through the ductus arteriosus. B. Right-to-left shunt through the ductus arterious resulting from pulmonary vascular pressure exceeding aortic pressure.

oxygen levels improve and pulmonary congestion decreases, reducing the level of ventilatory support needed. Improvement in patient condition following administration of PGE_1 depends on the degree of ductal patency before the drug is given, with patients having total ductal closure showing the most dramatic improvements.

Diagnosis Diagnosis of a PDA involves both clinical symptoms and laboratory data. The most common indication of a PDA is a loud grade I to grade III systolic murmur heard at the upper-left sternal border. Some describe the murmur as sounding like a washing machine.

Positive identification of a PDA is made by ultrasound in which the ductus arteriosus is visible between the aorta and pulmonary artery. Advances in Doppler have made it possible to gauge the direction and velocity of blood in the heart by using colors. Typically, blood going one direction is red and that going the opposite direction is blue; however, a wide variety of hues is possible as direction and velocity changes. This process, called **color flow mapping**, can aid in detecting the direction of blood flow through the ductus. In the absence of color flow mapping, the direction of blood flow through the ductus can be determined using oxygen and noninvasive monitors.

A right-to-left shunt through a PDA is indicated when low arterial oxygen levels do not change with increases in F_iO_2. Placement of a pulse oximeter or $TcPO_2$ monitor preductally on the right arm and another postductally on the abdomen or lower extremities shows the higher preductal oxygen level, further indicating a right-to-left ductal shunt.

Left-to-right shunting is indicated by signs of congestive heart failure and pulmonary edema. The chest x-ray will show cardiomegaly with increased pulmonary vascularity.

Treatment Treatment of a PDA is limited to those patients who show associated signs and symptoms. At the first sign of symptoms, usually the appearance of a significant murmur, a fluid restriction of <120 mL/kg/day is started. A continuation of the murmur along with bounding pulses, active precordium, and an unimproved or deteriorating respiratory status indicate additional treatment with the diuretic furosemide (Lasix). The benefit of digoxin for the treatment of PDA in the preemie is questionable.[19]

The symptomatic infant of less than 1000 grams requires closure of the PDA either surgically or by the administration of indomethacin (Indocin).[20] Indomethacin is used to block prostagladin production in the ductus, allowing the smooth muscle to constrict. Two dangerous side effects of indomethacin administration are a constriction of renal vasculature with ensuing reduction in renal function and a reduction in platelet adhesion, leading to potential bleeding.

Symptomatic infants weighing over 1000 grams are placed on the previously mentioned fluid restriction for 48 hours. If ventilator parameters improve during that time, fluids are gradually increased. If the patient's condition worsens again, or if there was no improvement during the 48-hour trial, then methods to close the ductus should be considered.

Early closure of the PDA may decrease the incidence of BPD by reducing the amount of time spent on the ventilator.

Atrial Septal Defect (ASD) The most common type of ASD is an incompetent foramen ovale (Figure 8–5). This defect is called an osteum secundum defect and usually involves a failure of the tissue flap to cover the foramen, allowing the movement of blood between atria. Openings in the atria can also occur in the upper and lower atrial septum. Defects in the lower septum are often associated with clefts in the mitral or tricuspid valves.

Diagnosis A majority of ASDs are symptomless and go undetected. Severe ASDs may result in left-to-right shunting with resultant right ventricular overload; however, this is uncommon. There may also be an increase in atrial arrhythmias as the patient matures.

Ventricular Septal Defect (VSD) Defects in the ventricular septum, seen in Figure 8–6, may be isolated, or may occur with other cardiac defects. VSDs are classified according to where they are located when looked at from the right ventricle.

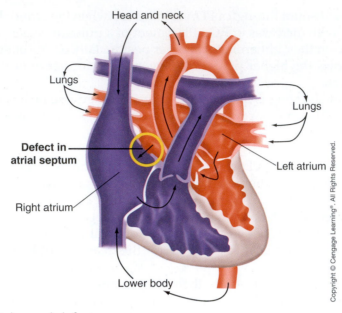

FIGURE 8–5. Atrial septal defect.

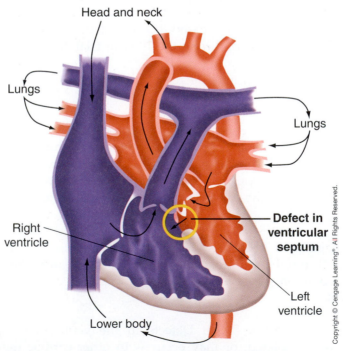

FIGURE 8–6. Ventricular septal defect.

In the presence of normal pulmonary vascular resistance, a VSD leads to left-to-right shunting of blood from left ventricle to right ventricle.

As pulmonary resistance increases, as occurs with RDS, the left-to-right shunting may be minimal. Small VSDs may go unnoticed and be asymptomatic.

Diagnosis and Treatment Diagnosis of a VSD is usually made by two-dimensional ultrasound. Treatment is usually withheld, unless the patient demonstrates a failure to thrive or congestive heart failure that does not respond to treatment. In these cases, the VSD is surgically closed by suture or patch.

Tetralogy of Fallot This combination of defects is the most common cause of cyanotic cardiac disease. The four defects that make up tetralogy of Fallot, pictured in Figure 8–7, are: 1) VSD, 2) an overriding aorta, 3) hypertrophy of the right ventricle, and 4) obstruction to flow through the pulmonary artery.

Cyanosis is caused by decreased blood flow through the pulmonary artery and the resultant passage of venous blood into the aorta. Arterial pH and $PaCO_2$ values are typically normal with decreased PaO_2 in proportion to the amount of pulmonary artery obstruction. On the chest x-ray, the heart has been described as looking like a boot, with normal lung markings.

Diagnosis and Treatment Ultrasound is normally used to diagnose this disorder. The echocardiogram can detect the overriding aorta as well as the presence of the VSD. Cardiac catheterization is used to verify the diagnosis and to differentiate between pulmonary atresia, which has many of the same symptoms. Surgical repair includes closure of the VSD and relief of the pulmonary outflow obstruction.

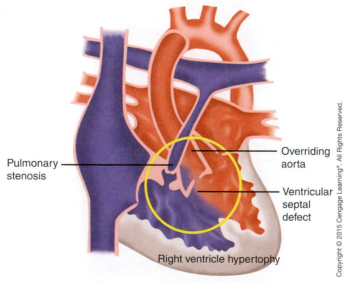

Pulmonary stenosis

Overriding aorta

Ventricular septal defect

Right ventricle hypertophy

FIGURE 8–7. Tetralogy of Fallot.

Complete Transposition of the Great Vessels In this defect, the aorta arises from the right ventricle and the pulmonary artery arises from the left ventricle. Blood flow leaving the right ventricle is passed through the body and returns to the right atrium. Oxygenated blood from the pulmonary system enters the left atrium, the left ventricle, and is then passed through the pulmonary artery into the lungs again, as shown in Figure 8–8. Without an abnormal opening between the two systems, life is not possible.

Mixing of the two blood flows occurs through an ASD, a PDA, or through a VSD. The degree of cyanosis is usually profound with this defect, but may be minimal if a large shunt is present. The patient will often show signs of congestive heart failure. Blood gases show normal or slightly elevated arterial $PaCO_2$, normal or slightly acidotic pH, and an extremely low PaO_2 that is unaffected by oxygen administration.

Diagnosis and Treatment Cardiac ultrasound is very useful in diagnosis, and cardiac catheterization verifies the diagnosis. **Balloon septostomy** which uses a balloon catheter to widen the atrial or ventricular septal defect is frequently required during the cardiac catheterization to improve mixing of the two blood flows.

Surgical correction involves either the dissection of the aorta and pulmonary artery with reattachment to the correct ventricle or the redirection of atrial blood flows to the opposite ventricles. Administration of prostaglandin E_1 may be used to keep the ductus arteriosus open and improve oxygenation.

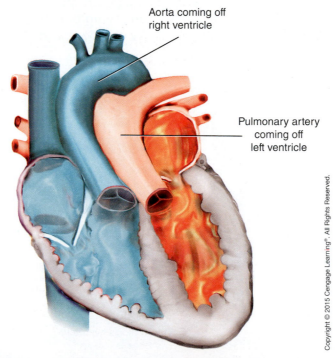

Aorta coming off
right ventricle

Pulmonary artery
coming off
left ventricle

FIGURE 8–8. Complete transposition of the great vessels.

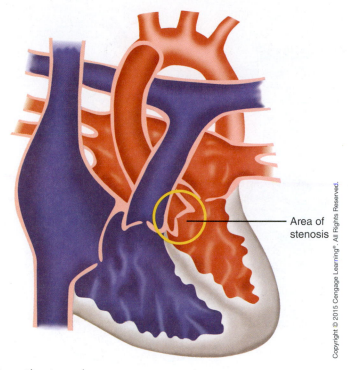

Area of
stenosis

FIGURE 8–9. Subaortic stenosis.

Subaortic Stenosis This cardiac defect involves stenosis either at the aortic valve, above it, or below it, illustrated in Figure 8–9, causing an obstruction to the outflow from the left ventricle. The cardinal findings in this defect are secondary to the reduction in cardiac output. The neonate has cool pale skin secondary to poor perfusion and diminished peripheral pulses. Severe stenosis may cause a dramatic decrease in blood pressure also.

Diagnosis and Treatment Diagnosis is mainly accomplished by cardiac catheterization. A pressure difference of 50 mmHg between the left ventricle and the aorta shows significant involvement. On ultrasound, the aortic valve appears thickened with an enlarged left ventricle and diminished stroke volumes. Blood gas values are typically normal. The chest x-ray will show a cardiomegaly, but is otherwise unremarkable. The only treatment for this defect is surgical intervention to repair the stenotic valve.

Coarctation of the Aorta Coarctation of the aorta, seen in Figure 8–10, involves a constriction of the aorta that severely restricts blood flow. It can occur anywhere on the aorta from the aortic root to the abdominal aorta but most commonly occurs near the entry of the ductus arteriosus into the aorta.

The location of the stricture and the presence of other anomalies determine the clinical signs the patient demonstrates. The most common anomalies associated

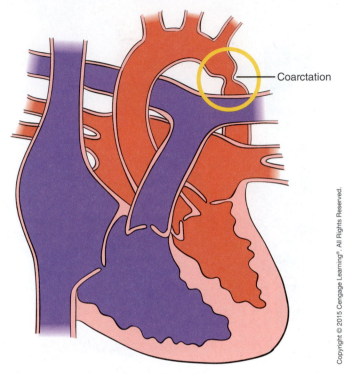

Coarctation

FIGURE 8–10. Coarctation of the aorta.

with coarctation of the aorta are PDA, VSD, and a defective aortic valve. Signs of this disease are associated with a decrease in cardiac output. The coarctation causes an increase in the pressure the left ventricle has to contract against to eject blood, called **afterload**. This leads to left heart enlargement and increased pressures previous to the defect. With a coarctation distal to the aortic arch, it is possible to measure higher systolic pressures in the upper extremities than the systolic pressure in the lower extremities. CXR findings show cardiomegaly and increased vascular markings indicating pulmonary venous obstruction. Blood gases are typically normal and nondiagnostic.

Diagnosis and Treatment Positive diagnosis is made by visualization of the stricture via ultrasound and followed up with cardiac catheterization. Treatment is surgical repair of the aorta by using the left subclavian artery to patch the aorta and increase its diameter. Prostaglandin E_1 is used to maintain ductal patency and increase blood flow to the descending aorta.

Tricuspid Atresia Tricuspid atresia, shown in Figure 8–11, results from a complete agenesis of the tricuspid valve between the right atrium and ventricle. The result is that no blood flows between the two. The venous blood is therefore shunted through the foramen ovale or an ASD into the left atrium. Blood flow to the lungs must come from either a PDA or a VSD. The right ventricle and pulmonary artery may be

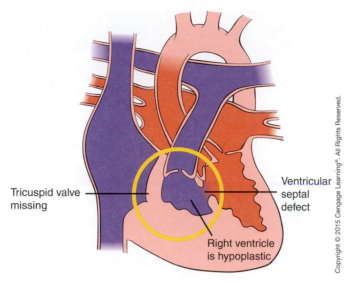

Tricuspid valve
missing

Ventricular
septal
defect

Right ventricle
is hypoplastic

FIGURE 8–11. Tricuspid atresia.

hypoplastic if a large PDA exists. Cyanosis is present when there is a significant compromise in pulmonary blood flow. Blood gases show normal pH and $PaCO_2$. PaO_2 may be near normal in the presence of a large VSD or PDA, or may be tremendously low if there is little blood flow to the lungs.

Diagnosis and Treatment On ultrasound the tricuspid valve is not seen, and color flows will show atrial shunting and the presence of a PDA or VSD. Immediate treatment involves cardiac catheterization with a balloon septostomy to improve mixing in the atria. Permanent treatment involves the surgical creation of a connection between the right atria and pulmonary artery or right ventricle (**Fontan procedure**), and the closure of any septal defects.

Anomalous Venous Return The defect termed anomalous venous return, presented in Figure 8–12, involves the return of pulmonary venous blood to the right atrium instead of the left atrium. An ASD must be present in order for the neonate to survive. These patients are typically cyanotic to some degree. The pH and $PaCO_2$ are near normal, with the level of PaO_2 depending on the degree of pulmonary blood flow. Ultrasound is usually nondiagnostic for this disease. Immediate cardiac catheterization with a balloon septostomy should be performed to increase intra-atrial mixing. Surgical correction is then needed to reimplant the pulmonary veins into the left atria.

Truncus Arteriosus Truncus arteriosus (Figure 8–13) is a defect in which one large vessel arises from both right and left ventricles over a large VSD. The large vessel gives rise to the pulmonary arteries, the coronary arteries, and the systemic arteries and has one valve at its origin.

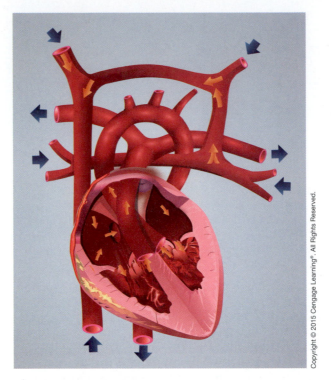

FIGURE 8–12. Anomalous venous return.

Cyanosis is usually present to some degree due to the pulmonary and systemic blood flows arising from a common vessel. Minimal cyanosis indicates adequate pulmonary perfusion. Blood gases may be normal or may show a decreased PaO_2 when pulmonary perfusion is decreased. On the chest x-ray, there are typically increased lung vasculature markings secondary to the increased pulmonary pressures.

Diagnosis and Treatment Echocardiography is useful in diagnosis, and the presence of only one valve helps differentiate this condition from tetralogy of Fallot. Cardiac catheterization is used to verify the diagnosis. Surgical treatment involves separating the pulmonary artery from the large vessel, closing the VSD, and placing a valve between the right ventricle and pulmonary artery. Prognosis is poor with this defect, having a 40% to 50% mortality rate.

Hypoplastic Left Heart Syndrome This syndrome involves several anomalies, including coarctation of the aorta, hypoplastic left ventricle, and aortic and mitral valve stenosis or atresia (Figure 8–14). These lesions lead to a diminished blood flow through the left ventricle and lead to an obligatory left-to-right atrial shunt and a right-to-left ductal shunt. Constriction of the ductus arteriosus leads to rapid hypotension and shock.

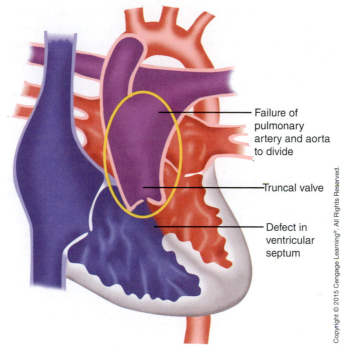

Failure of
pulmonary
artery and aorta
to divide

Truncal valve

Defect in
ventricular
septum

FIGURE 8–13. Truncus arteriosus.

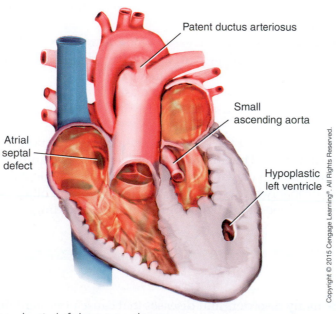

Patent ductus arteriosus

Small
ascending aorta

Atrial
septal
defect

Hypoplastic
left ventricle

FIGURE 8–14. Hypoplastic left heart syndrome.

Diagnosis and Treatment Diagnosis of hypoplastic left heart syndrome is based on physical signs and laboratory data. Physically, the patient appears ashen and grayish as a result of hypoperfusion. A nonspecific systolic murmur may be heard. Signs of congestive heart failure, such as bounding pulses, an active precordium, and an enlarged liver, may be present.

Laboratory diagnosis is made by echocardiogram and cardiac catheterization showing a small left ventricle, abnormal aortic valve, and small ascending aorta.

There is no current medical treatment for hypoplastic left heart syndrome. The only chance for survival is a risky surgical procedure.[20]

RESPIRATORY CARE OF THE PATIENT WITH CARDIAC DEFECTS

The various cardiac defects discussed differ in how they affect the pulmonary system. Cardiac defects either reduce blood flow to the lungs or increase pulmonary blood flow. Defects that reduce pulmonary flow include tricuspid atresia and tetralogy of Fallot. Defects that increase blood flow include VSD, coarctation of the aorta, subaortic stenosis, PDA, and anomalous venous return.

In neonates with decreased pulmonary blood flow, lung compliance is typically increased. The use of too high ventilatory pressures further compromises blood flow and worsen V/Q ratios. Changing the frequency of ventilation instead of inspiratory pressures will help keep mean airway pressure low and still meet ventilatory needs. Cautious use of oxygen is also required in these patients as high PaO_2 will increase the chance of the closure of the PDA, which may be the only source of pulmonary blood flow in these patients.

In contrast to patients with decreased blood flow, increased pulmonary blood flow decreases the lung compliance. In these patients, higher ventilatory pressures and PEEP are required to maintain adequate V/Q ratios. The higher pulmonary blood pressures are less affected by the increases in ventilatory pressures in these patients. Oxygen must also be used judiciously in these patients if the cardiac defect involves a necessary PDA.

A recent study evaluated the change in pulmonary function following the successful closure of a PDA. The authors concluded there is significant improvement in compliance and other ventilatory parameters in those patients with a successful closure.[21] It can probably be assumed that correction of the other heart defects that increase pulmonary blood flow would result in similar findings.

SUMMARY

While there are many disorders and diseases that cause persistent illness in the perinatal period, this chapter has summarized those that are most likely to be seen.

The fetus is susceptible to infection transplacentally or by the organism ascending through the birth canal. During delivery, the fetus may come in contact with infected maternal blood, secretions, or lesions. Following delivery, the risk of hospital-acquired infection from personnel or equipment becomes a problem.

Bacterial infections are often acquired by the ascending route and lead to pneumonia, and less often, urinary tract infections and sepsis. Chorioamnionitis is a bacterial infection of the amniotic tissue and its presence indicates a high risk of fetal infection.

Viruses are unique in that they can lead to fetal malformation if acquired during certain developmental stages. In particular, rubella, CMV, and herpes can cause a great deal of problems in the developing fetus. Rubella affects the fetus in the first 5 months of gestation and causes cardiac defects, growth retardation, and hearing loss. CMV also affects the fetus during the early gestational period, causing brain and liver damage, growth retardation, and microcephaly. Herpes viruses are passed to the fetus during delivery, by contact with active genital lesions. Herpes may lead to severe neurologic problems, bleeding disorders, and liver problems. Prevention of infection in the mother is the only method of treatment often available, as little can be done once the damage has occurred.

A virus for which many volumes have been and will be written is HIV. This one virus has caused a significant portion of viral related morbidity and mortality and continues to defy methods of prevention and treatments. While the virus itself is not the cause of morbidity and mortality, by destroying the immune system, the patient becomes a victim of one of several opportunistic infections, such as *Pneumocystis jirovecii* pneumonia, Kaposi's sarcoma, and yeasts. As this virus continues to resist all attempts to control it, it will continue to play a major role in patient care efforts for the unforeseeable future. It is incumbent on the respiratory therapist to be fully aware of the current preventive measures and treatments to competently take care of these patients. Above all, the respiratory therapist must treat these patients with the same care and dignity as any other patient and, in addition, be aware of the special psychosocial needs of this special group.

Toxoplasmosis, a protozoan organism, affects the fetus during the last trimester of pregnancy and leads to severe neurological and hepatic disorders. The fetus obtains some immunity transplacentally from the mother. The IgG antibody is the only one small enough to be passed transplacentally. It provides the fetus immunity to certain diseases that the mother has acquired immunity to. The IgM antibody is produced by the fetus around the 30th week of gestation. An increased level of IgM in the neonate is an indication that an infective process is present. The IgA antibody is produced by the neonate at about 1 month of life. Mainly a secreted antibody, it is found in the secretions of the gut, and respiratory tree. IgA is also found in breast milk and may aid in the protection of the gastrointestinal tract from bacterial invasion. The IgE antibody is the allergic response antibody and provides protection against environmental antigens. The last antibody, IgD, is present in serum tissue. Its exact role has yet to be determined.

Several anomalies can affect the respiratory tract during fetal growth and development. Because the trachea and esophagus arise from the same germinal tissue, several defects can occur with either, or both. The most common type of anomaly is an atresia of the upper esophagus with an accompanying fistula between the lower esophagus and trachea. Other possible anomalies include esophageal atresia without any fistula, a normal esophagus and trachea with a fistula connecting the two ("H" type), lower esophageal atresia with the upper esophagus attaching to the trachea, and both upper and lower esophageal attachments to the trachea. Choanal atresia is a tissue blockage located at the posterior nasal chamber. Because neonates prefer to nose breath, this blockage can cause respiratory distress. Finally, Pierre-Robin sequence (micrognathia) causes respiratory distress because of airway occlusion by the tongue. In this syndrome, the mandible fails to develop appropriately, causing the oral cavity to be too small for the normally developed tongue.

Cardiac defects are not uncommon, affecting 1 out of every 100 deliveries. Failure of the ductus arteriosus to close following delivery leads to the shunting of blood away from the lungs and difficulty in maintaining oxygenation. Another cardiac defect that leads to shunting is a defect in the atrial septum. Because of higher pressures in the left atrium, blood shunts from the left atrium to the right. Ventricular septal defects allow blood to shunt from the left ventricle to the right. One of the most well-known defects is tetralogy of Fallot. The tetrad of defects are ventricular septal defect, an overriding aorta, hypertrophy of the right ventricle, and pulmonary valve obstruction. Transposition of the great vessels occurs when the aorta arises from the right ventricle, and the pulmonary artery arises from the left ventricle. Coarctation of the aorta, involves a constriction of the aorta, which severely impedes blood flow. In tricuspid atresia, blood flow between the right atrium and right ventricle is interrupted, and shunting through the foramen ovale occurs. Anomalous venous return involves the return of pulmonary blood flow to the right atrium instead of the left. In truncus arteriosus, one large vessel acts as both the aorta and pulmonary artery. Finally, hypoplastic left heart syndrome is seen when outflow from the left ventricle is impeded by coarctation of the aorta and stenosis of the aortic valve. Respiratory care of these patients depends on an understanding as to whether the defect causes an increase or decrease of blood flow to the lungs. As changes occur, the respiratory therapist must be ready to adjust ventilator settings to compensate for changes in compliance.

POSTTEST

1. A 30-year-old female is admitted to the high-risk delivery area at 5:00 pm with premature contractions. She weighs 210 lbs and is estimated to be at 30 weeks gestation. Her history is positive for hypertension and possible drug use. Her amniotic membranes ruptured yesterday at around noon while she was exercising. Which historical item carries the highest risk of infection to the fetus?

    a. the mothers' weight
    b. the mother's hypertension
    c. the mother's drug use
    d. the rupture of the membranes

2. During a prenatal class, a couple has a question about prenatal screening for strep. The mother is at 33 weeks gestation and recently moved from another city and lost her OB/GYN. Your recommendation is:
   a. She should receive a blood screening test for the presence of strep A and B.
   b. No screening is recommended at this time.
   c. She should get a rectal and vaginal swab to check for strep B.
   d. She should get screened only if she is symptomatic.

3. You are called to the delivery of a fetus in distress. The maternal history is positive for HIV. Which of the following tests would be the quickest to test the neonate for the HIV infection?
   a. ELISA
   b. Western blot
   c. PCR
   d. P24 antigen

4. You are examining a 40-week neonate who has had some nasal flaring and expiratory grunting. While assessing the red reflex of the eyes, you note the presence of cataracts bilaterally. What is the most likely agent this patient was infected with?
   a. rubella
   b. CMV
   c. toxoplasmosis
   d. herpesvirus Type I

5. You are called to assess an infant with suspected PCP infection. The patient is on 30% oxygen, and blood gases show a PaO_2 of 118 mmHg, and a PCO_2 of 45 mmHg. The barometric pressure is 760 mmHg. What degree of PCP illness does this patient have?
   a. none
   b. mild
   c. moderate/severe
   d. severe

6. You are entering a room to obtain an arterial blood gas from a neonatal patient. Which of the following standard precautions applies?
   a. You do not need to wash your hands as long as you are wearing gloves during the procedure.
   b. You should wash your hands only after removing your gloves following the procedure.
   c. You should wash and use an alcohol-based cleanser only prior to putting on gloves.
   d. You should wash your hands prior to putting on the gloves and again after removing the gloves.

7. An infant is found to have immunity against pneumococcus. The most likely source of this immunity is:
   a. Secretory IgA from breast milk
   b. natural immunity from IgD
   c. IgE from previous exposure to pneumococcus
   d. transplacentally from IgG

8. After starting feedings on a newborn, the baby develops immediate respiratory distress with coughing, choking, and vomiting. A tracheaesophageal anomaly is suspected. Which of the following is most likely?
   a. upper esophageal atresia with a lower tube fistula
   b. esophageal atresia with no fistula
   c. an "H-type" fistula
   d. an upper and lower attachment of the esophagus to the trachea

9. While performing a ventilator check on a 34-week neonate, you auscultate the chest and note a Grade III systolic murmur. It is loudest over the left upper sternal border. The most likely cause of the murmur is:
   a. atrial septal defect
   b. patent ductus arteriosus
   c. ventricular septal defect
   d. tetralogy of Fallot

10. You are called stat to the delivery room to assess a cyanotic term neonate. You supply 100% oxygen to the patient with no change to the cyanosis 1 hour later. A chest x-ray is obtained and shows normal lung markings, but the cardiac silhouette is shaped like a boot. The most likely diagnosis is:
    a. patent ductus arteriosus
    b. ventricular septal defect
    c. tetralogy of Fallot
    d. atrial septal defect

11. Indomethacin is given to treat which of the following heart anomalies?
    a. PDA
    b. VSD
    c. ASD
    d. hypoplastic left heart

REFERENCES

1. Brown AS, Derkits EJ. Prenatal infection and schizophrenia: a review of epidemiologic and translational studies. *Am J Psychiatry* 67:261–2801, 2009.
2. Meyer U, Yee BK, Feldon J. The neurodevelopmental impact of prenatal infections at different times of pregnancy: the earlier the worse? *Neuroscientist.* 13(3): 241–256, June 2007.
3. Brown AS. Epidemiologic studies of exposure to prenatal infection and risk of schizophrenia and autism. *Dev Neurobiol.* 72(10): Apr. 5, 2012.
4. Preventing Infections in Pregnance, Centers for Disease Control and Prevention. http://www.cdc.gov/pregnancy/infections.html
5. Schrag SD, et al. Prevention of Perinatal Group B Streptococcal Disease. http://www.cdc.gov/mmwr/preview/mmwrhtml/rr5111a1.htm
6. Recommended Prevention Services. Centers for Disease Control and Prevention. http://www.cdc.gov/hiv/prevention/programs/pwp/rpc.html

7. Shannon L. Clinical perspectives and current trends of HIV infection in the newborn and child. *Neonatal Network.* 14:21–34, 1995.

8. Goedert JJ, et al. Mother-to-infant transmission of human immunodeficiency virus type I: association with prematurity or low anti-gp 120. *Lancet.* 2:1351–1354, 1989.

9. Connor EM, et al. Reduction of maternal-infant transmission of human immunodeficiency virus type I with zidovudine treatment. Pediatric AIDS clinical trials. *N Engl J Med.* 331:1173–1180, 1994.

10. Kuhn L, et al. Maternal-infant HIV transmission and circumstances of delivery. *Am J Public Health.* 84:1110–1115, 1984.

11. Recommendations for Use of Antiretroviral Drugs in Pregnant HIV-1-Infected Women for Maternal Health and Interventions to Reduce Perinatal HIV Transmission in the United States. Clinical Guidelines Portal. http://aidsinfo.nih.gov/guidelines/html/3/perinatal-guidelines/148/mechanisms-of-action-of-antiretroviral-prophylaxis-in-reducing-perinatal-transmission-of-hiv

12. AIDSinfo Drug Database. http://aidsinfo.nih.gov/drugs

13. Schleiss MR. Pediatric Cytomegalovirus Infection http://emedicine.medscape.com/article/963090-overview

14. Harrison GJ. Neonatal herpes simplex virus infection: management and prevention. *UpToDate.* 2013. http://www.uptodate.com/contents/neonatal-herpes-simplex-virus-infection-management-and-prevention.

15. Wright WF. (1–3)-β-D-Glucan assay. A review of its laboratory and clinical application http://www.medscape.com/viewarticle/752221.

16. http://www.cdc.gov/HAI/settings/outpatient/outpatient-care-gl-standared-precautions.html

17. MacDonald MG. editor, *Avery's Neonatology: Pathophysiology and Management of the Newborn.* 6th ed. Philadelphia, PA: JB Lippincott Co., 2005.

18. Pierre Robin Sequence. International Craniofacial Institute. http://www.craniofacial.net/conditions-pierre-robin.

19. Cloherty JP, et al. *Manual of Neonatal Care.* 7th ed. Philadelphia, PA: Lippincott, 2011.

20. Gardner SL, et al. *Merenstein and Gardner's Handbook of Neonatal Intensive Care.* 7th ed. St. Louis, MO: CV Mosby Co., 2011.

21. Stefano S, et al. Closure of the ductus arteriosus with indomethacin in ventiltaed neonates with respiratory distress syndrome: effects on pulmonary compliance and ventilation. *Rev Resp Dis.* 143:236, 1991.

BIBLIOGRAPHY AND SUGGESTED READINGS

Centers for Disease Control and Prevention. *Guide to Infection Prevention for Outpatient Settings: Minimum Expectations for Safe Care*, May 2011.

Greenfield RA (ed.). *Pediatric HIV Infection* March 2013, Medscape Reference http://emedicine.medscape.com/article/965086-overview.

Krist AH, Crawford-Faucher A. Management of newborns exposed to maternal HIV infection *Am Fam Physician*. 65(10):2049–2057, May 15, 2002.

Lambert EC, Canent RV, Hohn AR. Congenital cardiac anomalies: a review of conditions causing death or severe distress in the first month of life. *Pediatrics*. 37(2):343–335, February 1, 1966.

Mayo Clinic. Congenital heart defects in children. Slide Show. http://www.mayoclinic.com/health/congenital-heart-defects/CC00026.

Stegmann BJ, Carey JC. TORCH infections. Toxoplasmosis, other (syphilis, varicella-zoster, parvovirus B19), rubella, cytomegalovirus (CMV), and herpes infections. *Curr Womens Health Rep*. 2(4):253–258, Aug. 2002.

World Health Organization. Treatment of children living with HIV. 2013. http://www.who.int/hiv/topics/paediatric/en/index.html.

The Pediatric Patient

A baby is something you carry inside you for nine months, in your arms for three years, and in your heart till the day you die.

—*Mary Mason*

CHAPTER 9

Techniques of Pediatric Resuscitation and Stabilization

OBJECTIVES

Upon the completion of this chapter, the reader should be able to:

1. Describe the steps in pediatric advanced life support (PALS) for each of the following scenarios:
   a. Pulseless arrest
   b. Bradycardia
   c. Tachycardia
2. Describe the anatomic and physiologic differences between an adult and child and discuss how they relate to trauma care.
3. List and describe each of the steps involved in the primary survey.
4. When given patient responses, determine an appropriate Glasgow Coma Score.
5. Describe the secondary survey and the purpose of each step.
6. Regarding shock, describe each of the following:
   a. Pathophysiology
   b. Types
   c. Treatment
7. Define near drowning and describe its pathophysiology and initial respiratory management.
8. Compare and contrast epiglottitis and croup with regard to their presentation and treatment.
9. Describe the factors that make children prone to foreign body aspiration.
10. Describe the diagnosis and treatment of hydrocarbon aspiration.
11. Regarding the inhalation of smoke and chlorine, describe the diagnosis, monitoring, and treatment of each.
12. Compare and contrast first, second, and third degree burns.
13. When provided with areas on a child's body that are burned, calculate the amount of body surface area involved.
14. Describe the evaluation and management of the burn patient.
15. Using the Parkland formula, calculate the amount of fluid resuscitation when given the patient weight and surface area burned.

16. Describe the etiology and treatment of neck injuries in the pediatric population.
17. When given a diagram of a cross section of the skull, the student will label the anatomical landmarks.
18. Discuss and describe the pathophysiology of primary and secondary head injury.
19. Compare and contrast epidural hematoma and subdural hematoma regarding causes, signs, and symptoms.
20. Describe the goals of treatment of head injury and identify the specific strategies to achieve those goals.
21. Identify the four factors that have been identified that elevate the risk of sudden infant death syndrome (SIDS) in the prone position.
22. Describe the management of poisoning in the pediatric patient.
23. Describe anaphylaxis and discuss common causes and treatment.

KEY TERMS

adsorption	hemotympanum	pericranium
aponeurosis	hydrocyanic acid	periosteum
Battle's sign	intraosseous (IO)	raccoon eyes
contrecoup	mammalian dive reflex	rule of nines
coup	meninges	secondary drowning
decerebrate	narrow-complex	syndrome
decorticate	tachycardia	subglottic
glucocorticoid	near drowning	trabeculae
growing fracture	neurocranium	
hematoma	obtundation	

INTRODUCTION

Cardiac arrest is an uncommon occurrence in children, but it happens frequently enough to warrant a knowledge of the causes and treatment of arrest. When cardiac arrest does occur in the pediatric population, it is often the result of shock or progressive respiratory failure. Cardiac arrest is the final stage in a progressive downward spiral that starts with hypoxemia, acidosis, and hypercapnea, eventually leading to bradycardia and profound hypotension.

Causes of emergency situations in the pediatric population are numerous. In all age groups, acute illness requiring emergent care may be precipitated by preexisting conditions, such as a genetic defect or asthma. Prior to the development of the ability to crawl, newborns may be subject to trauma, starting with accidental neglect such as an infant left alone in the bathtub or not being placed in a car seat. When the infant learns to crawl and then walk, it opens up an entire new world full of possibilities. During this time, the infant is still susceptible to accidents due to neglect; however, they are also now vulnerable to self-inflicted injury and trauma. As their skills advance, so do the opportunities for injury.

A major focus during this time should be on education and prevention. Parents and caretakers must be knowledgeable of the safety precautions needed for their particular infant. The old adage, "An ounce of prevention is better than a pound of cure" certainly applies to this patient population. Checklists are available to help educate parents and caregivers in creating a safe work and home environment.[1] Prevention education includes reducing the risk of SIDS; preventing motor vehicle, bicycle, pedestrian, and firearm injuries; and prevention of drowning, burns, and choking.[2] As respiratory therapists, our role is primarily in the care of the patient following an injury; however, we can and should take an active role in the educational aspects of prevention. This chapter will review pediatric advanced life support and some of the more common causes of injury and trauma in the pediatric populations that will require respiratory care during both the acute and chronic phases.

PEDIATRIC ADVANCED LIFE SUPPORT

The American Academy of Pediatrics provides training in Pediatric Advanced Life Support (PALS), and it is highly recommended that any health care provider who will work with the pediatric population receive that training.[3,4] This section will offer a review of the techniques involved in the resuscitation and stabilization of a pediatric patient in cardiac arrest; *it is not a substitute for the training*.

PALS differs from basic life support (BLS) in that BLS is typically designed for a single rescuer, whereas PALS assumes the resuscitation will take place in an environment, such as a hospital emergency room, where a team of rescuers will each perform a focused task, and as a team they will work to revive and stabilize the patient.

BLS Considerations

Because so many cardiac events in pediatrics involve hypoxia, it is essential that chest compressions and ventilation with 100% oxygen be started immediately. If a bag/mask is not readily available, then chest compressions are started while the second person prepares for ventilations. High-quality chest compressions are done at a rate of at least 100 per minute at a depth at least one third of the AP diameter of the chest and allowing complete recoil of the chest after each compression. Interruptions in compressions and excessive ventilation are to be avoided. Chest compressions are best delivered with the victim on a firm surface. While compressions and ventilation are proceeding, other rescuers are retrieving the AED or defibrillator, gaining vascular access, and preparing medications and calculating dosages.

Monitoring

When an arrest occurs with a hospitalized patient, the rescuers can take advantage of any monitors in use on the patient to improve the quality of the chest compressions. On patients with an arterial catheter, the arterial wave form can be watched to assess compression quality. The aim is to achieve higher amplitudes on the wave form, indicating good arterial blood flow. Changes in hand position and depth of compressions can alter the wave pattern, thus, helping the rescuers achieve the best circulation. If available, an end-tidal CO_2 monitor can also be used to evaluate the chest compressions. Rescuers are always watching for signs of the return of spontaneous circulation (ROSC), and both the arterial pressure wave and the end-tidal CO_2 monitor waveform can be used to assess for ROSC.

Airways

During resuscitative efforts, it is important to maintain a patent airway. Both oro- and nasopharyngeal airways are used to help maintain an open airway by keeping the tongue from occluding the posterior pharynx. Oropharyngeal airways should only be used in unresponsive patients without a gag reflex, but nasopharyngeal airways may be used in patients with a gag reflex. The proper size is important to prevent pushing the tongue into the airway if it is too small, or occluding the airway if it is too big.

Oxygen

Until ROSC is achieved, the rescuers should use 100% oxygen during the resuscitation. Once ROSC is achieved, the oxygen is titrated to maintain a saturation of at least 94% using a pulse oximeter. This helps to avoid hyperoxia.

Bag-Mask Ventilation

In most cases, oxygenation and ventilation can be adequately maintained with the use of a bag and mask for short periods of time. It is important to use the correct sized mask and assure that it is properly positioned on the patients face. Additionally, the rescuer must maintain an open airway while using the bag-mask in order for it to be effective. When using the bag-mask, the rescuer should only use enough force and tidal volume to cause a visual rise in the chest. On a nonintubated patient, two ventilations of one second each are delivered after 30 compressions. If the patient is intubated, ventilations are given at a rate of 1 breath every 6 to 8 seconds with no interruption of chest compressions. The rate of ventilations is slightly higher at 1 breath every 3 to 5 seconds if the patient has a perfusing heart rhythm but is not breathing. If enough rescuers are available, a two-person bag-mask ventilation may be more effective than one person. While one rescuer compresses the bag, the other maintains the airway and the mask using two hands. One of the possible complications of bag-mask ventilation is gastric inflation. This complication can be minimized by using just enough pressure to cause a visible chest rise, applying cricoid pressure in the unresponsive patient, and placing an oro- or nasogastric tube.

Endotracheal Intubation

Due to differences in anatomy, endotracheal intubation in a pediatric patient requires special training. The placement of an advanced airway, such as an endotracheal tube greatly improves the security of ventilation and reduces the risk of gastric inflation and aspiration. In addition to the skill required to perform the intubation, the rescuer must have a knowledge of tube sizes, securing the tube, and verifying tube position.

Advanced skills

A successful resuscitation includes the administration of medications intravenously. Vascular access is an essential skill and is challenging to achieve in children during an emergency. Peripheral IV access is an acceptable method if it can be done quickly. **Intraosseous (IO)** access is a safe and effective method to deliver medications to children. It also provides a quick method for access when vascular access may be compromised. If IV or IO access is not possible, certain medications can be administered via the endotracheal tube.

Medications

Medications used during pediatric resuscitation include adenosine, amiodarone, atropine, calcium, epinephrine, glucose, lidocaine, magnesium, procainamide, sodium bicarbonate, and vasopressin.

Overview of PALS Algorithms

The PALS algorithms are similar to those for BLS in that they give the rescuer a decision making tree for various forms of cardiac arrhythmias.[5] The algorithms are available through the American Heart Association PALS web site.

Pulseless Arrest Regardless of the type of rhythm or lack thereof, when an unresponsive child is found, the rescuer always initiates the algorithms by calling for help and requesting an AED and activating the emergency response system. CPR is then started immediately with oxygen, if it is available. The cardiac rhythm is determined if using an ECG monitor, or if an AED is being used, the device will indicate whether the rhythm is "shockable" or "not shockable." Shockable rhythms are ventricular fibrillation and rapid ventricular tachycardia and nonshockable rhythms are asystole and pulseless electrical activity (PEA). The highest survival is seen when high-quality CPR is started early with minimal interruptions. CPR should be continued up until the shock is delivered and then resumed immediately following shock delivery. Chest compressions and ventilations are given for two minute intervals followed by a recheck of the cardiac rhythm and throughout the rescue, all involved should be searching for and treating any reversible causes of the arrest.

Bradycardia Bradycardia is a heart rate that is less than the lower limit of normal for the child's age. Generally, it is accepted that bradycardia is any heart rate less than 100 bpm in the first 3 years of life, less than 60 bpm in the 3 to 9 year old, and less than 50 bpm in the 9- to 16- year-old patient. These rates are those that typically result in hemodynamic compromise. This algorithm starts with assessing and supporting a patent airway, breathing, and circulation. Oxygen is administered, an ECG is attached, and vascular access is achieved. The overall goal in the face of bradycardia is to assess and reassess the patient for signs of cardiopulmonary compromise. Often, the establishment of adequate ventilation and oxygenation will restore a normal heart rate, in which case the patient is monitored and evaluated. Any time the heart rate drops below 60/minute with signs of poor perfusion in the presence of effective ventilation with oxygen, CPR is initiated. After 2 minutes, the patient is reevaluated for persistence of bradycardia and cardiopulmonary compromise. The rescuer is always checking for adequate ventilation and oxygenation. If bradycardia persists despite adequate ventilation, oxygenation and chest compressions, medications and/or transcutaneous pacing are initiated.

Tachycardia Tachycardias are divided into **narrow-complex**, in which the QRS complex is less than 0.09 seconds, and wide-complex, where the QRS complex is greater than 0.09 seconds. The rhythm is then further defined from the ECG as sinus tachycardia, in which P waves are present and normal before each QRS complex, or supraventricular, in which P waves are either absent or abnormal. In the presence of a narrow-complex tachycardia, the rescuers search for and treat any reversible causes and monitor the patient. In the presence of supraventricular tachycardia, the ECG is continuously monitored. Vagal stimulation is attempted if the patient is hemodynamically stable. In infants and young children, this is done by applying ice to the face, being careful not to occlude the airway. In older children, valsalva maneuvers or carotid massage can be used. Pharmacologic cardioversion with adenosine can be very effective at converting supraventricular tachycardias; however, it must be used only with expert consultation in infants.

Synchronized cardioversion with sedation using a defibrillator is used if the patient is hemodynamically unstable or if adenosine is ineffective.

A wide-complex tachycardia typically originates in the ventricles, but could be supraventricular. In hemodynamically stable patients, wide-complex tachycardia is treated with adenosine, electric cardioversion with sedation, and amiodarone. In the hemodynamically unstable patient, electric cardioversion is recommended.

TRAUMA CARE

Accidents are the leading cause of death between ages 1 and 24.[6] Statistics from the Centers for Disease Control and Prevention (CDC) show that a majority of non-fatal injuries are caused by falls and most deaths are related to vehicle related accidents (Figure 9–1). Age breakdown shows that most fall injuries occur in younger patients, 1 year of age or less, while vehicle accidents are more likely to affect the teenage

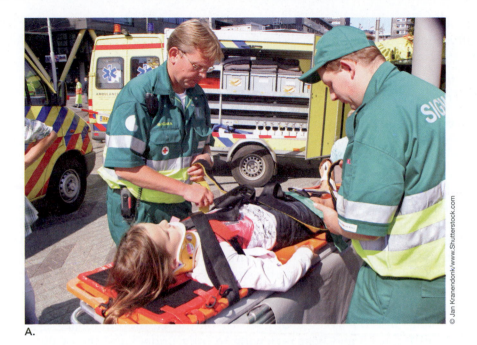

A.

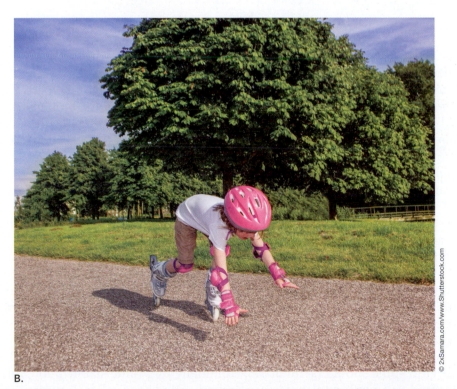

B.

FIGURE 9–1. A. Many traumatic injuries in older children, particularly teens, are the result of traffic accidents. B. Traumatic injuries in younger children are often from falls.

population. Specifically, the leading cause of injury death in children younger than 1 is suffocation. Drowning accounts for the most injury deaths in ages 1–4, and motor vehicle accidents for those aged 5–19.[7]

Anatomic and Physiologic Considerations

When dealing with trauma in the pediatric population, it is important to understand the differences in both the psychological and the physiological responses between a child and an adult. Because children are smaller anatomically than adults, any trauma affects a greater portion of their body surface area. Additionally, the smaller amount of fat, tissue, and muscle provide less protection allowing deeper injury with external trauma. Because of these issues, one must always assume the presence of internal injury even in the absence of external signs.

A child's head is larger in proportion to its body than that of an adult. This accounts for the high number of head injuries as well as a source of heat loss. Adding to the potential for injury is the relative shortness of the neck which not only hinders a good examination, but also increases the risk of trauma from sudden movements and external forces.

Anatomic and physiologic differences of the cardiopulmonary system are covered in Chapter 5 and bear reviewing to fully understand the evaluation of a trauma patient.

Trauma Assessment Successful resuscitation and management of a pediatric trauma patient begins before the arrival of the patient. Ideally, all of the trauma team members are alerted and are made aware of the details of the patient and the extent of injury in anticipation of the arrival. Each team member is assigned a given task and the emergency physician takes on the role of team leader. All on-call services should be alerted, including radiology, lab, surgery, specialists, and the intensive care areas. All resuscitation equipment should be checked to ensure it is present and working properly, including airway maintenance, IV lines, and fluids. Knowing the approximate age and/or weight of the patient will help prepare appropriate medication dosages and equipment.

Primary Survey Upon arrival of the patient, the initial primary survey is performed by assessing and managing the child's airway, cervical spine, breathing, and circulation. Additionally, the patient is assessed for disability (Mental/Neurologic function). The primary survey and initial resuscitation should occur within the first 5 minutes of arrival. One of the team members should obtain a history from the parents or emergency medical services personnel if possible (e.g., type of trauma, speed of the vehicle, height of the fall, restraints or safety equipment used, and whether other people were injured).

The first step is to assess the child's airway while protecting the cervical spine. The cervical spine should be immobilized initially by in-line stabilization, followed by the rapid and gentle application of a properly fitted hard collar. Traumatic injuries of the cervical spine are uncommon in children; however, always assume there is a cervical spine injury until examination and radiographs prove otherwise. The typical standard of care is to immobilize the neck in the presence of any trauma where there is a risk of spinal injury. The spine immobilization is left in place until the absence of injury is confirmed following standard hospital protocols.

Securing the airway occurs simultaneously while stabilizing the cervical spine. The jaw-thrust maneuver is the recommended method of opening the airway when cervical injury is suspected. Any obstruction such as secretions, blood, or vomitus should be removed with suction. If the jaw-thrust is inadequate at maintaining the airway, the placement of an oral-pharyngeal or nasopharyngeal airway is indicated.

During the initial primary survey, it is of utmost importance to maintain patient thermoregulation. Lying on the ground, being wet, being placed on a backboard are all common with trauma, and all contribute to heat loss. By the time the patient reaches the emergency department, his or her temperature may have become dangerously low if precautions are not taken. Once in the emergency room, warm blankets are used to cover the patient and exposure is limited to those areas where access is needed. Thermoregulation is covered in more detail in Chapter 6.

The second step in the primary assessment is to assess breathing. As a general standard, the patient should be placed on an oxygen mask with a 10-liter/minute oxygen flow. It is also essential that a pulse oximeter be placed on the patient. Assessment of the patient's breathing is done by observing the work of breathing, the effectiveness of breathing, and watching for any signs of inadequate respiration such as lowered heart rate or diminished mental status. The work of breathing can be assessed quickly by the use of accessory muscles and the presence of an elevated respiratory rate. Breathing effectiveness is assessed by the patient's oxygen saturation, presence and quality of breath sounds, and adequate chest expansion. Spontaneous breathing is considered acceptable if the patient is able to maintain normal oxygen saturations and carbon dioxide levels. The use of an end-tidal monitor can greatly facilitate the assessment. If it is determined that breathing is inadequate, the team must exclude a tension pneumothorax and then provide positive pressure ventilation with a bag-mask device, and consider intubation. Once positive pressure ventilation is started, a large orogastric tube is placed to prevent gastric distention.

The third level of the primary assessment is circulation. Initially, this is done by attaching a cardiac monitor, which should be done in the field or as soon as the patient arrives, checking the pulse rate, skin color, capillary refill time, and blood pressure. The effects of inadequate circulation may be observable as an increased respiratory rate, skin pallor, and a diminished mental state. When these signs are correlated with a decreased blood pressure, the probability of inadequate circulation is high. IV or intraosseous (IO) access should be established quickly in order to boost blood volume and elevate blood pressure. Any external hemorrhage must be stopped using direct pressure.

Disability is next assessed. Disability refers to the mental state, or neurological function, of the patient. Note whether the child is alert and responds to voice commands. Quickly assess neurological status by noting the response to a painful stimulus. Pain response can be determined by squeezing an earlobe and observing the reaction. A normal response would be to immediately cry and retract from the

Table 9–1

THE PEDIATRIC GLASGOW COMA SCALE

Eye Opening Response	< 1 year
4	Spontaneous
3	To shout
2	To pain
1	None

Verbal Response	0 to 2 years
5	Babbles, coos appropriately
4	Cries but is inconsolable
3	Persistent crying or screaming in pain
2	Grunts or moans to pain
1	None

Motor Response	< 1 year
6	Spontaneous
5	Localizes pain
4	Withdraws to pain
3	Abnormal flexion to pain (decerebrate)
2	Abnormal extension to pain (decorticate)
1	None

pain where a muted response may be no more than flexion or extension of the limbs. Pupillary size and reaction are also noted as part of the assessment. Assigning a Glasgow Coma Score using the Pediatric scale (Table 9–1) can help to quantify the level of consciousness.

Secondary Survey Once the patient is stabilized and the primary survey is completed, a secondary survey is done. During the secondary survey, the child is continuously monitored for airway, breathing, circulation, and mental state. Any deterioration requires a return to the primary survey with measures taken to rectify the problem. Prior to starting the secondary survey it is important to develop a rapport with the patient. Being at the head offers a great opportunity to offer reassurance and explain what is happening. As possible, try to involve the parents and allow them to also comfort the child. Thermoregulation is of high importance during this time, so as much as possible, keep the child covered and only remove clothing judiciously. The sudden removal and disappearance of a child's favorite clothing may add to his or her distress.

The physical examination during the secondary survey essentially entails a complete head-to-toe examination. In particular the respiratory therapist is carefully examining the upper airways, including the nose, mouth, pharynx, and larynx for any signs of fracture, bleeding, or obstruction. Additionally, the trachea is examined for signs of deviation possibly indicating a pneumo- or hemothorax. The dilation of neck vessels may indicate an increase in intrathoracic pressure. The chest is carefully examined for signs of rib or clavicle tenderness, equal chest movement, and quality of breath sounds. The heart is also auscultated for volume of heart sounds and the presence of murmurs. The examination is continued to include the abdomen, the upper and lower extremities, and neuromuscular function. Any movement of the child must be done while protecting the cervical spine. Throughout this examination, the child is assessed for bruising, bleeding, lacerations, deformities, and tenderness, all of which may indicate the presence of additional underlying injury.

SHOCK

The physiologic condition called shock involves the inability of the body to deliver necessary nutrients to the tissues and, at the same time, the inability to remove the waste products of metabolism. The lack of oxygen delivery results in hypoxia at the tissue level and leads to anaerobic metabolism. An alteration in the acid-base status follows, and if it is not reversed, cell dysfunction and death occur.

Shock is classified as compensated, decompensated, and irreversible. Compensated shock refers to a condition of adequate cardiac output and tissue perfusion; however, the blood flow is maldistributed. Decompensated shock occurs when cardiac output and other compensatory mechanisms are not adequate to perfuse the tissues and severe cellular damage follows. As the name implies, irreversible shock is the condition in which tissue perfusion is so extreme that cell death occurs and recovery is unlikely.

Pathophysiology

The pathophysiology of shock covers all organ systems. Initially, mental status is altered as hypoxia, electrolyte, and acid-base disorders worsen. Myocardial dysfunction along with the loss of vascular tone leads to cardiovascular compromise. As blood pressure and tissue perfusion decrease toxic wastes build up and worsen the condition. The work of breathing increases leading to fatigue and respiratory failure. Lowered perfusion leads to acute kidney injury and possible kidney failure. Blood shunting away from the gut results in ischemic injury to the bowels. The release of inflammatory mediators worsens the shock by increasing capillary permeability, worsening myocardial contractility, and pulmonary vasoconstriction.

Types of Shock

Eight types of shock have been identified each one with its particular etiology and pathophysiology.

Respiratory In respiratory shock, trauma to the respiratory tract leads to a reduction in oxygen and carbon dioxide exchange. Shock results when the cells do not receive enough oxygen to support metabolism.

Neurogenic Neurogenic shock occurs when injury or trauma to the central nervous system damages nerve impulses to blood vessels. The lack of innervation results in vessel dilation and loss of vascular tone. The result is a precipitous drop in blood pressure.

Hypovolemic/Hemorrhagic Hypovolemic shock occurs following a loss of intravascular volume. Causes include severe gastroenteritis, fluid loss from severe burns, and blood loss. The loss of volume results in decreased cardiac output and, if not reversed, eventual organ failure.

Septic The introduction of infective organisms into the circulatory system and the subsequent release of their toxins causes an inflammatory response that can lead to septic shock. Initially, the patient shows alterations in respiratory rate, heart rate, and white blood cell count. As the shock advances mental status is impaired, peripheral perfusion decreases, and blood pressure drops.

Anaphylactic Anaphylactic shock results from a reaction to a substance to which the patient is allergic. An outpouring of histamine results in a loss of vascular tone from the dilation of blood vessels throughout the body. This results in a maldistribution of intravascular volume and tissue hypoxia.

Cardiogenic Although rare in the pediatric population, the failure of the heart to adequately pump leads to cardiogenic shock. In adults the most common cause is MI and in children dysrhythmias and congenital lesions that impede left ventricular outflow.

Metabolic Another type of shock occurs with some type of metabolic disruption, such as hyper- or hypoglycemia.

Psychogenic Psychogenic shock is typically seen in the presence of overwhelming emotional factors and is related to a sympathetic response causing a temporary decrease in cerebral perfusion. The drop in perfusion results in syncope and is typically very temporary.

Treatment The overriding goal for treating shock is the restoration of perfusion and oxygenation. Perfusion is returned by increasing cardiac output with fluid resuscitation and the use of pressor agents to strengthen the heart contractions. Ventilation and oxygenation are achieved by maintaining the airway, providing ventilator support, and 100% oxygen delivery. In the presence of blood loss, volume support via packed red blood cells and fluid replacement is initiated immediately to prevent complications of hypovolemic shock. One of the most important aspects in the management of shock is the rapid recognition of underlying conditions and their treatment. A good history and physical exam can help to quickly identify possible causes of shock and allow early intervention.

NEAR DROWNING

The term "**near drowning**" indicates surviving an underwater suffocation at least temporarily. This is in contrast to "drowning" in which the patient dies secondary to underwater suffocation. The World Health Organization defines drowning as "the process of experiencing respiratory impairment from submission/immersion in liquid." Typically, the victim of near drowning is unconscious and frequently suffers subsequent consequences that may lead to death. Another phenomenon seen with near drowning is labeled **secondary drowning syndrome**. In this syndrome, which occurs in roughly 5% of near drowning cases, there is a deterioration of pulmonary function following the loss or inactivation of surfactant. This leads to failing gas exchange and eventual pulmonary failure.[8]

The two most susceptible age groups are adolescents and children under age 5. Younger victims typically fall into buckets, bathtubs, or swimming pools, whereas adolescents typically drown in lakes, rivers, and the ocean. In both age groups, males are more likely to drown than females.

Pathophysiology

The urge to breathe is influenced by hypoxemia but probably more so by hypercapnia. Once submerged, both hypoxia and hypercapnia quickly progress until the patient attempts to take a breath. Water entering the larynx causes laryngospasm that effectively prevents water from entering the lungs. Water can then enter the esophagus and the stomach. If water does enter the lungs, secondary drowning, previously discussed, can occur. As the hypoxemia continues secondary damage to the organs begins to occur. The heart and brain are very susceptible to anoxia and are frequently the most damaged. Ventricular fibrillation and asystole as well as other arrhythmias are common. In the brain, anoxia leads to the death of brain cells. The presence of arrhythmias along with the hypoxemia leads to further brain damage and eventual brain death.

One exception appears when a victim is suddenly submersed in ice water. A phenomenon called the **mammalian dive reflex** causes a rapid slowing of metabolism and a shunting of blood away from the extremities and to the brain, heart, and major organs. There are cases of victims surviving up to an hour or more of submersion in these conditions.

Initial Respiratory Management

As with all trauma's, the ABCs are followed when caring for the near drowning patient. Upon arrival to the emergency department, the patient is placed on a cardiac monitor and pulse oximeters. The patient should receive 100% oxygen and, additionally, assisted ventilation if needed. The lungs are auscultated carefully to determine adequacy of air movement. The presence of wheezing or stridor is treated appropriately with aerosolized beta adrenergics. An arterial blood gas should be drawn as soon as possible. Hypoxemia in the face of 100% oxygen indicates the need for CPAP or PEEP. Additionally, the presence of apnea, vomiting, or an unstable airway indicates the need to intubate the patient. A chest x-ray should be obtained as quickly as possible to check for atelectasis and/or early signs of ARDS. An NG tube should be placed not only to relieve the stomach from any swallowed water, but also to avoid gastric dilation from the resuscitation.

Hypothermia must be anticipated in the near drowning patient. Further hypothermia is prevented by removing wet clothing and providing core rewarming with warmed IV fluids, heat lamps, and warmed blankets.

In the presence of suspected hypoxic cerebral damage, it is recommended that arterial carbon dioxide levels be kept in the normal range as there are no studies that show improved outcomes in patients who were hyperventilated.[9, 10,11] In the absence of neck injury, the head can be elevated to help control increased intracranial pressures (ICP).

PULMONARY EMERGENCIES

A patient who is presenting with any degree of respiratory compromise is in distress even if they appear and act normal. This section will look at those causes of respiratory compromise that frequently lead to emergency situations.

Upper Airways

Emergencies related to upper airway obstruction involve a blockage of the trachea, larynx, or pharynx.

Epiglottitis A true emergency, epiglottitis is an infection that involves not just the epiglottis but the surrounding tissues as well (Figure 9–2). Rapid inflammation of these tissues can cause a complete blockage of the trachea and subsequent asphyxia. Epiglottitis is traditionally associated with *H. influenza*; however, it can also be caused by several other bacteria and viruses. The use of vaccines against *H. influenza* has greatly reduced the incidence of epiglottitis. Of interest, it is thought that George Washington died of this malady.[12]

Presentation The classic presentation of epiglottitis is the acute onset of sore throat, fever, and difficulty swallowing (dysphagia) that progresses to respiratory distress. Due to the pain associated with swallowing as well as a compromise to

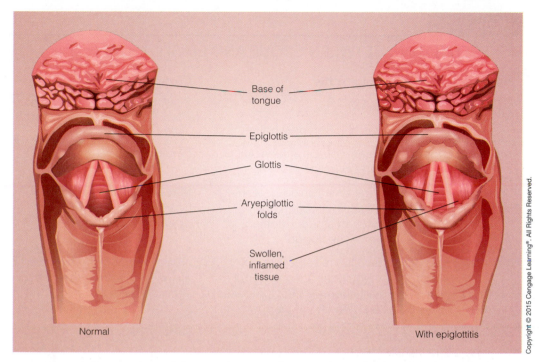

Base of tongue

Epiglottis

Glottis

Aryepiglottic folds

Swollen, inflamed tissue

Normal

With epiglottitis

FIGURE 9–2. Inflammation of the epiglottis and aryepiglottic folds as seen in epiglottis.

the swallowing mechanisms, the child often leans forward with the mouth open and allows the saliva to drool from the mouth. As the disease progresses, the voice becomes muffled and the patient appears "toxic." Stridor, if present, is often mild.

It is of utmost importance to consider epiglottitis in the differential of any child with upper airway signs. Unrecognized, airway obstruction and subsequent respiratory arrest is a high risk. Early recognition allows for interventions that can avoid a catastrophic outcome. The patient with epiglottitis may present with symptoms similar to croup, making it important to differentiate between the two. Table 9–2 contrasts the diagnostic differences between the two.

Examination and Treatment Keeping the child calm is of utmost importance as any agitation can lead to a rapid deterioration of the patient. As much as possible the parents should be kept close to reassure and help reduce the child's anxiety. Invasive procedures, such as an IV, should be delayed until the airway is secured. Both a cardiac monitor and pulse oximeters are placed on the patient upon admission to the emergency room. Oxygen should be provided via cannula or mask. From the time of arrival, the patient should be in constant visual contact with medical staff. An AP and lateral x-ray of the neck can show swelling of the soft tissues. The classic description of the swollen epiglottis as seen on the lateral neck x-ray is the "thumb sign" (Figure 9–3). Patients who have a suspected pneumonia should also have a chest x-ray done. None of these should be done if they lead to patient agitation.

Table 9–2

DIFFERENTIATING BETWEEN CROUP AND EPIGLOTTITIS

Presentation	Epiglottitis	Croup
Age	2–6 years	6 months–3 years
Rate of onset	Rapid (often only hours)	Slow (2–3 days)
Infectious origin	*Haemophilus influenzae* Type b (bacterial)	Parainfluenza virus
Clinical presentation	High fever, anxious, leaning forward, drooling, low pitched stridor, muffled voice, no cough	May be afebrile or febrile; hoarse, barky cough; tight upper airway stridor
X-ray examination	Swollen, edematous epiglot- tis (thumb sign), and *supra- glottic* structures seen on lateral neck film	Narrowing of the subglottic *airway (hourglass) seen on* A-P neck film
Seasonal incidence	Any season	Usually winter

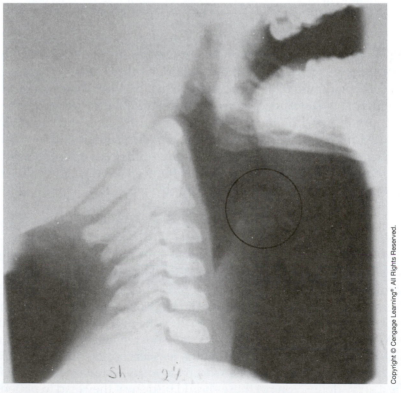

FIGURE 9–3. The "thumb sign" of epiglottis seen on a lateral neck radiograph.

From the time of arrival, preparations should be made for immediate intubation and ventilation in the event of acute loss of airway. This includes any travel away from the emergency department. Additionally, an otolaryngologist, anesthesiologist, or general surgeon trained to perform emergency tracheostomy should be on standby until the airway is established. Once epiglottitis is suspected, the patient is taken to the operating room for securing the airway. Intubation in a controlled environment, such as the operating room, is preferred due to possible need to perform a tracheostomy. Evidence shows increased mortality and morbidity when intubation is not performed; however, there have been reports of successful "watch and wait" strategies, primarily with older pediatric patients who were able to better tolerate their secretions.[13] This approach however, is to be used only with extreme caution. If respiratory arrest occurs before the airway can be secured, use of a bag-mask with slow, long ventilations is recommended. If the airway cannot be established, a needle cricothyroidotomy may be lifesaving.

Once the airway is established, the patient is transported to the intensive care unit and antibiotics are initiated that cover the most likely organisms. The patient is sedated for the duration of intubation and may require mechanical ventilation. The patient is then continuously monitored for a reduction in swelling and edema, at which point extubation can occur. Following extubation, the patient should be monitored for 1 to 2 days prior to discharge.

Croup (Laryngotracheobronchitis) *Croup* is the name given to a group of inflammatory diseases that affect the **subglottic** area of the larynx. Three primary disorders fall in the category of croup. The most common manifestation of croup is laryngotracheitis. Spasmodic croup and laryngotracheobronchitis are less common manifestations seen in pediatric populations.

Diagnosis Laryngotracheitis is the result of a viral organism, with parainfluenza virus accounting for 75% of all croup cases. RSV, influenzas, and *Mycoplasma pneumoniae* cause the remaining 25% of croup cases.

The onset is that of a common cold, with runny nose, cough, fever, and upper airway congestion. The onset of croup symptoms is much slower than is seen in epiglottitis, usually 3 to 4 days. The patient typically wakes in the night, with a tight, barky cough. The patient has upper airway stridor on inspiration and expiration and is in a degree of distress relative to the amount of airway obstruction. An anterior-posterior neck x-ray shows the narrowing of the airway at the level of the larynx. The trachea on these patients has been described as an hourglass, a pencil, and a steeple (Figure 9–4).

Spasmodic croup is an apparent allergic response that results in the sudden onset, usually at night, of a barky cough, shortness of breath, and stridor. The symptoms last for several hours and then subside. The distinguishing factor is in the history. The patient with spasmodic croup is typically healthy, with no signs of upper respiratory infection. There is also a frequent familial history of spasmodic croup and asthma.

Laryngotracheobronchitis is the name given to a bacterial superinfection of laryngotracheitis. As the name suggests, this category of croup involves not only the upper airway structures, but progresses to the bronchial airways and structures.

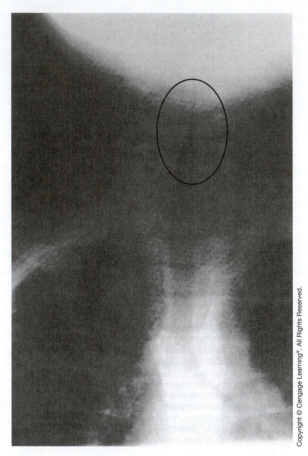

FIGURE 9–4. An A-P neck radiograph showing the narrowing of the larynx. Notice the appearance of a steeple or an hourglass.

Treatment Mild cases of croup may be successfully monitored and treated at home with room humidifiers, adequate hydration, and close observation. However, any sign of distress such as retractions, increased respiratory rate, and nasal flaring are indications for the need of medical intervention.

Because of its viral origin, common croup is treated by support and administration of drugs to reduce the subglottic swelling until the infection subsides. Primary medical treatment involves the nebulization of racemic epinephrine, 0.2–0.5 mL mixed with 2.5 mL of normal saline. Racemic epinephrine causes local vasoconstriction on the swollen tissues and reduces the edema.

If the stridor continues after the treatment, the patient is hospitalized and medication nebulizer treatments are continued as needed every 1 to 2 hours to relieve the airway occlusion. The treatments are then weaned to every 4 to 6 hours as the symptoms subside.

Steroids are often given, with Decadron being the popular choice due to its long half-life (36 to 72 hours) and because it is much more potent than hydrocortisone.[14]

Patients with severe obstruction of the airway may benefit from the use of an oxygen/helium gas mixture to provide oxygenation. Further treatment involves the use of cool mist tents to further reduce swelling and administer any necessary oxygen.

Severe manifestations of croup, such as labored breathing, decreased breath sounds, retractions, and worsening blood gases, may require intubation and the institution of mechanical ventilation. The use of **glucocorticoid** therapy for the treatment of croup has been strongly supported. In particular, nebulized budesonide has been shown to provide prompt clinical improvement in patients with mild to moderate croup.[15]

Although it is not usually a life-threatening disease, any disease that causes swelling of the airway must be closely monitored for signs of worsening condition. The patient who appears to be at rest and comfortable may be semi-comatose from exhaustion and the inability to ventilate. The nature of mist tents, with their high output of aerosol, further inhibits the ability to adequately visualize the patient. Because of these factors, the croup patient must be monitored for breath sounds, respiratory rate, and the presence of retractions at least every 4 hours until the airway blockage is clear.

Foreign Body Obstruction There are several reasons why children are vulnerable for foreign body obstruction. First and foremost is the physiology of development in which oral exploration is a major stage during early life. The narrowness of the airway, which makes even small objects potential airway obstructors is another factor. Finally, aspiration of gastric contents is a common result of reflux in the newborn infant.

The pathologic result of aspiration is air trapping and tissue damage secondary to hydrocarbon aspiration. Air trapping is the result of the ball-valve effect, in which the aspirated object advances deeper into the airway during inspiration, as the airway dilates, and then becomes trapped during exhalation, when the airway collapses back to its original size. The result is the trapping of air behind the object, leading to hyperexpansion of the lung, reduced ventilation, and possible pneumothoraces.

Hydrocarbons The aspiration of hydrocarbons, such as gasoline, oils, turpentine, and kerosene, cause toxic damage to the epithelial lining of the lung called chemical bronchitis. Absorption of these toxic liquids into the blood leads to central nervous system disorders and toxic cardiomyopathies and hepatosplenomegaly. Chemical bronchitis leads to inflammation, edema, atelectasis, mucosal necrosis, and, if aspirated deeply, the formation of hyaline membranes. It is also thought that the aspiration of hydrocarbons may be a factor in the development of Goodpasture syndrome.[16]

Diagnosis and Treatment The diagnosis of foreign body aspiration is made primarily on the history. The patient has a sudden onset of a dry, hacking cough. The patient may have been observed eating the object before the onset of symptoms. If the object is inhaled deeply into the tracheobronchial tree, the coughing may subside somewhat.

Chest x-ray examination may show air trapping distal to the obstruction during expiration. Hydrocarbon aspiration is probable when the symptomatic patient is found near an open container of hydrocarbon liquid and the patient has the strong odor of the liquid on their breath.

Treatment of an aspirated foreign body involves measures to remove the object. Chest physiotherapy may help dislodge the object from the airway. Severe cases may require the use of a bronchoscope to retrieve the object.

Treatment of hydrocarbon aspiration is nonspecific and consists mainly of support. However, if the substance has been swallowed, vomiting should not be induced. As symptoms dictate, the patient is given oxygen and bronchodilators, or intubation and mechanical ventilation are performed.

Inhalation of Noxious Gases

In our modern society, there is a constant danger of exposure to gases and vapors that pose a danger to the pulmonary system. This section will look at some of the more common sources of noxious gases.

Smoke Inhalation Smoke inhalation is a broad category that covers a range of noxious gases produced in a fire. Most deaths in fires result from the inhalation of these noxious fumes, not from burns. Modern furniture and building materials give off many acids and aldehydes in their smoke when burned. These include carbon monoxide, sulfur dioxide, hydrochloric acid, phosgene, and hydrocyanic acid.

Carbon monoxide and hydrocyanic acid are absorbed into the bloodstream and cause serious toxicities in the blood and tissues. Carbon monoxide binds the carrying sites on the hemoglobin molecule, making it impossible for the red blood cell to carry oxygen at those sites. High levels of carbon monoxide lead to widespread tissue hypoxia and eventual death. Of interest, pulse oximetry has been found to be unreliable in estimating O_2 saturation in CO-exposed patients.[17]

Hydrocyanic acid is chemically changed into cyanide, which prevents the uptake of oxygen from the blood by the tissues and leads to rapid death. The other gases and particles found in smoke damage the epithelial lining of the tracheobronchial tree, resulting in airway obstruction from edema, necrosis, sloughing of necrotic epithelium, and bronchospasm. Airway damage may also occur from thermal injury; however, thermal injuries are usually confined to the upper airways.

Diagnosis Any patient who presents with a history of being involved in a fire should be suspected of having suffered smoke inhalation. The patient with significant carbon monoxide poisoning may complain of headache, nausea, and vomiting with COHb levels of 20% to 30%. As the COHb climbs above 40%, the patient begins losing sensorium and becomes comatose.

Diagnosis is made by analyzing the carbon monoxide level of arterial blood with a CO oximeter.

Signs and symptoms of airway damage may be present immediately or may be delayed for hours. The patient shows signs of ever-increasing respiratory distress, with tachypnea, retractions, and cyanosis. As the airway obstruction increases, aeration decreases, widespread atelectasis forms, and the patient's status diminishes quickly.

Treatment The treatment of any patient with smoke inhalation and carbon monoxide poisoning is immediate application of 100% oxygen, preferably under pressure. In room air, the half-life of COHb is 5 hours, declining to 90 minutes in 100% oxygen. Hyperbaric oxygen administration reduces the half-life to less than 30 minutes.

Hyperbaric oxygen administration is the treatment of choice when the COHb is greater than 25%. If hyperbaric oxygen administration isn't available, or is only available at lower levels, oxygen is administered by a tight-fitting, non-rebreathing mask. The addition of a nasal cannula running at 5 lpm to 6 lpm will help increase the F_iO_2.

The hypoxia that results from carbon monoxide poisoning often affects the heart. Therefore, all smoke inhalation patients should have continuous ECG monitoring to observe for signs of myocardial damage.

Pulmonary edema is a frequent finding in patients suffering from carbon monoxide poisoning and smoke inhalation. This necessitates the frequent assessment of breath sounds and monitoring of the respiratory status.

The victim of carbon monoxide/smoke inhalation is at risk for development of RDS. This requires the respiratory therapist to monitor the patient's status closely and be prepared for quick intervention if necessary.

Monitoring and Treatment Patients without obvious, immediate airway damage are monitored closely for signs of worsening respiratory status. When respiratory failure is apparent, the patient is intubated and mechanically ventilated to maintain oxygenation and ventilation.

Antibiotics are given to combat lung infections that take advantage of the damaged tissues. Meticulous attention to proper aseptic techniques will help in preventing hospital-acquired pneumonias. Attention is also given to adequate fluid and electrolyte balance, especially if the patient is suffering from skin burns, which tremendously increases water losses. Bronchoscopy may be needed to remove the epithelial debris that clogs the airways.

Nebulized bronchodilators, followed by chest physiotherapy, are helpful in maintaining the patency of the airways.

Mechanical ventilation is required on the comatose patient to establish an airway and administer oxygen. Ventilator parameters must be set at the lowest levels to achieve oxygenation and ventilation with correct I:E ratios to prevent possible air trapping and barotrauma. In addition, hypocarbia must be avoided because of the left shift of the oxyhemoglobin dissociation curve in the presence of alkalosis.

Chlorine Inhalation Chlorine is a greenish-yellow gas that is extremely irritating to the mucous membranes and skin. In the pediatric patient, inhalation is commonly the result of accidents at swimming pools, where the chlorine is used to disinfect the water. Chlorine is also found in a variety of household cleaning agents.

The injury to the respiratory tract following chlorine inhalation follows four phases. In phase 1, from zero to 6 hours following exposure, choking and coughing are present to some degree, but diminish following removal from the site. Minimal wheezing and slight oropharyngeal redness are present.

Phase 2 occurs between 6 hours and 8 days with the onset of pharyngeal and pulmonary edema, inflammation, and plugging of the bronchi with mucus. Atelectasis develops, as does significant respiratory distress from the combination of upper airway edema and lower airway blockage from sloughing epithelium and tissue debris.

Treatment at this point is mainly supportive, with intubation or tracheostomy often necessary. Large tubes are preferable to assist in the aspiration of airway debris. Mechanical ventilation is started when signs of impending respiratory failure are present. High levels of oxygen may be needed to treat hypoxemia. The use of bronchodilators helps reduce any bronchospasm that may be present.

Phase 3 occurs during weeks 1 to 4 with a gradual improvement in pulmonary function. Phase 4 occurs after the fourth week, with further improvements in airway function and in blood gas status.

BURNS

Thermal burns are a common cause of death in children in the United States. Sequelae such as renal failure, sepsis, pulmonary complications, and severe scarring pose significant additional problems to the burn injury. One of the most common causes of burn injury is scalding especially in the population less than 3 years old.

First-Degree Burns

When only the epidermis is involved, a burn is classified as first degree. The skin becomes erythematous, but no blisters form. Sunburn is a common type of first degree burn. These burns heal within 1 week and rarely require treatment beyond symptomatic relief.

Second-Degree Burns

When a burn extends beyond the epidermis to the superficial dermis, it is called a "partial-thickness," or second-degree, burn. The skin becomes edematous, blistered, erythematous, and painful to the touch. In a true second-degree burn, the dermal appendages are preserved and allow for healing and regeneration.

Third-Degree Burns

When the burn destroys the dermis and dermal appendages, it is considered a "full-thickness," or third-degree, burn. The skin appears to be charred, with a whitish color and a leathery feel. Sensation is lost.

Body Surface Area

The area of body surface affected by the burn is an important part of the assessment and work-up. In adults, the "**rule of nines**" is used to estimate body surface area involvement, however, this typically does not work in children due to the tremendous variation in size. Figure 9–5 illustrates a method of determining body surface area percentages in pediatric patients.

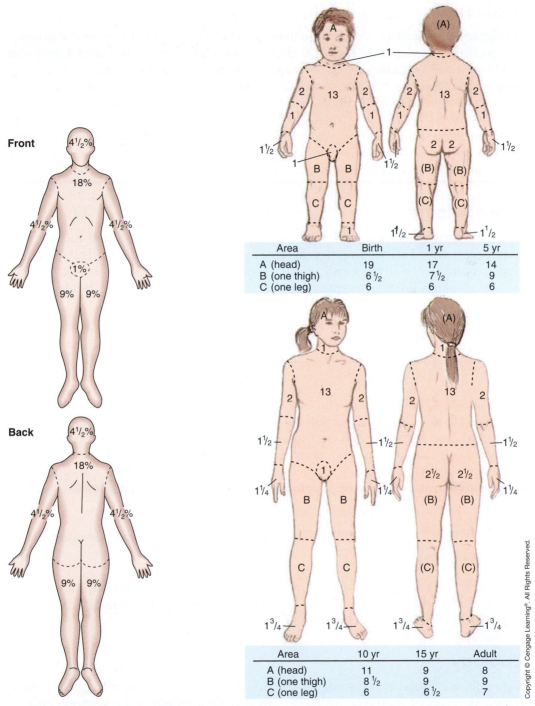

Front

4½%

18%

4½%   4½%

1%

9%   9%

Back

4½%

18%

4½%   4½%

9%   9%

Area	Birth	1 yr	5 yr
A (head)	19	17	14
B (one thigh)	6 ½	7 ½	9
C (one leg)	6	6	6

Area	10 yr	15 yr	Adult
A (head)	11	9	8
B (one thigh)	8 ½	9	9
C (one leg)	6	6 ½	7

FIGURE 9–5. A method of determining body surface area percentages in pediatric patients.

Evaluation

A primary assessment is done immediately to stabilize the patient. After stabilization has occurred, a secondary survey is done to completely assess the burn injury and its extent. Labs, including a CBC, hematocrit, electrolytes, and renal function tests are drawn to establish a baseline. A urinalysis, especially the specific gravity, can help assess hydration status. Additionally, an arterial blood gas, chest x-ray, and ongoing pulse-oximetry are used to manage the patients' pulmonary status. Criteria for hospitalization include: burns greater than 10% in a child; any burn in the very young; any full-thickness burn; burns to the face, neck, hands, feet or perineum; circumferential burns; inhalation injury; and associated trauma or significant pre-burn illness.[18]

Management

Once the airway is secured and breathing/ventilation is established the focus of treatment is aimed at maintaining adequate tissue perfusion. While fluid resuscitation remains controversial, most institutions have adopted the Parkland formula (below), which calculates fluid requirements for burn patients over a 24-hour period.

TBSA burned (%) $\times$ Wt (kg) $\times$ 4mL
Give 1/2 of total requirements in 1st 8 hours, then give 2nd half over next 16 hours.
Example: 40 kg patient with burns over 20% of the body
$20 \times 40 \times 4 = 3200$ mL

While the Parkland formula gives an estimation of fluid requirements, it is important to monitor urine output and maintain a urine flow of 1 mL/kg/h.

Initial care of the burned area involves covering the burned areas with sterile saline soaked dressings at room temperature. Hypothermia is a high risk, especially with the pediatric burn patient. Avoiding drafts can help reduce the amount of evaporative heat loss. Tetanus prophylaxis is also mandatory in all cases.[19]

SPINAL CORD INJURIES

Although not a common malady among children, spinal cord injuries do occur in infants and children, and an understanding of the pathophysiology involved is important for the respiratory therapist.

Etiology

Injury to the spinal cord is related to various accidents. Sudden hyperflexion or hyperextension of the neck during an automobile accident is a common cause of injury. Falls from trees, horses, and during sports are another cause of spinal injury. Injuries to the spine may occur in the neonate during breech deliveries. Gunshot wounds and stabbings are other possible causes of spinal cord injury.

Of most interest to the respiratory therapist are those injuries that affect the muscles of ventilation. The diaphragm is innervated by the phrenic nerve, which arises from the cervical plexus. The fourth cervical nerve is the main contributor to this plexus, with the third and fifth cervical nerves making secondary contributions. Injuries at or above this level result in loss of the use of the diaphragm and the need for long-term ventilatory assistance.

The intercostal muscles are innervated by the intercostal nerves, which arise from the 1st through the 11th thoracic vertebrae. Loss of these nerves by cord injury is not as devastating as a loss of the phrenic nerve; however, the patient will lose a portion of the pulmonary reserve when the intercostal nerves are damaged.

Treatment The three goals of management of spinal cord injuries are: (1) preservation of neurologic function and prevention of further neurologic deteriorations, (2) maximization of neurologic recovery, and (3) prevention of intercurrent nonneurologic complications.

The role of the respiratory therapist in the early stages of the injury is to manage the ventilatory status of the patient and prevent pneumonias through vigorous pulmonary toilet and maintenance of the airway. In the later stages of the injury, the respiratory therapist is vital in the rehabilitation of the pulmonary system. This is done by using deep breathing, assisted coughing techniques, and exercises that strengthen the diaphragm.

HEAD INJURY

It is estimated that head injuries in children aged 1–19 lead to over 600,000 hospitalizations a year. Of those injured, roughly 22,000 deaths result. Eighty percent of children with multiple trauma have severe head injury as compared to adults in which only 50% have severe head injury.[20] Several basic concepts in the care of head injuries may help to reduce morbidity and mortality in these patients.

Head Anatomy

There are several layers of soft tissue, tendon, fascia, and bone that comprise the anatomy of the head (Figure 9–6). Starting at the outermost level is the scalp. The scalp is composed of five layers. The first three layers of the scalp are connected and move in unison. The first layer is the skin, which contains the hair follicles and sebaceous glands. The skin of the scalp is very well vascularized which accounts for the amount of blood lost when it is lacerated. The next layer is also very vascular and makes up the connective tissue layer. Cutaneous nerves also permeate the connective tissue layer. Just beneath this layer is the **aponeurosis** which is a broad tendon sheath that serves as an attachment for the forehead and temporal muscles. The free movement of the first three layers over the cranium is due to the next layer, which consists of loose areolar tissue in a spongy layer. This layer also has potential spaces that can distend with blood or fluid in the event of injury. The final layer is the **pericranium**, which is connective tissue and forms the external **periosteum** of the **neurocranium**.

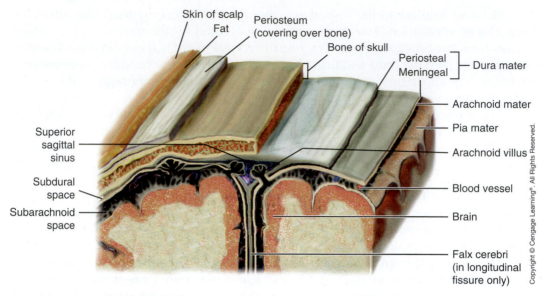

Skin of scalp
Fat
Periosteum
(covering over bone)
Bone of skull
Periosteal
Meningeal } Dura mater
Arachnoid mater
Pia mater
Superior
sagittal
sinus
Arachnoid villus
Subdural
space
Blood vessel
Subarachnoid
space
Brain
Falx cerebri
(in longitudinal
fissure only)

FIGURE 9–6. Layers of the skull.

The cranium is the skeletal portion of the head. The portion that protects the brain is called the neurocranium. The internal surface of the neurocranium is covered with a membranous covering called the **meninges**, composed of three layers. The dura mater is the thick external fibrous layer and itself is composed of two layers, the external periosteal layer and the internal meningeal layer. The arachnoid mater is the thin intermediate layer and the pia mater is the internal layer. The pia mater is delicate in comparison to the other layers and contains vasculature. Between the arachnoid and pia mater is the subarachnoid space which is filled with cerebrospinal fluid. The subarachnoid space is framed by **trabeculae**; small bridges of fibroblasts that have the appearance of a spider web. The subdural space between the dura and arachnoid mater is not a true space, but can become a fluid filled space as a result of trauma. The brain lies just beneath the pia mater.

Head trauma can result in fractures and bleeding that can occur in several areas. Tears in the middle meningeal artery result in blood accumulation between the dura and the cranium, forming an epidural **hematoma** also called a subdural hematoma. Subarachnoid hemorrhage is usually the result of the rupture of an aneurysm but may be associated with cranial fractures and cerebral lacerations.

Pathophysiology

When dealing with closed head injuries, it is important to understand there are two mechanisms that damage the brain. First is the primary insult, or the injury that occurs at the moment of the accident. How badly the brain is damaged is determined by the intensity of the blow. Primary injuries are related to the physical impact of the brain against the cranial bone, resulting in fractures and contusions.

Secondary injuries are the result of the primary injury. They include hypoxia, hypotension, and hypercarbia, which worsen the brain ischemia, and associated swelling, and hematomas, which may cause herniation of the brain. The effect of the secondary injuries is to damage areas of the brain that may not have been affected by the primary insult. Eventually, the entire brain becomes involved, resulting in high morbidity and mortality. Treating and preventing secondary insults are a vital part of treating head-injured patients.

Often, a comatose pediatric patient with signs of brain stem injury has not suffered irreversible damage but can still recover if proper treatment of ICP is initiated quickly.

Specific Head Injuries

Injuries to the scalp are common and may bleed profusely due to the abundant vascularization. Significant blood loss can occur from even relatively small lacerations. With all head injuries, including lacerations, the skull must be examined thoroughly for the presence of a fracture. In the presence of a skull fracture, there may or may not be brain injury and conversely, the absence of a skull fracture does not rule out a brain injury. In infants and children, the phenomenon of a "**growing fracture**" is occasionally seen. Typically, in children under 2 years of age, the fracture is associated with a tear in the dura. Brain growth at this age is rapid, and the growing brain can lead to an extrusion of brain tissue through the fracture, called a leptomeningeal cyst, and subsequent "growing fracture,"

Epidural hematomas (Figure 9–7) are often occult in children. Most are associated with a skull fracture and require rapid diagnosis and surgical intervention to lessen mortality and morbidity. Signs and symptoms are as they are in adults and include altered mentation, headache, and vomiting.

Subdural hematomas (Figure 9–8) are less common in children than in adults. Shaking and impact injuries are common causes as they are typically of the

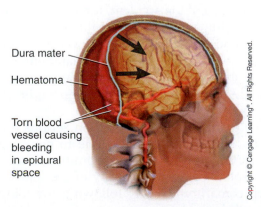

Dura mater

Hematoma

Torn blood vessel causing bleeding in epidural space

FIGURE 9–7. Epidural hematoma.

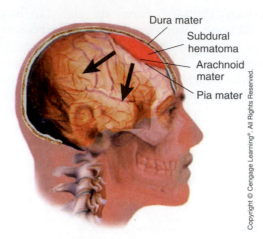

Dura mater

Subdural
hematoma

Arachnoid
mater

Pia mater

FIGURE 9–8. Subdural hematoma.

acceleration-deceleration type. Subdural hematomas are typically more indolent than epidural hematomas and manifest as lethargy, irritability, and vomiting.

Fracture of the basilar skull can occur anywhere along the base of the skull and present with cerebrospinal fluid from the nose and **hemotympanum** (blood behind the tympanic membrane). Late findings include periorbital ecchymosis, also called "**raccoon eyes**" and auricular ecchymosis, also called "**Battle's sign**."

Brain contusion is essentially a bruise occurring in the brain parenchyma and can either be a **coup** or **contrecoup** injury. A coup injury occurs at the site of injury whereas a contrecoup injury occurs at a site away from the injury.

Treatment

The overriding goal of treating a head injury is to prevent any secondary injury to the brain, which includes hypoxemia, ischemia, and increased ICP. Treatment of a head injury must begin at the site of the accident, if recovery is to be expected. The most important aspect of treating a head-injured patient is to maintain and protect the airway from aspiration and to provide adequate ventilation and oxygenation. Endotracheal intubation is the method of choice for maintaining the airway of the severely injured patient. Intubation should only be carried out by trained personnel who are able to intubate and/or ventilate without hyperextending the head and possibly exacerbating a neck injury.

Diffuse swelling of the brain is the most common serious finding following a severe head injury, and its treatment is the keystone to neurologic recovery. The signs of cerebral edema, **obtundation**, sweating, vomiting, and bradycardia, may occur rapidly or slowly, depending on the severity of the injury. The most severe injuries present in a deep coma immediately following the injury. There is often evidence of **decorticate** and **decerebrate** posturing, (Figure 9–9) abnormal pupillary responses, and apnea. The diagnosis of brain swelling is confirmed by CT scan, which shows a decrease in the size, or even a total loss of the ventricles.

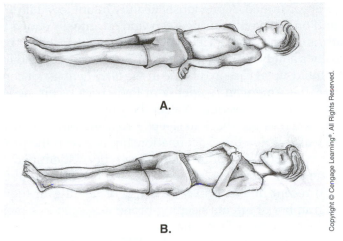

FIGURE 9–9. A. Decerebrate posturing B. Decorticate posturing.

Immediate treatment of the brain swelling is essential with prompt access to neurosurgical intervention being the priority. Hypoxemia and hypercarbia must be avoided, as they both cause an increase in cerebral blood flow and ICP. Mechanical ventilation is provided and arterial blood gases are closely followed in order to maintain arterial oxygen and carbon dioxide levels at normal levels. In the event the ICP continues to rise, hyperventilating the patient to lower the arterial carbon dioxide can assist in decreasing the ICP to safer levels.[21]

Continuous monitoring of the $PaCO_2$ and PaO_2, by transcutaneous monitors, pulse oximetry, or end-tidal CO_2 will help the respiratory therapist adjust the ventilator as needed to maintain the desired parameters. Maintenance of brain perfusion is the overriding goal during the initial treatment of head injury. Blood perfusion to the brain is calculated by subtracting intracranial pressure from the mean arterial pressure. Monitoring those pressures requires the placement of an arterial line as well as ICP monitor. An indwelling Foley catheter to measure urine output can help provide an indirect measurement of cardiac output as well as help assess fluid status. Ideally, a state of mild dehydration can help reduce ICP and edema.

Suctioning should be done only as needed and should be done quickly to avoid increasing peak inspiratory pressures. Levels of positive end-expiratory pressures should be kept at a minimum, if used at all.

Medications used to help prevent secondary brain injury include diuretics, antiseizure medications, and coma-inducing drugs. Additionally, the head of the bed is elevated to 30°.

SUDDEN INFANT DEATH SYNDROME

Although much time and effort has been spent in the study of sudden infant death syndrome (SIDS), it remains a relatively unknown entity and accounts for the highest number of deaths in infants of less than 1 year old. The diagnosis of SIDS is not made until an autopsy is performed. A previously healthy infant less than 1 year of age who dies suddenly and unexpectedly during sleep, and on autopsy shows no apparent reason for the death, is diagnosed as a victim of SIDS. Many researchers believe that problems with the baby's ability to wake up (sleep arousal), and the inability for the baby's body to detect a build-up of carbon dioxide in the blood are major contributors.[22]

In April 1992, the American Academy of Pediatrics recommended that infants not be placed in the prone position to sleep because of the association with SIDS; this initiative is known as the "back to sleep" program. Since then, SIDS rates have dropped dramatically. While the exact relationship between the prone position and SIDS has not been determined, four factors have been identified that elevate the risk of SIDS in the prone position. They are: (1) the use of natural fiber mattresses, (2) swaddling (3) recent illness, and (4) the use of heating in the bedroom.[23] The reduction in the number of infants sleeping prone was seen as a major contributing factor in a SIDS decline rate in Tasmania.[24]

Recently, risk factors associated with SIDS have been extensively studied. Traditional risk factors include black race, low birth weight, prematurity, 5-minute Apgar score less than 7, male gender, low maternal age and education level, multiple births, and maternal smoking. When examined statistically, the only risk factor independently associated with SIDS was maternal smoking.[25] This link between maternal smoking, passive smoke exposure, and SIDS has been corroborated in other studies.[26, 27, 28] A list of risk factors is shown in Table 9–3.

Table 9–3

SIDS RISK FACTORS

Sleeping on the stomach

Being around cigarette smoke while in the womb or after being born

Sleeping in the same bed as their parents

Soft bedding in the crib

Multiple birth babies (being a twin, triplet, etc.)

Premature birth

Having a brother or sister who had SIDS

Mothers who smoke or use illegal drugs

Being born to a teen mother

Short time period between pregnancies

Late or no prenatal care

Living in poverty situations

Several other factors that play a role in SIDS have been proposed. They include the following: increased levels of interleukin-6 in the cerebrospinal fluid[29], surfactant abnormalities[30]; anaphylaxis[31]; variability in organ weights[32]; gastroesophageal reflux[33], abnormal pulmonary inflammatory response[34], maternal cocaine use[35], and basement membrane thickening of the vocal cords.[36]

SIDS usually hits during winter and at night, and the most common ages are 2 to 4 months with males being affected more frequently than females. Even with knowledge of risk factors, it remains impossible to identify those infants who will die of SIDS. The incidence of SIDS remains at approximately 2 out of every 1000 births and continues to frustrate attempts to establish its cause.

The common event in all SIDS deaths is a quiet cessation of breathing during sleep. It is apparent that SIDS is a complex, multifactorial disorder that at the present time has no cure.

POISONING

Poisoning deaths in the pediatric population have dropped significantly in the past few decades thanks largely to heightened awareness by parents, child-resistant packaging, and more aggressive and sophisticated treatments. While a majority of poisonings are by ingestion, inhalation, injection and contact poisonings can also occur. Perhaps the most important step in the management of accidental poisoning is a complete and accurate history of the ingestion, including the toxin or medication, how much was taken and the time of exposure. If the history is inadequate or incomplete, assume the worst.

When doing an examination on a poisoned pediatric patient, there are often clues to help identify the nature of the poison. Specifically, alterations of heart rate, respiratory rate and effort, blood pressure, and temperature can help with the diagnosis. A good neurologic exam, watching for signs of reduced consciousness and a change in the pupillary response can aid in identifying the toxin. Additionally, a toxicology screening can help in identification of the toxin; however, it does have limitations. In particular, if a medication with a short half-life is ingested, the screen may be negative if too long of a time has passed since ingestion. A urine screen may be helpful due the fact that drug metabolites continue to be excreted following ingestion for several days.

Management

The immediate care of the poisoned patient is to support the airway, breathing, and circulation. Most patients who are not critically ill can be safely managed using activated charcoal. Activated charcoal works best when given soon after the ingestion. The charcoal binds to the toxin (**adsorption**) and allows it to pass through the GI tract without being absorbed into the circulatory system. Evacuation of the toxin can be achieved with syrup of ipecac; however, this method is contraindicated in children less than 6 months of age and in those who have ingested hydrocarbons, acids and alkalis, or sharp objects. Additionally, any patient in a coma or with a history of seizures should not receive ipecac. Cathartics such as sorbitol, magnesium citrate, and magnesium sulfate are used to induce diarrhea. Gastric lavage can remove toxins from the stomach by repeated flushing of a large-bore orogastric tube with sterile saline.

ANAPHYLAXIS

Anaphylaxis is essentially a "whole-body" allergic reaction that is rapid in onset and may cause death.[37] Various tissues in the body release histamine and other inflammatory mediators that lead to swelling of the airways and GI tract. Hypotension occurs from a dilation of the vasculature and maldistribution of the blood volume. The patient can become lethargic and confused as the process continues. Anaphylaxis is most commonly caused by foods, medicines, and insect envenomations. Common foods causing anaphylaxis include nuts, milk, fish, shellfish, soy, wheat, and eggs. While any medication can trigger an allergic reaction, the most common causes are the β-lactam antibiotics, sulfa, anticonvulsants, aspirin, and NSAIDs. Bee and wasp stings account for most allergic reactions to envenomations. Other causes include latex, exercise, x-ray contrasts, and idiopathic.

Symptoms of an allergic reaction and anaphylaxis include hives, skin and eyes itching, and swelling of the lips, tongue, or face. As the process worsens, the patient begins to wheeze and has difficulty breathing, appears confused, complains of being dizzy and lightheaded, and complains of abdominal pain and cramping with diarrhea. If vital signs are taken, the patient will have tachycardia and hypotension.

The mainstay of treatment for anaphylaxis is epinephrine administered IM. Additionally, antihistamines, both H1 and H2, as well as corticosteroids are included in the treatment plan.

SUMMARY

The resuscitation and stabilization of pediatric patients is a skill all respiratory therapists must be proficient in. While the primary role is to maintain oxygenation and ventilation, it is equally important to recognize the signs, symptoms, and causes of pediatric cardiac arrest and trauma. While unusual in children, cardiac arrest can and does occur, making its recognition essential for all who work in pediatrics. Education of the parents and caretakers can greatly reduce the risk of most causes of cardiac arrest and trauma.

It is highly recommended that all respiratory therapists be trained in pediatric advanced life support (PALS) as offered by the American Academy of Pediatrics. The proper application of chest compressions, airway maintenance, monitoring, and the provision of adequate ventilation are skills that are critical when working to reverse the effects of cardiac arrest. When possible, training should be obtained to perform pediatric tracheal intubation. Part of the PALS training is the training to administer lifesaving medications either via IV or IO access. The use of algorithms allows the team to consistently and effectively identify and treat various life threatening arrhythmias.

Trauma care in a pediatric patient begins before the patient arrives in the emergency department. Anticipation by the trauma team avoids any last second surprises. Patient assessment begins with the primary survey. The purpose of the primary survey is to quickly assess the airway, breathing, circulation, and cervical spine and stabilize the patient. Once the primary survey is complete and the patient is stabile, the secondary survey is done. A thorough head to toe exam is done to look for any injury that may not have been apparent in the primary survey.

Shock can be caused by several events and must be quickly identified and treated to avoid serious complications or death. The fascination children have with water may lead them get into trouble quickly. Near drowning is not uncommon in the pediatric population, and understanding the pathophysiology behind the injury allows proper assessment and management for the most favorable outcome. Obstruction of the upper airway from infectious causes, as in epiglottitis and croup, can lead to dire consequences if not identified and managed appropriately. An understanding of the presenting signs and symptoms will allow for a quick differentiation between the two with appropriate treatment. Children are also susceptible to airway obstruction from foreign bodies and chemicals. Small items that typically would not block an adult airway can totally obstruct the trachea in a pediatric patient. Additionally, the inhalation of hydrocarbons, noxious gases, and smoke can quickly create an emergency situation.

In young children, thermal injury is a common cause of death with scalding being one of the most common sources of injury. An understanding of the different degrees of burns and the evaluation and management of each is a vital skill for the respiratory therapist working with pediatric patient populations.

When working with children who have been involved in a traumatic accident, the care of the spinal cord becomes of paramount importance. An understanding of the etiology of the injury as well as its management is critical. Head injuries are a major cause of hospitalizations in children and result in many deaths. Knowledge of the anatomy of the skull helps one to locate and identify injuries to the brain as well as the vasculature and bony structures. The pathophysiology of head injury includes both primary and secondary injuries. Treating and preventing those secondary insults are a vital part of the management of head injury.

Despite all the research that has been done, frighteningly little is known about SIDS and it remains the leading cause of death between the ages of 1 month to 1 year. While little is known about the etiology of this disorder, much has been learned about how to reduce the risk of SIDS.

Deaths from poisonings have dropped significantly in the past few decades. This drop can be attributed to an aggressive education of parents, child-resistant packaging, and new sophisticated treatment options. The management of poisoning, while not in the immediate purview of the respiratory therapist, can affect the respiratory system and, thus, must be understood to work with these patients.

POSTTEST

1. You are called STAT to a room on the pediatric wing of the hospital during a day shift. You find a 2 year old who is unresponsive to any stimulus. The patient is not breathing and there is no palpable pulse. Which of the following is the next appropriate step?
   a. Shout for help and activate the EMS.
   b. Begin mouth to mouth ventilations.
   c. Apply an ECG or AED to evaluate the heart rhythm.
   d. Begin chest compressions at a rate of 60/minute.
2. You are asked to evaluate a 3-year-old patient with tachycardia. You are assessing the patients ECG and notice that the QRS complex is 0.125 ms in length. The patient is showing signs of cardiopulmonary compromise. The next step in the evaluation is:
   a. begin chest compressions
   b. perform vagal maneuvers
   c. synchronized cardioversion
   d. consider the use of adenosine
3. You are covering the emergency department during your shift when a 5-year-old patient arrives following a fall from a ladder. The first step in the primary survey of this patient is:
   a. Assess the cardiac rhythm.
   b. Maintain an adequate airway while mobilizing the cervical spine.
   c. Establish IV access.
   d. Check the patient's mental status.
4. While performing a Glasgow Coma Score on a 9-month-old car accident victim, you note that she opens her eyes to pain, cries persistently and withdraws in response to pain. Her coma score is:
   a. 5
   b. 7
   c. 9
   d. 11
5. A 4-year-old patient has a 4-day history of vomiting and diarrhea. He is lethargic and does not respond well to verbal stimulus. His skin is cool to the touch and pale. You suspect he is in shock. What is the most likely type of shock in this patient?
   a. hypovolemic
   b. respiratory
   c. neurogenic
   d. cardiogenic

6. A 6-year-old girl was found by her family in a neighborhood pond. CPR was started immediately. Upon arrival at the emergency department, CPR is still being performed, and she is intubated and being bag ventilated. She is still in her wet clothing. Which of the following is the most appropriate step at this point:
   a. Remove her wet clothing and warm her as soon as possible.
   b. Obtain a chest x-ray.
   c. Establish IV access.
   d. Place a cardiac monitor.

7. You are performing a pulmonary examination on a 7-year-old male patient with a history of sore throat, fever, and dysphagia. He is lying on the gurney and you note a large amount of drool coming from the corner of his mouth. The next step in the evaluation of this patient would be:
   a. Make arrangements for the patient to be taken to the operating room to establish an airway.
   b. Visualize the oropharynx with a tongue depressor.
   c. Establish IV access.
   d. Give the patient a small volume nebulizer treatment with racemic epinephrine.

8. You are caring for a 8-month-old patient diagnosed with croup. He has been receiving nebulized racemic epinephrine Q4–6 hours with mild relief from the symptoms. The pediatrician asks you what else might be done to help improve the symptoms. Your recommendation is:
   a. chest physiotherapy
   b. increase the percent of oxygen the patient is receiving
   c. add decadron to the treatment
   d. change the nebulized medication to albuterol

9. While treating a 9-year-old male who was rescued from a burning house, you note that the pulse oximeter is reading 95% saturation. The patient is on a simple oxygen mask running at 6 lpm. With this information, what is the best course of action?
   a. Ninety-five percent is an adequate saturation; nothing needs to be done.
   b. It is likely the pulse oximeter reading is not valid. A blood gas should be drawn to assess the patient's oxygenation status.
   c. The oxygen should be turned up to at least 10 lpm.
   d. The patient should be intubated to protect the airway from the inevitable swelling.

10. A 10-year-old female is brought into the emergency department following an accidental burn at home. She has second-degree burns over the left anterior arm and palm, and her left anterior upper thigh. She weighs 70 pounds. What percent body area is involved?
    a. 1%
    b. 5%
    c. 9%
    d. 18%

11. Using the Parkland formula, what would be her fluid needs?
    a. 1.1 liters
    b. 2.14 liters
    c. 3.21 liters
    d. 4.3 liters
12. A 12-year-old boy is brought to the emergency room following an accident on his bike in which he went over the handlebars and hit his head on the pavement. He was not wearing a helmet. He was reportedly confused at the scene. What type of head injury is he likely to have?
    a. epidural bleed
    b. subarachnoid bleed
    c. intraventricular bleed
    d. subdural bleed
13. "Battle's sign" is indicative of which of the following?
    a. increased intracranial pressure
    b. basilar skull fracture
    c. intraventricular bleed
    d. cerebellar hemorrhage
14. Of the following, which is not linked to an increase in the risk of SIDS in the prone position?
    a. the use of natural fiber mattresses
    b. swaddling
    c. recent illness
    d. the use of a humidifier/vaporizor in the bedroom
15. Which of the following is an example of adsorption in the treatment of poisoning?
    a. ipecac
    b. activated charcoal
    c. sorbitol
    d. lavage

REFERENCES

1. BLS for Healthcare Providers. Channing Bete Company. South Deerfield, MA: AHA, 2010.
2. PALS Provider Manual. Channing Bete Company. South Deerfield, MA: AHA, AAP, 2010.
3. Pediatric Advanced Life Support. South Deerfield, MA: American Heart Association, 2010.
4. Kleinman ME, et al. Pediatric Advanced Life Support: 2010 American Heart Association Guidelines for Cardiopulmonary Resuscitation and Emergency Cardiovascular Care. http://pediatrics.aappublications.org/content/126/5/e1361.full. 2010

5. Kleinman, M.E. et.al. Pediatric Advanced Life Support: 2010 American Heart Association Guidelines for Cardiopulmonary Resuscitation and Emergency Cardiovascular Care.

6. Medline Plus. Death among children and adolescents http://www.nlm.nih .gov/medlineplus/ency/article/001915.htm.

7. Heron M. Deaths: Leading Causes for 2010. National Vital Statistics Reports, CDC. http://www.cdc.gov/nchs/data/nvsr/nvsr62/nvsr62_06.pdf.

8. Peam JH. Secondary drowning in children. *Br Med J.* 281(6248):1103–1105, Oct. 25, 1980.

9. Paul RL, et al. Intracranial pressure responses to alterations in arterial carbon dioxide pressure in patients with head injuries. *J Neurosurg.* 36:714–720, 1972.

10. Muizelaar JP, et al. Adverse effects of prolonged hyperventilation in patients with severe head injury: A randomized clinical trial. *J Neurosurg.* 75:731–739, 1991.

11. Obrist WD, et al. Cerebral blood flow and metabolism in comatose patients with acute head injury. *J Neurosurg.* 61:241–253, 1984.

12. http://emedicine.medscape.com/article/763612-overview.

13. Felter, RAF. Emergent management of pediatric epiglottitis. http://emedicine. medscape.com/article/801369-overview#a1.

14. Levin D, et al. *Essentials of Pediatric Intensive Care.* 2nd ed. St. Louis, MO: Quality Medical Publishing, Inc., 1997.

15. Klassen ME. Nebulized budesonide for children with mild-to-moderate croup. *N Engl J Med.* 331:285, 1994.

16. Goodpasture syndrome. PubMed Health. http://www.ncbi.nlm.nih.gov/ pubmedhealth/PMH0001197/. 2013

17. Buckley RG, et. al. The pulse oximetry gap in carbon monoxide intoxication. *Ann Emerg Med.* 24(2):252–255, Aug. 1994.

18. World Health Organization. Management of burns. http://www.who.int/ surgery/publications/Burns_management.pdf.

19. World Health Organization. Management of burns. http://www.who.int/ surgery/publications/Burns_management.pdf.

20. Strange GR, et al. Head trauma. *Pediatric Emergency Medicine: A Comprehensive Study Guide.* 2nd ed. New York: McGraw-Hill, 2002.

21. Ibid.

22. Sudden infant death syndrome. PubMed Health http://www.ncbi.nlm.nih .gov/pubmedhealth/PMH0002533/. 2011

23. Ponsonby AL, et al. Factors potentiating the risk of sudden infant death syndrome associated with the prone position. *N Engl J Med.* 329:377, 1993.

24. Dwyer T, et al. The contribution of changes in the prevalence of prone sleeping position to the decline in sudden infant death syndrome in Tasmania. *JAMA.* 273:783–789, 1995.

25. Taylor JA, Sanderson M. A reexamination of the risk factors for the suddeen infant death syndrome. *J Pediatr.* 126:887–891, 1995.

26. DiFranza JR, Lew RA. Effect of maternal cigarette smoking on pregnancy complications and sudden infant death syndrome. *J Fam Pract.* 40:385–394, 1995.

27. Klonoff-Cohen HS, et al. The effect of passive smoking and tobacco exposure through breast milk on sudden infant death syndrome. *JAMA*. 273:795–798, 1995.

28. Fleming PJ. Understanding and preventing sudden infant death syndrome. *Curr Opin Pediatr*. 6:158–162, 1994.

29. Vege A, et al. SIDS cases have increased levels of interleukin-6 in cerebrospinal fluid. *Acta Pediatr*. 84:193–196, 1995.

30. Masters IB et al. Surfactant abnormalities in ALTE and SIDS. *Arch Dis Child*. 71:501–505, 1994.

31. Holgate ST, et al. The anaphylaxis hypothesis of sudden infant death syndrome (SIDS): mast cell degranulation in cot death revealed by elevated concentrations of tryptase in serum. *Clin Exp Allergy*. 24:1115–1122, 1994.

32. Siebert JR, Haas JE. Organ weights in sudden infant death syndrome. *Pediatr Pathol*. 14:973–985, 1994.

33. Freed GE, et al. Sudden infant death syndrome prevention and an understanding of selected clinical issues. *Pediatr Clin N Am*. 41:967–990, 1994.

34. Howat WJ, et al. Pulmonary immunopathology of sudden infant death syndrome. *Lancet*. 343:1390–1392, 1994.

35. Fox CH. Cocaine use in pregnancy. *J Am Board Fam Pract*. 7:225–228, 1994.

36. Shatz A. Age-related basement membrane thickening of the vocal cords in sudden infant death syndrome (SIDS). *Laryngoscope*. 104:865–868, 1994.

37. Tintinalli, Judith E. *Emergency Medicine: A Comprehensive Study Guide (Emergency Medicine [Tintinalli])*. New York: McGraw-Hill, 2010, pp. 177–182.

BIBLIOGRAPHY AND SUGGESTED READINGS

Fleegler, E and Kleinman, M. "Guidelines for pediatric advanced life support" Feb. 2014. UpToDate. http://www.uptodate.com/contents/guidelines-for-pediatric-advanced-life-support

APLS: The Pediatric Emergency Medicine Resource. 2012 Jones & Bartlett Learning LLC, American Academy of Pediatrics, and American College of Emergency Physicians. http://www.aplsonline.com/default.aspx

Pediatric Educatin for Prehospital Professionals, 3rd. ed. 2013 American Academy of Pediatrics and Jones & Bartlett Learning. http://www.peppsite.com/

King, C. and Henretig, F.M. "Textbook of Pediatric Emergency Procedures" 2008. Philadelphia, Lippincott Williams & Wilkins.

Polin, R.A, Fox, W.W. and Abman, S.H. "Fetal and Neonatal Physiology, 4th ed. 2011. Amsterdam. Saunders/Elsevier

Harries, M. "ABC of Resuscitation Near Drowning" BMJ 2003; 327: `1336

OBJECTIVES

Upon completion of this chapter, the reader should be able to:

1. List at least seven anatomic and physiologic differences between a pediatric patient and an adult.
2. Describe the terms "chief complaint" and "differential diagnosis" and how they are used to arrive at a diagnosis.
3. Define and describe a "well-child" visit and how it differs from an ill-child visit.
4. Describe the steps in taking a history during a well-child visit and an ill-child visit.
5. Explain the general concepts of physical examination in pediatric patients.
6. When given appropriate data, calculate a patient's status using an appropriate growth chart.
7. Discuss and describe strategies used during the physical examination of an infant and child that will help make the encounter safe and less stressful for the patient.
8. Describe how to perform a general assessment on a pediatric patient.
9. Describe and explain the performance of a head-to-toe examination for each body system.
10. List three goals to be achieved when examining the pediatric pulmonary system. Include a description of how each goal is assessed.
11. Define the term "anticipatory guidance" and list resources that are available to help in the education of parents.
12. List the indications and contraindications for performing a pulmonary function testing (PFT) on a pediatric patient.
13. Describe the special requirements needed when assessing pulmonary function on the pediatric patient.

KEY TERMS

alae nasi
anticipatory guidance
chief complaint (CC)
differential diagnosis
  (DDx)

Erb's point
hyperpnea
hypoventilation
petichiae
pleural effusion

purpura
red reflex
scoliosis

INTRODUCTION

Proper respiratory care of the pediatric patient begins with a firm understanding of the anatomic and physiologic differences between pediatric and adult patients, as discussed in the beginning of this chapter. That understanding is used along with a physical assessment to diagnose respiratory problems and help plan and implement a course of treatment. Certain problems (particularly airway emergencies in young children) and specific cardiopulmonary diseases or abnormalities are unique to pediatric patients because of these anatomic and physiologic differences.

ANATOMIC AND PHYSIOLOGIC DIFFERENCES

When assessing a pediatric patient, it is important for the provider to have an understanding of the anatomic and physiologic differences between an adult and a child. Children are not just "small adults." We will first compare general differences and then look at specific body areas.

Compared to adults, children have a proportionately larger body surface area (BSA). Additionally, smaller patients have a greater ratio of BSA to skin surface area. As in neonates, the increase in BSA can lead to an increase in insensible water loss and thermoregulation problems. Two important body functions, the basal metabolic rate and minute ventilation, both parallel the BSA. The skin of a child is immature and less keratinized, making it more prone to trauma and the absorption of chemicals. Children also have immature blood-brain barriers and a greater receptivity to the central nervous system (CNS). Due to this, medications and agents that affect the CNS often produce more symptoms in the pediatric population. Dehydration can affect children more quickly than adults. An increase in the frequency of diarrhea and vomiting leads to a higher risk of dehydration.

Upper Airways

One of the most obvious anatomical differences between an adult and child is the tongue. The pediatric tongue is proportionally larger than the adult and takes up more space in the oropharynx. The tongue of a child is more prone to occlude the upper airway and often makes ventilation difficult with any degree of airway swelling.

The trachea in the child is narrower and easier to collapse due to an immaturity of the tracheal rins. Hyperextension and hyperflexion of the neck may lead to an occlusion of the trachea. The narrowness of the trachea makes any swelling a high risk for airway occlusion.

The epiglottis in the pediatric patient is larger proportionally and is U-shaped. This makes it more difficult to perform intubations. Some find it easier to intubate children using a straight laryngoscope blade rather than a curved blade. With the straight blade, it is often easier to lift the child's epiglottis, allowing better visualization of the trachea.

A child's larynx is higher and more anterior anatomically than the adults, at about the level of the first or second vertebrae, as opposed to the adult's, which is at the fourth or fifth cervical vertebrae.

In the adult, the left mainstem bronchus is at a more severe angle, making aspiration often occur on the right. In the child, both mainstem bronchi have less of an angle, making aspiration equally likely to occur on either side. Figure 10–1 shows the major anatomic and physiologic differences.

PHYSICAL ASSESSMENT OF THE PEDIATRIC PATIENT

Medical care of pediatric patients usually begins with caregivers concern for signs and/or symptoms that are predictive of impending malady or distress. It is investigated by the recognition of a "chief complaint" that directs attention to the need for further evaluation or treatment and proceeds with a thorough history obtained about the patient.

History

Typically, the medical history starts with the **chief complaint (CC)**. The CC is a concise statement that describes the symptom or condition that is the reason for the encounter. It is from the CC that a **differential diagnosis (DDx)** is first formed. A DDx is a list of all the potential problems that could be causing the reported symptoms and signs. It allows the provider to then use a process of elimination through the history and physical examination to arrive at the most likely cause. The CC could also simply be a well-child check, in which there are no symptoms present.

Any physical examination should begin with a thorough evaluation of the patient's history. An accurate DDx starts with and depends on an accurate history. One of the first things learned in medicine is, "Listen carefully to your patient. They are telling you the diagnosis."

Well-Child Visits

The concept of a well-child visit is based on the anticipated and expected reaching of milestones, both physical and developmental, from birth through adolescence.

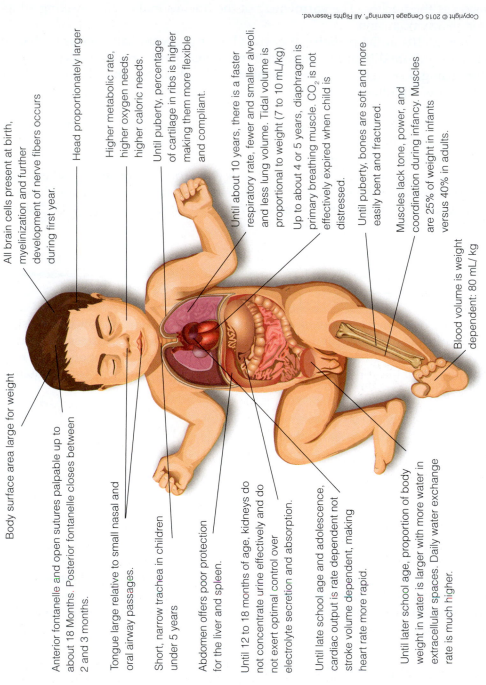

All brain cells present at birth, myelinization and further development of nerve fibers occurs during first year.

Head proportionately larger

Higher metabolic rate, higher oxygen needs, higher caloric needs.

Until puberty, percentage of cartilage in ribs is higher making them more flexible and compliant.

Until about 10 years, there is a faster respiratory rate, fewer and smaller alveoli, and less lung volume. Tidal volume is proportional to weight (7 to 10 mL/kg)

Up to about 4 or 5 years, diaphragm is primary breathing muscle. CO_2 is not effectively expired when child is distressed.

Until puberty, bones are soft and more easily bent and fractured.

Muscles lack tone, power, and coordination during infancy. Muscles are 25% of weight in infants versus 40% in adults.

Blood volume is weight dependent: 80 mL/ kg

Body surface area large for weight

Anterior fontanelle and open sutures palpable up to about 18 Months. Posterior fontanelle closes between 2 and 3 months.

Tongue large relative to small nasal and oral airway passages.

Short, narrow trachea in children under 5 years

Abdomen offers poor protection for the liver and spleen.

Until 12 to 18 months of age, kidneys do not concentrate urine effectively and do not exert optimal control over electrolyte secretion and absorption.

Until late school age and adolescence, cardiac output is rate dependent not stroke volume dependent, making heart rate more rapid.

Until later school age, proportion of body weight in water is larger with more water in extracellular spaces. Daily water exchange rate is much higher.

FIGURE 10–1. Anatomic and physiologic differences between a child and an adult.

These visits are timed and occur more frequently when development happens most quickly. During the visit, a complete physical examination is done as well as an assessment of growth and development. Another important part of the visit is parent education regarding things such as safety, nutrition, sleep, and other health issues. The National Institutes of Health maintains a web site called MedlinePlus for patients and their families. One of the many sites covers well-child visits and is an excellent resource for providers and families.[1] For a well-child visit, the following areas should be investigated during the history taking.

- Development and growth
- Medical history
- Nutritional status

Development and Growth Normally, questions look at developmental changes that are ongoing, normative, and expected. These changes usually occur in an orderly fashion in a manner that allows for individual variation.[2] The parents are questioned about their perception of their child's growth and development.

- Does anything seem to be out of proportion or missing?
- Does the child compare to others of similar age as far as language, emotions, psychological development, coordination, and growth?

Medical History In general, a good history should review the medical history since the last visit. Things like previously diagnosed problems as well as illnesses that didn't require a visit to the office should be included. How has the child been acting? Is he/she active, or tired and lethargic?

Nutritional Status The historical importance of the baby's nutritional status cannot be overemphasized. Nutritional status includes what the baby is eating and drinking and how much. Is the intake at appropriate portions and nutritionally sound?

History Taking on an Ill Patient

The history of pediatric patients may also include a review of maternal and early childhood tendencies that may indicate the relation to the current illness. When assessing the history of the respiratory system, several questions need to be addressed. The line of questioning is particularly important for the respiratory therapist to accurately assess the current condition. Correlations to any anomaly are dependent upon the recognition of particular signs and symptoms relating to knowledge of common disorders affecting children. Open-ended questioning, then, follows a general to specific path which confirms or detours the respiratory therapist's suspicions about the condition being investigated. Depending on the age of the patient, questions may need to be addressed to the parents to obtain meaningful and accurate information.

1. *Is the current illness an acute or chronic process?* The aim here is to determine when the symptoms appeared. Chronic problems, especially in younger patients, point to congenital problems or abnormalities. Chronic symptoms may also indicate long-term diseases such as cystic fibrosis or asthma.

2. *Are there signs of a concurrent infection?* Typical signs of infection include a fever, purulent discharges from the eyes and nose, or sputum from the nose or lungs, and swelling of the lymph nodes in the neck.

3. *If the patient has been treated for the current problem before, what was the effect of prior treatments?* This information can save a lot of time if it is known how the child has reacted to previous treatments and regimes.

4. *Have other members of the family had similar symptoms?* The presence of similar symptoms in other family members may indicate hereditary diseases such as cystic fibrosis. It may also show the presence of an infection that is being passed among family members.

5. *What is the character of the cough?* A cough is the most common patient sign with the least diagnostic value and must be thoroughly investigated. A tight, barky cough may be caused by an upper-airway disease, such as croup or epiglottitis, or could indicate a foreign body obstruction. A cough may be productive or nonproductive. Expectoration does not have to occur for the cough to be productive. A productive cough is usually defined as one in which rhonchi or crackles are heard, indicating the presence of material in the tracheobronchial tree. A dry nonproductive cough may be from an allergy, virus, or foreign body aspiration. In younger pediatric patients, a cough that is associated with swallowing suggests aspiration into the tracheobronchial tree secondary to tracheoesophageal fistulas.

6. *What is the pattern of breathing?* Acute onset of breathing difficulty, shown by increased respiratory rate, retractions, and labored breathing, without fever, points toward an airway obstruction. If accompanied by chest pain, a pneumothorax, fractured ribs, or a **pleural effusion** may be present. Chronic patterns of labored breathing are evidence of lung or cardiac anomalies. In asthma, labored breathing may only be present during an attack.

7. *Is there a history or evidence of wheezing?* Wheezing is frequently associated with asthma. However, it can be heard whenever airway obstruction is present. It is typically loudest during expiration. Any persistent audible wheezing with an acute onset points to a foreign body lodged somewhere in the tracheobronchial tree. If the child is asthmatic, it is important to determine what medications have been given and how the asthma has reacted in past occurrences.

8. *Is cyanosis present?* Presence of cyanosis is almost always the result of some degree of hypoxemia. It is most frequently defined as having 5 gms% of deoxygenated hemoglobin. The exception is a cold patient, where cyanosis may be secondary to peripheral circulatory stasis, not hypoxemia. Cyanosis that persists in spite of oxygen administration signifies a right-to-left shunting of blood.

9. *Does the patient complain of chest pain?* Obviously, this will only pertain to the older pediatric patient who can verbalize. Possible causes of chest pain are many. Causes are ruled out or diagnosed by the use of a chest x-ray, location and to the severity of the pain, and/or recent history of infection or trauma. Potential sources of chest pain include the esophagus, diaphragm, chest wall, pericardium, parietal pleura, and the lung itself.

10. *What is the nature of the sputum?* When possible, a history of the color, amount, consistency, and odor of sputum will help in diagnosing lung disorders. Large amounts of thick, clear, or purulent secretions may be caused by cystic fibrosis. Foul-smelling secretions may show a lung abscess or an acute bacterial process. Blood may be present in community-acquired pneumonia or in bronchiectasis.

11. *What is the growth pattern of the patient?* Some respiratory diseases may produce failure to thrive, so called because of the failure of the patient to grow and develop normally. Careful attention to growth and development are important to assess for potential anomalies.

12. *What is the patient's environment?* The environment includes not only the physical surroundings, but also the social and emotional characteristics of the surroundings. The presence of stressors in any of the above aspects of the environment may help diagnose the source of the respiratory problem.

Concepts of Physical Examination in Pediatric Patients

Whether an examination is being done on a well child, or an ill one, the setting of the examination is always an important consideration. First and foremost is safety. For the younger patients, the area must be child-proofed, that is, anything that is in the reach of the child must be secured and safe. All items on countertops or trays must be secured to prevent the child from pulling them onto his/her head. Electrical outlets should be properly protected. A safe environment also involves having a parent/guardian present at all times during the exam. A good examination requires a pleasant and comfortable environment with strong lighting, warm inviting colors and decorations that will help calm the child's nerves. If possible the temperature should be slightly warmer than that needed for adults. For younger children, age appropriate toys are useful to help reduce anxiety and act as wonderful distractors. For the older patients, appropriate books and magazines can also provide a diversion while waiting.

The examination starts with the standard measurements of weight, height/length, head circumference, and vital signs. Each measurement is plotted on a growth chart which compares the infant's size to that of others the same age. While it's easy to fixate on the percentile the baby is at, it is more important to follow the trend of steady growth from visit to visit. Examples of growth charts for boys and girls, ages 2 to 20 years are shown in Figure 10–2.

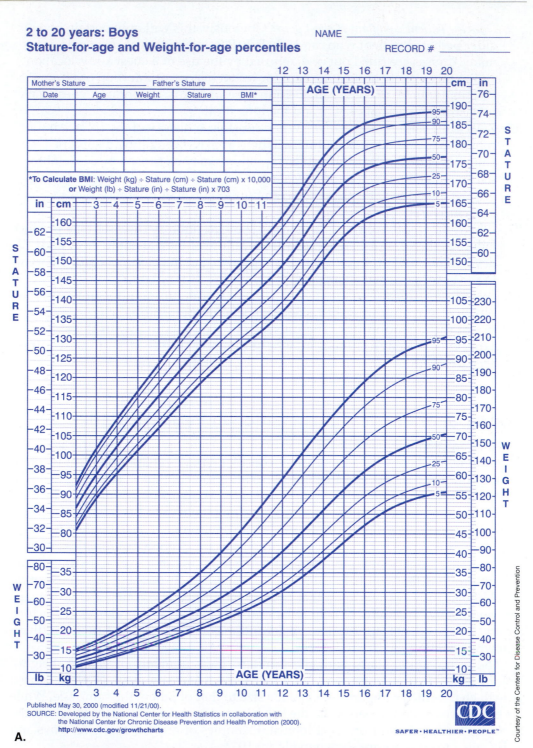

2 to 20 years: Boys
Stature-for-age and Weight-for-age percentiles

NAME _____

RECORD # _____

FIGURE 10–2. A. Growth chart for boys.

Published May 30, 2000 (modified 11/21/00).
SOURCE: Developed by the National Center for Health Statistics in collaboration with
the National Center for Chronic Disease Prevention and Health Promotion (2000).
http://www.cdc.gov/growthcharts

Courtesy of the Centers for Disease Control and Prevention

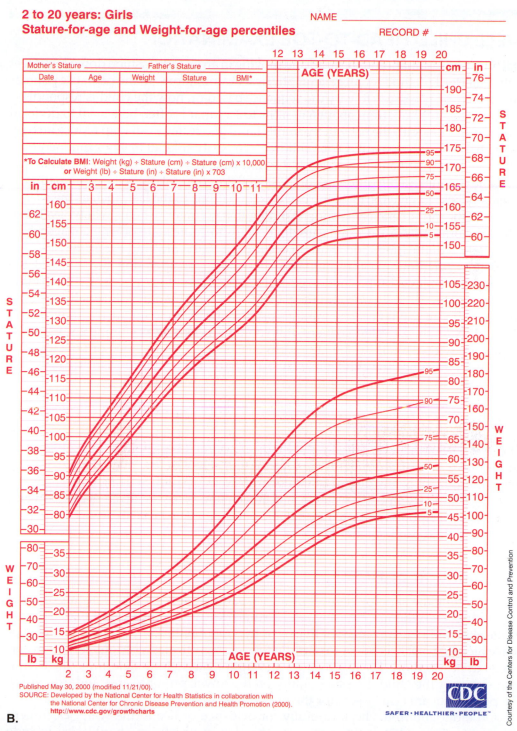

2 to 20 years: Girls
Stature-for-age and Weight-for-age percentiles

NAME _____

RECORD # _____

FIGURE 10–2. B. Growth chart for girls.

Published May 30, 2000 (modified 11/21/00).
SOURCE: Developed by the National Center for Health Statistics in collaboration with
the National Center for Chronic Disease Prevention and Health Promotion (2000).
http://www.cdc.gov/growthcharts

Courtesy of the Centers for Disease Control and Prevention

WELL CHILD HEAD-TO-TOE EXAMINATION

Starting the examination at the head and moving in an orderly fashion down to the feet is the standard method for all general physical examinations. In the pediatric population, it may be necessary to vary the sequence based on how the child is responding. For younger children, from about 6 months to 1 year, it is often beneficial to perform the examination with the baby in a parent's lap. This strategy can help reduce anxiety in the baby and the parent. Older children can easily tolerate being examined on a table, but be sensitive to bare skin on the cold table covering. A warmed blanket on the table can make a big difference on how well the child tolerates the examination. It is usually best to save the most intrusive examinations to the last, such as the examination of the mouth and ears. Understanding that younger patients will typically cry when the oral and/or ear exams are done, helps to coordinate other exams, such as auscultation of the lungs and heart, to occur prior to the oral and ear exams.

Before performing the examination, take into consideration the age and the developmental level of the child. Age and developmental variations will determine how you approach the exam and the patient. The examination will usually go more smoothly if you can take a few minutes prior to the exam to interact with the child. Depending on the age of the patient, this could be as simple as jingling a set of keys, or playing with a small stuffed animal, to conversing about school, or hobbies with an older child. Once the child gets above a year of age, it is important to do everything possible to maintain their modesty during the examination.

General Assessment

The first part of the well-child exam is to do a general assessment of the patient. You should take note of the general appearance, the behavior, the overall state of wellness, and if there is any degree of illness or distress present. Starting with the body, look for symmetry in body features and movement. Note the facial expression and the patient's responsiveness to his/her surroundings. The facial expression and posture of the child can help identify pain.

Examination of the Skin

Next examine the skin for signs of cyanosis, pallor, and jaundice. Note any areas of skin redness (erythema), bruising, and birthmarks. Assess the overall pigmentation of the skin and note any areas of hyper- or hypopigmentation. Any evidence of capillary bleeding, such as **purpura** or **petichiae**, often indicates a serious condition and needs to be acted on. The skin texture and turgor can help to determine the hydration status of the child. Pressing lightly on the lower pre-tibal area and examining the periorbital area can assess for the presence of any edema.

On older children, check carefully for evidence of lice in the scalp. Document any areas of dry skin and/or eczema. The skin examination should also include looking for any signs of trauma or signs of abuse.

Examination of the Head, Eyes, Ears, Nose, and Throat (HEENT)

The first part of the HEENT exam is to visually inspect the head and face for symmetry, noting any irregularities in the shape, size, or location of the ears, eyes, nose, and mouth. Visually examine the neck for irregularities such as a deviation of the trachea, an enlarged thyroid, or enlarged lymph nodes. The next step is to palpate the skull for any irregularities or tender areas. Palpate gently over the eyes, ears, and sinuses to assess any discomfort. The eyes should be examined with a light to check for proper pupillary response and alignment. The **red reflex**, the reflection of light off the retina, should be visible and unclouded. Depending on the age of the patient, the visual acuity should be determined. For younger patients, it may be necessary to use a custom eye chart with animals or shapes, rather than the traditional Snellen chart. The ears should be examined with an otoscope to check for any cerumen impaction in the external canal. Additionally, hearing can be checked by rubbing the fingers, or rattling keys, or a bell. Younger patients will turn toward the source of the sound whereas older children can be asked if they can hear the rubbing or rattling. The nares are examined for patency and, if possible, an examination of the anterior nasal cavities can assess for any blockage or growths. An examination of the mouth looking for abnormalities in tooth growth, palate, and oropharynx is then done. Inspection is done of the mucosa and gingivae for moisture content. Evidence of dental caries is also noted. Large tonsils can occlude the airway if swollen; therefore, it is important to note the size of the tonsils to help with parental education in the event of future tonsilar swelling. Palpation of the neck is done next to check for any masses. In older children, lymph nodes should be palpated in the anterior and posterior cervical chain as well as under the chin in the submental areas.

Examination of the Pediatric Pulmonary System

When examining the pulmonary system of the pediatric patient, there are three primary goals to achieve: 1) to evaluate and localize the disease, if one is present; 2) to observe for adequacy of gas exchange; and 3) to determine the nature of the patient's ventilations. Each of these areas will be reviewed separately.

Localization of the Disease Much of the information gathered while taking the history will help in determining the location of the disease. The respiratory therapist will then use additional information to either prove or disprove its presence, that is, confirm suspicions to the presence of an anomaly. A chest radiograph is an excellent source of determining location and extent of the disease. Areas of infection or consolidation will appear as white areas on the radiograph. Air trapping, secondary to aspiration of foreign bodies or mucus plugging, will appear as a dark, hyperaerated area distal to the plugging.

Chest radiographs should never be used alone to diagnose, but only to verify what is already suspected. Thus, the respiratory therapist should already have an idea of what the disease process is from the history and physical examination.

The chest radiograph is then used to confirm if the disease is actually present and where it is located. Some diseases may not be detected by chest radiograph, but the information is still important in ruling out other causes of the related signs or symptoms. Chest radiographs and their interpretation are covered in more detail in Chapter 16.

Auscultating breath sounds may also be helpful in determining the location of disease processes. Figure 10–3 shows the location of the various lung segments as they relate to the exterior thorax. Breath sounds should be evaluated with an appropriately sized stethoscope, warmed before placing it on the chest. You should begin auscultation at the apices and slowly work down, carefully comparing similar segments in both lung fields. Check for equal aeration bilaterally. The presence of adventitious sounds such as wheezes, crackles, rhonchi, or stridor in a certain segment or lobe of either lung helps localize the disease to that site.

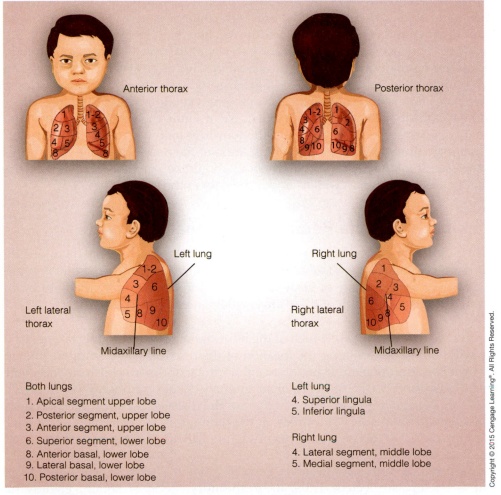

Both lungs
1. Apical segment upper lobe
2. Posterior segment, upper lobe
3. Anterior segment, upper lobe
6. Superior segment, lower lobe
8. Anterior basal, lower lobe
9. Lateral basal, lower lobe
10. Posterior basal, lower lobe

Left lung
4. Superior lingula
5. Inferior lingula

Right lung
4. Lateral segment, middle lobe
5. Medial segment, middle lobe

FIGURE 10–3. The lung segments and their relationship to the exterior thorax.

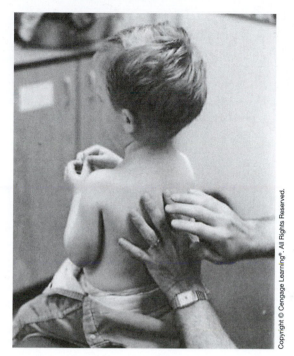

FIGURE 10–4. Percussion of the thorax to assess the location of consolidation or other lung processes.

Percussion of the chest is another adjunct in assessing the location of the disease process (Figure 10–4). Involved lung areas will usually have a dull percussion note over the area of involvement. Hyperaerated areas, including pneumothoraces, will have a high-pitched, tympanic, or hyper-resonant quality.

Palpating the trachea at the sternal notch gives clues to changes in thoracic pressures (Figure 10–5). The trachea normally sits midline in the neck as it enters the thorax. The presence of atelectatic or consolidated alveoli may cause the trachea to deviate toward the involved side. This deviation is the result of a slight hyperinflation of the unaffected lung and the collapse and tension of the affected lung. In the presence of a pneumothorax, tension pneumothorax, severe air trapping, or hyperinflation, the trachea will deviate away from the involved lung for the same reason as mentioned above.

Assessing Adequacy of Gas Exchange Adequacy of gas exchange is best determined by obtaining and analyzing an arterial blood gas sample. Physical signs of hypoxia include tachycardia, tachypnea, cyanosis, labored breathing, and/or a deteriorating mental state.

Signs of hypercarbia include a rapid bounding pulse, confusion or drowsiness, muscular twitching, and, in severe cases, coma. Any patient who has diminished breath sounds and any of these symptoms should be started on oxygen therapy

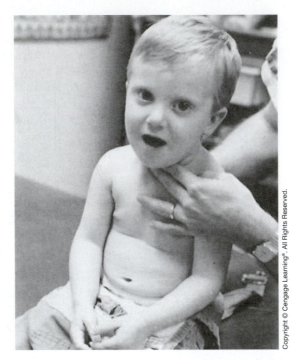

FIGURE 10–5. Palpating the sternal notch to assess the position of the trachea.

and a blood gas drawn immediately to evaluate the extent of hypoxemia (or tissue hypoxia), or hypercarbia.

Pulse oximeters or transcutaneous monitors are also invaluable in helping assess the adequacy of gas exchange. Their use does not, however, eliminate the need to perform arterial blood gas evaluations rather to trend suspected inadequacy of gaseous exchange.

Determining the Nature of Ventilations The last part of the physical examination of the pulmonary system involves determining the nature of the pediatric patient's ventilations. This includes evaluating the rate, depth, rhythm, and ease of breathing.

Rate The respiratory rate (the presence or absence of tachypnea) is a good indicator of distress. An elevated rate is usually secondary to decreased lung and chest wall compliance or difficulty breathing. The difficulty is in ascertaining a normal respiratory rate for an individual pediatric patient. The normal respiratory rate falls rapidly during the first years of life, leveling off during late adolescence and early adulthood. The respiratory rate is often higher when the patient is awake and slows during sleep. After age 1, any resting quiet respiratory rate above 40 should be investigated further. As the child reaches 5 years and above, a resting rate above 35 is cause for concern and should be followed up to assess its underlying cause.

Depth The depth of ventilation may be difficult to assess. Extremes are easily detected, but assessment between the two extremes requires unyielding practice and careful observation. The normal breath should have some chest expansion accompanied by abdominal movement. As the breath becomes significantly more shallow, the chest and abdominal movements decline. Shallow breathing that results in hypercapnea, termed **hypoventilation**, usually results from metabolic alkalosis, paralysis of the diaphragm, or CNS disorders. Overtly deep breathing with or without an increasing frequency, called **hyperpnea**, is found in patients with metabolic acidosis, fever, severe anemia, and in deadspace-producing diseases

Rhythm The last area of assessment is the child's rhythm of breathing. Normal quiet breathing is regular, pausing slightly at end-expiration and interrupted only by an occasional sigh. Any apnea or irregular rhythm in the breathing witnessed in the pediatric patient is abnormal and should be investigated further. Either of these abnormalities could be associated with neurologic problems such as hypoxic-ischemic insults.

Ease of Breathing The effort of breathing is divided into two categories: labored and normal breathing. The presence of labored breathing, indicated by tachypnea, hyperpnea, or retractions, may be an objective sign of airway obstruction. Retractions may occur intercostally, substernally or suprasternally, and subclavicularly or supraclavicularly. As the airway obstruction worsens, retractions increase in severity. Flaring of the **alae nasi**, the external opening of the nose, is also a sign of labored breathing.

Examination of the Heart

The art of listening to the heart takes years of practice to hone. Understanding heart sounds is beyond the scope of this text so the focus will be on a basic cardiac examination. The first part of the exam is to assess the rate and rhythm of the heart. This can be done simply by palpating the radial or brachial artery. A basic auscultation of the heart can then be done by placing the stethoscope at approximately the 3rd intercostal space of the left sternal border. This position, also called **Erb's point**, is a good area to hear all the valves (Figure 10–6). Listen carefully for the first and second heart sounds (S1 and S2). Make a note of any sounds heard other than S1 and S2, which could be a murmur and an indication of a valve abnormality. It is important to note the volume and duration of the abnormal sound as well as when it is heard in the cycle.

Abdominal Examination

The abdomen is best examined with the patient in a supine position. As with the examination of the other body systems, the examination of the abdomen starts with a visual inspection. Note the shape and size of the abdomen and the presence

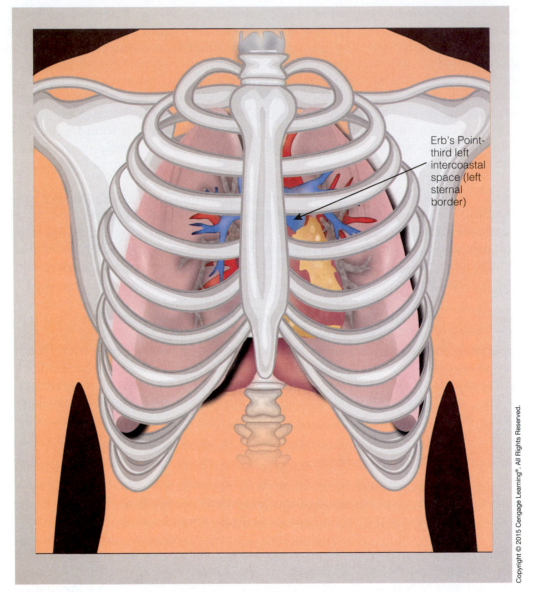

Erb's Point-
third left
intercoastal
space (left
sternal
border)

FIGURE 10–6. Location of Erb's point.

of any asymmetry. Auscultation is then done with the stethoscope placed over each of the four quadrants. Abdominal quadrants are imaginary lines vertically and horizontally through the umbilicus and labeled the right and left upper quadrants and the right and left lower quadrants (RUQ, LUQ, RLQ, LLQ) (Figure 10–7). Listen for the presence or absence of bowel sounds in each quadrant. Following auscultation, the abdomen can be gently palpated to check for tenderness or

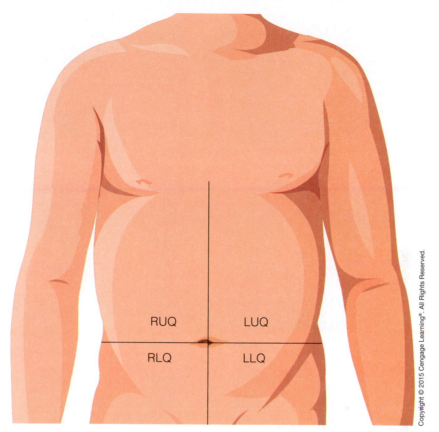

FIGURE 10–7. Abdominal quadrants.

rigidity. Gently pressing over the four quadrants can help determine the presence of any masses.

Musculoskeletal Examination

The initial visual assessment of the child, done at the beginning of the examination, should have noted any asymmetry in the musculoskeletal system. At this point the examination typically focuses on range of motion (ROM) and strength. The major joints are tested for their ROM by having the patient go through the cardinal movements of flexion, extension, adduction, abduction, and rotation. Major muscle groups are checked against resistance and any variation between groups is noted. Checking the spine for scoliosis, which is an abnormal curvature of the spine from side to side (Figure 10–8), is done simply by positioning the patient in front of you, facing away and bending to touch the toes. The spine is visualized and palpated and any right or left deviation is noted. The gait of the child is then observed for any limp or deviation in the alignment of the feet.

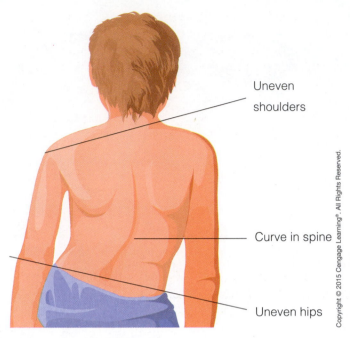

Uneven shoulders

Curve in spine

Uneven hips

FIGURE 10–8. Characteristics of scoliosis.

Neurological Evaluation

The neurological evaluation can be quite involved and often requires a lot of practice to detect subtle deficiencies. Essentially, the neurological exam can be broken down into three areas: mental and cognitive status, balance and coordination, and cranial nerves. Cognition involves the processes of attention and memory, reasoning, and decision making. The mental status exam typically incorporates those attributes as well as things such as appearance, mood, and behavior. Although many aspects of the mental exam are observational, cognition can be tested in several ways. For example, memory can be assessed by giving the child two or three words and then asking them to recall the words after an interval of time. Keep in mind the age and maturity of the patient and use words that are appropriate based on those criteria. In older, school-age children, attention and concentration can be assessed by the use of serial sevens, in which the child is asked to count backward from 100, or another appropriate number, by sevens. Alternatively, the child can be asked to spell a 4- or 5-letter word backward. Reasoning can be a difficult thing to assess in children. In adults, asking the patient to interpret a proverb is a reasonable assessment tool; however, children lack the insight into the deeper meaning of proverbs. An alternative could be to give the child a simple story and ask the child to determine if the story makes sense or is nonsensical.

There are several ways to test balance and coordination. For younger patients, tossing a ball to them and seeing if they can catch is a means of assessing hand/eye coordination. A more complex exam for older children might be to have them touch their nose, then your finger as you move it slowly in front of them. Having the child stand on one leg or to stand still with both eyes closed can be done to assess balance.

Testing the twelve cranial nerves is beyond the scope of this chapter; however, in quick review, they include testing smell, vision, eye movements, facial sensation, muscle use, tongue movement, vocalization, and neck and shoulder strength. More advanced neurological testing involves sensation and reflexes.

ANTICIPATORY GUIDANCE

In its common use, the term **anticipatory guidance** refers to educating parents about what to expect in the first months and years of their child's life as far as promoting health and safety.[3] Most practices include handouts that are given to the parents at each visit that are age specific. The handouts cover health issues, including immunization schedules, safety issues, and general tips on helping the child progress mentally and physically into adolescence. Since 2002, the American Academy of Pediatrics has been involved in the Bright Futures initiative with the aim of "prevention and health promotion for infants, children, adolescents, and their families.[4] The Bright Futures web site contains a large amount of material and resources for providers and families. One of their valuable resources is their *Clinical Guide*, which includes a chapter on anticipatory guidance.[5] This chapter covers the areas of bicycle helmet use, strategies to help children with media, obesity issues, interviewing, and tobacco smoke exposure and cessation.

PEDIATRIC PULMONARY FUNCTION TESTING (PFT)

Pulmonary function tests that are done on pediatric patients yield a wealth of information if taken the time to perform. Measurement of expiratory flow curves is helpful in the diagnosis of early obstructive disease. For example, the flow measurements at small lung volumes (V_{max} 25) may be decreased before a decrease in spirometer values can be appreciated.[6]

Provocation of bronchospasm is possible in many children with asthma by having them exercise, especially in cool air. Bronchospasm may also be provoked with the use of antigens and *methacholine* aerosolization. The benefit of these types of pulmonary function tests is to determine the cause and extent of childhood asthma.

The diagnosis and progression of cystic fibrosis is aided by the close following of FVC and FEV_1 measurements. Less than expected increases in both values as the child grows is a typical finding in obstructive lung disease.

Pulmonary function tests are helpful in following the patient with bronchopulmonary dysplasia (BPD) following hospital discharge. The patient is tested over time to evaluate the status of the lung disease. Future problems with exercise intolerance or hyperreactive bronchospasm may be avoided in these patients. Pulmonary function testing can also help differentiate between the deconditioned patient and those with bronchospastic disease as causes of exercise intolerance.

The performance of pulmonary function tests on pediatric patients, including those in their teens, is mainly dependent on the cooperation and maturity of the subject. Age is not always predictive of patient maturity. For example, two 5-year-old patients may be opposite in their ability to follow commands and cooperate and so will have vastly different results.

Special Requirements

Assuming that the patient is cooperative and able to follow commands, the performance of pulmonary function tests on pediatric patients is basically the same as on adults. There are, however, a few special requirements that must be considered.

Accuracy of Equipment Although the equipment is not different from that used for adults, it should be accurate at low volumes and flows. Desired accuracy should be ±3% of the reading, or 30 mL, whichever is greater, for volumes. Accuracy for flows should be ±5% or 0.1 liter per second, whichever is greater.[6]

Training It is important that the person performing the test understand children. They must have a high level of patience to teach the patient the proper techniques. The person and the environment must be friendly so the patient will be at ease and not be frightened.

Interpretation of Results Before any attempt is made to interpret results, the patient effort must be verified as being acceptable. There should be no artifacts from coughing, slow onset, or early termination of the maneuver. To be considered acceptable, the patient should produce three forced vital capacity maneuvers that are within 10% of the best effort.[6] Comparison of measured values must also be made to suitable pediatric references and standards and not to regressed adult values.

Determination of Total Lung Volume Where there is no evidence of severe airway obstruction, nitrogen washout and helium dilution are generally reliable for the determination of total lung capacity and residual volume. A body plethysmograph may also be used, but may not be tolerated as well by the patient. Young patients may not be able to tolerate the confining nature of the plethysmograph, making accurate measurements difficult.

DLCO Tests The diffusing capacity of carbon monoxide (DLCO) is rarely done on the pediatric patient for three main reasons: 1) smaller lung volumes necessitate smaller washout volumes when obtaining helium and carbon monoxide plateau concentrations; 2) it is difficult to get a 10-second breath hold from the patient; and 3) there is a low incidence of interstitial lung disease in the pediatric group.[6]

Indications

The indications for performing a PFT on a pediatric patient are the same as for an adult. They include the following:

1. To investigate patients with signs and symptoms that suggest pulmonary disease
2. To monitor patients with known pulmonary disease for progression and response to treatment
3. To investigate patients with a disease that may have respiratory complications
4. To perform a preoperative evaluation
5. To evaluate a patient at risk for lung disease

Contraindications

Contraindications to performing a PFT on a pediatric patient are few and include:

1. Active pulmonary bleeding
2. Recent ophthalmic surgery
3. Current pneumothorax

ARTERIAL BLOOD GAS ANALYSIS

Finally in the pediatric patient where pulmonary function measurements are not possible, an arterial blood gas may be helpful in diagnosing respiratory symptoms. In many lung diseases, the arterial PaO_2 and $PaCO_2$ will change before changes in lung function are noted.

SUMMARY

Assessment of the pediatric patient starts with an understanding of the anatomic and physiologic differences between children and adults. Those differences frequently manifest themselves during illness, when the pediatric patient acts and responds differently than the adult would to the same illness. These differences go beyond just size, but are also seen with metabolism, and other basic bodily functions. Anatomic and physiologic differences frequently lead to the child reacting very differently to medications, or to stressors common during illness. This understanding also prepares the respiratory therapist to anticipate potential problems that may occur and take actions to alleviate them early, or prevent them entirely.

The assessment always starts with a thorough medical history. The history typically starts with the primary concern, called the chief complaint, Additionally, any other medical history that is pertinent must be discussed and its role in the current problem considered. During the medical history, the practitioner develops a list of possible causes, called the *differential diagnosis*. From that differential, the use of physical exam and laboratory findings help to narrow the list down to the most probable etiology. During the history, information is gained that gives the provider an in-depth look into the health of the patient. Important clues are gained that will help decide if the disease is acute or chronic, if there are signs of other issues, or if it is an inherited issue. Specific to the respiratory therapist, this chapter reviews a thorough pulmonary history and physical exam of the cardiopulmonary system as well as a head to toe examination covering the other body systems.

Well-child visits are an essential part of the health care of the pediatric patient. These visits are designed to assess the growth and developmental milestones. Areas assessed include physical as well as neurological development. Additionally, this time is used to educate parents and caregivers regarding safety issues, nutrition, sleep, and other health issues. The term "anticipatory guidance" is discussed and refers to the planned education of parents and caregivers regarding the expectations of growth and development as well as age specific immunization schedules and safety issues.

Pulmonary function testing (PFT) in children can yield a wealth of information; however, pulmonary function in children can also be difficult to measure. This chapter reviews the use of PFTs in the pediatric population and how that information is used in the overall diagnosis and treatment of pulmonary diseases.

POSTTEST

1. A 4-year-old is brought to the emergency department after aspirating a peanut. The patient is currently in no respiratory distress. The most likely area for the peanut to be is:
   a. in the left mainstem bronchus
   b. in the right mainstem bronchus
   c. in the trachea
   d. It could be in the right or left mainstem bronchi.
2. You are seeing a 2-year-old patient in the outpatient clinic. While taking a history, the mother states that she brought the child in due to a fever, which was 102°F at home. The mother states that the baby has a history of "ear tubes" and has had a cough for the past week. The baby is current on his immunizations. Which of these historical items is the chief complaint?
   a. the history of "ear tubes"
   b. fever
   c. immunization status
   d. presence of a cough × 1 week

3. Which of the following is an example of a well-child visit?
    a. A child is brought to the office to follow-up on test results.
    b. A 5-month-old is brought to the health department for immunizations.
    c. A 1-year-old is brought to the clinic to check whether developmental milestones are being met.
    d. A worried mother calls to ask about a change in her daughter's eating habits.
4. While taking a medical history, which of the following questions would typically be asked during an ill-child visit?
    a. How long has the fever been present?
    b. How does your child interact with other children his age?
    c. Do you have any concerns about your child's ability to concentrate?
    d. Are you using an appropriate car seat for your child?
5. While performing an assessment on a pediatric patient, you note that the baby is extremely fussy and uncooperative. Which of the following would most likely help calm the patient and allow for a better exam?
    a. Play some music in the background.
    b. Darken the room.
    c. Give the patient some food or drink.
    d. Have the patient sit on his/her parent's lap.
6. Using the graph in Figure 11–1, calculate the stature for age percentile of a 9-year-old male who is 54 inches tall.
    a. 20th percentile
    b. 30th percentile
    c. 50th percentile
    d. 75th percentile
7. During a physical examination of a 3-month-old child, you note some asymmetry between the right and left arm. This discovery would most like occur during which part of the physical exam?
    a. the general assessment
    b. the cardiopulmonary examination
    c. the neurological examination
    d. the skin examination
8. To auscultate the cardiac sounds, which of the following locations is recommended?
    a. 5th intercostal space, mid-clavicular line
    b. 3rd intercostal space, left sternal border
    c. 2nd intercostal space, right sternal border
    d. any location over the heart
9. While assessing a 6-year-old pediatric patient, you discover that the patient has a rapid bounding pulse, confusion, and muscular twitching. Which of the following is suspected?
    a. hypoxia
    b. hypokalemia
    c. hypercarbia
    d. hypocarbia

10. With regard to the examination of the pulmonary system of the pediatric patient, which of the following is not one of the three primary goals?
    a. to evaluate and localize the disease, if one is present
    b. to observe for adequacy of gas exchange
    c. to determine the nature of the patient's ventilations
    d. to assess the patency of the airways
11. Which of the following is an example of anticipatory guidance?
    a. jelping parents select an appropriate bike helmet for their child
    b. talking to parents about what is causing their child's fever
    c. painting the walls of the exam room a soothing color
    d. having a parent present at all times during an examination
12. Of the following, which is not a contraindication to perform a pulmonary function study on a 7 year old?
    a. active pulmonary bleeding
    b. recent infection
    c. recent ophthalmic surgery
    d. current pneumothorax

REFERENCES

1. http://www.nlm.nih.gov/medlineplus/ency/article/001928.htm
2. Rakel, RE et al. *Textbook of Family Medicine*, 8th ed. Elsevier, 2011.
3. http://www.yourpediatrician.com/antic.htm
4. http://brightfutures.aap.org/
5. http://brightfutures.aap.org/pdfs/Preventive%20Services%20PDFs/Anticipatory%20Guidance.PDF
6. Eisenberg JD, Wall MA. Pulmonary function testing in children. *Clin Chest Med.* 8:661–667, 1987.

BIBLIOGRAPHY AND SUGGESTED READINGS

Drutz JE. The pediatric physical examination: General principles and standard measurements *UpToDate, 2012.* http://www.uptodate.com/contents/the-pediatric-physical-examination-general-principles-and-standard-measurements.

Immunizations and developmental milestones. *Centers for Disease Control, 2013.* http://www.cdc.gov/vaccines/parents/downloads/milestones-tracker.pdf.

Physical examination benchmarks. *University of Washington Dept. of Pediatrics.* http://www.washington.edu/medicine/pediatrics/students/current/third-year/core-materials/physical-examination-benchmarks.

Well-child care: A check-up for success. *Healthychildren.org, American Academy of Pediatrics.*

Well-child visits. *National Institutes of Health MedlinePlus.* http://www.nlm.nih.gov/medlineplus/ency/article/001928.htm.

CHAPTER 11

Continuing Care of the Pediatric Patient

OBJECTIVES

Upon the completion of this chapter, the reader should be able to:

1. Describe the rationale for screening pediatric patients for hypertension.
2. Using the Tanner maturity scale, estimate the level of sexual maturity of a patient when given the physical characteristics.
3. List the typical screening tests used in the pediatric population.
4. Describe the reason for nutritional deficiencies in pediatric and adolescent patients.
5. Compare and contrast each of the following:
   a. Autistic disorder
   b. Asperger syndrome
   c. Pervasive developmental disorder
6. Identify and describe the three types of attention deficit/hyperactivity disorder (ADHD).
7. Use the Pediatric Symptoms Checklist to identify behavioral and emotional problems in school-aged children.
8. Identify the recommended vaccines for ages 0–18.
9. Identify the common sleep interrupters.
10. Describe the physical causes of obstructive sleep apnea.
11. Describe the signs of oppositional defiant disorder and conduct disorder.
12. Compare and contrast anorexia nervosa and bulimia.
13. List the symptoms of eating disorders in adolescents.
14. Identify a febrile infant at low-risk for serious bacterial infection using the Rochester Criteria.
15. List the complications of acute otitis media (AOM).

KEY TERMS

anorexia nervosa	bulimia nervosa	pica
attention-deficit/ hyperactivity disorder (ADHD)	global developmental delay	pyrogens rapid eye movement (REM)
autism spectrum disorders (ASDs)	intratemporal otorrhea	Tanner scale

INTRODUCTION

Caring for the pediatric patient requires an understanding of common disorders that may interfere with or play a role in the respiratory care of the patient. This chapter will briefly review some of the more common medical and psychological issues found in the pediatric patient, ultimately assisting the respiratory therapist to become a better provider.

GROWTH AND DEVELOPMENT

The care of the pediatric patient requires an understanding of normal growth and development. Physical and developmental growth typically takes place in an orderly progression. Chapter 10 reviews the "well-child exam" along with the expected growth patterns during childhood.

One of the more threatening aspects of child and adolescent health is an alarming increase in hypertension. There has been an increase in the prevalence of childhood hypertension since 1988[1]. Increasing obesity rates seem to be a factor in this rising prevalence. Uncontrolled hypertension leads to end-organ damage along with cardiovascular risk and should, therefore, be screened for in all children aged 3 and older and in younger patients with certain high-risk health concerns.[2]

Children grow and mature at different paces. To help follow normative growth patterns, growth charts, as described in Chapter 10, are essential tools. While physical growth typically follows a predictable course, puberty has a tremendous variation among adolescents. Puberty in both males and females is a time of significant growth. To help in the assessment of the sexual maturity that accompanies puberty, the **Tanner scale**[3] utilizes the changes in the male genitalia, pubic hair presence and distribution, and female breast development and pubic hair growth patterns to stage the level of maturity.

The Tanner scale follows the changes in maturity using a visual comparison chart along with a descriptive explanation (see Tables 11–1 through 11–3).

Part of the assessment of the pediatric patient involves preventative care, which includes screening for the early detection of possible health issues. Typical screening tests include hearing and vision, lead toxicity, iron deficiency anemia, and tuberculosis.

Table 11–1

SEXUAL MATURITY RATING (SMR) FOR FEMALE GENITALIA

Developmental Stage	Description
Stage I 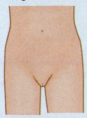	**Preadolescent Stage** (before age 8) No pubic hair, only body hair (vellus hair)
Stage II 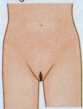	**Early Adolescent Stage** (ages 8 to 12) Sparse growth of long, slightly dark, fine pubic hair, slightly curly and located along the labia
Stage III 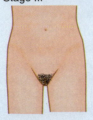	**Adolescent Stage** (ages 12 to 13) Pubic hair becomes darker, curlier, and spreads over the symphysis
Stage IV 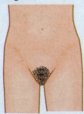	**Late Adolescent Stage** (ages 13 to 15) Texture and curl of pubic hair is similar to that of an adult but not spread to thighs
Stage V 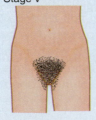	**Adult Stage** Adult appearance in quality and quantity of pubic hair; growth is spread to inner aspect of thighs and abdomen

Table 11–2

SEXUAL MATURITY RATING (SMR) FOR FEMALE BREAST DEVELOPMENT

Developmental Stage

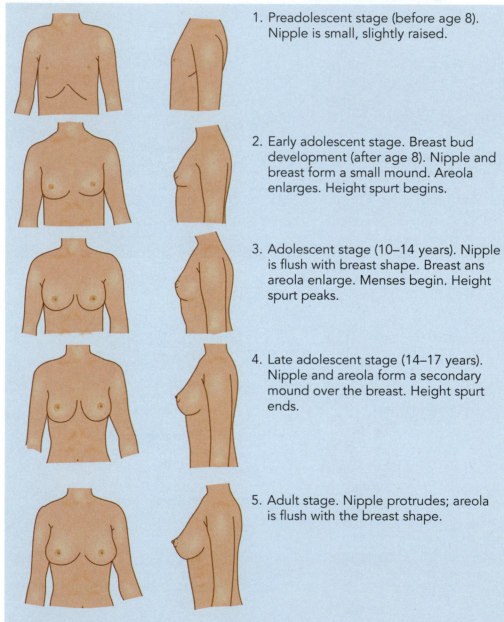

1. Preadolescent stage (before age 8). Nipple is small, slightly raised.

2. Early adolescent stage. Breast bud development (after age 8). Nipple and breast form a small mound. Areola enlarges. Height spurt begins.

3. Adolescent stage (10–14 years). Nipple is flush with breast shape. Breast ans areola enlarge. Menses begin. Height spurt peaks.

4. Late adolescent stage (14–17 years). Nipple and areola form a secondary mound over the breast. Height spurt ends.

5. Adult stage. Nipple protrudes; areola is flush with the breast shape.

Table 11–3

SEXUAL MATURITY RATING (SMR) FOR MALE GENITALIA

Developmental Stage	Pubic hair	Penis	Scrotum
	No public hair, only body hair (vellus hair)	Preadolescent; childhood size and proportion	Preadolescent; childhood size and proportion
	Sprase growth of long slightly dark, straight hair	Slightly or no growth	Growth in testes and scrotum; scrotum reddens and changes texture
	Becomes darker and coarser; slightly curled and spreads over symphysis	Growth, especially in length	Further growth
	Texture and curl of pubic hair is similar to that of an adult but not spread to thighs	Further growth in length; diameter increases; development of glans	Further growth; scrotum darkens
	Adult appearance in quality of pubic hair; growth is spread to medical surface of thighs	Adult size and shape	Adult size and shape

Nutrition is an essential aspect of proper growth and development. Infants require around 120 kcal/kg/day to meet their basal metabolic requirements along with the energy needed for growth.[4] While malnutrition remains a problem in the United States, there has been a shift to inappropriate nutrition, which focuses on an imbalance between calories and nutrients, leading to obesity. In adolescence, there is a greater risk for nutritional deficiencies due to the frequent missing of meals, fast foods, increased snacking, and fad diets.

BEHAVIORAL DEVELOPMENT

Behavioral development is similar to growth in that it typically occurs following a predictable course; however, like growth, there is tremendous variability. Measured along with behavioral development is neurodevelopment. These two areas overlap and are normally categorized into language development, fine and gross motor skills, personal and social development, and cognitive skills. Developmental delays can occur in any one or any combination of these areas and are estimated to have a prevalence of around 10%.[4] Tables and charts showing developmental milestones are used to identify delays and are utilized during well-child examinations. When there is a significant delay in two or more of the examined areas, it is termed a **global developmental delay**. Developmental disabilities that cause significant social, communication, and behavioral challenges are termed **autism spectrum disorders (ASDs)** and include "classic" autism, or autistic disorder, Asperger syndrome, and pervasive developmental disorder not otherwise specified (PDD-NOS). It is estimated that 1 in 88 children has been identified with ASD.[5]

One of the most common neurobehavioral disorders of childhood is **attention-deficit/hyperactivity disorder (ADHD)**. Children with ADHD have trouble paying attention and controlling their impulsive behaviors. They can also be overactive. It is estimated that between 3% and 7% of school-aged children have ADHD.[6] Three types of ADHD have been identified: predominantly inattentive type, predominantly hyperactive-impulsive type, and combined type. The cause(s) and risk factors that lead to ADHD are still unknown; however, it is believed that genetics plays a major role.[6] One tool used to help identify behavioral and emotional problems in school-aged children is the Pediatric Symptom Checklist. The checklist is shown in Figure 11–1.

Asperger syndrome is similar to autism, but there are also important differences. Children with Asperger syndrome typically function better than do those with autism. In addition, children with Asperger syndrome generally have normal intelligence and near-normal language development, although they may develop problems communicating as they get older.[7]

The term PDD-NOS refers to children who have significant problems with communication and play, and some difficulty interacting with others, but are too social to be considered autistic. It's sometimes referred to as a milder form of autism.[7]

Child's Name _____ Record Number _____

Today's Date _____ Filled Out by _____

Date of Birth _____

Pediatric Symptom Checklist

Emotional and physical health go together in children. Because parents are often the first to notice a problem with their child's behavior, emotions or learning, you may help your child get the best care possible by answering these questions. Please mark under the heading that best fits your child.

Never Sometimes Often

	(0)	(1)	(2)
1. Complains of aches/pains 1	____	____	____
2. Spends more time alone 2	____	____	____
3. Tires easily, has little energy 3	____	____	____
4. Fidgety, unable to sit still 4	____	____	____
5. Has trouble with a teacher 5	____	____	____
6. Less interested in school 6	____	____	____
7. Acts as if driven by a motor 7	____	____	____
8. Daydreams too much 8	____	____	____
9. Distracted easily 9	____	____	____
10. Is afraid of new situations 10	____	____	____
11. Feels sad, unhappy 11	____	____	____
12. Is irritable, angry 12	____	____	____
13. Feels hopeless 13	____	____	____
14. Has trouble concentrating 14	____	____	____
15. Less interest in friends 15	____	____	____
16. Fights with others 16	____	____	____
17. Absent from school 17	____	____	____
18. School grades dropping 18	____	____	____
19. Is down on him or herself 19	____	____	____
20. Visits doctor with doctor finding nothing wrong 20	____	____	____
21. Has trouble sleeping 21	____	____	____
22. Worries a lot 22	____	____	____
23. Wants to be with you more than before 23	____	____	____
24. Feels he or she is bad 24	____	____	____
25. Takes unnecessary risks 25	____	____	____
26. Gets hurt frequently 26	____	____	____
27. Seems to be having less fun 27	____	____	____
28. Acts younger than children his or her age 28	____	____	____
29. Does not listen to rules 29	____	____	____

FIGURE 11–1. Pediatric Symptom Checklist.

(continues)

30. Does not show feelings 30	____	____	____
31. Does not understand other people's feelings 31	____	____	____
32. Teases others 32	____	____	____
33. Blames others for his or her troubles 33	____	____	____
34. Takes things that do not belong to him or her 34	____	____	____
35. Refuses to share 35	____	____	____

Total score _____

Does your child have any emotional or behavioral problems for which she/he needs help? ( ) N ( ) Y

Are there any services that you would like your child to receive for these problems? ( ) N ( ) Y

If yes, what services?_____

FIGURE 11–1. (*continued*)

IMMUNIZATION

Control and prevention of childhood infectious diseases is achieved by the use of immunizations. Prior to widespread immunization, thousands of children were killed or disabled yearly by common infectious diseases. Current vaccines for persons aged 0–18 include hepatitis A and B, rotavirus, diphtheria, tetanus, pertussis, haemophilus influenza, pneumococcus, polio, influenza, measles, mumps, rubella, varicella, HPV, and meningococcus. Current immunization schedules for children can be found at the Centers for Disease Control and Prevention web site.[8]

BEHAVIORAL PROBLEMS

In addition to autism and ADHD, previously discussed, there are some behavioral problems that contribute to the continuing medical care of the child.

Sleep Problems

Sleep is initiated following natural patterns and cycles and consists of two well understood stages: **rapid eye movement (REM)** and non–rapid eye movement (non-REM). In adults, non-REM sleep makes up the first four stages, each lasting from 5 to 15 minutes. It is during non-REM sleep when body restoration takes place. In adults, REM sleep occurs roughly 90 minutes after the onset of sleep with the first stage lasting about 10 minutes and each subsequent stage getting longer until the final stage, which can last up to an hour. During REM sleep, the eyes move rapidly in different directions, thus the name.

The amount of sleep needed varies by age with newborns needing 16–18 hours per day, adolescents needing 8–9 hours per day, and adults needing 7–8 hours.[9,10] Sleep problems in children are common and are divided into problems involving an abnormal polysomnography test and problems that are behavioral.[11] In addition to possibly causing behavior problems, a lack of sleep has been tied to slower reaction times and an increase in accidents and injuries. Indications are that American children get less sleep than children in other societies, and this appears to be worsening.[12]

Infants less than 6 months of age typically spend half of their sleep time in active REM sleep, in contrast to adults, who spend only 20% of sleep time in REM sleep. Additionally, infants enter sleep at an active REM level, whereas adults don't enter REM until approximately 90 minutes into sleep.[11] Childhood sleep patterns approach those of adults after 6 months of age.

Any evaluation of sleep problems should include a consideration of sleep interrupters, such as pain, chronic itching, asthma, gastroesophageal reflux disease (GERD), and obstructive sleep apnea. Other issues that can occur to interrupt sleep are sleep refusal and night terrors. Sleep refusal may simply be oppositional, or it could be related to needs and fears. Night terrors arise during a sudden partial arousal from the deepest non-REM sleep.[4] Essentially, part of the brain is awake and the other part is still asleep. In this sleep/wake state, the child does not respond to any efforts to comfort them, resulting in a serious impact on the parents.

Obstructive Sleep Apnea Obstructive sleep apnea is at one extreme of a continuum of breathing difficulties that occur during sleep. At the other extreme is frequent loud snoring. It is estimated that 2% to 4% of all children are affected by obstructive sleep apnea.[13] Physiologically, sleep apnea acts as would choking, with a drop in the heart rate, a rise in blood pressure, brain function arousal, hypoxemia, and disrupted sleep. Physical causes include enlarged tonsils and adenoids, obesity, lower jaw and tongue abnormalities, and neuromuscular deficits.

Untreated, obstructive sleep apnea can lead to social problems, behavioral and learning disorders, enuresis, growth shunting, obesity, and an increased risk of hypertension and other cardiopulmonary problems.[13] Up to 25% of children diagnosed with ADHD may also have symptoms of obstructive sleep apnea.[14]

Oppositional Defiant Disorder (ODD)

It is not unusual for children to go through phases of oppositional behavior that fall into a "normal" pattern. The first occurs between 18 and 24 months and is affectionately called the "terrible twos." During this time, the oppositional behavior is related to a developing autonomy. The second occurrence may be seen during the teenage years when there is another move toward an autonomous identity and a separation from the parents. These episodes typically last less than 6 months. Additionally, all children show oppositional behavior from time to time, especially when hungry, tired, or upset. In contrast, children with ODD exhibit oppositional and defiant behavior chronically. Children with ODD show frequent temper tantrums, excessive arguing, and deliberate attempts to upset people, mean and hateful talking, and revenge seeking.[15]

Conduct Disorder

Conduct disorder is a group of behavioral and/or emotional problems that lead to a disregard for rules and socially unacceptable behaviors. Conduct disorder is more prevalent in males where it often manifests as aggression. The aggression can be directed toward people or animals. The typical patient bullies and threatens others and often initiates physical fights. They can be physically cruel to people and animals. Additionally, the aggression may be played out as a destruction of property or stealing.[16] In females, the disorder is often displayed as covert behaviors such as crimes and prostitution.[4] Of major concern with this disorder is the high rate of mortality, which may approach 50%.

EATING DISORDERS

Anyone who has worked with children knows how difficult feeding can be. Most of the time, the issues are minor and self-limited. When an eating disorder leads to malnutrition, it can become a medical problem requiring intervention. One of the key features of this disorder is the often used phrase, "failure to thrive." Typically, the child fails to gain appropriate weight over a period of time. Although many patients diagnosed as failure to thrive have gastrointestinal, endocrinologic, or neurologic issues, up to half are caused by psychosocial issues.[4]

One bizarre eating disorder, known as pica, involves the intake of non-foods such as hair, dirt, animal droppings, and paint. At issue is not just a vitamin and mineral deficiency, but possible poisoning with heavy metals.

Two of the better known eating disorders are anorexia nervosa and bulimia nervosa. While both problems are seen in boys and girls, there is a higher prevalence in adolescent girls.[17] Both disorders involve a distortion of body image and a preoccupation with food. The typical patient is a perfectionist and high achiever, however, suffers from low self-esteem. The symptoms of anorexia nervosa are manifest as a refusal to eat in a relentless pursuit to become thin. In contrast, the symptoms of bulimia nervosa exhibit as a binging on large quantities of high-caloric food, which then may be followed by self-induced vomiting or use of laxatives to "purge" the body. Symptoms of eating disorders are shown in Table 11–4.

Table 11–4

SYMPTOMS OF EATING DISORDERS IN ADOLESCENCE

Insomnia

Skipping a majority of meals

Dental caries and erosion of tooth enamel

Loss of hair and/or nail dystrophy

Constipation

Frequent weight taking

Unusual eating habits

Extreme exercise habits

Unusual hyperactivity

PEDIATRIC FEVER

The traditional definition of fever is a rectal temperature above 100.4°F or 38°C. Above most other symptoms, the presence of fever continues to be one of the most common concerns of parents and is one of the most common reasons for visits to the office or emergency department. In and of itself, fever is not problematic unless it reaches high levels (greater than 107°F or 41.6°C) and persists at that high level.[18]

Fever is a response to endogenous proteins (**pyrogens**) that raise the temperature set-point in the hypothalamus. Endogenous pyrogens are produced by phagocytotic leukocytes and released into the general circulation. Fever can accompany many conditions, including infection, malignancy, autoimmune disorders, metabolic diseases, medications, chronic inflammation, CNS disorders, and exposure to high environmental temperatures. In most instances, pediatric fever is caused by viral infections that are mostly self-limiting.[19]

Younger infants have a greater probability of serious bacterial infection accompanying fevers above 38°C (100.4°F) than do older infants and children, therefore, a more aggressive approach is needed to evaluate and manage young infants.[20] One method proposed to help identify febrile infants at low risk for serious bacterial infection is the "Rochester Criteria"[21].

ACUTE OTITIS MEDIA

Acute otitis media (AOM) follows only upper respiratory infections as the most common disease of childhood. It is also the most common cause for pediatric visits to the doctor's office.[22] AOM occurs when fluid accumulates in the middle ear, leading to inflammation secondary to bacterial infection. Eustachian tube dysfunction is a leading cause of AOM. Additionally, in children, the eustachian tube is smaller and more level than adults, making it difficult for fluid to drain out of the middle ear. In the presence of upper respiratory infection (URI), the eustachian tubes can become inflamed and blocked with mucus, furthering the problem. AOM typically occurs recurrently throughout childhood with one third of children having six or more episodes by age 7.[23]

Variations of AOM include otitis media with effusion in which fluid accumulates behind the tympanic membrane and remains after the acute phase of the infection and chronic suppurative otitis media, which occurs when the inflammation of the middle ear persists beyond 6 weeks. Chronic suppurative otitis media is frequently associated with **otorrhea**, which is drainage into the external ear canal.

Complications of AOM are divided into **intratemporal** and an intracranial type (Table 11–5). Intratemporal relates to complications in the structures of the ear in contrast to intracranial which occur within the brain and its structures.

Table 11–5

COMPLICATIONS RELATED TO ACUTE OTITIS MEDIA (AOM)

Intratemporal
  Hearing loss (conductive and sensorineural)
  Perforation of the tympanic membrane
  Chronic suppurative otitis media
  Cholesteatoma
  Tympanosclerosis
  Mastoiditis
  Petrositis
  Labyrinthitis
  Facial paralysis
  Cholesterol granuloma
  Infectious eczematoid dermatitis

Intracranial
  Meningitis
  Subdural empyema
  Brain abcess
  Extradural abscess
  Lateral sinus thrombosis
  Otitic hydrocephalus

Source: Waseem, M (ed). *Otitis Media*. Medscape Reference, 2013. http://emedicine.medscape.com/article/994656-overview.

In 2004, the American Academy of Pediatrics and the American Academy of Family Physicians identified three specific criteria that must be present in order to diagnose AOM. This was an attempt to decrease the amount of antibiotic use in the treatment of AOM. The three criteria are: 1) acute onset of symptoms; 2) presence of fluid in the middle ear; and 3) signs and symptoms of inflammation. These guidelines did not have the anticipated effect in reducing the rate of antibiotic use, resulting in the American Academy of Pediatrics convening a committee in 2009 to update the guidelines.[22] Highlights from the committee include that a bulging tympanic membrane is more highly specific to AOM and should be used in diagnosis. Additionally, the committee recommended that AOM should not be diagnosed if a middle ear effusion is not present. A third change is an extension of the "wait-and-see" approach to certain children younger than 2 years old.[23]

THERMOREGULATION

The most common occurrence of hypothermia in the pediatric population occurs during trauma and the subsequent care of the patient. Following a traumatic injury, the child is often exposed to accelerated heat loss from lying on the cold ground and exposure. Open wounds and blood loss add to the loss of heat. Hypothermia is exacerbated by inherent ineffectiveness of heat production in the child and the added exposure from the injuries and resuscitation. Physiologically, children have a high body surface area to weight ratio along with a relatively low amount of fat. This combination places the child at a higher risk of hypothermia. In the presence of an injury to the central nervous system, the patient may lose the ability to shiver and the ability of the body to detect heat loss may be impaired.

Once emergency care arrives, further heat loss can occur if precautions are not taken, by the removal of clothing in the presence of cooler environmental temperatures. Placing the child on a cold backboard enhances conductive heat loss. Additionally, placing the patient in a supine position further exposes more body surface area to the colder environment. The administration of non-warmed IV fluids can lead to a more rapid core cooling. The use of sedatives and muscle relaxants can also inhibit the shivering response. All of these factors can and should be mediated when dealing with the pediatric trauma patient.

SUMMARY

Continuing care for the pediatric patient requires the provider to have an understanding of the common health concerns facing this population. During this time of life, it is important to monitor and measure the growth and development of the patient, as compared to established norms. One health issue that is becoming more prevelant in children is hypertension. A similar trend is seen with obesity, which appears to play a role in the increasing number of children with hypertension.

Sexual development is another essential part of the growth of the child. The Tanner scale is used to assess sexual maturity in both males and females and is helpful to the health care provider as decisions regarding health care are made. Other aspects of assessment include preventative care, such as nutrition, and behavioral development. Some of the more well-known behavioral disorders seen in children are the ASD, ADHD, and Asperger syndrome. Other variations of these three disorders can be subtle to assess.

Vaccines have effected a huge advance in the reduction of many formerly devastating childhood infectious diseases. Immunization schedules follow an established standard, and updated versions are available through the CDC. Many children struggle with sleep problems, and many do not achieve the amount of sleep needed for optimal health. Children in American society appear to get less sleep than in other societies, and this issue appears to be getting worse. A sleep issue may be the result of an anatomic or physiologic concern, such as obstructive sleep apnea. Causes include enlarged tonsils and adenoids, obesity, abnormalities with the tongue and/or jaw, and neuromuscular problems.

Oppositional defiant disorder, conduct disorder, and eating disorders are other groups of behavioral and emotional problems that can be frustrating for parents and health care providers to confront and deal with. An understanding of the disorders is the beginning of learning how to help the patient with these conditions. Pyrogens are naturally occurring proteins that raise the temperature set point in the hypothalamus and lead to fever. Pediatric fevers can be frightening to parents; however a majority of them are harmless and simply a reaction to a viral infection. One proposed method to help determine if the child is at low risk for serious bacterial infection is the Rochester Criteria.

Infection and/or fluid accumulation in the middle ear leads to AOM, which is another illness commonly seen in childhood. While complications are rare, an understanding of the pathophysiology of this condition is important to avoid them. Finally, the issue of thermoregulation in the pediatric patient is discussed as it relates to common health issues as well as those that can occur during emergency care.

POSTTEST

1. Which of the following health risks is a primary reason to recommend screening of children for hypertension?
    a. Hypertension can lead to obesity.
    b. Hypertension may lead to end-organ damage and increases cardiovascular risk.
    c. Hypertension in childhood frequently leads to asthma.
    d. Hypertension and sleep apnea are the leading cause of premature death in children.

2. Examination of a 13-year-old female reveals dark, coarse pubic hair extending from the labia to the mons pubis. The breasts show enlargement of the tissue with no contour separation. This patient's Tanner stage of development is:
   a. stage I
   b. stage II
   c. stage III
   d. stage IV
   e. stage V
3. Which of the following tests is recommended for pediatric health screening?
   a. lead toxicity
   b. skin examination
   c. blood glucose
   d. cholesterol levels
4. Of the following, which is not typically associated with Asperger syndrome?
   a. Patients typically function better than do those with autism.
   b. Patients generally have normal intelligence.
   c. Patients have near-normal language development.
   d. The age of diagnosis is typically when the patient reaches puberty.
5. Sleeping problems have been linked to which of the following?
   a. behavior problems
   b. obesity
   c. hypertension
   d. increase in childhood illnesses
6. A parent confides in you that her 6-year-old daughter has been eating dirt recently. This is an example of:
   a. anorexia nervosa
   b. bulimia nervosa
   c. pica
   d. conduct disorder
7. According to the Rochester Criteria, which of the following infants with a fever would not be at high risk for a serious bacterial infection?
   a. The infant appears generally well.
   b. The infant recently finished a course of antibiotics for otitis media.
   c. The infant was hospitalized 6 months earlier for severe croup.
   d. The infant was born at 32 weeks gestation.
8. Which of the following is not one of the three specific criteria that must be present in order to diagnose AOM?
   a. acute onset of symptoms
   b. presence of fluid in the middle ear
   c. signs and symptoms of inflammation
   d. diminished hearing

9. You are called to the emergency room to maintain the airway of a 9-year-old boy who was involved in a bicycle accident. When you arrive, you find that the boy is on a backboard in his underwear. Which of the following would help prevent the most common avoidable risk in this situation?
   a. use 100% oxygen
   b. cover the patient in a warm blanket
   c. replenish body fluids by starting an IV drip
   d. constantly monitor HR and BP

REFERENCES

1. Din-Dzietham R, et al. High blood pressure trends in children and adolescents in national surveys, 1963 to 2002. *Circulation.* 116(13):1488–1496, 2007.
2. Falkner, B. Chair, The fourth report on the diagnosis, evaluation, and treatment of high blood pressure in children and adolescents. *Pediatrics.* 114:555, 2004.
3. The American College of Obstetricians and Gynecologists. *Tool Kit for Teen Care*, 2nd ed. http://www.acog.org/~/media/Departments/Adolescent%20Health%20Care/Teen%20Care%20Tool%20Kit/TannerStaging2.pdf?dmc=1&ts=20130610T1735528268
4. Rakel RE, Rakel DP. *Textbook of Family Medicine*, 8th ed. Philadelphia, PA: Elsevier Saunders, 2011.
5. Centers for Disease Control and Prevention. Autism spectrum disorders, Aug. 2012. http://www.cdc.gov/ncbddd/autism/index.html
6. Centers for Disease Control and Prevention. Attention-deficit/hyperactivity disorder (ADHD), Apr. 2013. http://www.cdc.gov/ncbddd/adhd/index.html.
7. Health Center WebMD. Autism spectrum disorders, 2013. http://www.webmd.com/brain/autism/mental-health-aspergers-syndrome.
8. Centers for Disease Control and Prevention. Immunization schedules, http://www.cdc.gov/vaccines/schedules/index.html.
9. WebMD. Sleep problems in children, 2012. http://www.webmd.com/sleep-disorders/guide/children-sleep-problems.
10. WebMD. Stages of sleep: REM and non-REM sleep, 2012. http://www.webmd.com/sleep-disorders/excessive-sleepiness-10/sleep-101
11. Thiedke CC. Sleep disorders and sleep problems in childhood. *Am Fam Physician.* 63(2):277–278, Jan. 15, 2001.
12. Dahl RE The impact of inadequate sleep on children's daytime cognitive function. *Semin Pediatr Neurol.* 3(1):44–50, 1996.
13. American Academy of Otolaryngology-Head and Neck Surgery. Fact Sheet: Pediatric Sleep Disordered Breathing/Obstructive Sleep Apnea, 2011.
14. American Sleep Apnea Association. Children's Sleep Apnea, 2012.
15. Am Acad Child Adol Psych. Children with Oppositional Defiant Disorder. Facts for Families. #72, Mar. 2011.

16. Am Acad Child Adol Psych. Conduct Disorder: Facts for Families. #33, May 2012.
17. Am Acad Child Adol Psych.Teenagers with Eating Disorders: Facts for Families. #2, May 2008.
18. Ferry R. Fever in children. Emedicinehealth, 2010. http://www .emedicinehealth.com/fever_in_children/article_em.htm.
19. Hay WW, et al. (eds). *Current Diagnosis and Treatment Pediatrics*. 21st ed. New York: McGraw-Hill, 2012.
20. Luszczak M. Evaluation and management of infants and young children with fever. *Am Fam Physician*. 64(7):1219–1227, Oct. 2001.
21. Jaskiewicz JA, et al. Febrile infants at low risk for serious bacterial infection— an appraisal of the Rochester criteria and implications for management. Febrile Infant Collaborative Study Group. *Pediatrics*. 94:390–6, 1994.
22. Waseem M (ed). Otitis Media. Medscape Reference, 2013. http://emedicine .medscape.com/article/994656-overview.
23. Martin BN, et al. *Practice Guideline Insights: New Methods for Diagnosis and Treatment of Acute Otitis Media*. Medscape Education Clinical Briefs, Feb. 2013. http://www.medscape.org/viewarticle/782368

BIBLIOGRAPHY AND SUGGESTED READINGS

Centers for Disease Control and Prevention, Attention-Deficit/Hyperactivity Disorder (ADHD). April 2013. http://www.cdc.gov/ncbddd/adhd/index.html.
Centers for Disease Control and Prevention. Growth Charts. http://www.cdc.gov/ growthcharts.
Hay WW, et al. (eds). *Current Diagnosis and Treatment Pediatrics*. 21st ed. New York: McGraw-Hill, 2012.
Marcdante D, et al. *Nelson Essentials of Pediatrics*. Philadelphia, PA: Elsevier Saunders, 2011.
Marquardt N. (ed). *Pediatrics Board Review Series*. Baltimore: Lippincott, Williams & Wilkins, 2005.
Medline Plus. *Normal Growth and Development*. Bethesda, MD: U.S. National Library of Medicine and the National Institutes of Health, 2013.
Osborn LM (ed). *Pediatrics*. Philadelphia, PA: Mosby, Inc., 2005.
Rakel RE, Rakel DP. *Textbook of Family Medicine*, 8th ed. Philadelphia, PA: Elsevier Saunders, 2011.

CHAPTER 12

Pediatric Diseases Requiring Respiratory Care

OBJECTIVES

Upon completion of this chapter, the reader should be able to:

1. Describe the characteristic signs and symptoms, disease pathophysiology, and treatment of the following disorders:
   a. Acute respiratory distress syndrome (ARDS)
   b. Asthma
   c. Cystic fibrosis
2. Compare and contrast progressive spinal muscular atrophy of infants (Werdnig–Hoffman paralysis), juvenile spinal muscle atrophy (Kugelberg–Welander disease), and muscular dystrophy.
3. Identify the causative organisms, accompanying signs of the disorder, and treatment of the following:
   a. Guillain–Barré syndrome
   b. Tetanus
   c. Botulism
4. Describe the common etiology and diagnosis of myasthenia gravis.
5. Identify and explain the manifestations of Reye's syndrome, its pathophysiology, and treatment. List and describe the five staging criteria for Reye's syndrome.
6. Describe, for each of the following infectious diseases, the causative organisms, symptoms, diagnosis, and treatment of:
   a. Pneumonia
   b. Bronchiolitis

KEY TERMS

azoospermia	decorticate	intrinsic
bronchiolitis obliterans organizing pneumonia (BOOP)	doll's eye reflex	intussusception
	electromyography	leukotrienes
	extrinsic	muscarinic
decerebrate	inotropic	oculocephalic

INTRODUCTION

To a worried parent, there is not much scarier than having a sick child. An understanding of the nature, causes, and treatment of common maladies can go a long way in helping the respiratory therapist to be not only a highly qualified practitioner, but also a reassuring presence for the family of the patient.

VENTILATORY DISEASES

In the pediatric patient, ventilatory diseases are manifest by the inability to utilize oxygen or eliminate carbon dioxide. Normally, about 250 mL of oxygen is consumed by the cells and 200 mL of carbon dioxide is produced each minute during internal (aerobic) respiration producing the energy for daily functions. The lungs sole purpose is to exchange oxygen and carbon dioxide over a large surface area such that physiologic processes are maintained and able to thrive. Any interruption in this process produces deficiencies that can be evaluated by an arterial blood gas analysis.

Acute Respiratory Distress Syndrome (ARDS)

ARDS afflicts patients of all ages, including children. Despite advances in understanding and treatment of the disease, mortality remained near 50% before the protective lung strategy (PLS) outlined in the National Heart Blood and Lung Institute's ARDSnet protocol in 1999.[1,2] Although the incidence and mortality of ARDS declined by 25% by employing elements of its use, ventilator management in respiratory distress and acute lung injury (ALI) remains fraught with a variety of strategies that vary with individual patient presentations and weaning protocols. New technology continues to advance the field and strategies such as airway pressure release ventilation (APRV), high frequency oscillatory ventilation (HFOV), and the use of nitric oxide are receiving further attention. Respiratory therapists are required to keep abreast of the current research and developments that drive the field forward. A strategy that appears productive may not always work in a particular circumstance that requires a respiratory therapist to have knowledge to develop a "repertoire" of strategies to fall back upon. Although considerable research has broadened our understanding of the pathophysiology of this pervasive disease, the key elements that initiate and potentiate ARDS have yet to be fully defined. Patient outcomes are only improved

Table 12–1

POSSIBLE MEDIATORS OF LUNG INJURY

Neutrophils
Platelets
Leukotriene-B$_4$
Platelet-activating factor
Bacterial peptides
Macrophage-derived chemotactic factor
Oxygen radicals
Proteolytic enzymes
Phospholipase products
Endotoxin
Kallikrein
Interleukin-1
Coagulation factors

by early recognition and intervention before the triggering factors are allowed to evolve. Table 12–1 lists the possible mediators of lung injury that can lead to ARDS.[3]

Pathophysiology The classic inflammatory condition seen with ARDS results in a severe mismatch between ventilation and perfusion due to progressively "leaky pulmonary capillaries" from a causative injury. Capillary leak leads to the characteristic hallmarks of the disease to include pulmonary hypertension, reduced lung compliance, hypercarbia, tissue hypoxia, acidosis, tissue necrosis, progressive atelectasis, and pulmonary infiltrates (ground glass appearance) outlined on an x-ray. These conditions are perpetuated in a vicious cycle of refractory hypoxemia, advanced hypercarbia, and worsening acidosis. If the cycle is not interrupted, death ensues. ARDS is the result of either direct or indirect injury to the pulmonary system. Examples of direct injury are infection (sepsis), aspiration pneumonitis, near drowning, and fat or air embolism. Indirect injuries may include chest wall trauma, burns or complicated abdominal or thoracic surgery. Table 12–2 lists mechanisms that have been associated with the onset of ARDS.

   ARDS has been divided into four distinct phases that follow the pathogenesis of the disease.[3] In the first phase, the patient becomes dyspneic and tachypneic from latent pulmonary capillary leak into the interstitial space surrounding a small number of the alveoli. In this phase, the chest x-ray may appear normal and the patient's

Table 12–2

POSSIBLE TRIGGERING MECHANISMS OF ARDS

- Shock

- Thoracic trauma

- Pulmonary contusion

- Severe head injury

- Pulmonary embolism (fat, blood, or air)

- Aspiration syndrome

- Near-drowning

- Extensive burns

- Sepsis

- Diffuse pulmonary infection

- Transfusion of large amounts of stored blood

- Oxygen toxicity

- Disseminated intravascular coagulation

- Prolonged cardiopulmonary bypass

- Narcotic drug overdose

oxygenation status and saturation is normal. The second phase occurs within 12 to 24 hours characterized by interstitial edema. It is during this phase that alveolar damage begins and diffuse infiltrates begin appearing on the chest x-ray.

Research suggests that there are numerous pathways leading to the alveolar damage associated with ARDS. One study by Sivan and associates demonstrates that concept.[4] Several inflammatory pathways are activated in the lungs of the ARDS patient. The challenge is to determine which factors are primary causes of ARDS and which are secondary responses to the initial insult.

Commonly seen changes include an increase of proteinases of neutrophilic origin in the alveoli, components of the complement, kinin-forming, coagulation; and fibrinolytic cascades, and a change in pulmonary surfactant. These changes cause a fibrotic process (hyaline membrane formation) in the lungs, similar to normal wound healing, that leads to impaired gas exchange in that affected alveoli fold back on themselves and collapse, resulting in a need for extended care. Patients who survive ARDS appear to be those who have minimal fibrotic changes in the lungs.

As the pathological processes for ARDS advances, phase 3 begins. During this phase, a larger portion of alveolar/capillary membranes are overwhelmed with fluid, resulting in accumulation in the alveoli and distal airways. Damage to the alveoli also results in a decrease in surfactant production in alveolar type II cells causing progressive alveolar collapse and a subsequent reduction in lung compliance. This is the result of the increasing surface tension required to keep alveoli open with diminishing surfactant. During phase 3, respiratory failure develops with worsening hypoxemia, hypercarbia ($PaCO_2$ greater than 60 mmHg), and acidosis. Diffuse infiltrates appear on the chest x-ray along with the development of air bronchograms. Mechanical ventilation with high F_iO_2 and PEEP is often initiated at this point. It is possible that alveolar damage is increased by the high oxygen and positive pressure mechanical ventilation (barotraumas).[3] The fourth phase is described as progressive respiratory failure, fibrosis of the lungs, and recurrent, resistant pneumonias. Whether all of these changes occur in the pediatric patient is still being evaluated.

A study that evaluated the role of vitamin E levels in the development of ARDS was outlined by Richard and associates.[5] They concluded that the development of ARDS is associated with vitamin E deficiency and an enhancement of plasma lipoperoxidation. They also concluded that the vitamin E deficiency is a probable consequence of malnutrition making the healing process difficult in patients requiring extended care.

Signs and Symptoms Symptoms (subjective data) in the early stages of the disease are expressed by the patient as anxiety and by acute shortness of breath (dyspnea). Signs are objective measures of respiratory distress indicated by inspiratory crackles, increased respiratory rate, retractions, and possible expiratory grunting observed in infants or small children. The patient may also have signs of pulmonary edema such as frothy pink secretions as alveoli become overwhelmed by fluid. Those patients who have conditions that predispose them to the development of ARDS should be carefully monitored for early recognition of the syndrome.

Initially, compensatory mechanisms to interrupt respiratory failure include hyperventilation, which causes hypocapnia and respiratory alkalosis. As the disease progresses, arterial oxygenation begins to worsen, leading to hypoxemia (low PaO_2), eventually becoming resistant (refractory) to oxygen therapy. As pulmonary insufficiency develops, the arterial PCO_2 rises and the patient becomes acidotic. Compliance begins to worsen as the lungs become stiff. Crackles and rhonchi become more apparent during the advanced stages of the disease.

As compliance drops, physiologic deadspace increases leading to decreased alveolar ventilation and a rise in minute ventilation. Intrapulmonary shunting increases and may exceed 20% or more of the cardiac output.[6] The chest x-ray becomes progressively worse, with diffuse, uneven infiltrations throughout both lung fields, eventually described as reticulogranular or a "ground glass" appearance.

Treatment Treatment of ARDS is aimed at supporting the injured lungs (using low stretch protocols) to maintain normal physiologic function, that is, giving them time to heal. Early intervention may result in less severe lung injury with a shorter hospital course of treatment and fewer complications. Hudson (1990) outlined three strategies for early treatment of ARDS: 1) correction of physiologic derangements, 2) suppression of alveolar inflammation, and 3) the prevention of complications.[7] Additionally, it is crucial to resolve the source of infection, either medically or surgically, to reduce the inflammatory response.

The correction of physiologic derangement is achieved by several methods. As the patient begins to progress into respiratory failure, the patient is generally intubated and mechanical ventilation is initiated to reverse the hypoxemia and hypercapnia. Research by Kallet advocates a role for spontaneous breathing although its efficacy may not be well tolerated in children.[8] Moderate to high levels of PEEP may also be needed to keep alveoli open and bring the functional residual capacity back up to normal, thus improving oxygenation and ventilation. Although, Hudson indicated that early application of PEEP does not reduce the incidence of ARDS or alter the course of the disease.[7]

There is growing concern that mechanical ventilation causes further lung injury in the ARDS patient, worsening the course of the disease.[3] Nonconventional support therapies, such as HFOV and ECMO, are possible answers to reducing lung injury. However, these modes are not without their own downsides. APRV and HFOV, with/or without nitric oxide seems to be the most promising modes of therapy at this time.

The success in the use of artificial surfactant on neonates has sparked interest in this mode of therapy for victims of ARDS. To date, few studies have been performed, but those that have been done show promise.[3] Questions remain regarding the best surfactant to use, amount, and best delivery method. In virtually all studies done, there was short-term oxygenation improvement and decreased incidence of pneumothoraces observed with its use.

Another technology, nitric oxide, may prove to be beneficial in the treatment of ARDS. Its main benefit is the ability to reduce pulmonary hypertension, while not causing systemic hypotension. Much research remains to be done, however, before nitric oxide is used as a treatment for ARDS.

The reduction of lung edema is another factor in the early treatment of ARDS. This has been accomplished by the use of diuretics, vasoactive and positive **inotropic** agents that improve cardiac contractility. Another approach is the use of terbutaline to enhance the clearance of alveolar edema by epithelial cells; however, this technique has not yet been applied to humans.[9] One hazard with the use of diuretics is the potential of lowering cardiac output and impairing tissue oxygenation. Careful consideration must be used when evaluating the maintenance of circulating fluid status in patients with ARDS.

The administration of prostaglandin E_1 (PGE_1) has also been reported to increase survival in ARDS patients. A study by Russel, however, has shown that the use of PGE_1 does not alter the outcome.[10]

The use of anti-inflammatory drugs, such as corticosteroids and nonsteroidal anti-inflammatory drugs (NSAIDs) has not been shown to decrease the onset or the severity of ARDS. Additionally, the use of antiprotease, antioxidants, platelet-activating factor antagonists, and specific antibodies against toxic inflammatory agents is being investigated for potential use in the treatment of ARDS.

Aerosolized bronchodilators may reduce airflow resistance and improve oxygenation and ventilation in the ARDS patient. V/Q mismatch that is associated with ARDS has been shown to be improved by the use of Almatrine. Although not yet available in the United States, it appears to be helpful in the treatment of pulmonary vasoconstriction associated with ARDS.

The most common and severe complication of ARDS are concomitant infections from invasive use of lines, tubes, and monitoring systems. Two strategies being studied to reduce infections include the use of sucralfate to prevent gastric bleeding and selective decontamination of the digestive tract (SDD). Studies have demonstrated a lower incidence of pneumonia in ARDS patients treated with sucralfate. This reduction may be due in part to a prevention of bacterial proliferation by maintaining gastric acidity and the direct antimicrobial effect of sucralfate.

SDD involves the prevention of aerobic colonization of the upper airway and gut, allowing anaerobic organisms to remain. This is done by the selective use of gram-positive IV antibiotics and simultaneous topical and oral administration of tobramycin, polymyxin E, and amphotericin. Studies involving SDD are being conducted in Europe, and further research in these areas remains to be done.

Asthma

Asthma is a hyperreactive airway disorder in which a patient's airway spasms and constricts, swells, and pours secretions into the lumen of the bronchus in response to various irritants or triggers. The result is moderate to severe airway obstruction, shortness of breath, and dyspnea that may be life threatening (status asthmaticus).

Asthma is the most common pediatric disease, affecting 5% to 10% of children, and the most frequent cause of hospitalization of pediatric patients in the United States.[11] Over 500,000 hospitalizations which result in over 4,000 deaths in the United States can be specifically attributed to asthma.[12] The incidence of asthma in the adult population is 3% to 5% (about 25 million Americans), with half of all patients acquiring the disease before age 10.[13] Asthma affects 1 in 12 school-aged children in the United States.[14] It affects twice as many boys than girls prior to puberty when girls outnumber boys after puberty with symptoms associated with asthma. Despite all that is known about asthma and its treatment, the mortality rate continues to climb.

The World Health Organization (WHO) estimates that over 180,000 people die each year from symptoms associated with asthma. One of the most commonly encountered diseases in clinical medicine, asthma confounds simple definitions as multiple and various triggers precipitate symptoms. Although the exact etiology of the disease is elusive and specific triggers are described to influence different patients to various degrees, several factors that precipitate acute attacks have been identified. They are listed in Table 12–3.

Experts generally categorize asthma into two types which partly explain the most common exposures. **Extrinsic** or allergic asthma is a common variety of asthma that develops with exposure to specific allergenic substances such as dusts, mites, animal dander, molds, yeasts, and fungi. Atopy is described in which hypersensitivity to an antigen mediates an IgE antibody reaction in the airway. This produces

Table 12–3

FACTORS THAT PRECIPITATE ACUTE ASTHMA SYMPTOMS

1. Allergens
   a. Molds
   b. Pollens

2. Outdoor irritants
   a. Smoke
   b. Air pollution

3. Indoor irritants
   a. Animal danders
   b. Dusts

4. Exercise

5. Viral infections

6. Foods

7. Emotions

8. Aspirin and related drugs

the characteristic inflammatory response characterized by the degranulation of mast cells in the tracheal mucosa. The end result is edema, swelling, cellular infiltration, epithelial damage, and bronchospasm observed in allergic asthma reactions. Additionally, exposures such as occupational sensitivity to paint, resins, organic dusts, agricultural work, or in plastic manufacturing are also included in extrinsic characteristics associated with asthma hypersensitivities.

Intrinsic or nonallergic asthma, on the other hand, is associated with respiratory tract infections, emotions, exercise, or airway cooling that results in cholinergic hyperreactivity and bronchoconstriction experienced in an asthma attack. Inflammation of the airway follows similar pathologic pathways described in allergic asthma although patients demonstrate no evidence of an IgE mediated reaction they are not atopic.

Much research has been performed on the mediators, atopy, and treatment of asthma. One study found that secondhand cigarette smoke aggravates asthma in children. Another study found a high incidence of reactive airway disease in infants who suffered bronchopulmonary dysplasia as neonates.[11]

Pathophysiology The course of asthma includes two phases. In the acute phase, the presence of triggering stimuli on the airway causes the rupture or degranulation of the mast cell. The mast cell contains several chemical mediators that are released upon its rupture. These mediators include histamine, **leukotrienes** (formerly called slow-reacting substance of anaphylaxis or SRS-A), eosinophilic chemotactic factor of anaphylaxis (ECF-A), and prostaglandins. These mediators affect the smooth muscle of the tracheobronchial tree and result in bronchospasm, vasodilation, edema, increased secretions, and an accumulation of eosinophils.

The second phase of the asthma attack is the inflammatory phase of the disease. Following the initial acute response, mediators are released by eosinophils, neutrophils, macrophages, and lymphocytes. These mediators initiate the inflammatory response by swelling and in bronchoconstriction of the airways.

As resistance to flow in the airways increases, work of breathing increases concurrently. Resulting ventilation and perfusion mismatches worsen blood gases and further deteriorate the patient's respiratory status. Because the airways are narrower during expiration, air trapping results in an increased FRC. As a result, more negative intrapleural pressure is needed to maintain the same tidal volume and, thus, work of breathing increases.

The narrowing of airways is unevenly distributed throughout the lungs and results in wide V/Q imbalances. V/Q mismatching leads to hypoxemia, which causes the patient to hyperventilate and become hypocarbic and alkolotic. The changes in respiratory function lead to derangement of both cardiovascular and metabolic function. The patient becomes dehydrated secondary to a decreased ability to take fluids and increased insensible loss from tachypnea and fever, if present. Lactic acidosis results from a combination of hypoxemia, dehydration, and increased metabolism caused by tachypnea. Hypocarbia limits the conservation of bicarbonate by the kidney and leads to metabolic acidosis.

After a time, the patient begins to exhaust from the energy spent attempting to maintain ventilation. The $PaCO_2$ begins to rise, and the patient enters acute respiratory failure, the terminal phase of illness.

There appears to be two distinct onset patterns to asthma, sudden onset, and the more common, slow onset. Immunohistologically, it has been observed that patients with sudden-onset fatal asthma had higher numbers of neutrophils and less eosinophils in the airway mucosa, raising the possibility that the mechanisms of inflammation and airway narrowing are completely different from those seen with slow-onset asthma.[15]

Signs and Symptoms The patient suffering the effects of an asthmatic attack will often have a history of wheezing and shortness of breath mingled with periods of no symptoms at all. Many times the patient has a long history of hospital visits for evaluation and treatment. A complete, thorough history is crucial to treat the asthmatic patient adequately. The success or failure of previous treatments is helpful in developing an appropriate plan. Patients often relate their history and treatment patterns accurately and respiratory therapists are advised to heed regimes that have been successful in prior visits. The presence of dehydration and concurrent infection can also be detected by careful attention to the history.

Physical signs depend on the degree of the attack. A mild attack presents as a dry hacking cough, with little presence of wheezing. Patients suffering a moderate attack will have a productive cough, tachypnea, audible wheezes, tachycardia, and possible cyanosis illustrating the severity of the attack. The patient with a severe attack has diminished breath sounds from lack of ventilation, retractions, may develop rapid, shallow respiration, and may be stuporous or lethargic from hypoxia and hypercapnia in the late stages of the disease.

Arterial blood gas results may be used to classify acute asthma attacks into four stages of severity. In stage 1, the blood gases are within normal limits. In stage 2, the $PaCO_2$ begins to decrease and the pH becomes alkalotic. There may or may not be signs of hypoxemia in stage 2. Stage 3 shows a normal $PaCO_2$ and pH in a fatigued, hypoxemic patient. These patients should be admitted to the ICU and observed closely. Stage 4 depicts those patients with a high $PaCO_2$, a low pH, and a low PaO_2. These patients require immediate intubation and mechanical ventilation with high flow and rapid respiratory rates.

Additional blood tests may reveal eosinophilia and increased polymorphonuclear leukocytosis. The IgE levels may also be elevated in atopic asthma.

The measurement of peak expiratory flows helps to determine the extent of airway obstruction and the responsiveness to bronchodilator therapy.

There are several causes of wheezing that have been misdiagnosed as asthma that should be ruled out whenever asthma is suspected. Those disorders most frequently misdiagnosed as asthma include left ventricular failure, endobronchial lesions, vocal cord dysfunction, and **bronchiolitis obliterans organizing pneumonia (BOOP)**.

Treatment The primary treatment of an asthma attack is avoiding the precipitating factors that trigger the attack. In the presence of an active attack, oxygen is nearly always indicated to treat hypoxemia. The PaO_2 should be kept above 55 mmHg, if possible. Hypoxemia is often underestimated in the asthmatic patient due to compensatory hyperventilation, and under no circumstances should oxygen be withheld based on observation alone. The use of pulse oximetry may be helpful in assessing which patients require an arterial blood gas at presentation to the hospital. In a study by Carruthers and Harrison, they found that an oxygen saturation greater than 92% at presentation to the hospital suggested that respiratory failure is unlikely and an arterial blood gas may not be necessary.[16] They point out, however, that other parameters must be continually monitored and assessed in all asthmatic patients and arterial blood gases must be done whenever clinically indicated, regardless of the SpO_2.

The use of an 80:20 mixture of helium:oxygen (heliox) has been shown to be effective at reducing pulsus paradoxus and improving peak expiratory flow rates in acute asthmatics.[17] Pulsus paradoxus is an abnormal decrease in systolic pressure seen during inspiration. In asthma, its presence is indicative of severe disease. The use of heliox may also diminish the tendency of inspiratory muscles to fatigue and thus improve the patient outcome.

Asthma is a multifactorial process that often requires the use of multiple drugs in its treatment. The treatment of asthma is best understood when the mechanics of airway regulation are understood. The tone of airway smooth muscle is maintained and regulated by three elements in the autonomic nervous system: the sympathetic

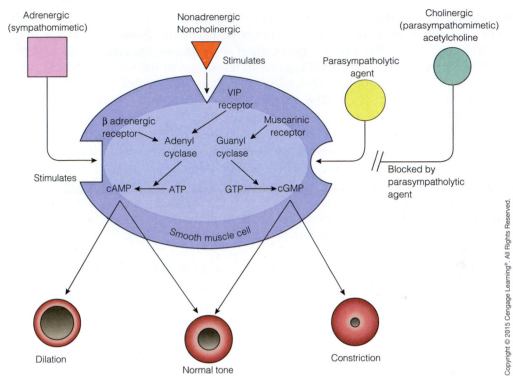

FIGURE 12–1. Regulation of airway smooth muscle tone.

(adrenergic), parasympathetic (cholinergic), and the nonadrenergic noncholinergic system (NANC) (see Figure 12–1). In addition, these nerves regulate mucus secretion, vascular permeability, blood flow, and the release of mediators from mast cells.[18]

The Nonadrenergic Noncholinergic System (NANC) While little is known about the NANC system, it is apparent that it plays a significant role in maintaining the airways. The NANC is believed to be the primary nervous system that inhibits bronchial smooth muscle contraction. The transmitters involved in the NANC system have not been positively identified but vasoactive intestinal peptide (VIP) and peptide histidine methanol appear to be the primary mediators. When the VIP receptors are stimulated, ATP is converted to cAMP by adenyl cyclase, resulting in bronchodilation. While VIP is a powerful bronchodilator, it has yet to be used successfully as an aerosol. It has been suggested that the hyperreactive airways seen in asthma are the result of a defect in the NANC system.

The Sympathetic System The exact role of the sympathetic system in maintaining airway tone is not completely understood. While the smooth muscle of the airways has little, if any, sympathetic innervation, the airways themselves have an abundance of sympathetic β_2 receptors in the small peripheral airways. It is well known that stimulation of these β_2 receptors leads to bronchodilation, but the exact mechanism by which that occurs is poorly understood. The mechanism is similar to that of VIP receptors, in that stimulation of the β_2 sites causes the conversion of ATP to cAMP with the increase in cAMP leading to relaxation of the smooth muscle.

The Parasympathetic System

The Parasympathetic System The parasympathetic system is the main system controlling airway smooth muscle and mucus secretion. The main receptor of the parasympathetic system is the muscarinic receptor, which is stimulated by the transmitter acetylcholine. Muscarinic receptors are found almost exclusively in the large central airways. When the muscarinic receptor is stimulated, GTP is converted to cGMP by guanyl cyclase. The increased level of cGMP causes contraction of the bronchial smooth muscle, increased mucus secretion in the airways, and the release of mast cell mediators. These mediators lead to the inflammatory response with edema, increased muscle spasm, and mucus secretion into the airways.

Agents Used to Treat Asthma

Agents Used to Treat Asthma Most drugs used to treat asthma are given by aerosol. This allows direct placement of the drug at the site of the problem, and allows for rapid onset of action. Based on the understanding of airway physiology (just reviewed) there are three main drug categories used to treat asthma.

Sympathomimetics (β_2-Adrenergic Agonists)

Sympathomimetics (β_2-Adrenergic Agonists) The most commonly used medications are the sympathomimetic agents, those drugs that stimulate the β_2-adrenergic sites. In addition to causing bronchodilation, these drugs also have been shown to inhibit mast cell degranulation, reduce the permeability of the pulmonary vasculature, and improve the mucociliary transport of secretions.[18]

One of the oldest β_2 drugs used to treat asthma is epinephrine. Epinephrine, and two of its synthetic derivatives, isoproterenol, and isoetharine, were the standard medications used for many years. While providing rapid bronchodilation, these drugs have a limited duration, and often cause tremors, palpitations, and anxiety. For these reasons, newer medications that have a longer duration of action and fewer side effects have been developed. These medications include: bitolterol (Tornalate®), metaproterenol (Alupent®, Metaprel®), terbutaline (Brethine®, Bricanyl®), fenoterol (Berotec®), albuterol (salbutamol in Europe; Proventil®, Ventolin®), pirbuterol (Maxair®), carbuterol (Bronsecur®), procaterol (Pro-Air®), salmeterol xinafoate (Serevent®), and formoterol. All catecholamine derivatives have proven to be effective mediators in reversing bronchoconstriction observed in acute asthma. These drugs are often termed "rescue" medications. However, it cannot be overstated that asthma is largely a disease resulting in inflammation and sympathomimetics merely treat the symptoms (wheezing) associated with asthma and not the underlying problem. For that reason, many asthma controllers have combined the use of an inhaled corticosteroid with a bronchodilator in an effort to control repeated asthma attacks.

Parasympatholytics (Anticholinergics)

Parasympatholytics (Anticholinergics) Drugs in this category are chemically similar to the neurotransmitter acetylcholine in that they actively bind to the muscarinic receptors. The difference, however, is that as an antagonist, these drugs do not stimulate any continuation of the nerve impulse, effectively blocking its transmission. The prototype parasympatholytic drug is atropine. Other drugs used in this category are derivatives of atropine and include atropine methonitrate, glycopyrrolate (Robinul®), ipratopium bromide (Atrovent®), and oxitropium bromide (Oxivent®). Two new long-acting anticholinergics have recently been introduced, tiotropium (Spiriva®) and aclidinium bromide (Tudorza®) At present, both of these medications only have an indication for COPD in adults; however, future studies may find a use for them in the pediatric population.

Use of Sympathomimetics and Parasympatholytics As understanding of lung physiology and asthma progresses, therapeutic drug treatment also progresses. In particular, the discovery that sympathetic innervation is mainly in the small peripheral bronchioles, and parasympathetic innervation mainly in the large airways, has led to the theory that it may be advantageous to deliver a parasympatholytic drug first, followed by a sympathomimetic.[19] By delivering the parasympatholytic drug first, the large airways are opened, allowing better penetration of the sympathomimetic drug to the peripheral airways.

Traditionally, aerosolized bronchodilators are given as a treatment that lasts 10 to 15 minutes, every 3 to 4 hours. A novel method of treating acute exacerbations of asthma, is the use of continuous aerosol therapy.[20] Fairly high doses of albuterol given by continuous aerosol have been shown to be safe and effective.[21]

Salmeterol xinafoate, one of the newer long lasting sympathomimetics, has been shown to be more effective when given twice daily, then albuterol administered 4 times daily.[22] The use of extended release oral theophylline in conjunction with an aerosolized sympathomimetic has also been shown to reduce asthma symptoms.[23] The result of longer dosing with the use of newer drugs, or by combination therapy, may improve patient compliance and reduce the need for more frequent treatment. Of interest to note, are studies indicating that MDI therapy using a spacer is at least as efficacious, if not superior to nebulizer therapy.[24, 25]

Of major concern with the use of the sympathomimetic drugs is the possibility of overuse, resulting in asthma that is nonresponsive to treatment. This resistant asthma is thought to be the result of too frequent administration of inhaled β_2-adrenergic drugs causing rebound bronchoconstricton. Another theory is that too frequent use desensitizes the β_2 sites, making them increasingly less responsive to the medication. To offset this possibility, it has been suggested that asthmatic patients only use these medications on an "as needed" basis, treating only as their symptoms warrant.[26] However, a study by Chapman and associates showed that regular treatment with salbutamol resulted in less frequent asthma symptoms and did not appear to lead to worsening attacks.[27] There is still much to be understood regarding the treatment of asthma. The most prudent counsel may be to use the medication only as directed and seek medical help if asthma symptoms do not respond.

Corticosteroids Corticosteroids have been shown to suppress the release of inflammatory mediators and are thus the drug of choice in the treatment of the inflammatory phase of asthma.[28]

Prophylactic reversal of airway hyperreactivity is best accomplished by the use of corticosteroids. Common steroids used include beclomethasone dipropionate, fluticosone (Flovent) triamcinolone acetonide (Azmacort), flunisolide (Aerobid), and budesonide (Pulmocort). There are many who advocate that steroids should be the drug of choice when treating asthma or used when the beta-agonists do not work.[28] A study by Salmeron and associates demonstrated that the use of inhaled beclomethasome dipropionate, 1500 µg/day, maintained optimal pulmonary function in asthmatic patients uncontrolled by albuterol and theophylline.[29] The rationale is that bronchial hyperreactivity is directly related to the degree of inflammation and that by treating the inflammation, the disease can be better controlled. Some have advocated changing the name to chronic eosinophilic bronchitis to indicate the inflammatory nature of the disease.

Other Medications to Treat Asthma If mast cell degranulation is prevented, the inflammatory processes of asthma are averted. Two drugs, cromolyn sodium (Intal®) and Nedacromil (Tilade®) stabilize the mast cell and prevent its degranulation. It is used as a prophylactic treatment for asthma.

Interestingly, aerosolized furosemide, a diuretic drug, has been shown to provide bronchodilation in children with mild asthma.[30] Anti-inflammatory drugs have shown some success in treating asthma, in particular, methotrexate and gold salts.[28]

Research is focusing on new medications aimed at treating the various aspects of asthma.[31] Cysteinyl leukotrienes released from the mast cell, and the immunoresponsive cells, cause bronchoconstriction, increased capillary permeability, and increase mucus secretion. Drugs aimed at blocking cysteinyl leukotriene receptors, and at inhibiting their production have been developed—Montelukast (Singulair®), Zafirlukast (Accolate®), and Pranlukast (Ultair®)—pending FDA approval. Drugs targeting platelet activating factor (PAF), and thromboxanes are being investigated. Drugs that inhibit lymphocyte-derived cytokines and augment cAMP are currently being investigated.

In the presence of purulent sputum, fever, or chest x-ray infiltrates, antibiotics are indicated.[32] Adequate hydration should be maintained, because asthmatics are frequently dehydrated, complicating the nature of the asthma. Conversely, excessive hydration may precipitate pulmonary edema in the asthmatic patient. Fluid administration should be based on clinical and laboratory indices of hydration. Although, it may be argued that humidification of the airway may help to loosen mucous plugs. Additionally, epinephrine is often given subcutaneously during moderate and severe attacks. It has powerful bronchodilatory effects, but also has dangerous side effects.

Decreased breath sounds with no wheezing may be an ominous sign, indicating respiratory failure. The definition of respiratory failure in an asthmatic is a refractory hypoxemia (PaO_2 <60mmHg on F_iO_2 of 0.5) or hypercarbia ($PaCO_2$ >40 mmHg). These patients are often the victims of status asthmaticus, also known as acute severe asthma. Status asthmaticus is a severe asthmatic attack that is refractory to sympathomimetic therapy. These patients require immediate attention and hospitalization.

The patients in status asthmaticus were started on continuous intravenous isoproterenol and aminophylline. The rate of administration was gradually increased until the desired effect was achieved or the heart rate reached 200 beats per minute.[33] Constant cardiac monitoring was necessary to monitor for dysrhythmias. This method is no longer used due to the side effects but illustrates measures necessary to reverse life threatening illness. The accepted therapy consists of a continuous albuterol aerosol delivered at a rate of 10 to 50 mg/hr. Care must be taken to monitor for signs of hypokalemia in continuous albuterol administration due to intracellular shift of the sodium potassium pump. Terbutaline has also been shown to be safe and effective delivered at a rate of 1 to 12 mg/hr as a continuous aerosol.

If the bronchodilators and aminophylline are not successful in relieving the symptoms, the patient should be intubated and ventilated mechanically. Sedation and paralysis are important to facilitate the intubation and ventilation and to reduce oxygen consumption. Pancuronium is the drug of choice for paralysis since both succinylcholine and tubocurarine are associated with histamine release.[32] Heliox may be necessary to overcome the obstruction and facilitate ventilation of the patient.

Due to the increased resistance of the airways and the potential for airtrapping, short inspiratory times and long expiratory times may be needed (if ventilatory support is needed) to provide adequate ventilation and avoid complications associated with barotrauma.

Several studies have investigated various novel techniques in treating status asthmaticus. Johnston and associates showed a significant improvement in status asthmaticus when the inhalational anesthetic isoflurane was given.[34]

Another study concluded that patients who have suffered at least one episode of asthma induced respiratory failure are at a high risk of developing repeated episodes of respiratory failure.[35] Special attention should be paid to those patients in an attempt to avoid subsequent bouts with respiratory failure.

Magnesium sulfate ($MgSO_4$) has also been used via infusion as a bronchodilator in severe asthma that does not respond to conventional therapy. The bronchodilatory effects have been reported to last up to 2 hours; however, no controlled studies have been done to support these data.

Heliox has been shown to improve gas exchange in severe asthma by decreasing the turbulence of the gas flow due to the properties of the helium.

Cystic Fibrosis (CF)

Cystic fibrosis is a hereditary disease (autosomal recessive) that affects all exocrine glands and leads to dysfunction in their secretions. Cystic fibrosis occurs in about 1 in 2000 live births, affecting mainly the Caucasian population where it is 8 times more prevalent than in Black populations. Cystic fibrosis is characterized by three clinically observable disorders: pulmonary disease, pancreatic insufficiency, and elevated sweat chloride concentrations.

The disease is passed to offspring as a Mendelian recessive trait, depicted in Figure 12–2 with both parents being carriers of the disease. Each offspring has a 25% chance of having CF, a 25% chance of being clear of the gene, and a 50% chance of

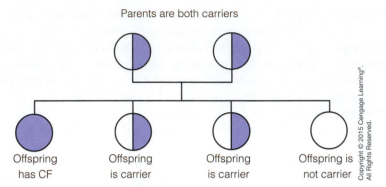

Parents are both carriers

Offspring has CF
Offspring is carrier
Offspring is carrier
Offspring is not carrier

FIGURE 12–2. Mendelian recessive trait. With both parents being carriers of the gene, each offspring has a 25% chance of having the trait, a 25% chance of not having the trait, and a 50% chance of being a carrier of the trait.

being a carrier. A defective CF gene has been localized as a part of chromosome 7 that accounts for the majority of CF cases. It is only recently that the actual gene has been identified. The mutation that has been identified (delta F508) is only found in 68% of CF patients' chromosomes. It is estimated there are 10 to 12 additional mutations that cause CF. Another mutation (A455E) is associated with preserved pancreatic function and milder pulmonary disease.[36] Identification of these defective genes makes gene therapy an attractive treatment. With gene therapy, the defective gene is replaced by a normal gene, hopefully bringing with it a reversal of the disease process. Because the gene mutation is easily expressed, the target is accessible, and the results easily verifiable, replacement of the CF gene mutation by gene therapy is encouraging.[37]

With improved understanding of the disease, the median survival age has steadily increased well into middle age.

Pathophysiology Early in the development of the disease, the pancreas of the patient with CF dilates, fills with secretions that become hardened, and soon atrophies and becomes fibrotic. The resultant lack of bile secretion into the intestine from the pancreatic insufficiency leads to malabsorption and malnutrition, despite a voracious appetite. The stools become bulky and hardened. Newborns with CF may present with an obstruction of the bowel with thickened meconium, known as a meconium ileus.

As the disease progresses, the lungs become involved in 98% of patients.[38] The pulmonary glands begin secreting a thick, viscous mucus that plugs the airways and leads to airway obstruction and chronic infections. Inflammation of the airways has been detected in patients as young as 4 weeks, indicating that the mechanisms initiating lung disease in CF begins very early in the disease.[39] Once the lung injury occurs, the patient becomes susceptible to bacterial pneumonias. Younger CF patients are commonly infected with *Staphylococcus aureus*, whereas mucoid *Pseudomonas aeruginosa* or *Serratia marcescens* is more prevalent as the patient gets older. Of interest to note is a study that sought to investigate why survival of females with CF is less than that of males. It was found that females contracted mucoid *P. aeruginosa* 1.7 years earlier than males. That earlier acquisition may contribute to the poorer survival of female patients.[40] Another bacteria causing pneumonia in CF patients, *Burkholderia cepacia*, is also associated with poor outcomes.

Other respiratory complications include chronic rhinosinusitis, nasal polyposis, pneumothorax, and hemoptysis. Cor pulmonale is often present as a result of chronic hypoxia and resultant increased pulmonary vascular resistance.

Death is often a result of hypoxia, which follows ever-worsening pulmonary congestion and infection, lung parenchyma and airway destruction, and cor pulmonale.

Diagnosis A majority of patients with CF are diagnosed in childhood, but a few are not diagnosed until their mid to late teens. Late diagnosis is often due to either a lack of pulmonary manifestations or a previous misdiagnosis of the disease. A report by Dankert-Roelse and coworkers suggests that early diagnosis and appropriate treatment of CF may prevent serious deterioration and death at a young age and may reduce the extent of early irreversible lung damage.[41]

The most reliable diagnostic indicator of CF is the determination of sweat chloride levels. Ninety-eight percent of patients with CF have sweat chloride levels greater than 60 mEq/L. The basic defect in the sweat glands is an inability to reabsorb sodium and chloride ions. The defect is not structural, but is related to altered membrane transport mechanisms of both ions. The sample is usually obtained by stimulating the sweat glands of the forearm, collecting the sample, and analyzing the chloride content. There are a few rare conditions that can cause a false-positive sweat chloride. For this reason, a definitive diagnosis of CF is only made when a positive sweat test is accompanied by at least one of the following: a clinical history of respiratory tract infection, symptoms of pancreatic insufficiency, or a documented family history of CF.

Conversely, a normal sweat chloride test does not rule out CF altogether. It is possible for a patient to have classic intestinal and respiratory symptoms and still have normal sweat electrolytes. Some patients with the CF gene mutation who also had mild manifestations of the disease, have been found to have normal sweat chloride values.[42, 43] Additionally, sweat chloride levels may be normal in very young CF patients. In light of these possibilities, any patient having chronic lung congestion, pancreatic insufficiency, failure to thrive, or respiratory colonization with *Pseudomonas*, should be suspected as having CF despite the presence of normal sweat chloride results.

Screening for CF is another possible tool to aid in the diagnosis; however, widespread screening may be impractical due to the high number of false positives and false negatives. One such screening program, the measurement of immunoreactive trypsinogen, is described by Roberts and associates.[44]

The chest x-ray of the CF patient may appear normal at the onset of the disease, gradually showing bronchiectatic changes, hyperinflation, and air trapping as the disease progresses. The x-ray often shows bilateral upper lobe infiltrates and peribronchial thickening. The x-ray may also show a pneumothorax from a ruptured lung bleb.

The pulmonary function tests of a CF patient show a restrictive pattern early in the disease, progressing to an obstructive pattern with hyperinflation of static pulmonary volumes later in the clinical course. It has been suggested that a restrictive pattern late in the disease correlates with a poor prognosis; however, a recent study by Ries and associates concluded that a restrictive pattern in CF does not necessarily indicate more severe disease and may actually be reversible in some.[45] Whenever PFT studies are done on CF patients, it is important to consider the within-subject variability that occurs within the day, from day to day, and from week to week. This is done by predetermining the variability of the individual, rather than using group data.[46]

On physical examination, the patient presents with a chronic cough, possible nasal polyposis, and chronic sinusitis. The patient may have nonrespiratory signs such as **intussusceptions** (the prolapse of one segment of bowel into the lumen of another segment), intestinal obstruction, idiopathic pancreatitis, or obstructive **azoospermia**, the lack of spermatozoa in the semen. The stools are often foul-smelling, oily, and high in fat and protein content. In the later stages of the disease, the chest may become barrel-shaped and the patient may have digital clubbing.

Treatment Until a cure is found for CF, treatment is aimed at improving long-term survival and improving the quality of life. Because CF affects many body systems, treatment is a multidisciplinary effort. Treatment is focused not only on the respiratory system, but dietary and psychosocial areas as well.

Treatment of CF is often best handled at centralized facilities or CF clinics due to the need for various health care workers. The comprehensive plan of treatment by the team is to monitor the patient's condition, modify the therapy as needed, and hospitalize the patient as needed.

The treatment of pulmonary disease associated with CF makes up the bulk of therapy. Treatment is aimed at reducing infections and removing thick, viscous secretions.

As with all pulmonary diseases, oxygen is used on CF patients to relieve hypoxemia and improve the ability of the patient to exercise. The improvement of hypoxemia additionally slows the onset of cor pulmonale in the CF patient.

The treatment of pulmonary infections is handled on an acute or chronic basis. Acute antibiotic therapy consists of a combination therapy with an aminoglycoside and a broad-spectrum penicillin. Gentamicin, which is effective against *P. aeruginosa*, is the most common aminoglycoside used. The dosage of gentamicin used is often twice the normal dosage. This is because of an increase in the body clearance of aminoglycosides in patients with CF and a need for higher serum concentrations for adequate penetration into the thick pulmonary secretions. The penicillins with the best activity against *P. aeruginosa* are piperacillin, ticarcillin, azlocillin, and mezlocillin. Ceftazidime, a cephalosporin, has shown excellent results in CF infections.

The aerosolization of antibiotics has been suggested as a method of combating pulmonary infections. Short-term, high-dosage administration of aerosolized tobramycin was found to be safe and efficacious in treating stable CF patients infected with *P. aeruginosa*.[47]

Long-term antibiotic therapy is used on CF patients with severe pulmonary disease or who require frequent hospitalizations. Long-term therapy usually consists of oral antibiotics such as dicloxacillin, tetracycline, cotrimoxazole, cephradine, and chloramphenicol.

Bronchodilator therapy may be helpful in some CF patients, although many CF patients exhibit negative effects following bronchodilator therapy. It is, therefore, recommended that each CF patient receive a pulmonary function study before and after bronchodilator therapy to determine if the patient will respond favorably.

Several studies have been done to evaluate various bronchodilators and their effectiveness in treating patients with CF. Improvement in PFT results were seen in patients receiving large doses of inhaled salbutamol and ipratropium bromide in one study.[48] Delayed, but significant, improvement in PFTs was also seen in patients treated with inhaled theophylline.[49]

Other aerosolized drugs have been studied and shown to be helpful in treating the pulmonary symptoms of CF. Mucolytic type drugs that alter the adhesiveness of CF mucus, including human DNase I (rhDNase) and distearoyl phosphatidylglycerol, have been shown to improve pulmonary function.[50–53] An older mucolytic agent, acetylcysteine (Mucomyst®) is of limited clinical use and has been shown to cause bronchospasm. For this reason, it is not recommended for use with CF patients. Wetting agents such as saline and sodium bicarbonate may be helpful, but they are not used as first-line treatments. Agents that alter the ionic fluxes in the epithelium of the airways, such as amelioride and uridine 5'-triphosphate have been shown to increase mucus clearance and retard the decline in lung function.[51,54,55] Inhalation of the corticosteroid budesonide (Pulmocort®) has shown to induce a small, but significant, improvement in the pulmonary status of patients with CF.[56]

Because the inflammatory response to the chronic infections associated with CF contributes to lung destruction, the use of anti-inflammatory therapy has been proposed. In one study, high dose ibuprofen, taken consistently for four years, was shown to significantly slow the progression of lung disease in CF patients.[57]

A proven management tool in clearing the thickened bronchial secretions of CF is chest physical therapy (CPT). CPT modalities, discussed in Chapter 13, include traditional CPT (percussion, vibration, and postural drainage), positive expiratory pressure (PEP) therapy, autogenic drainage, forced expiratory technique (FET), high-frequency chest percussion, and exercise. Much controversy persists over which method is best at clearing secretions. Using statistical methodology, a review of numerous studies regarding CPT showed that traditional CPT combined with exercise provided the best improvement in FEV_1.[58] Another similar review found traditional CPT and exercise effective, but included PEP therapy as an effective management tool.[59] When traditional percussion is used, there appears to be no difference between manual and mechanical percussion.[60]

Conventional mechanical ventilation in the CF patient presents special problems. With increased airway obstruction and frequent bacterial infections, the long-term prognosis is reduced once a CF patient is placed on mechanical ventilation.

These problems are substantially reduced by the use of noninvasive ventilatory techniques. Noninvasive positive-pressure ventilation via nasal mask has been shown to be effective at providing ventilation.[61] Another useful noninvasive procedure to treat the CF patient is nasal CPAP, which has shown to reduce respiratory disturbances and improve oxygen saturation during sleep.[62]

Dietary treatment of CF consists of supplying lipase, protease, and amylase to aid in the digestion of fats, proteins, and carbohydrates. Additionally, patients with CF are given twice the normal amount of protein and calories in their diet to maintain proper growth.

Finally, as a last modality of treatment for those patients with severe lung disease and cor pulmonale, heart-lung transplant is offered as a viable option. The cost involved in transplant is similar to that of medical treatment for the same patient, and mortality appears to be low following the procedure.[63]

Typically, patients are referred for transplant late in the course of their disease. The rate of successful transplants may increase if patients were referred earlier in the course.[64]

NEUROMUSCULAR DISORDERS

There are several neuromuscular disorders that either primarily or secondarily affect the pulmonary system. Most often, the disease affects the muscles of ventilation, making breathing difficult, if not impossible, for the patient. The various diseases affect the muscles in one of four ways: 1) defects in the muscle itself; 2) a defect in the transmission of nervous impulses to the muscle; 3) a defect in the peripheral motor and sensory nerves; or 4) a defect in the central nervous system.

Spinal Muscular Atrophies

Diseases included in this category are identified by a progressive weakness in the skeletal muscles, gradually leading to their wasting away. These diseases are caused by a progressive degeneration of the anterior horn cells of the spinal cord and are often inherited as autosomal-recessive traits.

Progressive Spinal Muscular Atrophy of Infants (Werdnig–Hoffmann Paralysis)

This disorder is usually manifest at birth, with its most apparent feature being an inactive, (or nonvigorous) term neonate. It is the most common and most severe form of the spinal muscular atrophy diseases.

The infant lies in a frog-like position with limited movement of the arms and legs. Breathing is diaphragmatic and presents with sternal retractions often present. The cry and cough are weak, and there may be a pooling of secretions in the upper pharynx. The neonate has an alert appearance and sensation and intellect are within normal limits.

The disease is diagnosed with **electromyography**, a test which evaluates the electrical activity of skeletal muscles. When done on these patients, it typically shows a denervation pattern. Confirmation of the disease is made by muscle biopsy. Death is usually the result of respiratory failure or pulmonary infection from the inability to protect the airway by aspiration of food.

Juvenile Spinal Muscular Atrophy (Kugelberg–Welander Disease) In contrast to Werdnig–Hoffmann paralysis, Kugelberg–Welander disease appears later in childhood or adolescence, and it has a slower progression. Some of the first muscles affected are in the pelvic girdle, with the arms and legs involved later. It is rare for victims of this disorder to have severe complications, and many have a normal life span.

Muscular Dystrophies

Muscular dystrophies are the largest group of muscle diseases that affect children. They all exhibit progressive, symmetrical weakness and wasting of skeletal muscles. The basic defect in these diseases is a degeneration of the muscle fibers. The most severe and most common type of muscular dystrophy seen in children is pseudohypertrophic (Duchenne) muscular dystrophy. Duchenne's muscular dystrophy usually appears during the child's third year. It first appears as a difficulty in running, riding a bicycle, or climbing stairs. A later manifestation of the disease is difficulty in walking, with an apparent abnormal gait. The name pseudohypertrophy is derived from an enlargement of the calves, thighs, and upper arms from fatty infiltration.

As the disease progresses, profound muscular atrophy occurs with ambulation becoming almost impossible. In its terminal stages, the muscles of ventilation, particularly the diaphragm, are affected.

Acquired Neuromuscular Disorders

Problems categorized as acquired neuromuscular disorders are those that are acquired after delivery and are typically caused by infective organisms.

Infectious Polyneuritis (Guillain–Barré Syndrome) Guillain–Barré syndrome is characterized by a fairly rapid muscle weakness that usually begins in the legs and ascends upward in a symmetrical fashion. It may affect the respiratory muscles to the point that mechanical ventilation is required.

The cause of Guillain–Barré is unknown, but it has been linked to certain viral diseases, including infectious mononucleosis, hepatitis, influenza, and cytomegalovirus.

Affected muscles become flaccid and sensory changes may also be present. As the disease ascends, muscle weakness also ascends and affects the abdominal muscles, diaphragm, chest muscles, and possibly the muscles of the larynx and pharynx. The result of this degree of involvement is the inability to ventilate adequately to remove secretions and potential swallowing difficulty and aspiration.

Tetanus Tetanus is a preventable neuromuscular disease caused by the endotoxin *Clostridium tetani*. It is acquired through a wound in the skin, particularly puncture wounds and burns. The disease is a result of a defect in the transmission of nerve impulses at the neuromuscular junction. In the neonate, infection may occur if delivery occurs in contaminated surroundings. Tetanus spores are found in soil and dust and are more prevalent in rural areas.

Incubation is generally less than 14 days, but may be longer, depending on the severity of the contamination. Initial symptoms are a progressive stiffness and tenderness of neck and jaw muscles. Progression of the disease causes rigidity of the abdominal and limb muscles. The patient has difficulty swallowing and is extremely sensitive to external stimuli. The slightest stimulus causes convulsive contractions that last from seconds to minutes.

As the disease progresses, the patient suffers from laryngospasm and tetany of the respiratory muscles. The patient is then predisposed to aspiration of retained secretions, pneumonia, and atelectasis.

The disease is best prevented by proper vaccination with the tetanus toxoid or antitoxin. These immunizations maintain protective antibodies for roughly 10 years and should be a part of a child's well-baby care.

Botulism Botulism is the result of ingestion of food contaminated with the *Clostridium botulinum* organism. The most common source is improperly prepared home-canned foods. Symptoms appear quickly, usually 12 to 36 hours following ingestion. The pediatric patient shows weakness, dizziness, headache, difficulty in speaking, and vomiting. As the disease progresses, the respiratory muscles become paralyzed with possible atelectasis, aspiration, and pneumonia. The patient must be monitored closely for signs of respiratory failure.

Infants can acquire botulism from the ingestion of the spores of *Clostridium botulinum.* Although there is no common source of the organism, *Clostridium botulinum* has been found in honey and, therefore, it should not be given to infants. The infant patient becomes constipated and lethargic and feedings are poorly tolerated.

Treatment consists of administration of botulism antitoxin (which is controversial in infants) and general supportive measures.[65]

Other Causes of Neurologic Disorders

Neurological disorders arising from sources other than an acquired cause are also seen in the pediatric population. Although uncommon, an understanding of their manifestations and treatments is important for the respiratory.

Myasthenia Gravis Although it is relatively uncommon in childhood, myasthenia gravis may appear in two forms: neonatal and juvenile. Transient neonatal myasthenia gravis occurs in infants of mothers who may not be aware they have the disease. There is general weakness, with depressed neurologic signs and a weak cry. Persistent neonatal myasthenia gravis is indisgtinguishable from the transient variety. It occurs in infants whose mothers do not have the disease.[65]

Juvenile myasthenia gravis is identical to that seen in adults. It usually appears after 10 years of age. Initial symptoms are paralysis of the optic muscles followed by difficulty in swallowing and speaking. There is also a generalized muscle weakness that is more pronounced following exercise and less pronounced following rest.

Diagnosis is made by observing the response following administration of anticholinesterase drugs. Two common drugs used are endrophonium (Tensilon®) and neostigmine (Prostigmin®). Following administration of the drug, muscle strength returns and lasts roughly 5 minutes.

Reye's Syndrome Reye's syndrome is a toxic encephalopathy first reported in 1963. It affects children from 2 months to adolescence, but the most common age group is 6 to 11 years. The etiology of Reye's syndrome is unknown, but most instances follow a viral illness. Many viruses have been implicated in the etiology of Reye's syndrome including parainfluenza, Epstein–Barr, coxsackie, mumps, rubella, adenovirus, herpes simplex, polio, influenza A and B, and varicella. Influenza A and B and varicella are most frequently associated with the onset of Reye's syndrome.

There may be an association between the ingestion of aspirin during the initial stages of illness and the occurrence of the syndrome. Because of this, the American Academy of Pediatrics has recommended that aspirin should not be used on children with varicella or suspected influenza.

Pathophysiology and Manifestations The two most affected organ systems in Reye's syndrome are the brain and the liver. The disease apparently affects the mitochondria of the cells, as electron microscopy reveals large and swollen mitochondria in the brain and in liver tissue. The result in the liver is a net reduction in the enzymes that converts ammonia to urea, leading to hyperammonemia. Liver dysfunction is also manifest by the presence of elevated SGOT, SGPT, and LDH enzymes levels. The diagnosis of Reye's syndrome is often accomplished by performing a percutaneous liver biopsy. The biopsy reveals swelling of hepatocytes with minimal inflammatory response. Prothrombin levels are also diminished in patients exhibiting signs of Reye's syndrome causing excessive bruising and/or an inability to clot blood. A majority of patients also have a drop in blood sugar levels below 50 mg/dl, with reduced insulin levels. The child initially presents with symptoms of an upper respiratory viral infection or chicken pox. During the apparent recovery stage of the viral infection, the child develops recurrent vomiting and worsening CNS function.

Progression of the disease is variable, ranging from a few hours to a few days. Changes in sensorium deteriorate from lethargy in the early stages to coma. The patients may also become hyperexcited, with arms and legs thrown about. As brain damage worsens, the patient enters a state of **decorticate** posturing, with flexed upper extremities (contraction toward the body's core) and extended lower extremities. The patient then begins more omnious signs, such as **decerebrate** posturing, where both upper and lower extremities are extended, muscle flaccidity, apnea, circulatory collapse, and death.

Treatment The progression of the disease, as well as potential prognosis and evaluation of therapies are all evaluated by the use of a staging system that follows the course of Reye's syndrome. The five stages are listed in Table 12–4.

Table 12–4

STAGING CRITERIA FOR REYE'S SYNDROME

Stage I—Vomiting, lethargy, and drowsiness; liver dysfunction; Type I EEG, follows commands, brisk pupillary reaction.

Stage II—Disorientation, combativeness, delirium, hyperventilation, hyperactive reflexes, appropriate responses to painful stimuli; evidence of liver dysfunction; Type I EEG, sluggish pupillary reaction.

Stage III—Obtunded, coma, hyperventilation, decorticate rigidity, preservation of pupillary light reaction and vestibulo–ocular reflexes (although sluggish); Type II EEG. Vestibulo–ocular reflexes produce eye movement that is opposite to head movement, which preserves images on the center of the visual field of the eye.

Stage IV—Deepening coma, decerebrate rigidity (arms extending away from the body), loss of **oculocephalic** reflexes, large and fixed pupils, loss of **doll's eye reflex**, loss of corneal reflexes; minimal liver dysfunction; Type III or IV EEG, evidence of brain stem dysfunction. The oculocephalic reflex tests the integrity of the brainstem. In a normal exam, as the patient's head is moved from side to side, the eyes lag behind the head movement and then assume midline. The doll's eye reflex is also a test for brainstem function. A normal test consists of moving the patient's rapidly to the side, the eyes deviate in the opposite direction. Obviously, these maneuvers are contraindicated if there is any possibility of neck injury.

Stage V—Seizures, loss of deep tendon reflexes, respiratory arrest, flaccidity; Type IV EEG, usually no evidence of liver dysfunction.

Successful treatment of Reye's syndrome requires early detection and an aggressive approach to treatment. The progression of the disease and appropriate treatment are determined by the stage that the disease manifests. Stage I disease requires supportive care, correction of hypoglycemia and acid-base disorders, and control of cerebral edema. The patient in stage II requires more aggressive monitoring. Special attention is focused on blood glucose level, coagulation studies, blood chemistries, and temperature. The patient should be made as comfortable as possible. Respiratory care procedures such as CPT and suctioning may require sedation to prevent patient agitation.

Stages III through V are treated aggressively in the intensive care unit. The patient is electively intubated to protect the airway, preceded by the administration of thiopental and either succinylcholine or pancuronium to facilitate intubation. The patient is maintained in a pharmacologic paralysis to allow mild hyperventilation. The brain swelling is treated as described previously under head injuries.

Additional respiratory care procedures includes appropriate pulmonary toilet to avoid pulmonary complications. The maintenance of analgesia is important because pain and anxiety may increase the intracranial pressure. A device to monitor intracranial pressure is placed, with the goal of maintaining the pressure less than

20 mmHg. Dialysis or blood transfusions may be necessary to reduce blood ammonia levels.

Mortality rates have dropped from initial reports of 80% to more recent reports of 20%, probably due to early diagnosis and aggressive treatment. Recovery is rapid and without long-term effect in the presence of early diagnosis and treatment. The child may awaken disoriented and frightened, with no recollection of the hospitalization. Those who work with the recovering child must take steps to lessen the fear and confusion that may be present.

INFECTIOUS LUNG DISEASES

Infectious lung diseases include acquired infections or inflammatory processes throughout the lung paranchyma and tracheobronchial tree. Pleural inflammation, effusions, and exudative processes in the thorax can complicate many diagnoses requiring respiratory care of the pediatric patient.

Pneumonia

Pneumonia is the most common serious infection that occurs in newborn infants. As a cause of death in neonates, it is second only to hyaline membrane disease in frequency.[66] Pneumonia may be acquired while the infant is still in utero. Infection of the amniotic fluid leading to congenital pneumonia is additionally a cause of premature labor.

Three factors that favor in utero infection are: 1) prolonged rupture of the amniotic membranes, usually more than 24 hours; 2) prolonged labor, even in the presence of intact membranes; and 3) excessive obstetrical manipulation. The most common causative organisms of perinatal infection are enteric organisms such as *E. coli* and group B streptococcus.

Postnatal pneumonia is most often caused by contamination of the neonate's airway by infected humidifier reservoirs, poor hand washing, and contaminated incubators and other equipment. The most common organisms causing postnatal pneumonia are *S. aureus* and *S. epidermidis*. Other organisms causing pneumonia include *Klebsiella pneumoniae*, type b *H. influenzae*, *P. aeruginosa*, and *Candida albicans*.

Nonbacterial organisms that cause pneumonia are acquired by contact with an infected birth canal or by hospital acquired infection. Those organisms acquired from the birth canal include herpes simplex virus, cytomegalovirus (CMV), *Chlamydia trachomatis*, and *Ureaplasma urealyticum*. Hospital acquired infections often include respiratory syncytial virus (RSV), rhinovirus, and enteroviruses.

Diagnosis The diagnosis of neonatal pneumonia is inexact, being based on the history, physical examination, chest x-ray results, and laboratory data. Symptoms of pneumonia often occur at birth, usually within 48 hours following delivery. The infant is tachycardic and shows signs of respiratory distress. Additionally, the infant may be flaccid, pale, and cyanotic. The amniotic fluid may appear foul smelling, indicating the presence of infection. The white blood count is not consistent and may be depressed below 5000 cells/mcL or elevated above 15,000 cells/mcL. Elevation of the patient's temperature is possible in term infants, whereas premature infants with pneumonia may be hypothermic.

The chest x-ray shows unilateral or bilateral streaky densities or consolidation in the perihilar region of the chest. Signs of a postdelivery pneumonia include an increasing tachycardia, poor feeding, and possible aspiration of feedings and lethargy.

Any infant who shows physical signs of pneumonia, or who is at risk of developing a pneumonia, is started immediately on broad-spectrum antibiotics to combat any potential infection. Clinical symptoms are treated as they appear, and blood gas values are closely monitored and treated aggressively.

Bronchiolitis

Bronchiolitis is a viral infection that leads to inflammation, swelling, mucous production, and bronchoconstriction in the bronchioles. Cell-to-cell transfer along the respiratory tract may lead to atelectasis and pneumonia in severe infections in young children. The disease has its highest mortality and morbidity among infants less than 6 months old and those suffering from congenital cardiac defects, BPD, cystic fibrosis (CF), and asthma. The most common causative organisms are RSV, causing approximately 75% of all cases, and the parainfluenza virus as well as *Mycoplasma pneumoniae*, rhinovirus, and adenovirus. RSV infection is highly contagious and requires extreme care in hand washing and other precautions to prevent hospital-acquired outbreaks.

Diagnosis Bronchiolitis begins as a typical upper airway infection with a runny nose, cough, and mild fever that lasts 2 to 3 days. With the onset of bronchiolar involvement, the cough worsens and the patient of less than 3 years begins showing signs of small airway obstruction and congestion. These signs include excessive nasal secretions, (substernal, intercostal, and supraclavicular) retractions, wheezing, rhonchi, crackles, and alveolar hyperinflation. Infants older than 3 years are seldom affected to the same degree.

Upon presentation of these symptoms, an RSV culture is obtained from the nasopharynx. It is important to rule out other pathologic processes such as cystic fibrosis and pertussis as part of the diagnostic workup. It has been suggested that infants with repeated bouts of bronchiolitis be considered to be asthmatic.

Treatment Patients of less than 4 months may need hospitalization to control fluid intake, nutrition, airway suction, and potential apnea. In those patients who require hospitalization, the level of distress and blood gas values determine the next step in treatment. Patients with severe distress, apnea, and worsening blood gas values can be treated with ribavirin, which has a specific antiviral activity against RSV. Benefits must outweigh the risks of the drug. While not recommended as a treatment for all bronchiolitis patients, ribavirin seems to benefit most the patient at high risk.[67] High-risk patients include those with a history of underlying disease, hypoxia, prematurity, young age, apnea, and pulmonary consolidation as seen on chest x-ray.[68] Ribavirin is given to the patient via a special small-particle aerosol generator called the Viratek SPAG-2 nebulizer.

Treatment is done for 12 to 18 hours per day for at least 3 days and no more than 7 days. Ribavirin can be safely administered to mechanically ventilated patients; however, it does not appear to affect the immediate outcome in these patients.[69]

Extreme care should be taken by the health care worker when administering ribavirin to avoid inhalation of the drug. Precautions regarding the delivery of ribavirin are detailed in Chapter 14.

Sympathomimetic drugs and theophylline may be used to help reduce the associated bronchospasm and improve ventilation until the infection clears.

Mechanical ventilation is instituted when arterial blood gases show impending respiratory failure, or in the presence of frequent and severe apnea. Mechanically ventilated patients with bronchiolitis must receive adequate lavage and suctioning to remove excess secretions. Care must be taken to avoid barotrauma by using low rates and pressures, as tolerated. This sometimes requires accepting higher than normal $PaCO_2$ levels (45–55 mmHg) and lower than normal pHs (7.30–7.35), allowing renal compensation.

Other treatments being proposed to treat bronchiolitis include alpha-interferon 2A, immunoglobulin A, both of which are still in the experimental stages.

Much work has been done to find a vaccine for RSV. At this time, an immunoglobulin that is specific for RSV has been approved as prophylaxis for patients deemed at high risk. Some of the criteria used in determining patients at high risk include: prematurity, chronic lung disease, body mass less than 5 kg, congenital heart disease, T-cell immunodeficiency, and lower socioeconomic status. The medication is called Synagis® (palivizumab) and is infused once per month during RSV season with a dosage of 15 mg/kg body weight.

Outcomes The long term effects of RSV infection is difficult to assess because the infection is universal in the first few years of life and as such, no uninfected control group exists.[70] One prospective study concluded that RSV bronchiolitis in the first year of life is an important risk factor for the development of asthma during the subsequent 2 years.[71]

SUMMARY

The list of pediatric diseases requiring respiratory care is extensive. In general, they can be divided into groups comprised of ventilatory diseases, neuromuscular disorders, and infectious lung diseases. Problems associated with inhalation of noxious gases and SIDS are covered in Chapter 9.

ARDS, as seen in the pediatric population, differs from RDS of the newborn. ARDS is predisposed by either direct or indirect trauma to the pulmonary system. ARDS is divided into four phases, starting with dyspnea and tachypnea, and worsening to pulmonary fibrosis, pneumonias, hypoxemia, hypercarbia, and acidosis. If intervention is not undertaken aggressively, death ensues.

Asthma continues to be a significant cause of respiratory distress in the pediatric population. The cause of asthma is complex and interrelated between many factors. Ideally, avoidance of triggering factors is of primary importance. Drug treatment is focused on preventing the release of inflammatory mediators, reversing of bronchospasm, and reduction of inflammation in the airways. Research focusing on newer, longer acting medications which prevent or slow the onset of asthma, are promising.

Cystic fibrosis is an inherited disorder that causes the mucus secreting glands of the pulmonary tree to produce extremely thick, viscous mucus. This, in turn, leads to chronic infections, lung damage, and eventual death. The diagnosis of CF is made by the presence of chronic lung congestion, pancreatic insufficiency, a failure to thrive, respiratory colonization with *Pseudomonas*, with or without elevated sweat chloride levels. Treatment is aimed at removing excessive secretions with CPT techniques, and aerosolized bronchodilators, mucolytics, and antibiotics. The goal is to reduce the number and severity of infections.

Neuromuscular disorders may be the result of atrophic disorders, muscular dystrophies, acquired disorders, and trauma. Respiratory care for these disorders varies from measures to prevent atelectasis and infection, in the case of paralytic disorders, to a reduction in cerebral blood flow, as with traumatic brain injuries.

Infectious lung diseases often require aggressive respiratory care to prevent unwanted complications. Pneumonias are treated with antibiotic therapy and also therapies aimed at removing excessive secretions and reinflating the atelectatic lung.

Bronchiolitis is a viral infection that has its most dire consequences on young patients with underlying illness, hypoxia, prematurity, young age, apnea, and pulmonary consolidation as seen on chest x-ray. Treatment with ribavirin is indicated for these patients at high risk. Other treatments include aerosolized bronchodilators, alpha-interferon 2A, immunoglobulin A, and RSV immune globulin.

POSTTEST

1. Which of the following is not considered one of the phases of ARDS?
    a. dyspnea and tachycardia
    b. progressive respiratory failure
    c. alveolar/capillary membranes become leaky
    d. significant barotrauma

2. Which of the following are possible strategies in the treatment of ARDS?
     I. maintain arterial PCO_2 below normal
     II. hyperventilation
     III. correct any physical derangements
     IV. suppress alveolar inflammation
     V. prevent complications
        a. I, III, V
        b. II, III, V
        c. III, IV, V
        d. I, II, IV, V

3. The release of mediators by eosinophils, neutrophils, macrophages, and lymphocytes is seen during:
     a. phase II of an asthma attack
     b. an exacerbation of ARDS
     c. Werdnig–Hoffman paralysis
     d. Guillain–Barré syndrome

4. The branch(es) of CNS that appear(s) to be primarily responsible for inhibiting bronchial smooth muscle contraction is (are) the:
     a. sympathetic
     b. parasympathetic
     c. nonadrenergic noncholinergic
     d. both a and c

5. Which of the following would be the drug of choice during the inflammatory stage of asthma?
     a. theophylline
     b. beclomethasone
     c. albuterol
     d. cromolyn

6. The most reliable diagnosis of cystic fibrosis involves:
     a. family history
     b. failure to thrive
     c. sweat/chloride levels
     d. evidence of pancreatic insufficiency

7. Which of the following are commonly used in the treatment of patients with cystic fibrosis?
     I. oxygen
     II. aerosolized antibiotics
     III. theophylline
     IV. mist tents
     V. CPT
        a. I, IV
        b. I, III, V
        c. II, III, V
        d. I, II, III, V

8. Which of the following is (are) inherited as autosomal-recessive traits?
    I. Kugelberg–Welander disease
    II. Duchenne–type muscular dystrophy
    III. Guillain–Barré syndrome
    IV. Werdnig–Hoffman paralysis
        a. I only
        b. I, IV
        c. II, III
        d. II, III, IV

9. Edrophonium (Tensilon) is used to diagnose which of the following?
    a. myasthenia gravis
    b. Guillain–Barré syndrome
    c. botulism
    d. Duchenne-type muscular dystrophy

10. Reye's syndrome is diagnosed by:
    a. patient history
    b. sputum culture and sensitivity
    c. CT scan
    d. liver biopsy

11. Which of the following would favor the development of an in utero fetal pneumonia?
    I. fetal asphyxia
    II. prolonged rupture of the amniotic membranes
    III. maternal exercise
    IV. excessive obstetrical manipulation
    V. prolonged labor
        a. I, II, III, V
        b. II, III, IV
        c. I, III, V
        d. II, IV, V

12. Which of the following organisms is the most likely to cause bronchiolitis?
    a. parainfluenza virus
    b. respiratory syncytial virus
    c. *Haemophilus influenzae*

REFERENCES

1. Press release: NHBLI Clinical trial stopped early: Successful ventilator strategy found for intensive care patients on life support. http://www.nih.gov/news/pr/mar99/nhlbi-15.htm.

2. Miller, Sagy. Pressure characteristics of mechanical ventilation and incidence of pneumothorax before and after the implementation of protective lung strategies in the management of pediatric patients with severe ARDS. *Chest.* 134(5):969–973, November 2008.

3. Heulitt MJ, et al. Acute respiratory distress syndrome in pediatric patients: redirecting therapy to reduce iatrogenic lung injury. *Resp. Care.* 40:74–85, 1995.

4. Sivan Y, et al. Adult respiratory distress syndrome in severely neutropenic children. *Pediatr Pulmonol.* 8:104–108, 1990.

5. Richard C, et al. Vitamin E deficiency and lipoperoxidation during adult respiratory distress syndrome. *Crit Care Med.* 18:4–9, 1990.

6. Idell S. The deadly danger of ARDS. *Emer Med.* 21:67–68, 70, 72, 1989.

7. Hudson LD. The prediction and prevention of ARDS. *Resp Care.* 35:161–173, 1990.

8. Kallet, RH. Patient-ventilator interaction during acute lung injury, and the role of spontaneous breathing: part 2: airway pressure release ventilation. *Respir Care,* (56)2:190–203, February 2011.

9. Maunder RJ, Hudson LD. Pharmacologic strategies for treating the adult respiratory distress syndrome. *Resp. Care.* 35:241–246, 1990.

10. Russel JA, et al. Physiologic effects and side effects of prostaglandin E_1 in the adult respiratory distress syndrome. *Chest.* 97:684–692.

11. Stachtiaris LE, Marino RV. The asthmatic child. *Emer Med.* 21:119–120, 123–124, 1989.

12. DesJardins T, Burton GG. Clinical manifestations and assessment of respiratory diseases. 6th ed. Maryland Heights, MO:Mosby/Elsevier, 2011.

13. Mitchell RS, et al. *Synopsis of Clinical Pulmonary Disease.* 4th ed. St. Louis, MO: CV Mosby Co., 1989.

14. Zahr LK, et al. Assessment and management of the child with asthma. *Ped Nurs.* 15:109–114, 1989.

15. Sur S, et al. Sudden-onset fatal asthma: a distinct entity with few eosinophils and relatively more neutrophils in the airway submucosa? *Am Rev Respir Dis.* 148:713, 1993.

16. Carruthers DM, Harrison BD. Arterial blood gas analysis or oxygen saturation in the assessment of acute asthma. *Thorax.* 50:186–188,1995.

17. Manthous CA, et al. Heliox improves pulsus paradoxus and peak expiratory flow in nonintubated patients with severe asthma. *Am J Respir Crit Care Med.* 151:310, 1995.

18. Howder CL. Antimuscarinic and β_2-adrenoceptor bronchodilators in obstructive airways disease. *Resp Care.* 38:1364–1388, 1983.

19. Mathewson HS. Combined drug therapy in asthma [editorial]. *Resp. Care.* 38:1340, 1993.

20. Colacone A, et al. Continuous nebulization of albuterol (salbutamol) in acute asthma. *Chest.* 97:693–697, 1990.

21. Fink JB, Jue PK. Humidity and aerosol therapy for pediatrics. In: Barnhart SL, Czervinske MP. *Perinatal and Pediatric Respiratory Care.* Philadelphia, PA: WB Saunders Co., 1995.

22. D'Alonzo GE, et al. Salmeterol xinafoate as maintenance therapy compared with albuterol in patients with asthma. *JAMA.* 271:1412, 1994.

23. Rivington RN, et al. Efficacy of Uniphyl®, salbutamol, and their combination in asthmatic patients on high-dose inhyaled steroids. *Am J Respir Crit Care Med.* 151:325, 1995.

24. Chou KJ, et al. Metered-dose inhalers with spacers vs Nebulizers for pediatric asthma. *Arch Pediatr Adolesc Med.* 149:201–205, 1995.

25. Lin YZ, Hsieh KH. Metered dose inhaler and nebuliser in acute asthma. *Arch Dis Child.* 72:214–218, 1995.

26. Spitzer WO, et al. The use of beta-agonists and the risk of death from asthma. *N Engl J Med.* 326:501–506, 1992.

27. Chapman KR, et al. Regular vs as-needed inhaled salbutamol in asthma control. *Lancet.* 343:1379, 1994.

28. Mathewson HS. Asthma and bronchitis: a shift of therapeutic emphasis. *Resp Care.* 35:273, 275, 277, 1990.

29. Salmeron S, et al. High doses of inhaled corticosteroids in unstable chronic asthma: a multicenter, double-blind, placebo-controlled study. *Am Rev Respir Dis.* 140:167–171, 1989.

30. Chin T, et al. Reversal of bronchial obstruction in children with mild stable asthma by aerosolized furosemide. *Pediatr Pulmonol.* 18:93, 1994.

31. Mathewson HS. New avenues of asthma therapy. *Resp Care.* 40:655–657, 1995.

32. Feinsilver SH. Respiratory failure in asthma and COPD. *Emer Med.* 21:90, 93–94, 96, 1989.

33. Zimmerman SS, et al. *Critical Care Pediatrics.* Philadelphia, PA: WB Saunders Co., 1985.

34. Johnston RG, et al. Isoflurane therapy for status asthmaticus in children and adults. *Chest.* 97:698–701, 1990.

35. Newcomb RW. Respiratory failure from asthma: a marker for children with high morbidity and mortality. *Am J Dis Child.* 142:1041–1044, 1988.

36. Gan KH, et al. A cystic fibrosis mutation associated with mild lung disease. *N Engl J Med.* 333:95–99, 1995.

37. Colledge WH, Evans MJ. Cystic fibrosis gene therapy. *Br Med Bull.* 51:82–90, 1995.

38. Burgess WR, Chernick V. *Respiratory Therapy in Newborn Infants and Children.* New York: Thieme-Stratton Inc., 1982.

39. Kahn TZ, et al. Early pulmonary inflammation in infants with cystic fibrosis. *Am J Respir Crit Care Med.* 151:1075, 1995.

40. Demko CA, et al. Gender differences in cystic fibrosis: *Pseudomona aeruginosa* infection. *J Clin Epidemiol.* 48:1041–1049, 1995.

41. Dankert-Roelse JE, et al. Survival and clinical outcome in patients with cystic fibrosis, with or without neonatal screening. *J Pediatrics.* 114:362–367, 1989.

42. Stewart B, et al. Normal sweat chloride values do not exclude the diagnosis of cystic fibrosis. *Am J Respir Crit Care Med 151.* 3(pt 1):899–903, 1995.

43. Highsmith WE, et al. A novel mutation in the cystic fibrosis gene in patients with pulmonary disease but normal sweat chloride concentrations. *N Engl J Med.* 331:974, 1994.

44. Roberts G, et al. Screening for cystic fibrosis: a four year regional experience. *Arch Dis Child.* 63:1438–1443, 1988.

45. Ries AL, et al. Restricted pulmonary function in cystic fibrosis. *Chest.* 94:575–579, 1988.

46. Cooper PJ, et al. Variability of pulmonary function tests in cystic fibrosis. *Pediatr Pulmonol.* 8:16–22, 1990.

47. Ramsey BW, et al. Efficacy of aerosolized tobramycin in patients with cystic fibrosis. *N Engl J Med.* 328:1740–1746, 1993.

48. Sanchez I. The effect of high doses of inhaled salbutamol and ipratropium bromide in patients with stable cystic fibrosis. *Chest.* 104:842, 1993.

49. Pan SH, et al. Bronchodilation from intravenous theophylline in patients with cystic fibrosis: results of a blinded placebo-controlled crossover clinical trial. *Pediatr Pulmonol.* 6:172–179, 1989.

50. Fuchs HJ, et al. Effect of aerosolized recombinant human DNase on exacerbations of respiratory symptoms and on pulmonary function in patients with cystic fibrosis. *N Engl J Med.* 331:637, 1991.

51. Harris CE, Wilmott RW. Inhalation-based therapies in the treatment of cystic fibrosis. *Curr Opin Pediatr.* 6:234–238, 1991.

52. Shah PL, et al. Medium term treatment of stable stage cystic fibrosis with recombinant human DNase I. *Thorax.* 50:333–338, 1995.

53. Shak S. Aerosolized recombinant human DNase I for the treatment of cystic fibrosis. *Chest.* 107:(2)(Suppl):65s–70s, 1995.

54. Tomkiewicz RP, et al. Amiloride inhalation therapy in cystic fibrosis. Influence on ion content, hydration, and rheology of sputum. *Am Rev Respir Dis.* 148:(4)(pt 1):1002–1007, 1993.

55. Wilmott RW, Fiedler MA. Recent advances in the treatment of cystic fibrosis. *Pediatr Clin N Am.* 41:431–451, 1994.

56. Van-Haren EH, et al. The effects of the inhaled corticosteroid budesonide on lung function and bronchial hyperresponsiveness in adult patients with cystic fibrosis. *Respir J Med.* 332:848, 1995.

57. Konstan MW, et al. Effect of high-dose ibuprofen in patients with cystic fibrosis. *N Engl J Med.* 332:848, 1995.

58. Thomas J, et al. Chest physical therapy management of patients with cystic fibrosis: a meta-analysis. *Am J Respir Crit Care Med.* 151:846, 1995.

59. Boyd S, et al. Evaluation of the literature on the effectiveness of physical therapy modalities in the management of children with cystic fibrosis. *Pediatr Phys Ther.* 6:70–74, 1994.

60. Bauer ML, et al. Comparison of manual and mechanical chest percussion in hospitalized patients with cystic fibrosis. *J Pediatr.* 124:250.1994.

61. Padman R, et al. Noninvasive positive pressure ventilation in end-stage cystic fibrosis: a report of seven cases. *Resp Care.* 39:736–739, 1994.
62. Regnis JA, et al. Benefits of nocturnal nasal CPAP in patients with cystic fibrosis. *Chest.* 106:1717–1724, 1994.
63. Scott J, et al. Heart-lung transplantation for cystic fibrosis. *Lancet.* 2:192–194, 1988.
64. Ciriaco P, et al. Analysis of cystic fibrosis referrals for lung transplantation. *Chest.* 107:1323–1327, 1995.
65. Hockenberry, MJ. et. al. *Whaley & Wong's Nursing Care of Infants and Children.* 9th ed. St. Louis, MO: Mosby, 2011.
66. Thibeault DW, Gregory GA. *Neonatal Pulmonary Care.* 2nd ed. Norwalk, Conn: Appleton-Century-Crofts, 1986.
67. Makela MJ, et al. Respiratory syncytial virus infection in children. *Curr Opin Pediatr.* 6:17–22, 1994.
68. Wang EE, et al. Pediatric investigators collaborative network on infections in Canada (PICNIC) prospective study of risk factors and outcomes in patients hospitalized with respiratory syncytial viral lower respiratory tract infection. *J Pediatr.* 126:212–219, 1995.
69. Meert KL, et al. Aerosolized ribavirin in mechanically ventilated children with respiratory syncytial virus lower respiratory tract disease: a prospective, double-blind, randomized trial. *Crit Care Med.* 22:566, 1994.
70. Long CE, et al. Sequelae of respiratory syncytial virus infections. A role for intervention studies. *Am J Respir Crit Care Med.* 151:1678–1680, 1995.
71. Sigurs N, et al. Asthma and immunoglobulin E antibodies after respiratory syncytial virus bronchiolitis: a prospective cohort study with matched controls. *Pediatrics.* 95:500–505, 1995.

BIBLIOGRAPHY AND SUGGESTED READINGS

Beachey W. *Respiratory Care Anatomy and Physiology* 3rd ed. St. Louis, MO: Mosby, 2013.

Chipps BE, et al. Alpha-2A-interferon for treatment of bronchiolitis caused by respiratory syncytial virus. *Pediatr Infect Dis J.* 12:653–658, 1993.

Cottrell GP. *Cardiopulmonary Anatomy and Physiology for Respiratory Care Practitioners.* Philadelphia, PA: FA Davis, 2001.

DeBruin W, et al. Acute hypoxemic respiratory failure in infants and children: clinical and pathologic characteristics. *Crit Care Med.* 20:1223–1234, 1992.

Des Jardins T. *Cardiopulmonary Anatomy and Physiology.* 6th ed. Clifton Park, NY: Cengage Learning, 2013.

Groothuis JR, et al. Respiratory syncytial virus (RSV) infection in preterm infants and the protective effects of RSV immune globulin RSVIG. Respiratory syncytial virus immune globulin study group. *Pediatrics.* 95:463–467, 1995.

Harwood R. *Exam Review and Study Guide for Perinatal/Pediatric Respiratory Care.* Philadelphia, PA: FA Davis, 1999.

Hess D. Neonatal and pediatric respiratory care: some implications for adult respiratory care practitioners. *Resp Care.* 36:489–513, 1991.

Pilbeam SP. *Mechanical Ventilation: Physiological and Clinical Applications.* 5th ed. St. Louis, MO: Mosby, 2012.

Steinbach S, et al. Transmissibility of *Pseudomonas cepacia* infection in clinic patients and lung transplant recipients with cystic fibrosis. *N Engl J Med.* 331:981, 1994.

Taussig LM, Landau LI. *Pediatric Respiratory Medicine.* 2nd ed. St. Louis, MO: Mosby, 2008.

Weltzin R, et al. Intranasal monoclonal immunoglobulin A against respiratory syncytial virus protects against upper and lower respiratory tract infections in mice. *Antimicrob Agents Chemother.* 38:2785–2791, 1994.

UNIT THREE

General Concepts of Clinical Medicine

Hugs can do great amounts of good——especially for children.
—*Princess Diana*

CHAPTER 13

Respiratory Care Procedures

OBJECTIVES

Upon completion of this chapter, the reader should be able to:

1. Discuss the indications for and hazards of oxygen therapy.
2. Describe, for each of the following, its role in oxygen delivery:
   a. Oxygen blenders and flowmeters
   b. Oxygen analyzers
3. Compare and contrast bubble and wick humidifiers.
4. Describe the indications, hazards, and approximate F_iO_2 for each of the following:
   a. Oxygen hood
   b. Oxygen cannula
   c. High-flow nasal cannula (HFNC)
   d. Simple oxygen mask
   e. Nonrebreathing mask
   f. Venturi mask
   g. Tent
   h. Incubator
   i. Resuscitation bags
5. List the indications for airway clearance.
6. List the contraindications of airway clearance therapy.
7. Briefly describe each of the following airway clearance techniques:
   a. Positive expiratory pressure (PEP)
   b. Forced exhalation technique (FET)
   c. Autogenic drainage
   d. High-frequency chest compression
   e. Flutter valve therapy

8. Describe the procedure for performing CPT including:
    a. Auscultation
    b. Postural drainage
    c. Percussion
    d. Vibration
    e. Removal of secretions
9. Describe the indications for and hazards of suctioning and the equipment used.
    a. Bulb suction
    b. Nasotracheal suction
    c. Suction catheter size selection
10. Review alterations in the procedure for suctioning when the patient's clinical signs indicate.
11. Discuss the following as they apply to aerosol delivery:
    a. Particle amount
    b. Particle size
    c. Particle characteristics
    d. Airway anatomy
    e. Ventilatory pattern
12. Discuss the advantages and disadvantages of each of the following:
    a. Small volume nebulizer (SVN)
    b. Metered dose inhaler (MDI)
    c. MDI spacer
    d. Dry powder inhaler (DPI)
    e. Ultrasonic nebulizer
    f. Continuous nebulizer
13. List the indications for aerosolized drug therapy.
14. Describe the equipment used to deliver aerosolized medications. Compare and contrast updraft nebulizers to mainstream nebulizers.
15. Discuss the procedure for placement of a medication nebulizer inline to a ventilator circuit.
16. List and describe the hazards of aerosolized medications.
17. Explain the techniques used to prevent ventilator malfunction when aerosolizing ribavirin into a ventilator circuit.

KEY TERMS

crackle	lavage	Trendelenburg
emesis	mainstream nebulizer	updraft nebulizer
epistaxis	reconcentration	wheeze
hydrophobic	reflux	
hydroscopic	rhonchus	

INTRODUCTION

Respiratory care procedures are performed in all areas of the hospital, from the delivery room to the NICU and intensive care units and the emergency room. In the neonatal and pediatric patient population, these procedures not only provide relief from the effects of pulmonary diseases, but they can also be lifesaving.

OXYGEN THERAPY

Oxygen is often a misunderstood drug. In the eyes of some, it is a wonder drug that can cure many problems. This misconception often leads to its misuse. The purpose of this section is to look at oxygen as a drug that must be used with as much precision and understanding as any other drug. Oxygen has side effects and complications that may further injure the lungs of the compromised patient. This section discusses those complications as well as the many methods and devices used to deliver oxygen to neonatal and pediatric patients.

Indications

The main indication for the administration of oxygen is the presence of hypoxemia in the patient. Hypoxemia is defined as a level of oxygen in the blood that is less than normal. Acceptable room air arterial PaO_2 for a neonate is 60 mmHg with a SpO_2 of 90%, whereas in the older pediatric patient a PaO_2 of less than 80 mmHg with an SpO_2 of 95% (55 mmHg at 5000 ft.) is considered hypoxic.

The diagnosis of hypoxemia is made by one of several methods. Actual measurement of the oxygen present in the arterial blood by arterial blood gas analysis is the most reliable source for determining hypoxemia. Transcutaneous monitoring and pulse oximetry offer rapid, noninvasive alternatives to diagnose the presence of hypoxemia. The methods of obtaining and interpreting blood gas results are covered in more detail in Chapter 16.

Hypoxemia may be suspected when the patient shows signs of respiratory distress. Those signs include retractions, expiratory grunting, nasal flaring, and central cyanosis. Acrocyanosis is normal in neonates during the first few hours after delivery and does not require supplemental oxygen to correct. A word of caution regarding the assessment of cyanosis—the skin will not appear cyanotic until 5 g/dL of hemoglobin become desaturated. It should be noted that by the time an infant becomes cyanotic, there may be a significant level of tissue hypoxia. Cyanosis should not be the primary indicator for the need of supplemental oxygen. The use of pulse oximetry and arterial blood gases are much more reliable and will show indications of hypoxemia before cyanosis is visually apparent. If the patient has low hemoglobin levels, there may be a significant level of hypoxemia present with no sign of cyanosis.

Hazards

The hazards associated with the use of oxygen are listed in Table 13–1. There is a strong correlation between high levels of arterial oxygen and the development of retinopathy of prematurity (ROP). Although other factors, such as prematurity, low birth weight, intraventricular hemorrhage, and sepsis, are also considered factors in the development of ROP, oxygen is suspected for playing a major role in its development. It is believed that high levels of oxygen cause vasoconstriction of the retinal and cerebral vessels. This constriction may lead to ischemia resulting in retinal scar tissue and possible retinal detachment. Chapter 7 discusses the development of ROP in more detail.

The toxic effects of oxygen are seen in the development of bronchopulmonary dysplasia (BPD). High levels of oxygen administered over a prolonged period may cause a breakdown and destruction of alveolar tissues, leading to a loss of surface area for gas exchange and pulmonary fibrosis. High levels of oxygen also cause a constriction of the cerebral vasculature, possibly reducing much-needed blood flow to a developing brain. Additionally, high levels of oxygen can cause nitrogen washout, resulting in absorption atelectasis. On the other end of the spectrum, if too little oxygen is delivered, the patient may continue to suffer the effects of hypoxemia.

With these hazards in mind, the goal of oxygen therapy is to maintain a PaO_2 that is high enough to avoid the dangers of hypoxemia, but also low enough to avoid complications such as ROP, BPD, and oxygen toxicity. Arterial PaO_2 of 50–70 mmHg are recommended to meet this criterion.

Another hazard that must be considered is the fire danger associated with oxygen use. Oxygen is not an explosive gas; however, it intensifies combustion to the point that a small spark or flame may instantly become an inferno. Instruction must be given to those who may work with or visit the patient that no type of flame of spark may be used in the presence of an oxygen-enriched environment. In all cases, whenever oxygen is in use, precautionary signs advising of the danger of combustion must be placed at the bedside and at the entrance to the room.

Table 13–1
HAZARDS OF OXYGEN USE
Retinopathy of prematurity
Oxygen toxicity leading to bronchopulmonary dysplasia
Cerebral vasoconstriction
Fire hazard

Equipment

We begin this section on oxygen equipment by examining those points that are common to all oxygen administration, expanding to common devices used to deliver the oxygen to the patient.

Oxygen Blenders and Flowmeters Oxygen can be delivered to patients via a flowmeter attached to a 100% oxygen source or via a flowmeter attached to an oxygen blender. Whenever a patient is placed on supplemental oxygen, regardless of the source, care must be taken to monitor the patient's oxygenation status. When a flowmeter is attached directly to a 100% oxygen source, determining the precise F_iO_2 being delivered is difficult. The use of an oxygen blender is highly recommended because it enables a more accurate and controlled delivery of oxygen. The oxygen blender is the usual starting point for the administration of various concentrations of oxygen. The blender is first connected to a 50-psi source of oxygen and air. These gases pass through a series of regulators to lower the pressure to a workable level and then they are mixed to achieve the desired concentration of air and oxygen. The desired oxygen level ordered by a physician will be set on the oxygen blender via a rotating dial. Any concentration of oxygen from 21% to 100% is possible. The blended gas is then passed to the exterior of the device, where a flowmeter is used to direct the proper flow of gas to the patient.

Three types of flowmeters are available. They are standard-flow, low-flow, and micro-flow flowmeters. Standard-flow flowmeters are most often used in adult patient populations and provide designated liter flows from 0 to 15 L/min. Low-flow flowmeters and micro-flow flowmeters are more often used in newborn and pediatric patient populations because they have the ability to provide more finely titrated liter flow. Low-flow flowmeters have maximum flow rates of 1–3 L/min in 0.1 L/min increments. Micro-flow flowmeters provide flow rates of less than 0.1 L/min in increments of 0.01 L/min.

Oxygen Analyzers Although most oxygen blenders indicate an approximate F_iO_2 on the mixture dial, few will be entirely accurate. If a precise oxygen percentage is desired, it is essential that an oxygen analyzer be placed in line with the oxygen delivery device, proximal to the patient, in order to monitor the precise oxygen percent being delivered. The only precaution is to place the analyzer in the system proximal to the humidifier, because the wet gas may cause erroneous readings. The analyzer should be calibrated to room air and 100% oxygen to ensure accuracy before being placed in the system. Thereafter, a calibration should be done at least every 8 hours, and possibly every 4 hours to ensure accuracy and prevent drifting.

Humidifiers After leaving the blender and before reaching the patient, the gas should pass through a humidification device. Gases are stored in a dry state and therefore require the addition of humidity before being administered to a patient. This is especially true of the intubated patient, whose normal humidification mechanism is being bypassed, and of infants who are placed on supplemental oxygen. Low flows of oxygen delivered via a cannula may not require humidification on older patients, because normal airway mechanisms provide adequate moisture to the gas. Younger patients may require humidification even at low flows due to smaller tidal volume to weight ratios and gas to tissue surface area ratios. The addition of humidity at high flows helps prevent drying of the airways, which leads to impairment of mucus cleaning, potential infection, and atelectasis.

Humidification devices fall into two classes: low flow and high flow. Low-flow humidity systems are usually designed for flows of 10 L/min or less. A low-flow system supplies a relatively small amount of humidity and does not heat the gas. These devices are classified as bubble or diffuser humidifiers. This type of humidifier allows the gas to bubble up through a reservoir of sterile water. The gas picks up water molecules as it rises to the surface (Figure 13–1). Oxygen cannulas and simple masks are examples of modalities that use the bubble humidifier.

High-flow systems, usually having flows greater than 10 L/min, are designed to provide a fully saturated gas at a desired temperature. Warmed, fully humidified gas delivery is essential for intubated patients for reasons previously mentioned. A warm, humid gas can also be invaluable in preventing evaporative heat loss in the small neonate. Varieties of this type of humidifier include large volume jet nebulizers, advanced bubble humidifiers, and passover humidifiers.

Large-volume jet nebulizers produce an aerosol by using Bernoulli's principle, which lowers the lateral pressure around the jet that draws water up a capillary

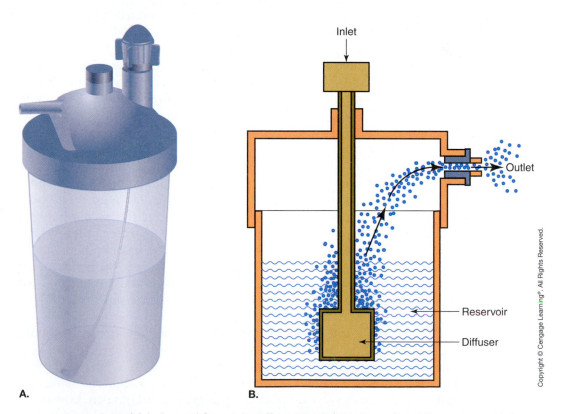

FIGURE 13–1. A. Bubble humidifier with diffuser. B. Schematic of a diffuser humidifier.

tube. When the water reaches the jet, the gas breaks it up into an aerosol, which is then carried with the gas to the patient. A heater is either attached to a steel plate at the bottom of the reservoir, or placed around the nebulizer orifice. Caution must be exercised when gas flow is interrupted through the nebulizer not to allow the water in the reservoir to overheat. Most jet nebulizers have a built-in air entrainment port, which allows various F_iO_2 to be achieved.

When using a jet nebulizer, it is important that the total flow meets or exceeds the patient's inspiratory flow demand. A continual stream of aerosol exiting the exhalation ports during inspiration ensures inspiratory flow demand is met.

Passover humidifiers use either a heated water-saturated wick or a heated chamber covered by a **hydrophobic** material (Figure 13–2). The wick is a material that absorbs water by capillary action. A heater surrounds the wick, and as it heats, the water evaporates. The source gas is then passed through the humidifier, over the wick where it picks up the heated water vapor, and out to the patient.

As the warmed humidified gas passes through the tubing that carries it to the patient, the cooler air surrounding the tubing cools the gas. This results in a rain-out

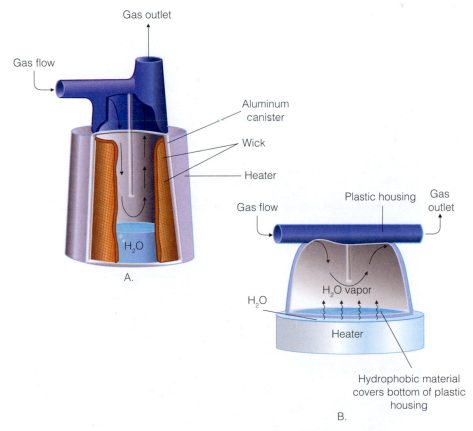

FIGURE 13–2. A. Cutaway view of a wick-type humidifier. B. A cutaway view of a hydrophobic humidifier.

or condensation of the molecular water on the walls of the tubing. This could pose a potential danger if the accumulated water were allowed to drain toward the infant. To prevent this, some type of collection device should be placed in the tubing at the lowest point between the humidifier and the patient.

Certain humidifiers resist the rain-out problem by placing a heated wire into the tubing. The wire keeps the gas at the desired temperature as it travels through the tubing, thus greatly reducing rain-out. These devices are most commonly found on ventilator circuits. When this type is used, the gas temperature is measured as it exits the humidifier and again at the patient interface. By keeping the distal gas temperature warmer than the humidifier temperature, the patient is given a more consistent humidity and temperature of gas, with less rain-out.

Oxygen Hood An oxygen hood is a clear, plastic hood that fits over the infant's head, shown in Figure 13–3. It provides an oxygen-enriched environment for the patient with relative ease and comfort. Oxygen hoods are generally used with F_iO_2 of less than 50%. A patient requiring more than 50% oxygen can be managed in a hood;

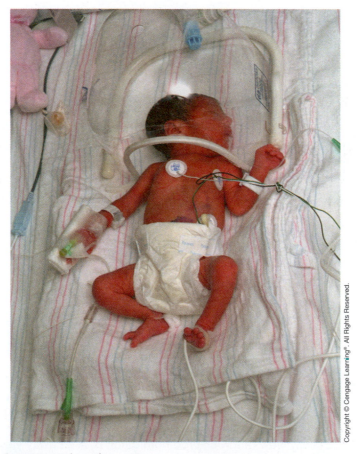

FIGURE 13–3. An oxygen hood.

however, it becomes difficult to maintain consistent concentrations above that level. This is due in part to the large neck opening and the less-than-tight seal around the edges of the hood, allowing ambient gas to dilute the hood gas.

An infant requiring high levels of oxygen should be closely assessed for signs of respiratory distress or other problems. An increasing F_iO_2 requirement is frequently the result of worsening respiratory status and may require more intensive measures than an oxygen hood can provide. Due to the layering effect of the oxygen in the hood, the F_iO_2 should be monitored at the level of the patient's face to ensure accurate readings.

There are some hazards associated with the use of an oxygen hood that pose potential problems. If the gas flow to the oxygen hood is too slow, there is a chance of CO_2 retention in the hood. According to Gale and associates, a flow of more than 7 L/min should be used to avoid this problem.[1] Although unlikely, it is also possible for the infant's breathing to become hampered by the face being pressed against the wall of the hood, or the neck opening being too tight and occluding the airway. This potential problem can be avoided with proper selection of hood size. High or low gas temperatures blown into the hood may cause the infant to overheat or become chilled. This could make thermoregulation of the patient difficult to maintain. To avoid thermoregulatory problems, gas temperatures should be maintained at temperatures equal to that within the incubator or the open warmer.

Oxygen Cannulas and Masks Oxygen cannulas can be used on patients in acute need of supplemental oxygen, or used on those patients with chronic oxygen need. Chronic oxygen use is often associated with BPD. Cannulas can also be used as a tool to wean the patient from an oxygen hood, gradually weaning the patient to room air. Flows used on the neonatal patient are usually less than 1 L/min. Higher flows may lead to nasal mucosal drying and **epistaxis** (nose bleeds) and should be used cautiously. Although the exact F_iO_2 delivered via a cannula depends on the patient's age, size, tidal volume, and respiratory rate, it can be estimated. At 0.25 L/min, the F_iO_2 will range from 24% to 27%. At 0.50 L/min, approximate F_iO_2 is 26% to 32%, and at 1 L/min, the F_iO_2 is roughly 30% to 35%.

Neonatal and pediatric cannulas are available from various manufacturers. The pediatric-sized prongs are shorter in length and smaller in diameter than their adult counterparts, due to the smaller size of the pediatric patient (Figure 13–4). The neonatal cannula has prongs that are even shorter and smaller, accommodating the even smaller neonatal nose and face. An option for the smaller patients is to cut off the prongs and position the resultant hole below the nasal openings.

The high-flow nasal cannula (HFNC) provides increased accuracy and effectiveness when delivering oxygen via a cannula. A benefit of HFNC may include a reduction in the patient's work of breathing. The nasopharynx is used as the reservoir and the increased flow of gas eliminates the entrainment of room air and allows the respiratory therapist to provide higher fractions of inspired oxygen. Some devices provide heated and humidified up to 99.9% relative humidity at normal body temp of 37°C. Selection of an appropriate cannula size that does not occlude the patient's nares is important. Patients should be monitored for gastric distension

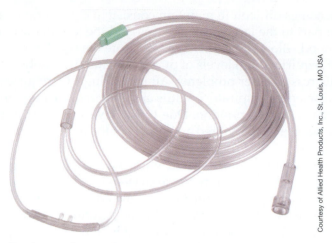

Courtesy of Allied Health Products, Inc., St. Louis, MO USA

FIGURE 13–4. A pediatric nasal cannula.

and overinflation of the lungs. These symptoms may be due to excessive pressure that has developed in the airway. Safety measures that include a pop-off may help reduce this risk. Patients should also be monitored closely in terms of breath sounds, oxygen saturation, vital signs, and breathing pattern.

The HFNCs may be used in some infant patients to provide an alternative to nasal continuous positive airway pressure (NCPAP). Studies have shown that the use of HFNCs at flow rates of 1–2.5 L/min can deliver positive distending pressures in premature infants similar to that of the distending pressures delivered by NCPAP. The increase in distending pressures at these flow rates has proven to be effective in the treatment of apnea of prematurity. As mentioned above, flow rates higher than 1 L/min in infants may cause complications related to excessive mucosal drying, therefore humidification of this device is essential.

The combination of a small patient and constant movement may make it difficult to keep an oxygen cannula in place. On such difficult patients, it may be helpful to attach the cannula to the face. This may be done with a tape designed to cover IV sites or cannula securing pads. The IV tape has good holding capabilities and can be used for fairly long periods without causing skin breakdowns. The cannula securing pads attach to the cheeks of the infant and have adhesive flaps that lift up to allow the cannula to be secured in place. These pads also allow for repeated adjustment of the cannula without pulling the adhesive base away from the skin.

Oxygen masks provide a higher percentage of oxygen than cannulas but are used infrequently because they are not tolerated as well by the small patient. Oxygen masks come in assorted designs, each devised for specific oxygen requirements. When used on a neonate, a simple oxygen mask will provide 60% to 80% F_iO_2 at 5 L/min when tight against the face. A loosely placed mask provides about 40% F_iO_2 at 5 L/min. On the older pediatric patient, liter flows of 6–8 L/min provide a range of 35% to 45%, depending on the size and age of the patient.

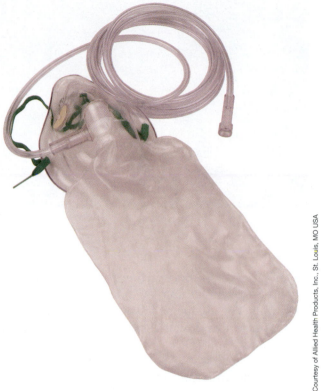

Courtesy of Allied Health Products, Inc., St. Louis, MO USA

FIGURE 13-5. A nonrebreathing oxygen mask.

Nonrebreathing masks are similar in design to the simple mask except for the addition of a reservoir bag to the bottom of the mask that has a one-way valve preventing exhaled gas to enter the reservoir bag. There are also rubber flaps over the exhalation ports that allow exhaled gas to exit the mask, but prevent entrainment of room air. This type of mask (Figure 13–5), if functioning properly, can provide 70% to 100% F_iO_2 at flows of 6–15 L/min. The liter flow should be sufficient to prevent complete deflation of the reservoir bag on inspiration.

Venturi masks (Figure 13–6) use various sized openings on a Venturi device to entrain room air and achieve precise oxygen concentrations in the mask. Common oxygen concentrations available with Venturi masks are 24%, 28%, 31%, 35%, 40%, and 50%. To achieve the desired F_iO_2, it is important to use the proper oxygen liter flow for the particular Venturi device. Total flow entering the mask is a combination of the oxygen flow and the entrained flow of room air. At a concentration of 24%, the entrainment ratio is 20:1. With oxygen flow of 4 L/min the total flow to the mask is 84 L/min. At a 50% concentration, the ratio is 1.75:1. With oxygen flow of 12 L/min total flow to the mask is 33 L/min.

Hazards present with the use of any oxygen mask include possible aspiration in vomiting patients, skin necrosis from a tight mask, low F_iO_2 if the mask is loose, and CO_2 retention in the presence of low total gas flow through the mask. Whenever

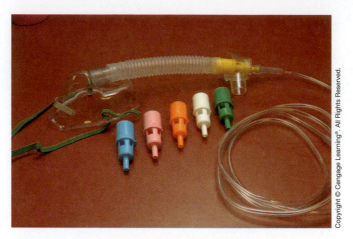

FIGURE 13–6. Venturi mask.

a mask is used, it must have an oxygen flow sufficient to flush out the patient's exhaled gases and prevent rebreathing CO_2. To avoid this problem, flows should not be set below 5 L/min. The exception to this is when masks are used on neonatal patients. In these circumstances, lower flows may be used because of the smaller tidal volumes.

Tents Tents are plastic enclosures that cover the entire patient. Tents come in various sizes to accommodate a variety of patient sizes. Tents most commonly provide an oxygen-enriched, cool mist to the patient environment for the treatment of laryngo-tracheobronchitis (croup) or other types of upper airway swelling. The internal environment of the tent is cooled from 5°C to 10°C below ambient temperature by the effects of evaporation or the use of a refrigeration unit. Due to the large size of the tent and the layering effect of the oxygen, F_iO_2 should be monitored near the patient's face to ensure accurate measurement. Generally, oxygen concentrations greater than 50% are difficult to achieve. Most devices will provide up to 40% oxygen.

There are several hazards associated with tent use. High-output nebulizers can create a fog inside the tent that makes it difficult to observe the patient. In severe cases of airway obstruction, it is vital to monitor the patient closely and watch for signs of distress. The presence of a thick mist may hamper this effort.

Because of its oxygen-enriched environment, a tent has a higher fire danger. All those working with tents, including parents and the patient, must be familiar with the dangers of flames or sparks in this environment. To avoid any possible problems, patients should not be given toys that create sparks.

Another possible hazard is that the high degree of moisture in the environment could potentially overhydrate the neonatal patient through the respiratory tract. Close monitoring for signs of overhydration should be observed in these patients.

Finally, although extremely unlikely, it is possible that the patient could become asphyxiated by an accidental lodging of the head between the mattress and the tent, or by a collapse of the tent onto the patient. Care should be taken when setting up

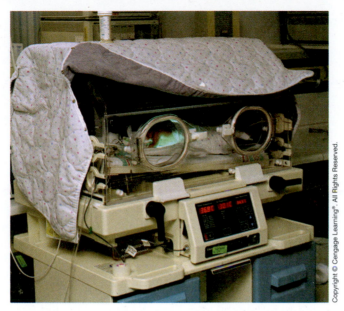

FIGURE 13–7. An incubator.

the internal or external framework of the tent. These hazards can be greatly lessened with proper setup, instruction, and observation.

Incubators Incubators provide a temperature-controlled and relatively quiet environment for the neonatal patient. Figure 13–7 illustrates an incubator. It is possible to provide the patient's oxygen needs directly into the incubator. Blended, warmed, and humidified oxygen can be delivered directly into the incubator to achieve the desired F_iO_2. Due to the previously mentioned effect of oxygen layering, the F_iO_2 should be measured near the patient's face.

The main problem encountered with this type of oxygen delivery is that the constant opening of the doors and portholes and the relatively large size of the incubator make it very difficult to maintain a consistent F_iO_2. Ideally, if the patient requires an F_iO_2 of higher than 25%, it may be more easily managed with an oxygen hood.

Resuscitation Bag Oxygen delivery via a resuscitation bag is most commonly used during neonatal resuscitation, emergencies or other short-term applications (Figure 13–8). Two types of bags are now in use: self-inflating and flow-inflating.

Self-inflating bags are very commonly used and require less skill than flow-inflating bags. They are designed to reinflate following decompression, thus not requiring a gas source to function. Because of this design, it is possible for the gas source to become disconnected and the provider to be unaware of it. The gas delivered to the patient is entrained in the bag on each reinflation. With a proper reservoir attached and sufficient oxygen flow, most self-inflating bags can achieve F_iO_2 of between 80% and 100%. Without a reservoir, or with inadequate flow rates, the F_iO_2 is unpredictable and not appropriate for most situations. Most self-inflating bags are

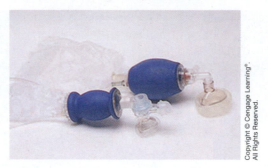

FIGURE 13–8. Self-inflating resuscitation bags.

not able to provide blow-by oxygen due to one-way valves that prevent rebreathing of exhaled gas from returning to the reservoir. The valve(s) only open during compression of the bag on inspiration.

Flow-inflating bags, on the other hand, have the advantage of providing the percentage of oxygen that is used to power them. F_iO_2 of 100% can be achieved simply by using pure oxygen to inflate the bag. Flow rates are adjusted to allow reinflation of the bag between breaths. Faster rates require higher flows, whereas in the self-inflating bag, the reinflation time remains constant regardless of rate. Flow-inflating bags allow for more control over pressures delivered to the airway, inspiratory time, and positive end expiratory pressure (PEEP). Because of their design, flow-inflating bags can be used to deliver blow-by oxygen and continuous positive airway pressure (CPAP) in spontaneously breathing patients. This device requires providers to have some level of skill to operate it correctly, including an understanding of flow adjustment and the need for a tight seal in order for the bag to function properly.

When using a resuscitation bag on a neonate or pediatric patient it is necessary to have some means of measuring the pressures delivered to the airway. Most resuscitation bags have either a port near the elbow attachment where a pressure manometer can be connected via a pressure line or a built-in pressure manometer that is part of the bag-mask assembly and is easily viewed by the provider. In the same general area, there is another port that is used for the entrainment of oxygen into the device.

Pressure masks come in a variety of sizes and shapes. The ideal mask should form a tight seal around the patient's mouth and nose, and not cover the eyes or hang over the chin. The seal should be able to be maintained with minimally applied pressure. When stocking a resuscitation area, it is suggested that a variety of mask sizes be available so an appropriate fit can be achieved.

AIRWAY CLEARANCE

One of the most widely studied aspects of respiratory care is that of airway clearance. Procedures and techniques have changed fairly dramatically from the early days where patients were hung over the edge of the bed and pounded on.

Normally, airway clearance relies on effective mucociliary action and an effective cough. Assistance in airway clearing becomes necessary when either of these two mechanisms dysfunction and result in mucus retention. As mucus increases in the airways, obstruction occurs and leads to air trapping, atelectasis, ineffective gas exchange, inflammation, and infection. Although there are several therapies that assist in airway clearance, the traditional treatment for increased mucus retention is chest physiotherapy (CPT), which consists of percussion, postural drainage, vibration of the chest wall, and secretion removal.

Indications

The need for airway clearance is based on careful assessment of the patient's pulmonary status. Indications are not specific to any age group but apply to any patient meeting the criteria. Indications are listed in Table 13–2. The indications for airway clearance can be effectively divided into four general categories: conditions that result in increased retention of secretions, diseases that produce excessive secretions, aspiration, and prophylaxis. Efficient removal of secretions during the course of a disease may help in preventing complications such as infection, air trapping, and barotrauma.

Airway clearance is especially necessary for the neonatal patient because of the small diameter of the airways. Any accumulation of secretions can lead to severe imbalances in ventilation/perfusion ratios. Once the neonate is intubated, the airway diameter is reduced even further by the endotracheal tube. Occlusion of the tube with secretions results in increased airway resistance and subsequent increases in ventilatory pressures if the patient is being ventilated on a volume control mode or

Table 13–2		
INDICATIONS FOR AIRWAY CLEARANCE		
Retained Secretions	*Excessive Secretions*	*Aspiration*
Atelectasis	Cystic Fibrosis	Meconium
RDS	Pneumonia	Foreign body
BPD	Asthma	
Intubation	Bronchitis	*Prophylaxis*
Ineffective cough mechanism	Bronchiectasis	Post extubation
Pain		
Paralysis		
Neuromuscular diseases		
Ciliary dyskinesia		

a decrease in delivered tidal volumes if the patient is being ventilated on a pressure-limited mode. Intubation disrupts the normal cough mechanism, making mechanical removal of secretions necessary.

Postoperative or posttrauma patients may be unable or unwilling to cough because of the pain involved. The cough mechanism may also be limited by paralytic or neuromuscular diseases. In any of these cases, the lack of effective coughing allows secretions to build in the airways. Finally, the inability of the cilia to beat in a coordinated fashion (dyskinesia) or total paralysis of the cilia, prevents the secretions from being moved up the airways to be removed.

There are several disease processes that cause the lungs to secrete an increased amount of mucus into the airways. With some diseases, such as cystic fibrosis, abnormally thick mucus makes removal even harder. Other diseases include pneumonia, asthma, bronchitis, and bronchiectasis.

Any aspiration, whether it is of meconium in a newborn, or a foreign body, should benefit from the use of airway clearance techniques.

Following extubation, several days may be required before the patient is able to produce an effective cough. During this time, assistance with airway clearance is prophylactic in preventing the build-up of secretions.

Contraindications and Hazards

Airway clearance therapy is not without detrimental side effects. Contraindications of treatment and postural drainage are listed in Table 13–3.

Hypoxemia that may occur during the treatment and the ensuing tracheal suctioning of the infant is a significant hazard. Hypoxemia is frequently associated with patient agitation and tracheal suctioning.

Table 13–3
CONTRAINDICATIONS OF AIRWAY CLEARANCE THERAPY
Pulmonary hemorrhage
Excessive agitation or hypoxemia during treatment
Feedings within the previous 45 minutes to 1 hour
History of reflux
Neonates of less than 1200 g birth weight or less than 32 weeks' gestation
History of intraventricular hemorrhage of greater than Grade I, or less than 7 days postbleed
Untreated pneumothorax
Congestive heart failure

Treatment should be stopped in patients who require more than a 25% increase in F_iO_2 to maintain an adequate PaO_2. The use of transcutaneous monitors and pulse oximeters can help reduce hypoxemic episodes during CPT and tracheal suctioning. By watching the infant's PaO_2 or saturation during the procedure, the respiratory therapist can increase F_iO_2 levels in response to patient hypoxemia.

Airway clearance often requires various movements of the patient. Water that has condensed in the tubing must be removed before the start of the treatment to prevent draining the water into the patient's airway.

Another hazard involves the use of postural drainage positions. The possibility of emesis and possible aspiration of feedings is of great concern. Placing the baby in a head-down position (**Trendelenburg**), especially following a feeding, and then percussing the infant, greatly increases the chance of **emesis** (vomiting) and potential aspiration. To prevent this, treatment should never be done within an hour following feedings. It is best done 15–20 minutes before feedings, when the chance of **emesis** is minimal. Postural drainage should never be done on patients with a history of **reflux**. If treatment is to be done, it should be performed with the infant in an upright position.

Postural drainage increases the intracranial pressure (ICP) when the patient is placed in the Trendelenburg position. The increase in ICP predisposes the early gestation baby to intraventricular hemorrhage (IVH). Studies have shown that infants of less than 1500 g are at a high risk for IVH.[2] It is therefore recommended that neonates of less than 1500 g not be placed in the Trendelenburg position because of the risk.

An additional concern involving preemies of less than 1200 g is the integrity of the skin. Percussion on these patients may cause skin damage that leads to edema, excoriations, and bruising.

Techniques

This discussion will begin with a look at several airway clearance techniques and end with a review of traditional CPT.

Positive Expiratory Pressure Positive expiratory pressure (PEP) therapy, developed in Denmark is now widely used in the United States. PEP therapy is done using a flow resistor and a mask or mouthpiece, through which the patient breathes in and out. As the patient exhales, a positive pressure is created in the airways. The pressure is monitored and adjusted, with pressures being either low (15–30 cm H_2O) or high (60–80 cm H_2O).

This inspiration/exhalation is done 10–20 times, and is followed by a forced exhalation technique (discussed next). These two techniques are repeated until secretions are expelled. The concept behind PEP therapy is to increase the transmural pressure of the airways and cause dilatation. Airway dilatation then allows gas to pass any obstruction and reach collapsed lung units. Allowing the gas to enter into previously occluded areas may improve oxygenation and ventilation and subsequently improve the mobilization of secretions toward the larger, central airways.

Forced Exhalation Technique Forced exhalation technique (FET), also referred to as a "huff cough," is used as an adjunct with other secretion removal techniques. FET is a way of modifying a patient's cough to avoid airway closure secondary to airway instability. It is performed by having the patient inhale slowly and then "huffing" forcefully 2–3 times. FET differs from a cough in that the glottis remains open during the "huff." FET combined with controlled breathing exercises is termed the active cycle of breathing (ACB) and consists of interspersing the FET with deep relaxed breaths. These relaxing breaths use diaphragmatic excursion to enhance lung volumes and promote an effective cough.[3] ACB is followed by a forceful cough to remove loosened secretions.

Autogenic Drainage Autogenic drainage is a technique in which the patient breathes at three different lung levels. In the first phase, the patient inhales a normal tidal volume and exhales midway into the expiratory reserve volume (ERV). This maneuver allows mucus lining the airways to loosen. At the next level, the patient inhales slightly above normal tidal volume and again exhales to mid-ERV. This allows for collection of the mucus from the periphery to the mid-central airways. For the third level, the patient inhales to near vital capacity and then exhales to the beginning of ERV. This maneuver is similar to a FET and allows removal of the secretions.

A distinct advantage to autogenic drainage is that it requires no equipment and can be done in any location and at any time. One disadvantage is that it may be difficult for the patient to properly learn and perform the technique.

High-Frequency Chest Compression The concept of this therapy is that by applying high-frequency oscillations to the chest wall, the vibrations are transferred to the airways. This results in improved gas liquid interface and improved mucus clearing. This therapy is provided by way of an inflatable vest that is worn by the patient . The vest is inflated and deflated extremely rapidly by a pump attached to it, resulting in the high-frequency oscillations.

Flutter Valve Therapy Flutter valve therapy is performed by having the patient exhale into a flutter device that contains a metal ball that rapidly moves toward and away from the path of exhalation (Figure 13–9). During the exhalation, the valve creates 10–20 H_2O of pressure as the ball flutters in the pipe, causing the oscillations that are transmitted to the airways. This device is position dependent and requires some coordination and understanding for the patient to perform the therapy effectively on their own.

Acapella Device This device combines the positive airway pressure from PEP therapy with high-frequency oscillations of flutter valve therapy. It also has a dial that allows for flow resister adjustment, altering the pressure required to exhale through it (Figure 13–10). The acapella is not position dependent, therefore it can be used by patients that have limited mobility or are unable to sit in full fowlers or dangle position in order to perform the therapy.

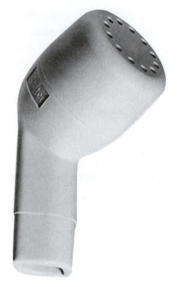

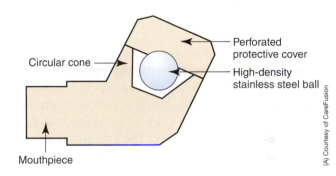

FIGURE 13–9. Flutter valve.

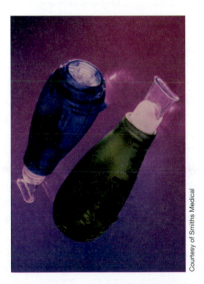

FIGURE 13–10. Acapella device.

Traditional Chest Physiotherapy The traditional method of performing chest physiotherapy consists of five techniques: auscultation, postural drainage, percussion, vibration, and removal of secretions.

Auscultation Auscultation involves listening to the sounds being produced in the lungs during the respiratory cycle. The respiratory therapist listens for sounds that may indicate the presence of airway secretions and/or reduced ventilation to a certain lung segment. Although the terminology for defining breath sounds is diverse, the definitions set forth by the American Thoracic Society (ATS) and the American College of Chest Physicians (ACCP) should be used. They recommend that a high-pitched continuous sound be called a **wheeze**, a continuous low-pitched sound be called **rhonchus**, and the term **crackle** for discontinuous sounds.[4] The presence of coarse crackles or rhonchus usually indicate the presence of airway secretions.

Postural Drainage Having auscultated the lung fields, the respiratory therapist determines the proper position for the patient to best facilitate drainage of the affected area. The patient is positioned in such a way that gravity is used to drain the site. This requires an understanding of the anatomy of the airways on the part of the respiratory therapist. Figure 13–11 illustrates the relationship of the segmental airways to the exterior thorax. The various positions used to drain each lung segment are illustrated in Figure 13–12.

The patient should be left in the position and the thorax should be percussed or vibrated for 2–5 minutes. If postural drainage is to be done alone, as in those patients who cannot tolerate percussion or vibration, the patient should remain in the position for 15–20 minutes.

Percussion Percussion is the rhythmic clapping on the thorax over the affected lung area to loosen secretions. Percussion on larger patients is done with the hands or with a mechanical percussor. The small size of the neonatal thorax prevents the use of hands for percussion and, thus, percussion is usually done with the aid of special devices. These devices may be obtained commercially (Figure 13–13) or can be made from resuscitation masks.

These cups are held between the fingers and percussion is achieved by the rhythmic up and down motion of the respiratory therapist's hand. A variation of the cup held in the fingers is the rubber cup attached to a plastic wand. The plastic wand is held between the thumb and index finger and percussion is done by a rhythmic movement of the wrist, similar to playing a drum. On the preemie, percussion may not be possible because of the fragility of the patient.

For larger patients, there are several commercially available mechanical percussion devices. These devices may be powered by compressed gas or electricity. One such pneumatic percussor is shown in Figure 13–14.

Percussion is done with enough force to produce a "popping" sound, but lightly enough to avoid trauma. Patients with BPD may have fragile bones and require special care when being percussed. Percussion is done over the rib cage to avoid damage to the liver or other abdominal organs. A light covering on the skin will reduce the chance of brushing and make the procedure more tolerable for the patient. Each area is percussed for 1–5 minutes as indicated.

Vibration Vibration differs from percussion in that it is a rapid, constant motion, rather than the rhythmic clapping. Vibration is used to help loosen secretions in the

Right lung		Left lung	
Upper lobe		**Upper lobe**	
Apical	1	Upper division	
Posterior	2	Apical/Posterior	1 & 2
Anterior	3	Anterior	3
Middle lobe		**Lower division (lingular)**	
Lateral	4	Superior lingula	4
Medial	5	Inferior lingula	5
Lower lobe		**Lower lobe**	
Superior	6	Superior	6
Medial basal	7	Anterior medial basal	7 & 8
Anterior basal	8	Lateral basal	9
Lateral basal	9	Posterior basal	10
Posterior basal	10		

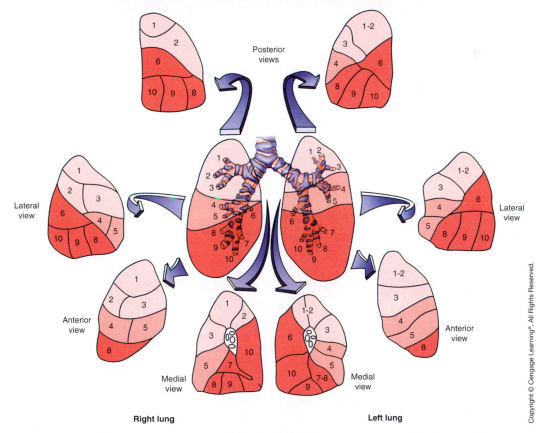

FIGURE 13–11. The relationship between the segmental airways and the external thorax.

airways and aid their mobilization. Vibration can be done with the fingertips by placing them on the thorax and rapidly shaking them. An easier method is to use a commercially available vibrator, designed to be used on small neonates, shown in Figure 13–15.

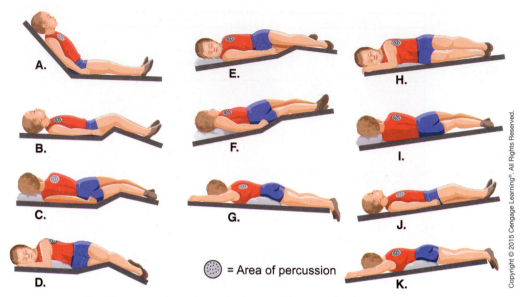

FIGURE 13–12. Positions used to drain the various lung segments. A. To drain the apical segments of the right and left upper lobes—torso elevated 30°. B. Drainage of the anterior segments of the right and left upper lobes—patient supine. C. Drainage of the posterior segment of the right upper lobe—patient prone, right side elevated 45°. D. Drainage of the posterior segment of the left upper lobe—head elevated 15°, left side elevated 45°. E. Drainage of the left lingular segment—head down 15°, patient lies on right hip, shoulders turned to lie flat on bed. F. Drainage of the right middle lobe—head down 15°, right side elevated 45°. G. Drainage of the apical segments of both lower lobes—patient prone. H. Drainage of the lateral basal segment of the left lower lobe—head down 39° left side elevated 45°. I. Drainage of the lateral basal segment of the right lower lobe—head down 30° right side elevated 45°. J. Drainage of the anterior basal segment of both lower lobes—head down 30° patient supine. K. Drainage of the posterior basal segments of both lower lobes—head down 30° patient prone.

Vibration is best done during expiration to allow gas flows to aid the movement of the secretions. As with percussion, care must be exercised when the vibration is done to ensure toleration by the patient.

Removal of Secretions At the completion of the postural drainage, percussion, and vibration, the patient is prepared for the removal of secretions. Older pediatric patients should be instructed to use FET.

Younger patients may need to be suctioned both orally and nasally. To avoid bradycardia secondary to hypoxemia, which may accompany suctioning, the nonintubated patient should be hyperoxygenated before performing the suctioning. This can be done via blow-by from the resuscitation bag, or by increasing the F_iO_2 to the oxygen delivery device being used.

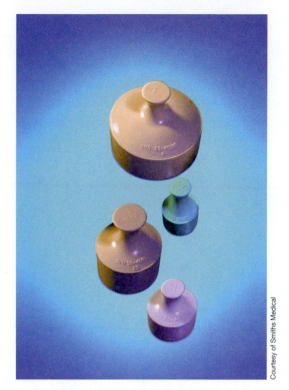

Courtesy of Smiths Medical

FIGURE 13–13. Palm cup percussors.

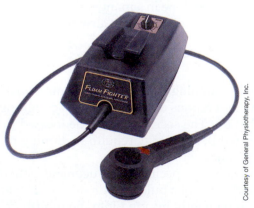

Courtesy of General Physiotherapy, Inc.

FIGURE 13–14. Flimm-Fighter percussor.

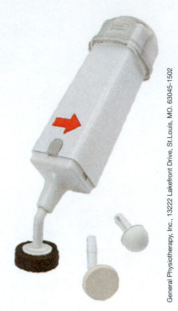

General Physiotherapy, Inc., 13222 Lakefront Drive, St.Louis, MO. 63045-1502

FIGURE 13–15. G5™ Neocussor™.

SUCTIONING

Many patients present with factors that promote the retention of airway secretions. The intubated patient has a decreased ability to remove airway secretions spontaneously and must be aided by the respiratory therapist. Secretions that block the airway increase resistance and subsequently increase work of breathing. As airway resistance increases, airflow is diminished and ventilation decreases.

Proper suctioning must be done in a manner that does not compromise the clinical status of the patient or the sterility of the airways.

Indications

Oral, nasal, or tracheal suctioning should be performed when the patient is unable to manage his/her own secretions due to ineffective coughing, excessive secretions, or endotracheal intubation. The secretions may be located in the trachea, pharynx, mouth, or nose. Intubated patients may require suctioning of the endotracheal tube (ETT) to preserve its patency.

Oral and nasal suctioning, specifically in neonatal patients, can often be effectively performed with the use of a bulb suction device. The base of the bulb suction device is compressed then gently inserted into the mouth or placed at the opening of the nares. Once in place, the pressure on the bulb is released creating suction to remove secretions that have accumulated in the focused area. The bulb suction device is removed from the patient and the secretions are removed from the device by abruptly compressing the bulb, forcing the secretions from the device. This process can be repeated in order to adequately clear the oropharynx or the nasopharynx. Aggressive suctioning with this device may result in mucosal damage, thus care should be used when inserting and applying suction. It is important to thoroughly clean the bulb suction device with soap and water following each use.

Suctioning through the ETT should be performed on an as-needed basis only, ranging from every hour to every 4 to 6 hours depending on the amount and consistency of pulmonary secretions. Clinically the patient may present with decreased chest excursion, and on auscultation coarse crackles and rhonchi may be heard. Occasionally, mucus may be seen in the ETT. Endotracheal suctioning is also indicated when a sputum culture or Gram stain is requested. These signs all indicate the need for tracheal suctioning. Suctioning should be done following a CPT treatment to remove any secretions that may have become dislodged and to prevent their aspiration back into the trachea.

Suctioning of the nose, mouth, and oropharynx is indicated to provide hygiene to the intubated patient. On the nonintubated patient, the same areas are suctioned to provide hygiene, as well as prevent aspiration of secretions and maintain airway patency. Oral and nasal suctioning can also be done to stimulate a cough. Due to its effect on the patient's ventilatory status, suctioning should be done at least 20 minutes before drawing a blood gas sample.

Equipment

The equipment needed to perform suctioning is listed in Table 13–4. Since bradycardia and hypoxemia often accompany suctioning, monitors that measure heart rate and oxygen status should be visually accessible to the person performing the procedure.

A stethoscope is necessary to access breath sounds before and after the suctioning. Noting the change in breath sounds is one means to indicate the effectiveness of the procedure.

A resuscitation bag and mask must be readily available at the bedside. In the event of a prolonged bradycardia that does not respond to stimulus, or in the case of an accidental extubation, a properly functioning resuscitation bag is essential. The F_iO_2 delivered to the bag should be set 10% above the current F_iO_2 before beginning the procedure. In the case of prolonged bradycardia, the F_iO_2 should be increased to 100% while bagging the patient.

When suctioning the ETT, the use of sterile saline lavage may become necessary. This procedure should be limited due to the risk of contamination of the saline port and the introduction of bacteria to the airway. The neonatal patient will require only a few drops, whereas the larger pediatric patient may require several milliliters of solution. In either instance the use of saline lavage while performing endotracheal suctioning should only be used to loosen or dislodge thick, tenacious secretions, not as a routine procedure. To prevent the necessity of saline lavage, respiratory therapists should be vigilant in providing adequate humidification and hydration to the patient. Adequate hydration will aid in thinning secretions and adequate

Table 13–4

EQUIPMENT NEEDED TO SUCTION

Cardiac, oxygen saturation, and/or transcutaneous monitors

Stethoscope

Resuscitation bag and mask with oxygen source and pressure manometer

Sterile saline for **lavage** (only if necessary to remove thick, tenacious secretions)

Sterile suction catheter kit with gloves (appropriately sized)

Suction regulator set at appropriate suction level

Water-soluble lubricant as needed

humidification of the airway will prevent drying of secretions in the presence of supplemental oxygen delivery or mechanical ventilation.

If the patient is to be suctioned nasally, the use of a water-soluble lubricant will facilitate the passage of the catheter into the nares. The lubricant should be opened and then squeezed onto a sterile field placed nearby. The sterile catheter should then be drawn through the lubricant before inserting it into the patient's nares. If an assistant is present, he or she may place the lubricant directly onto the catheter, being careful not to contaminate it.

A suction regulator set at −60 to −80 mmHg for neonates and −80 to −120 mmHg for pediatric patients and an appropriate collection canister are both required before suctioning.

The suction tubing that connects the catheter to the canister should be long enough to allow the procedure without pulling or kinking. The end of the tubing should be placed at a site that allows an easy connection to the suction catheter without breaking sterility.

The last piece of equipment is a suction catheter of the proper size. Table 13–5 shows the proper sizes for suction catheters used on neonates. The kit should contain at least one sterile glove, a sterile suction catheter, and a sterile water basin.

An alternative method of suctioning is the use of inline suction devices, which incorporate a suction catheter covered by a protective sheath and a patient connection "T-piece." The advantages to these types of suction devices are the ability to suction the patient without disconnecting the ventilator, less risk of contamination, and less overall cost.

Procedure

It is recommended that suctioning always be done with two people: one to perform the suctioning procedure, and the other to monitor the patient and provide support as needed.

Table 13–5

SELECTING SUCTION CATHETER SIZES

Intubated patients:

Endotracheal Tube (mm I.D.)	Suction Catheter (French)
2.5	5, 6
3.0	5, 6–8
3.5	8–10
4.0	8–10

Nonintubated patients:

Age	Suction Catheter (French)
Preemie	5, 6
Term newborn	5, 6–8
Newborn to 6 months	8–10

The first task in preparing the airway for suctioning is the preparation of the equipment. Select the appropriately sized suction catheter using Table 13–5 as a guide.

The technique of inserting the suction catheter into the ETT until resistance is felt may lead to trauma of the tracheal mucosa. To avoid possible injury, the suction catheter should be inserted only to the tip of the ETT.

The proper catheter insertion distance is determined by noting the cm mark on the exterior ETT, which corresponds to the level of the adapter (Figure 13–16). The adapter length, which is approximately 4 cm, is added to the cm mark on the ETT. This represents the distance from the tip of the ETT to the opening of the adapter and can then be used to determine the appropriate depth of catheter insertion. Once the insertion distance is determined, it should be noted and placed on a card near the patient's bedside to allow for consistency when suctioning.

Another means of determining the depth of advancing the suction catheter is lining up catheter measurements with the ETT measurements. Some suction catheters have cm markings on them. Lining up the centimeter markings with those on the outside of the ETT will ensure that the suction catheter has not passed the end of the ETT.

The vacuum pressure is now adjusted by occluding the opening of the suction tubing and adjusting the vacuum to the previously mentioned settings.

After washing your hands, auscultate the lungs to assess the presence of mucus in the airways and to serve as a guide to determine the adequacy of the suctioning. Before suctioning, the patient should be hyperoxygenated for 1 minute with an F_iO_2 10% to 15% higher than is currently being used. When a manual resuscitation bag is used, it is important to have a pressure manometer inline and to have it connected to an oxygen blender that will allow the provider to adjust the oxygen according to the needs of the patient during the procedure.

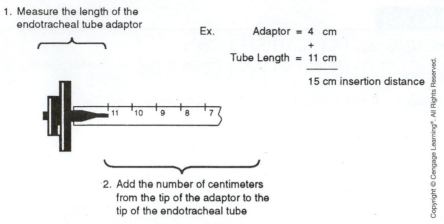

FIGURE 13–16. Method of determining proper insertion depth of a suction catheter.

After aseptically opening the package and donning the gloves, the catheter is removed from its protective package. When the patient is inside an incubator, the catheter should be wrapped around the hand or inside the clenched hand to protect it from being contaminated as the hand is inserted into the porthole. If a sterile inline suction catheter is being used, sterile gloving is not necessary but aseptic technique should be employed.

If the patient is to be lavaged, a few drops of sterile saline should be instilled into ETT, followed by two to three mechanical breaths. The suction catheter should now be inserted into the ETT to the predetermined distance, suction applied, and the catheter rotated and withdrawn. The entire suctioning procedure should not take more than 10 seconds, with a maximum of 5 seconds with suction applied. The procedure should be repeated as needed until the secretions have been removed. Careful monitoring of the vital signs will help prevent hypoxemia and bradycardia.

Hazards

Hazards associated with suctioning are listed in Table 13–6. The major hazard related to tracheal suctioning is bradycardia. Bradycardia is defined as a heart rate below 100 bpm. In the neonate, a heart rate below 100 bpm indicates lack of proper oxygenation and a decrease in cardiac output secondary to decreased contractility of the myocardium. It is, therefore, a serious hazard that requires rapid care by the respiratory therapist.

Bradycardia can be induced by way of two mechanisms. First, stimulation of the vagus nerve located in the trachea or in the oropharynx and nasopharynx can cause bradycardia. Vagal stimulation may be lessened by limiting the time that the suction catheter is in the trachea or pharynx. Insertion and removal of the suction catheter should last no longer than 10 seconds. It may be less hazardous to the patient to perform repeated, short-duration suctioning rather than one or two prolonged procedures.

Table 13–6

HAZARDS OF SUCTIONING

1. Bradycardia
   a. Vagal response
   b. Hypoxemia-induced

2. Hypoxemia

3. Mucosal damage

4. Atelectasis

5. Airway contamination

6. Accidental extubation

A second mechanism of bradycardia is hypoxia brought on by the tracheal suctioning. Hypoxia-induced bradycardia can be lessened by hyperoxygenating the infant before performing the procedure and by limiting the application of suction to 5 seconds.

As with many procedures done on neonates, suctioning produces a significant amount of stress to the patient. In addition to bradycardia and hypoxemia, suctioning causes an increase in the amount of arousal, stressful facial expressions, and an increase in autonomic activity. The effect of this psychological stress is not fully understood, but certainly is not helpful to the patient's well-being.

Other potential hazards of suctioning include mucosal damage, atelectasis, airway contamination, and accidental extubation. Mucosal damage may aid mucus plugging in the distal airways, leading to V/Q mismatches and worsening patient status, and may also lead to tissue swelling and edema, increasing resistance in the airway. Damage to the mucosa is reduced by regulating the insertion distance of the suction catheter as mentioned above.

AEROSOL THERAPY

Aerosolized medications can be delivered by one of several methods: the small volume nebulizer (SVN), which is run by a compressed gas source; the large volume nebulizer (LVN), also powered by compressed gas (both the SVN and LVN are jet nebulizers); the metered dose inhaler (MDI), powered by compressed gas; and the dry powder inhaler (DPI) in which the patient's inspiratory effort powers the delivery of medication.

The goal of treatment with aerosolized medications is to deliver an adequate amount of medicine to the desired sites in the pulmonary tree with a minimum of side effects. This being the case, an effective treatment depends on four factors: 1) the size and amount of particles produced, 2) the characteristics of the particles, 3) the anatomy of the airways, and 4) the patient's ventilatory pattern, none of which can be altered by the respiratory therapist. However, properly educating the patient in the use of the device may aid the patient in proper technique, improving medication delivery. Understanding the ideal situation for each factor can also aid the respiratory therapist in modifying the therapy accordingly.

Particle Amount and Size

Particle amount and size is dependent on the type of nebulizer used. Jet nebulizers are easy to use and in common use in many NICUs; however, one drawback is that particle size varies tremendously among nebulizers. When run continuously, much of the medication is lost during expiration, thus reducing the amount of drug available to the lungs. This can be reduced slightly with the addition of a reservoir that collects some of the aerosol produced during exhalation and makes it available on the next inspiration.

Particle Characteristics

The major characteristic of aerosol particles that affects deposition is its ability to take on additional water. This is called **hydroscopic** growth. These aerosols grow larger when added to an environment of high humidity, which makes them more likely to deposit higher in the airway. Other characteristics that determine aerosol deposition include the concentration and viscosity of the drug and the velocity at which it is delivered. More medication is delivered when the volume of diluents is increased.[5]

Studies have demonstrated that the lung deposition of aerosolized drugs delivered to intubated infants is only about one-twentieth of that in nonintubated adults and about one-tenth that of in intubated adults. The implication is that higher dosages are needed when delivering aerosolized drugs to an intubated infant in order to achieve a dose equivalent to that received by nonintubated patients.

Anatomy of the Airways

In general, the narrower the airway is, the greater the deposition of the medication. This is important in the neonatal and pediatric populations because their airways are narrow to begin with. Add to that the effect of bronchoconstriction, secretions, and the endotracheal tube, and the amount of drug reaching the terminal airways and alveoli is probably negligible.

Ventilation Pattern

Aerosol delivery is best enhanced when laminar inspiratory flow is employed, followed by a brief pause. For the patient, this requires a slow deep breath followed by an inspiratory pause. The timing of the aerosol is also important. Ideally, aerosol should be available from the onset of inspiration. This does not present a problem with continuous jet nebulization, but it can pose a problem when an MDI is used. If not activated at the proper time, the amount of delivered medication can drastically change. When giving an aerosol to a mechanically ventilated patient, it may aid aerosol deposition by lengthening inspiratory time, reducing flow rate and adding a short inspiratory pause at the end of inspiration.

Aerosolized drug delivery has limited use in the NICU setting. One reason for this limited usage is the unknown effects of the drugs and dosages on the neonate. With improved drugs and increased experience, however, aerosolized drugs are being used to a greater extent as part of the care of the premature infant.

In the case of the pediatric patient, aerosolized drugs have long been used in the treatment of several respiratory-related disorders. A problem exists regarding which is the best and most effective way to deliver the medication. An effective aerosol treatment requires a cooperative patient who can follow verbal commands. Unfortunately, very few infant and pediatric patients are cooperative enough to hold a mouth piece or allow the practitioner to hold a mask over the mouth and nose.

Nebulizers

The main advantage to the use of SVN therapy is that it requires little patient coordination. This makes it useful in very young patients. SVN therapy is also advantageous in acute distress or in the presence of reduced inspiratory flows and volumes. The use of SVNs allows modification of drug concentration and additionally allows the aerosolization of almost any liquid drug. Finally, SVNs are effective with minimal breath holding, which may be difficult for younger patients.

Major disadvantages to SVN therapy are: it is relatively expensive; it is less easily transported; both cleaning and preparation are required; the dose delivery is inefficient; it delivers a cold, wet aerosol when used with a mask or blow-by; and it provides a medium in which bacteria can grow. When used inline with a ventilator, jet nebulizers have additional drawbacks. The high humidity of the inspired gas may aid in the hydroscopic growth of the particle, resulting in deposition in the circuit or upper airway, again reducing the amount of drug delivered.

Large volume nebulizer (LVN) therapy is used when delivery of a medication is indicated over a long period of time. Continuous nebulizer therapy is used to treat acute recalcitrant asthma in which a SVN does not deliver enough medication to have an effect.

Continuous nebulizer therapy is most often used to deliver beta$_2$-agonists to patients suffering from severe asthma exacerbations. The dosage criteria should be determined after considering the type of continuous nebulization device, concentration of medication to be delivered, the size of the patient, and the patient's respiratory pattern.

Ultrasonic nebulizer (USN) therapy relies on a piezoelectric crystal that vibrates at high frequency, which creates sound waves that create waves resulting in droplet formation. Particle size of the droplets is determined by the wave frequency and the amplitude determines output. Large volume USNs are most commonly used for bland aerosol therapy or sputum induction. Small volume USNs are used to deliver medication. The benefit to using a small volume USN for aerosol drug delivery is the low residual drug volume as compared to SVNs. However, the cost of a small volume USN is higher than that of an SVN. Caution should be used to prevent bacterial growth in any USN and patients should be closely monitored for overhydration throughout the use of a USN.

Metered Dose Inhaler (MDI)

The advantages to the use of MDIs are that they are very portable, they provide efficient drug delivery, and they require a very short preparation and delivery time. An advantage to the use of MDIs inline with a ventilator is the resistance of the particles to hydroscopic growth due to accompanying surfactants.[6]

Disadvantages include: the difficulty of coordinating the breath and delivery of the drug, fixed drug concentrations, limited choice of drugs; possible reaction to the propellants used, the possibility of oropharyngeal impaction, and the possibility of aspiration of a foreign body. The use of spacers reduces the necessity of hand-breath coordination, and reduces the chance of oropharyngeal impaction.

Dry Powder Inhaler (DPI)

The advantages to using DPI devices include those mentioned with MDI devices; in addition, limited hand-breath coordination is needed, no propellants are used, and the drug doses are easily counted. Disadvantages to using DPI devices include: the limited number of drugs available, possible irritation of the airway from the dry powder, possible reaction to the carrier, it requires high inspiratory flowrates, some require loading before use, and it is less useful in the presence of acute obstruction.

Indications

Most aerosolized drugs fall into one of three categories: bronchodilators, mucolytics, and steroids. For a bronchodilator to be indicated, some degree of bronchoconstriction should be present. On the premature infant and the pediatric patient, this may be manifest by decreased breath sounds, decreased chest expansion, presence of wheezes and retractions, increased respiratory rate, nasal flaring, grunting, increasing ventilatory pressures, increasing F_iO_2 requirements, and an increasing $PaCO_2$.

Depending on the age and maturity of the pediatric patient, bronchoconstriction may also be verified by the results of pulmonary function studies. A decreased vital capacity and peak expiratory flow will help to diagnose bronchoconstriction.

The indication for the use of an aerosolized mucolytic is the presence of thick secretions that are difficult for the patient to expel. It is sometimes difficult to detect the difference between the presence of thick, copious secretions and bronchospasm.

The patient may or may not have loud rhonchi when auscultated. The patient may also show the same signs as the patient with bronchoconstriction. As mucus fills the airways, the effect is the same as a narrowing of the lumen, thus the similarity of signs.

Inhaled steroids are indicated when an inflammatory pulmonary process is present, such as BPD or asthma. While the exact mechanism of action is not known, steroids are thought to have antivasopressin effects, enhance surfactant production and β-adrenergic receptor function, stimulate antioxidant production, and improve pulmonary microcirculation.[6]

A patient who shows any of these signs is a candidate for aerosolized drug therapy. Once the treatment has been started, the respiratory therapist must evaluate the effectiveness of the treatment and watch carefully for any complications. The use of these drugs, their dosage, and their hazards are covered in detail in Chapter 14. Effectiveness of the treatment in the neonatal patient is indicated by improved breath sounds, increased chest expansion, and decreased signs of work of breathing.

Equipment

Most SVNs will work equally well using a mouthpiece, mask, or attached inline to a ventilator circuit. The most common nebulizer in use is the **updraft** type, which is used mainly in the vertical position. A tee piece is attached to the top of the nebulizer. The mouthpiece is inserted into one end of the tee piece, and a short length of aerosol tubing is placed on the opposite end of the tee to act as a reservoir. One study showed that the use of an expiratory reservoir significantly increased the amount of inhaled medication compared to the absence of a reservoir.[7]

For patients who require a mask, the setup is the same except that the mask is placed where the mouthpiece would be (Figure 13–17). Another possible use is to insert the top of the nebulizer into the bottom opening of an aerosol mask and either hold the mask over the mouth and nose or use the elastic strap to secure the mask to the patient's face (Figure 13–18).

One of the drawbacks of the **updraft nebulizer** is that it must be in a vertical position to nebulize properly. Fortunately, some of the newer nebulizers are designed to nebulize in a vertical or horizontal position. An updraft nebulizer can be used equally well in a pediatric ventilator circuit or a neonatal circuit. Adapters must be used to join the nebulizer to the circuit.

A less common type of SVN that is well adapted for use in the ventilator circuit is the **mainstream nebulizer**. The mainstream nebulizer has an advantage in that it does not require additional tubing to adapt it to the circuit. It is designed to be used in the horizontal position, which helps tremendously when it is used inside an incubator.

Use of an MDI requires an actuator device that triggers the canister and diverts the aerosol horizontally. To avoid the hazard of misaiming the device or holding it too close or distant, it is generally recommended that the MDI be used with a spacer device. The spacer is usually a chamber into which the medication is ejected, allowing the patient to then inhale the medication with less coordination needed.

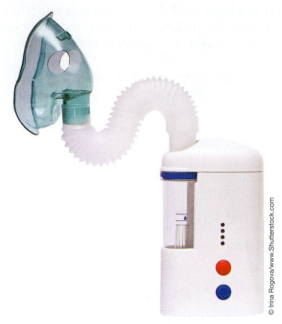

FIGURE 13–17. Nebulizer with attached mask.

Adapters also exist, which are placed inline with a ventilator circuit, allowing the MDI to be discharged directly into the circuit.

DPI therapy uses a special apparatus that dispenses the medication from a capsule or a blister packet as the patient inhales. Currently, there is no mechanism for using DPI therapy on patients being mechanically ventilated.

Considerations for Use on Intubated Patients

One of the biggest hazards associated with the use of aerosol delivery inline to the ventilator circuit is the potential increase in tidal volumes and peak pressures during ventilation. The problem the result of the necessity of providing 6 to 8 L/min of flow to properly nebulize the medication. Salyer and associates' recommended solution is to place the nebulizer at the humidifier outlet and nebulize during exhalation.[8] This allows the aerosol to fill the inspiratory limb of the circuit to be delivered to the patient with the next breath.

Another possible alternative is to reduce the ventilator gas flow proportionally to the flow being used to power the nebulizer. In addition to helping reduce tidal volumes and pressures, this may help prevent a buildup of inadvertent positive and expiratory pressure (PEEP) and the resultant increase in mean airway pressure. The additional flow added by an SVN is usually not enough to affect flow patterns in larger circuits such as those used in pediatric patients, and, subsequently, does not need compensation.

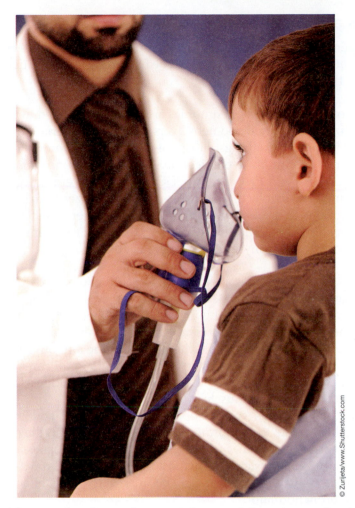

FIGURE 13–18. Holding mask in front of patient's face to deliver the medication.

When an SVN is used inline with a ventilator circuit, the cool gas of the nebulizer mixing with the warm gas of the humidifier leads to condensation. This may cause the medication to rain out in the tubing and not reach the patient. For this reason, it may be more effective to either bypass or turn off the humidifier during the treatment. Upon completion of the treatment, the humidifier should be promptly connected or turned back on.

If the humidifier is to be left on, the following concerns should be noted. Certain ventilator circuits have a distal temperature probe to measure gas temperature as it enters the patient. In these instances the nebulizer should be placed distally to the probe. A nebulizer that is placed proximally to the probe will cool the gas and cause the humidifier to intensify its heat output. When the nebulizer is removed, the gas temperature could potentially burn the patient's airways. By placing the nebulizer after the probe, the humidifier continues to maintain the proper heat output.

Hazards and Complications

Although aerosol therapy is a relatively safe procedure, there are certain conditions, described below in Table 13–7 that could be hazardous to the patient and require the attention of the respiratory therapist.

Infection Hospital acquired pneumonias are frequently linked to the use of contaminated nebulizers. Contaminated nebulizers can carry bacteria-laden aerosol into the sterile environment of the lungs. Hospital-acquired pneumonia can occur from the use of contaminated multiuse medication vials. Recommendations from the Centers for Disease Control and Prevention (CDC) for the prevention of hospital-acquired pneumonia include disinfecting and rinsing the nebulizer with sterile water following each treatment, or air-drying the nebulizer. Nebulizers must be replaced between patients with sterile ones and the respiratory therapist must ensure that only sterile fluids, dispensed aseptically, are used in the nebulizer.

Medication Side Effects As mentioned, specific drugs and their particular side effects are covered in Chapter 14. However, there are some conditions unique to the use of medication nebulizers that will be discussed here.

The nature of bronchodilators causes them not only to affect the smooth muscle of the airways but also to stimulate the heart and the smooth muscle of the vasculature. Early bronchodilators had very potent effects in all three areas. In contrast, modern bronchodilators minimally stimulate the heart and vessels, while having a strong effect on the smooth muscle.

The reaction to drugs varies depending on the size and maturation of each patient. For this reason, the respiratory therapist must watch the patient for changes in the cardiovascular system, muscle tremors, and nervousness. Nebulized mucolytics, especially acetylcysteine (Mucomyst®), may cause bronchospasm in certain patient groups, particularly asthmatics. Because of this side effect, acetylcysteine is given with a bronchodilator.

Table 13–7
HAZARDS ASSOCIATED WITH SVN THERAPY
Hospital acquired infection
Medication side effects
Drug reconcentration
Ventilator malfunction
Excessive noise

Drug Reconcentration Another potential hazard exists in the form of **reconcentration** of the nebulized drug. As the drug is nebulized, larger droplets return to the fluid reservoir. As the fluid reservoir gets lower, the concentration of the drug in the solution increases. Thus, toward the end of the treatment, the drug is in a higher concentration and could potentially produce more side effects.

Other Hazards It is possible that depositing medication on the ventilator expiratory valve may cause it to stick, resulting in hazardous PEEPs and inspiratory times. This problem can be minimized by placing a filter into the expiratory tubing to prevent the aerosolized medication from reaching the valve. Some nebulizers create a high level of noise that could potentially be harmful to the small preemie. To avoid problems with noise when used with that patient group, the nebulizer should be placed in the ventilator circuit outside the incubator.

Small Particle Aerosol Generators (SPAG)

The SPAG unit shown in Figure 13–19 is a unique device designed and intended for the administration of the drug ribavirin to treat respiratory syncytial virus. No other medication should be delivered through the SPAG unit and conversely, ribavirin should not be delivered through any other device. The administration of ribavirin, along with hazards and precautions, are covered in Chapter 14.

As mentioned, the SPAG unit is unique in its operation (Figure 13–19). Ribavirin is reconstituted in a large reservoir within the SPAG unit. Compressed gas enters the unit into a pressure regulator and is reduced to a working pressure of 26 psi. The gas is then fed to two separate flowmeters. One flowmeter supplies a gas flow to the nebulizer inside the reservoir. The nebulized particles exit the top of the reservoir and are met by flow from the other flowmeter. Together, the two flows enter

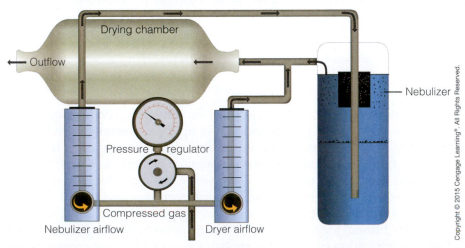

FIGURE 13–19. Small particle aerosol generator (SPAG).

a drying chamber. Inside the drying chamber, the nebulized particles undergo evaporation and are significantly reduced in size to between 1.2 and 1.4 microns. The particles then exit the drying chamber and are delivered to the patient. Ribavirin from the SPAG unit can be delivered to a mask, hood, tent, or ventilator circuit.

Because ribavirin can precipitate and accumulate on the walls of the ventilator tubing and the endotracheal tube, extreme care must be taken when administering the drug with mechanical ventilation. It is recommended that it only be used in this fashion by those who are familiar with this mode of delivery and with the ventilator. Several procedures have been shown to reduce risk associated with administering ribavirin via a ventilator. Suctioning of the ETT tube should be done every 1 to 2 hours and close monitoring of pressures be done every 2 to 4 hours. The use of a heated wire circuit may also reduce precipitation of the drug. One-way valves are used to prevent the drug from entering the humidifier or ventilator, and to prevent ventilator flow from entering the SPAG unit. The use of disposable exhalation valves, which are changed out every 4 hours, reduces the risk of clogging and excessive pressures. The flow of ribavirin from the expiratory circuit to the environment is slowed by the placement of bacteria filters in the expiratory circuit.

PRE- AND POSTASSESSMENT OF PATIENT

It is important to remember that all therapies require a thorough pre- and postassessment of the patient. The assessment of breath sounds, work of breathing, chest expansion, vital signs, oxygen saturation, patient history, and subjective data will provide a baseline evaluation to predicate the effectiveness of the therapy provided and the need for future therapy or the augmentation of therapy. Respiratory therapists should be vigilant in collecting a complete assessment before and after therapy in addition to reviewing the patient's chart for pertinent information that may affect or alter the course of treatment.

SUMMARY

When respiratory care first evolved, technicians were called on to bring oxygen tanks to the various floors. They then began setting up the oxygen tanks in the rooms and attaching the patients to masks and cannulas. As technologies in respiratory care evolved and the understanding of the pulmonary system increased, the respiratory therapist was the natural person to fill the new niche created. From simple beginnings, respiratory care has evolved into a highly technical and skilled profession with therapies, treatments, and procedures improving year by year. This chapter is a basic look at the traditional therapies and treatments done by the respiratory therapist.

The administration of oxygen is probably one of the most common procedures done on patients in the hospital. Neonates and pediatric patients are no exception.

Oxygen is delivered via any one of several methods and appliances, depending on the amount of oxygen and humidity needed by the patient.

One of the staples of respiratory care through the years is that of chest physiotherapy or CPT. New techniques have evolved to augment traditional CPT, which includes vibration, percussion, postural drainage, and removal of secretions. These new procedures include forced exhalation technique (FET), active cycle of breathing (ACB), positive expiratory pressure (PEP), autogenic drainage (AD), high-frequency chest compression (HFCC), flutter valve applications, and exercise.

Suctioning the patient's airway is a job that is frequently handed to the respiratory therapist. If done improperly, suctioning may lead to hypoxemia, bradycardia, and tracheal damage; therefore, the performance of suctioning must follow a strict guideline of proper timing, use of the proper size catheter, insertion to the proper depth, and for the proper time interval. Although following these guidelines does not guarantee an absence of side effects, they can at least be minimized.

Another traditional treatment modality used in respiratory therapy is the delivery of aerosolized medications. While the SVN remains the most common method of delivery, other delivery techniques such as MDIs and DPIs are increasing in popularity.

Studies have found MDIs to be as effective in aerosol delivery as the SVN, while being easier to administer, with fewer hazards and complications. A special nebulizer, the SPAG unit, is used exclusively to administer the antiviral drug ribavirin.

POSTTEST

1. Of the following, which are indicates for CPT?
   I. asthma
   II. atelectasis
   III. cystic fibrosis
   IV. prolonged bed rest
   V. ventilator care
      a. I, III, IV
      b. II, III, IV
      c. I, II, IV, V
      d. I, II, III, IV, V

2. To ensure maximum effectiveness, PEP should be followed by what technique?
      a. FET
      b. autogenic drainage
      c. high-frequency chest compressions
      d. CPT with postural drainage

3. Which of the following is not part of traditional CPT?
   a. postural drainage
   b. percussion
   c. hyperoxygenation
   d. removal of secretions
4. Which of the following modalities to administer aerosolized medication requires the least amount of patient coordination?
   a. MDI alone
   b. MDI with a spacer
   c. SVN
   d. DPI
5. Of the following, which are indications for aerosolized medication therapy?
   I. wheezing
   II. retractions
   III. increased respiratory rate
   IV. increased peak expiratory flow
   V. increasing F_iO_2 requirements
      a. I, III, IV, V
      b. II, IV
      c. II, III, V
      d. II, III, V
6. One advantage to the mainstream nebulizer is that:
   a. It is less expensive.
   b. It can be used horizontally.
   c. It produces smaller particle size.
   d. It can be reused.
7. Placement of a medication nebulizer in the ventilator circuit between the humidifier and the distal temperature probe may cause:
   a. overheating of the circuit when the nebulizer is removed
   b. malfunction of the nebulizer
   c. overhydration of the infant
   d. contamination of the ventilator circuit
8. Which of the following would be considered hazards of aerosol drug therapy?
   I. infection
   II. medication side effects
   III. drug reconcentration
   IV. overhydration
   V. intraventricular hemorrhage
      a. I, II, III, IV
      b. III, IV, V
      c. II, III, IV
      d. I, II, IV, V

9. Which of the following is not a disadvantage of MDI therapy?
    a. fixed drug concentrations
    b. not indicated in patients younger than 12 years
    c. possible reaction to the propellants
    d. possible oropharyngeal impaction
10. The *greatest* hazard associated with the aerosolization of ribavirin into a ventilator circuit is:
    a. medication may not reach the patient
    b. precipitation and accumulation of the drug on vent tubing and ETT
    c. malfunction of the oxygen analyzer
    d. patient may receive a lethal dose of the medication
11. While suctioning the endotracheal tube following a CPT treatment, the patient becomes bradycardic. Which of the following should the respiratory care practitioner do?
    a. continue the procedure, but shorten the duration of suctioning
    b. stop the procedure and order a stat chest x-ray
    c. when done, select a larger catheter and use less negative pressure
    d. stop the procedure, hyperoxygenate the patient, and shorten the duration of suction with subsequent attempts
12. The main indication for oxygen administration is:
    a. increasing altitude
    b. barotrauma
    c. hypoxemia
    d. hyperventilation
13. Which of the following is true regarding gaseous oxygen?
    a. It supports and intensifies combustion.
    b. It causes spontaneous combustion in plastics.
    c. It is the sole causative factor in the development of ROP.
    d. Its atmospheric concentration is higher at sea level.
14. A bubble humidifier is best used with what type of oxygen administration device?
    a. ventilator
    b. head box
    c. cannula
    d. incubator
15. A physician orders a pediatric patient to be on an F_iO_2 of 35%. Which of the following devices would best deliver the ordered F_iO_2?
    a. cannula at 3 L/min
    b. simple mask at 6 L/min
    c. nonrebreathing mask
    d. Venturi mask

REFERENCES

1. Gale R, et al. Accumulation of carbon dioxide in oxygen hoods, infant cots and incubators. *Pediatrics.* 60:454, 1977.
2. Avery GB, Fletcher MA, MacDonald MG. *Pathophysiology and Management of the Newborn.* 5th ed. Philadelphia, PA: JB Lippincott Co., 1999.
3. Lewis R. Chest physical therapy. In: Barnhard SL, Czervinske MP, eds. *Perinatal and Pediatric Respiratory Care.* Philadelphia, PA: WB Saunders Co., 1995.
4. Ward JJ. Lung sounds: easy to hear, hard to describe [editorial]. *Resp Care.* 34(1):17–19, 1989.
5. Fink JB, Jue PK. Humidity and aerosol therapy for pediatrics. In: Barnhart SL, Czervinske MP, eds. *Perinatal and Pediatric Respiratory Care.* Philadelphia, PA: WB Saunders Co, 1995.
6. Southgate WM. Aerosolized pharmacotherapy in the neonate. *Neonatal Network.* 14:29–36, 1995.
7. Pisut FM. Comparison of medication delivery by T-nebulizer with inspiratory and expiratory reservoir. *Resp Care.* 34:985–988, 1989.
8. Salyer JW, et al. The effect of continuous in-line nebulization on tidal volume during ventilation of an infant lung model [abstract]. *Resp Care.* 35:1121, 1990.

BIBLIOGRAPHY AND SUGGESTED READINGS

Aloan CA. *Respiratory Care of the Newborn: A Clinical Manual.* 2nd ed. Philadelphia, PA: JB Lippincott Co., 1997.

Andersen JB, Falk M. Chest physiotherapy in the pediatric age group. *Resp Care.* 36:546–554, 1991.

Bloom RS, Cropley C. *Textbook of Neonatal Resuscitation.* Dallas: American Heart Association/American Academy of Pediatrics, 1994.

Burton GG, et al. *Respiratory Care, a Guide to Clinical Practice,* 4th ed. Philadelphia, PA: JB Lippincott Co., 1997.

Dantzker DR, MacIntyre NR, Bakow ED. *Comprehensive Respiratory Care.* Philadelphia, PA: WB Saunders Co., 1995.

Goldsmith JP, Karotkin EH. *Assisted Ventilation of the Neonate.* 5th ed. Philadelphia: WB Saunders Co., 2010.

Hardy KA. A review of airway clearance: new techniques, indications, and recommendations. *Resp Care.* 39:440–452, 1994.

Hierholzer WJ, chairman. Guideline for prevention of nosocomial pneumonia: Centers for Disease Control and Prevention. *Resp Care.* 39:1191–1236, 1994.

Kacmarek RM. Ribavirin and pentamidine aerosols: caregiver beware [editorial]. *Resp Care.* 35:1034–1035, 1990.

Kacmarek RM, et al. *Current Respiratory Care.* Burlington, VT: BC Decker Inc., 1988.

McIlwaine M. Physiotherapy and airway clearance techniques and devices. *Paediatric Respiratory Reviews.* 7S:S220–S222, 2006.

McPherson SP. *Respiratory Therapy Equipment.* 9th ed. St. Louis, MO: CV Mosby Co., 2013.

Pilbeam SP. *Mechanical Ventilation: Physiological and Clinical Applications.* 5th ed. St. Louis, MO: Mosby, 2012.

Sreenan C, Lemke RP, Hudson-Madson A, Osiovich H. High-flow nasal cannulae in the management of apnea of prematurity: a comparison with conventional nasal continuous positive airway pressure. *Pediatrics.* 107:1081–1083,2001.

Shapiro BA, Peruzzi WT, Kozlowski-Templin R. *Clinical Application of Blood Gases.* 5th ed. St. Louis, MO: Mosby, 1994.

Taussig LM, Landau LI. *Pediatric Respiratory Medicine.* 2nd ed. St. Louis, MO: Mosby, 2008.

Tucker SM. *Pocket Guide to Fetal Monitoring and Assessment.* 7th ed. St. Louis, MO: Mosby, 2012.

CHAPTER 14

Pharmacology

OBJECTIVES

Upon completion of this chapter, the reader should be able to:

1. List and discuss the physiologic factors and mechanisms of drug transfer across the placenta.
2. Define a teratogenic substance and describe its actions on the fetus.
3. Discuss each of the following as it relates to neonatal pharmacokinetics. Include a description of the routes of absorption and the methods of distribution.
   a. Absorption
   b. Distribution
   c. Metabolism
   d. Excretion
4. Briefly describe how antibiotics work against bacteria, fungi, and viruses.
5. List the nine categories of antibiotics and at least one antibiotic from each category.
6. For each of the following cardiovascular conditions, describe at least one drug that is used in its treatment:
   a. Congestive heart failure
   b. Closure of the ductus arteriosus
   c. Pulmonary hypertension
   d. Hypotension
   e. Edema
7. List at least one drug from each of the following categories of respiratory medications. For each drug listed, describe briefly its indications and dosage:
   a. Sympathomimetic
   b. Parasympatholytic
   c. Steroid
   d. Antiviral
   e. Mucolytic

8. Describe at least one drug from each of the following categories. Include the indications and adverse effects:
   a. Anticonvulsant
   b. Steroid
   c. Sedative
   d. Paralytic
9. Describe the effects of maternal drug abuse on the fetus.

KEY TERMS

active transport	facilitated diffusion	pheochromocytoma
anuria	hydrolysis	pseudocholinesterase
beta-lactam	malignant hyperthermia	reduction
conjugation	ototoxic	simple diffusion
dyscrasias	oxidation	teratogens
extravasation	pharmacokinetics	ultrafiltration

INTRODUCTION

The study of pharmacology in the neonatal and pediatric populations is a complicated, intricate, and challenging subject. Therapeutic actions and adverse effects of many drugs may be quite different in neonates than in older children or adults. This is due to continuous changes that occur as the child develops, with respect to growth, and the associated pharmacodynamic responses.

Only 25% of all U.S. Food and Drug Administration (FDA) approved drugs are labeled as safe and effective in children. The available data for the remaining 75% of drugs are inadequate to allow for FDA approval in the pediatric population.

This chapter outlines many of the complicated and challenging factors associated with drug therapy in the neonatal and pediatric populations as well as defining therapeutic parameters for many of the drugs used in the treatment of neonates.

As technology improves, new medicines are constantly being added to the assortment used in neonatal and pediatric care. For this reason, it is impossible to provide an updated list of all drugs currently being used. It is strongly recommended that the respiratory therapist have at her/his disposal a current neonatal/pediatric pharmacologic manual for the latest information on drugs, dosages, and their uses.

PLACENTAL DRUG TRANSFER

Soranus of Ephesus during the second century A.D. wrote: "Even if a woman transgresses some or all of the rules mentioned (i.e., administration of drugs, sternutatives, pungent substances, and drunkenness, especially during the first trimester) and yet miscarriage of the fetus does not take place, let no one assume that the fetus has not been injured at all. For it has been harmed: it is weakened, becomes retarded in growth, less well nourished, and in general, more easily injured and susceptible to harmful agents; it becomes misshapen and of ignoble soul."[1] This shows an early understanding of the effects of maternal drug use on the fetus. This chapter begins by examining those factors that determine the effects of drugs on the fetus.

Physiologic Factors

Several factors should be kept in mind when considering the effects of drugs on the fetus. The extent to which drugs cross the placenta from the mother to the fetus varies, but many drugs reach concentrations in the fetus of 50% to 100% of the levels in maternal blood. The total amount of blood protein is less in the fetus and often results in more free drug, especially for drugs that are highly protein bound in the maternal blood.

Mechanisms of Placental Drug Transfer

The major mechanisms by which drugs cross the placenta are: **ultrafiltration**, **simple diffusion**, **facilitated diffusion**, **active transport**, and breaks in the placental villi. Ultrafiltration occurs as the placenta acts as a semipermeable membrane with maternal hydrostatic forces pushing drugs with low molecular weight through to the fetal side. Some substances readily pass through the placenta to the fetus by simple diffusion, which is often the result of a concentration gradient existing between the fetus and the mother. When the transfer of a drug across the placenta is aided by proteins in the membrane, it is called facilitated diffusion. Active transport occurs when the drug is moved across the placental membranes against the concentrations gradient. This process uses energy from ATP to accomplish. Drug transfer across the placenta is determined by the concentration difference across the placenta, the lipid solubility of the drug, the degree of ionization of the drug, and the molecular weight of the drug. Figure 14–1 outlines the process of drug transfer across the placenta.

Effects on the Fetus

Many drugs have been known to cause physical and/or mental developmental abnormalities in the embryo or fetus. These are known as **teratogens** or teratogenic substances.

Teratogens may cause spontaneous abortion, congenital malformations, intrauterine growth retardation, mental retardation, and carcinogenesis. The effects of teratogens are dependent on several factors. Those factors include the dose of drug that actually reaches the embryo or fetus, the length of exposure to the teratogen, the gestational age of the fetus at the time of exposure, and other drugs concurrently being taken by the mother.

Generally, the first trimester of pregnancy is the most critical time for teratogens to have an effect; however, drugs may also have teratogenic effects during the second and third trimesters.

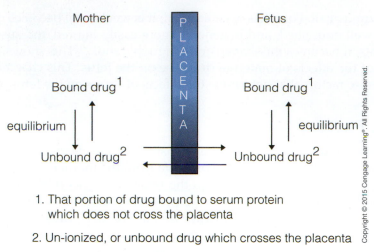

1. That portion of drug bound to serum protein which does not cross the placenta

2. Un-ionized, or unbound drug which crosses the placenta

FIGURE 14–1. Drug transfer across the placenta.

Drugs may have an adverse effect on labor and delivery if taken late in pregnancy. Additionally, the neonate is exposed to the drug, which could lead to prolonged exposure and toxicity.

It is important to remember that any drug, whether prescribed, or over-the-counter, has the potential of crossing the placenta and entering the fetal circulation. All side effects associated with that medication will also affect the fetus. For this reason, a thorough medical history is important as well as patient education to the mother at the commencement of the pregnancy to assure she understands the potential harm to her fetus.

NEONATAL PHARMACOKINETICS

Pharmacokinetics is a general term for the process by which drugs enter the body (absorption), are distributed throughout the system (distribution), are changed or altered from the original compound (metabolism), and eventually leave the body (excretion). This section will describe this process, with emphasis on the neonatal population (birth to one year).

Absorption

A drug may enter the system through a variety of mechanisms: through the gastrointestinal tract, intramuscularly, by topical absorption through the skin and respiratory tract, and through direct intravenous administration.

Gastrointestinal Tract The absorption of drugs from the gastrointestinal (GI) tract is often regulated by pH-dependent diffusion and gastric emptying time.

At birth, gastric pH is between 6 and 8 but falls to a pH of 1 to 3 in the first 24 hours after birth. This decrease is not present in premature neonates because of an immature acid-secreting mechanism. The pH then returns close to neutral, and there is no further acid secretion until the 10th and 15th day after birth. Normal adult values for GI acidity are reached by about 2 years of age. The difference in pH of the stomach for the neonate may affect the normal absorption of both basic and acidic drugs such as penicillins, phenobarbital, and phenytoin.

Gastric emptying time in the newborn infant may be as long as 6 to 8 hours and does not approach the adult values until 6 months of age. Many factors can influence the gastric emptying time, including gestational maturity, postnatal age, and type of oral feeding (human milk or formula), and unpredictable peristalsis in the newborn.

Intramuscular Administration The intramuscular absorption rate of drugs in the newborn is altered owing to many factors. Factors include variability in the blood flow to various muscles, a decrease in muscular contractions, and the low muscle mass in the neonate.

Skin The absorption of drugs through the skin of the newborn is greatly increased. Newborns generally have thin, well-hydrated skin, which allows for increased permeability and, therefore, enhanced drug absorption.

Respiratory Tract The combination of extensive vascularization, large surface area, and thin tissue separating the airway lumen and blood vasculature makes the respiratory tract ideally suited for absorption of drugs. Although most drugs administered to the respiratory tract have a topical effect, certain drugs used during resuscitation are purposely instilled into the lungs to achieve rapid systemic absorption. Drugs that may be given this route include lidocaine, atropine, epinephrine and naloxone.

Intravenous Administration Intravenous administration of drugs bypasses all of the previously described complications of drug absorption due to the drug being readily available in predictable amounts within the system. The effective dose of a drug can therefore be more accurately calculated.

Distribution

Following the absorption or injection of a drug into the bloodstream, it is distributed into interstitial, cellular, and extracellular fluids. The rate and extent of distribution are dependent on the physical and chemical properties of the drug.

Lipid-Soluble Drugs In general, lipid-soluble drugs that readily cross cell membranes are distributed throughout all fluid areas. Lipid-soluble drugs are distributed very rapidly into the heart, brain, liver, kidney, and other highly vascularized tissues and more slowly into muscle tissue and fat cells. Drugs that are less lipid soluble and that do not readily cross cell membranes may gather in tissues at higher concentrations than in plasma.

Many drugs are bound to plasma proteins (mostly plasma albumin), and their protein binding ability influences their activity throughout the system. Lipid-soluble drugs generally have a high affinity to be protein bound. Often, more than 90% of a lipid-soluble drug will be bound to plasma proteins. This leaves only 10% of unbound or free drug available to cross cell membranes and exhibit its maximal pharmacologic activity.

Binding to Serum Proteins Many drug interactions and toxicity reactions occur when drugs compete for binding to serum proteins, thus increasing the unbound portion of one or more of the drugs being administered. Several factors can significantly reduce the plasma protein binding of many drugs in the premature and full-term newborn. These include a reduced plasma protein concentration, a lower binding capacity of fetal serum albumin, a lower blood pH, and increased level of unconjugated bilirubin competing with the drug-binding sites. These are all factors to consider when calculating drug dosages for premature infants.

Volume of Distribution Another area for consideration when calculating dosages in premature infants is the volume of distribution. The volume of distribution is a proportional factor that relates the amount of drug in the body to the plasma concentration. The volume of distribution of many drugs in infants is different from adults for two main reasons. First, neonates have a decreased plasma protein binding capacity, and second, neonates have an increased extracellular fluid volume per kilogram of body weight. Extracellular fluid areas include the GI tract, the cerebrospinal fluid, aqueous humor, endolymph fluid, and joint fluids.

Extracellular fluid volume decreases from 50% of body weight in premature infants to 35% in 4- to 6-month-old infants, to 25% in 1-year-olds, and to 20% in adults. Total body water decreases from 86% in premature infants to 70% in full-term infants. This implies that the loading dose (on a mg/kg basis) of a water-soluble drug would decrease as the infant's age and weight increased.

Metabolism

Metabolism is the changing or alteration of the drug to a different form, either active or inactive, as the next step in the pharmacokinetic process. The primary site within the system where drug metabolism takes place is the liver; however, drug metabolism is also accomplished in other areas such as the plasma, kidney, and the gastrointestinal tract.

The liver produces many enzymes that aid the metabolism of drugs. In the premature and newborn infant, the ability of the liver enzyme system to mediate the metabolism of drugs is greatly reduced.

There are basically four types of drug metabolizing biochemical reactions that take place in the liver: conjugation, oxidation, reduction, and hydrolysis. Conjugation is the process of turning substances into a hydrophilic state, which allows their secretion. Oxidation and reduction are the processes of either adding (oxidation) or removing (reduction) an oxygen atom from the compound, effectively aiding its metabolism. Cytochrome P450 is the major enzyme in the liver responsible for these actions. Finally, hydrolysis is the process of adding a water molecule to a substance, which causes cleavage in the chemical bonds and aids in its degradation and removal from the body. The premature infant generally has a decreased ability for drug metabolism by all of these mechanisms, which is one of the factors that causes an increased half-life of the drug or drugs being administered. Half-life is the amount of time required to reduce a drug level to one half its initial value.

Several drugs, such as phenobarbital, have the effect of increasing the enzymatic activity of the liver. Exposure to these drugs may require the dosages of other drugs to be reevaluated.

Excretion

Because most drugs are poorly metabolized in the premature infant, the excretion of a drug is the most important factor in the termination of a drug's effects. Drugs can be eliminated from the body through various routes, including the kidneys (primary site of elimination), via biliary and fecal excretion, and through other body fluids such as sweat and saliva.

The renal function, both glomerular filtration rate (GFR) and tubular secretion, in premature and full-term infants is not completely developed at the time of birth. The renal function of infants does not achieve the same level as in adults until the child is between 6 months and 1 year of age. The creatinine clearance, as a measure of renal function, of full-term infants is generally 20 mL/min and increases to 60 mL/min by one month of age. In contrast, the creatinine clearance of premature infants (less than 34 weeks' gestation) is 16 mL/min and only increases to 40 mL/min by one month of age.

Drugs that are not extensively metabolized and are primarily excreted through the kidneys are, therefore, eliminated more slowly in premature infants and dosage adjustments must be made. Drugs that rely on the GFR for their effect (i.e., diuretics) may have to be increased due to the reduction in GFR.

MEDICATIONS

The study of pharmacology could be a lifetime study, especially when one considers that there are several thousand drugs available for use. To list each drug used in the neonatal/pediatric population could fill an entire volume. The approach to pharmacology in this chapter is to give the reader a general overview of therapeutics in the neonatal and pediatric populations. Antibiotic therapy makes up a large portion of therapeutics and, therefore, is treated differently from the other medications. An overview of antibiotic therapeutics is given, with the specific medications discussed in their groups so the reader can appreciate the role of antibiotics in the care of neonates, infants and children. Because they represent a smaller portion of drugs used, the other medications discussed are considered individually.

Antibiotics

A wealth of antibiotics is available for treating a variety of infections, and each year many new antibiotics become available. Therapeutics with antibiotics is a science in and of itself. Since the discovery of penicillin many years ago, antibiotic therapy has become complex and spread out with numerous drugs falling under various categories of drugs. Before using an antibiotic, there are three basic principles that must be observed: 1) Unless the situation is life-threatening, identify the infective organism whenever possible. Identification of the organism allows the respiratory therapist to use the appropriate antibiotic for which the organism is susceptible. 2) Always consider the pharmacologic and toxicologic aspects of the drug before it is started. 3) The response of the patient to the drug is extremely variable in the neonatal and pediatric population.

When using antibiotics, there are areas of consideration that the respiratory therapist must be aware of in anticipation of possible problems. Perhaps the biggest issue is the unwarranted use of antibiotics to treat every illness, particularly minor ones. Most parents are conditioned that their child will heal more quickly when an antibiotic is used. The respiratory therapist is in a position to teach parents the risks of antibiotic overuse, including the emergence of resistant organisms. Another special consideration in the pediatric population includes the ototoxic nature of the aminoglycosides. In general, there are risks to the use of antibiotics that require special consideration every time they are used. Depending on the antibiotic used, anywhere from 5% to 25% of patients will develop diarrhea.[2] *Clostridium difficile* is becoming a more frequent complication of antibiotic use, especially clindamycin, cephalosporins, and the fluoroquinolones.[3] Additionally, about 2% of patients receiving antibiotics will develop a skin reaction and 1 in 5000 will develop an anaphylactic reaction.[4, 5] Two related syndromes that are severe reactions are toxic epidermal necrolysis (TEN), and Stevens-Johnson syndrome. TEN has the highest mortality at 30–35%, with the mortality rate of Stevens-Johnson around 5–15%. Both have an incidence of around 1–3/million.[6]

Groups of antibiotics include the penicillins, cephalosporins, aminoglycosides, macrolides, quinolones, tetracyclines, sulfonamides, antifungals, and antivirals.

Penicillins Penicillin is one of the earliest discovered and most widely used antibiotic agents. Penicillin antibiotics are historically significant because they are the first drugs that were effective against many serious diseases.

Mode of Action Penicillins are **beta-lactam** antibiotics. The term beta-lactam refers to the chemical structure of the drug. The cell wall of the bacteria has several layers. The beta-lactam drugs penetrate the outer membrane through small canals in structures called porins. At the level of the cytoplasmic membrane, enzymes that are sensitive to the beta-lactams, called penicillin binding proteins (PBPs), are found. When the drug attaches to the PBPs, two processes kill the bacterial cell.

First, the attachment of the drug causes interference in cell wall synthesis, and second, the cell releases an enzyme that is autolytic and lyses the cell.

Classification and Uses There are four classifications of penicillins available. These are natural penicillins, penicillinase-resistant penicillins, amminopenicillins, and antipseudomonal penicillins.

The natural penicillins include penicillin G, which is combined with benzathine to provide a slow release of the drug. Penicillin G is used for gram-positive bacteria such as streptococci, and gram-negative coverage for pneumococci, *Haemophilus influenzae,* and gonococci. The second is penicillin V, which is acid-resistant and better tolerates oral administration. It has the same coverage as penicillin G, but is thought to be less active against gram-negative bacteria.

In an attempt to survive, some bacteria have developed the ability to produce an enzyme that inactivates the beta-lactam drugs. This enzyme is called penicillinase, or beta-lactamase. This class of penicillin is termed penicillinase-resistant penicillins. Several of the penicillin drugs are resistant to this enzyme and are effective against those bacteria that produce it. There are numerous reports, however, of bacteria, especially staphylococcus, that have become resistant to these antibiotics. *Staphylococcus aureus*, which has become resistant to methicillin, is called methicillin-resistant *Staphylococcus aureus*, or MRSA. Reports of resistance to this antibiotic have been documented. Any drug that is said to be effective against staphylococcus should be understood to not include MRSA.

The penicillinase-resistant group includes methicillin, nafcillin, cloxacillin, dicloxacillin, and oxacillin. These drugs are used almost exclusively to treat resistant strains of staphylococcus.

The aminopenicillins include ampicillin and amoxicillin. These drugs are used to treat gram-positive bacteria (except *S. aureus*), and gram-negatives such as *Shigella, H. influenzae, Salmonella, Proteus mirabilis*, and *Escherichia coli.* For use with bacteria that are producing beta-lactamase, ampicillin is combined with sulbactam, and amoxicillin is combined with clavulanic acid. These two chemicals inhibit beta-lactamase and prevent the drug from being inactivated by the enzyme. Group B streptococci frequently colonize the vaginal tract in healthy women. A neonate can acquire the organism either vertically while in utero or during delivery. The transmission rate from mothers colonized with group B strep to neonates delivered vaginally is approximately 50%; however, only 1%–2% of colonized neonates go on to develop invasive infection.[7] Although the infection rate is low, it is increased with premature delivery and prolonged rupture of the membranes. Currently, the approach is to treat culture-positive pregnant females prophylactically with penicillin or ampicillin initially.[8]

Antipseudomonal penicillins have been chemically altered to make them more useful against difficult bacteria such as pseudomonas. These drugs include azlocillin, mezlocillin, piperacillin, ticarcillin, and carbenicillin. For use with beta-lactamase producing bacteria, clavulanic acid is combined with ticarcillin and another anti-beta-lactamase drug, tazobactam, is combined with piperacillin. The addition of these chemicals makes the drugs useful against staphylococcus, enterococcus, and *Bacteroides fragilis.*

Cephalosporins The popularity of cephalosporins is based on their lower allergenic and toxicity risks as well as a broad spectrum of activity.

Mode of Action The cephalosporins are similar to the penicillins chemically in that they also have a beta-lactam ring and, thus, act on the bacteria in the same manner as the penicillins. Cephalosporins are often used in patients who are allergic to the penicillins. Their chemical structure makes them less susceptible to bacteria that produce beta-lactamase.

Classification and Uses The cephalosporins have been developed in generations (first, second, and third), with each successive generation of drugs becoming broader spectrum.

The first-generation cephalosporins are most active against gram-positive bacteria such as staphylococcus and streptococcus, and moderately active against gram-negative bacteria, such as *E. coli*, *Klebsiella*, and *Proteus*. These drugs are often used in surgical prophylaxis, especially before orthopedic and cardiovascular surgeries. Drugs in this category include cephalexin, cephalothin, cefadroxil, cephradine, cephapirin, and cefazolin.

Second-generation cephalosporins are more potent than first generations against gram-negative bacteria, while maintaining good gram-positive activity. Second-generation cephalosporins are often used to treat community acquired pneumonias. Penetration of the CNS is probably limited in these drugs. Drugs include cefaclor, cefamandole, cefoxitin, cefuroxime, cefonicid, ceforanide, cefmetazole, cefotetan, cefprozil, cefpodoxime, and loracarbef.

Third-generation cephalosporins possess the broadest spectrum and have the most potent activity against the gram-negative bacteria. Third-generation cephalosporins are further divided into those with pseudomonal activity and those without. The antipseudomonal drugs include ceftazidime and cefoperazone. Those without pseudomonal activity include cefotaxime, ceftizoxime, cefriaxone, and cefixime.

Other Beta-Lactam Drugs There are two other drug categories included with the beta-lactams, which are not penicillins or cephalosporins. Because of their broad activity, they are often humorously referred to as the "Gorillacillins." These drugs are the monobactams and the carbapenems. The monobactam drug, aztreonam, is effective against aminoglycoside- and cephalosporin-resistant gram-negative organisms. Its spectrum of activity is the same as the aminoglycosides, without the nephrotoxic (damage to the kidneys) and **ototoxic**, (damage to the auditory nerve and cochlea) side effects. The carbapenems, imipenem and meropenem, are synthetic agents that have broad-spectrum activity against gram-positive and gram-negative bacteria; they are also used to treat MRSA where it is resistant to vancomycin.

Aminoglycosides The aminoglycosides include gentamicin, kanamycin, neomycin, spectinomycin, streptomycin, amikacin, netilmicin, and tobramycin.

Mode of Action While not entirely understood, it is believed that the aminoglycosides inhibit bacterial protein synthesis by irreversibly binding the ribosomal subunits, thus "freezing" the elongation process.

Classification and Uses The aminoglycosides are considered the cornerstone of gram-negative bacterial infections. Aminoglycosides are often used in combination with other antibiotics to reduce the potential for resistance and to enhance the bacteriocidal activity. Uses include the treatment for gram-negative sepsis or bacteremia, pneumonias, and enterococcal infections.

Macrolides Drugs currently available in the macrolide group include erythromycin, clarithromycin, and azithromycin. Erythromycin is the prototype drug, while clarithromycin and azithromycin are newer-generation drugs.

Mode of Action The macrolides are similar to the aminoglycosides in that they bind to the ribosomal subunit of the bacteria. An important difference is that the bind is reversible, making them bacteriostatic instead of bacteriocidal.

Classification and Uses The macrolides have both gram-positive and gram-negative coverage. Organisms susceptible to macrolides include streptococcus and staphylococcus, *H. influenzae*, *Neisseria gonorrhoeae*, *N. catarrhalis*, *Legionella*, *Mycoplasma pneumoniae*, *Chlamydia pneumonia*, and *C. trachomatis*, *Mycobacterium*, and *Toxoplasma gondii*.

Hazards The major hazard associated with the macrolides is the inhibition of hepatic metabolism of certain drugs resulting in elevated serum concentrations and potential toxicities. These drugs include theophylline, carbamazepine, astemizole, terfenadine, and cisapride.

Quinolones This class of drug, also called 4-fluoroquinolones, includes ciprofloxacin, ofloxacin, lomefloxacin, norfloxacin, and enoxacin.

Mode of Action The quinolones inhibit DNA gyrase, the enzyme that nicks strands of DNA to promote the twisting or untwisting of the DNA strand, and then reseals the nicks. By inhibiting this enzyme, DNA replication is inhibited and the bacteria are effectively eliminated.

Classification and Uses In general, the quinolones are not used as first line agents. They are effective against staphylococcus, but have poor activity against streptococcus and because of this are generally not recommended for gram-positive infections. Gram-negative activity include *E. coli*, *Klebsiella*, *P. mirabilis*, *Morganella*, and *Pseudomonas* (if used combined with an aminoglycoside).

Hazards Quinolones inhibit hepatic enzymes and can cause increased serum levels, and possible toxicity in drugs that are hepatically metabolized. The quinolones are also extensively excreted renally, and the dose should be adjusted in patients with renal problems.

Tetracyclines and Chloramphenicol Drugs in this category include tetracycline, chlortetracycline, oxytetracycline, demeclocycline, doxycycline, minocycline, methacycline, and chloramphenicol.

Mode of Action The tetracyclines and chloramphenicol prevent protein synthesis at the level of the binding of transfer RNA/amino acid complexes to the ribosomes. This action disables the bacteria's ability to reproduce and, thus, makes tetracyclines bacteriostatic.

Classification and Uses All tetracyclines are active against most gram-positive cocci, and against many gram-negative bacilli. Mycoplasma and Chlamydia are also inhibited. The tetracyclines are often used as a substitute for patients who cannot tolerate, or are allergic to erythromycin. Chloramphenicol is the drug of choice to treat typhoid fever. It is also used to treat *H. influenzae*, *N. meningitidis*, and *S. pneumoniae* and is bactericidal against these organisms. Because choloramphenicol penetrates well into the eye and brain, it is effective at treating susceptible infections in those organs.

Hazards Tetracyclines should not be used in patients younger than 8 years old due to the fact that they can permanently stain the teeth. Hazards with choloramphenicol include: aplastic anemia, which has a low incidence but high mortality; dose-related bone marrow depression; and "gray baby syndrome," which is manifest as circulatory collapse in premature infants and neonates with doses in excess of 50 mg/kg/day or serum levels >20–25 mcg/mL.

Sulfonamides and Trimethoprim The sulfonamide, sulfamethoxazole, is given with trimethoprim, providing a raised activity level and widened spectrum of activity than when used alone. Other sulfonamides include sulfisoxazole, sulfadiazine, sulfamethizole, sulfadoxine, and sulfasalazine.

Mode of Action In order for a bacterium to reproduce, para-aminobenzoic acid (PABA) must be converted to folic acid. The steps in formation are first PABA, then dihydrofolate, tetrahydrofolate, and finally, folic acid. The sulfonamide drugs prevent the conversion of PABA to dihydrofolate, and trimethoprim prevents the conversion of dihydrofolate to tetrahydrofolate. The two, therefore, work synergistically to stop bacterial reproduction.

Classification and Uses The sulfonamides are used to treat various gram-positive and some gram-negative infections, such as *E. coli*, *Klebsiella*, *Proteus*, *Shigella*, *Xanthomonas maltophilia*, and *Nocardia*. Trimethoprim has activity against many gram-positive cocci, and most gram-negative rods.

Hazards Sulfonamides have been associated with acute hemolytic anemia, aplastic anemia, agranulocytosis, thrombocytopenia, and leukopenia. The sulfonamides also have a higher than normal rate of hypersensitivity reactions. Because a large percentage of trimethoprim is eliminated by the kidneys, the dosage must be closely monitored in patients with renal insufficiency.

Antifungals Fungal infections are commonly seen as an opportunistic skin infection, often occurring in areas that are warm and moist. These infections are usually treated with topical antifungals, but may require oral therapy if severe. Fungal infections of the blood and CNS carry a high risk of mortality and morbidity and must be treated aggressively with oral antifungal agents. The oral antifungals include amphotericin B, nystatin, flucytosine, ketoconazole, miconazole, griseofulvin, fluconazole, and intraconazole.

Mode of Action Most of the antifungals work by inhibiting enzymes in the cell membrane and binding membrane sterols, making them more permeable.

Classification and Uses Antifungals vary greatly in their ability to treat infections, and it is necessary to identify the organism before treating, to ensure coverage. In general, the antifungals are used to treat *Aspergillus, Candida, Blastomyces, Coccidioides, Cryptococci, Histoplasma, Leishmania,* and *Sporotrichum.*

Hazards One of the most common side effects seen with IV antifungals, especially amphotericin B, is the so-called "shake and bake" syndrome, consisting of chills, fever, headache, myalgias, hypotension, nausea, and vomiting. Chronic use of oral antifungals can lead to nephrotoxicity, thrombophlebitis, and anemia.

Antivirals Common antivirals include amantadine, rimantadine, acyclovir, famcyclovir, valacyclovir, vidarabine, zidovudine, ganciclovir, didanosine, and zalcitabine. Ribavirin, an aerosolized antiviral agent, is discussed in more detail below.

Mode of Action In order to understand how antivirals work, it is useful to review how viruses reproduce. When a virus attaches itself to a cell, it injects an enzyme messenger into the cell, which forces the cell to replicate the DNA of the virus. Chemically, the antiviral drug is similar to the amino acid thymidine. As the antiviral drug is placed in the DNA chain in place of the thymidine, further attachment of amino acids is blocked and, thus, the reproduction of the virus is stopped. It is for this reason that antiviral drugs are referred to as chain terminators.

Classifications and Uses Most of the antiviral drugs are used to treat HIV related illness. Other indications are herpes simplex infections, cytomegalovirus retinitis, varicella zoster, and influenza virus infections.

Hazards Each antiviral drug has its own side effects and hazards and many are dose related. Mild effects may include nausea and vomiting. More advanced hazards include phlebitis, CNS toxicity, depressed bone marrow function, convulsions, pancreatitis, and peripheral neuropathy.

Ribavirin Ribavirin is a broad-spectrum antiviral drug that is specifically used in the neonatal population for the treatment of bronchiolitis caused by respiratory syncytial virus (RSV). Ribavirin is delivered via a unique device called the small particle aerosol generator (SPAG). The use of this device is covered in Chapter 13.

Ribavirin comes as 6 g of a sterile powder that is reconstituted by adding 50 to 100 mL of sterile water with no additives. This solution is then transferred to a sterile

500 mL flask in the SPAG unit and further diluted with sterile water to a volume of 300 mL. This final concentration contains 20 mg of drug per mL. With this concentration, the SPAG unit delivers a mist of approximately 190 mg of ribavirin per liter. The dose delivered to the respiratory tract can then be estimated by using the equation in Table 14–1.

The dose and administration of ribavirin for the treatment of RSV is the same for ventilated and nonventilated patients. Treatment to ventilated patients is covered in Chapter 13. The mist from the SPAG unit is delivered to the patient via a hood, tent, or mask. When given via a hood or tent, the aerosol is delivered at a rate of 15 Lpm, and at 12 Lpm when delivered to a mask. The patient receives the aerosol continuously for 12–18 hours daily for 3–7 days. The exact length of treatment is determined individually for each patient and is based on the severity of illness, age of the patient, and the presence of underlying diseases.

Evidence from animal studies shows a potential for teratogencity with exposure to ribavirin. Additionally, no established data defining safe levels of exposure have been produced. Until studies show that exposure does not provide a risk, health care providers and visitors must protect themselves, and be protected from exposure to ribavirin. This is true especially for those females who are pregnant, or trying to become pregnant. The most frequent adverse effects reported are eye irritation, headache, nasal and throat irritation, pharyngitis, nausea, dizziness, fatigue, and rash.

The amount of environmental exposure varies tremendously depending on the method of delivery, length of exposure, number of patients being treated in a room, size of the room, room ventilation, administration schedules, and the integrity of the SPAG unit. To minimize environmental exposure, several precautionary measures have been devised. When a tent or hood is used, an outer hood or cover can be placed over the primary hood or tent. A vacuum tube is then placed in the space between the outer and inner covers. The idea behind this procedure is that any excess ribavirin delivered to the inner hood or tent, will escape to the space between the two covers. It is then evacuated through the vacuum tube to the outside, or through filters that remove the ribavirin. Other measures include requiring all who enter the room to wear gowns, gloves, goggles, and masks. Surgical masks do not filter the ribavirin. This makes the use of special, small particulate filter masks necessary.

Table 14–1

ESTIMATING RIBAVIRIN DELIVERY

TOTAL DOSE = MV × DOI × 0.19 × 0.7

MV = Minute Volume (liters)
DOI = Duration of inhalation (minutes)
0.19 = Concentration of ribavirin delivered
0.7 = Fraction of inhaled dose deposited in the respiratory tract

Except when immediate care is required, the SPAG unit should be shut off remotely, 10 to 15 minutes before entering the room. It is also recommended that ribavirin only be delivered in isolation rooms that are under negative pressure, have adequate air exchange, and vent to the outside.

Other Antibiotics Several other antibiotics exist that are not generally categorized. These include clinadamycin, lincomycin, vancomycin, and metronidazole. Clindamycin and lincomycin are limited for use with anaerobic infections and severe gram-positive infections. The primary use of vancomycin is in the treatment of MRSA, enterococci, and *Clostridia*. Metronidazole is very active against gram-negative anaerobes, amoebae, and *Trichomonas*.

Mucolytics Mucolytic drugs are designed to help loosen and clear the mucus from the airways by breaking up the sputum. Acetylcysteine (Mucomyst®) is the most commonly administered mucolytic. It is typically administered via aerosol, but oral forms also exist. It works by breaking the disulfide bonds in mucus, liquefying it and make it easier to expectorate. The aerosolized dose is typically 3 to 5 mL of a 20% solution administered three to four times daily. Alternatively, 6 to 10 mL of a 10% solution can be used.

Guiafenesin Guiafenesin is available over the counter and is found in many products marketed for cold relief. In addition to its mild mucolytic effect, it is also a mild antitussive. It is thought to work by increasing the volume and reducing the viscosity of mucus. Pediatric dosage of the immediate release formulation:

- Less than 2 years: 12 mg/kg/day orally in 6 divided doses
- 2 to 5 years: 50 to 100 mg orally every 4 hours as needed, not to exceed 600 mg/day
- 6 to 11 years: 100 to 200 mg orally every 4 hours as needed, not to exceed 1.2 g/day
- 12 years or older: 200 to 400 mg orally every 4 hours as needed, not to exceed 2.4 g/day
- Pediatric dose of the sustained release formulation:
  - 2 to 5 years: 300 mg orally every 12 hours, not to exceed 600 mg/day
  - 6 to 11 years: 600 mg orally every 12 hours, not to exceed 1.2 g/day
  - 12 years or older: 600 to 1200 mg orally every 12 hours, not to exceed 2.4 g/day[9]

Dornase Alfa (Pulmozyme®) Dornase alfa is a recombinant human deoxyribonuclease which is an enzyme that selectively cleaves DNA. The primary use of dornase alfa is in patients with cystic fibrosis. The recommended dose for use in most cystic fibrosis patients is one 2.5 mg single-use ampule inhaled once daily using a recommended nebulizer.

Other Expectorants Erdosteine, bromhexine and carbocisteine are mucolytics used primarily in other countries. They have a mechanism of action similar to acetylcysteine. Iodinated glycerol is another mucolytic used primarily outside of the United States.

Cardiovascular Medications

There are many types and combinations of cardiovascular medications. In the neonatal and pediatric populations, they are most often used to control the rate, rhythm, or strength of the cardiac cycle.

Adenosine Adenosine is a purine nucleoside and plays a role in energy transfer

Indications Adenosine is indicated for the acute treatment of sustained paroxysmal supraventricular tachycardia (SVT).

Dosages The starting dose for adenosine is 50 mcg/kg given intravenously rapidly over 1 to 2 seconds. The dose is then increased 50 mcg/kg every 2 minutes until sinus rhythm returns, for a total of 250 mcg/kg.

Effects Adenosine is the active metabolite of adenosine triphosphate (ATP). Its action consists of depressing sinus node automaticity and AV conduction. Response is expected within 2 minutes of the dose.

Adverse Effects and Precautions The most common adverse effects are flushing, irritability, and dyspnea, which normally resolve within 1 minute. Transient arrhythmias have been known to develop between the termination of SVT and normal sinus rhythm. Thirty percent of patients treated have a recurrence of SVT.

Atropine Atropine is a naturally occurring drug that functions as a parasympatholytic.

Indications Atropine is used in the reversal of severe sinus bradycardia, especially in the presence of parasympathetic influences (drugs, carotid sinus reflex).

Dosages Atropine is given at a dosage of 0.01 to 0.03 mg/kg intravenously over a 1-minute period. It can also be given via the endotracheal tube at 2 to 3 times the intravenous dose, followed immediately by 1 mL of normal saline (NS).

Effects Atropine is an anticholinergic drug. As such, it blocks the parasympathetic receptors, thus reducing the stimulation of the parasympathetic branch that is causing bradycardia.

Adverse Effects and Precautions Cardiac arrhythmias have been reported, often during the first 2 minutes following administration. Because of its effects on the gastrointestinal tract, abdominal distention, and esophageal reflux may be increased.

Epinephrine Also known as adrenaline, epinephrine is a powerful sympathomimetic hormone.

Indications Epinephrine is used during resuscitation for the treatment of acute cardiovascular collapse. It may also be used as a short-term treatment for cardiac failure that is resistant to other drugs. Additionally, it is used subcutaneously in the treatment of acute bronchospasm.

Dosages For bradycardia and hypotension, epinephrine is given 0.1 to 0.3 mL/kg of a 1:10,000 concentration.

Effects As a powerful sympathomimetic agent, epinephrine causes an increase in the rate and force of heart contractions, dilation of the bronchial smooth muscles, and constriction of the peripheral vasculature.

Adverse Effects and Precautions Arrhythmias such as premature ventricular contractions and ventricular tachycardia may be seen. The vasoconstrictive effect may lead to renal vascular ischemia.

Digoxin (Lanoxin®) Digoxin is derived from the foxglove plant and is categorized as a cardiac glycoside.

Indications Digoxin is indicated for use in atrial fibrillation, atrial flutter, paroxysmal atrial tachycardia (PAT), cardiogenic shock, and all degrees of congestive heart failure (CHF). Congestive heart failure is the primary indication for use in neonates.

Dosages An initial loading dose of digoxin (known as digitalization) is required to provide peak concentrations in the affected tissues and should be dosed as shown in Table 14–2.
   The maintenance dose of digoxin is 20% to 30% of the digitalizing dose per day divided into two doses given every 12 hours. For example, the loading dose for a 2-kg preterm infant should be 30 to 50 mcg with a maintenance dose of 3 to 7.5 mcg administered every 12 hours. The relative dose of digoxin in infants is higher than in adults. This is due to a decreased digoxin receptor binding affinity in the neonatal myocardium. Digoxin can be administered orally, intravenously, or intramuscularly.

Effects The effect of digoxin involves both a direct action on cardiac muscle and the specialized conduction system and indirect action on the cardiovascular system, which is mediated by the autonomic nervous system. The indirect actions effectively depress the sinoatrial (SA) node and prolong conduction to the atrioventricular (AV)

Table 14–2

INITIAL LOADING DOSE FOR DIGOXIN

Preterm infants: 15–25 mcg/kg
Full-term infants: 20–30 mcg/kg
1–24 months: 30–50 mcg/kg

node. Direct actions include increasing the force of myocardial systolic contraction, increasing the refractory period of the AV node, and increasing the total peripheral resistance.

Contraindications Digoxin is contraindicated in patients with ventricular fibrillation, ventricular tachycardia, or who are hypersensitive to the drug.

Adverse Effects and Precautions Common adverse effects include vomiting, anorexia, bradycardia, and arrhythmias. These adverse effects relate to the narrow range of therapeutic and toxic concentrations that occur within the body, and close monitoring of cardiac function and blood levels for the drug should be performed.

Indomethacin Sodium Trihydrate (Indocin® IV) Indomethacin is a nonsteroidal anti-inflammatory (NSAID) drug that inhibits the production of prostaglandins.

Indications Indomethacin is indicated to close a hemodynamically significant patent ductus arteriosus (PDA). Clinical factors used to decide on its use include patient weights between 500 and 1750 g and a persistent PDA following 48 hours of fluid restriction, diuretics, digoxin, and respiratory support. Clinically, a hemodynamically significant PDA is identified by the presence of the following: respiratory distress, continuous murmur, hyperactive precordium, and cardiomegaly.

Dosages Indomethacin is administered to neonates in three doses given at 12- to 24-hour intervals by the intravenous route only. Table 14–3 shows the recommended dosages by age.

   If closure or significant reduction of the ductus arteriosus occurs after 48 hours or more from completion of the first course of therapy, no further doses are necessary. If the ductus arteriosus reopens, a second course of one to three doses may be given as described in Table 14–3.

Contraindications Indomethacin is contraindicated in infants who have proven or suspected untreated infections, bleeding (particularly intracranial hemorrhage or

Table 14–3

RECOMMENDED DOSAGE OF INDOMETHACIN

Age at First Dose	Dosage (mg/kg)		
	1st	2nd	3rd
Less than 48 hours	0.2	0.1	0.1
2–7 days	0.2	0.2	0.2
Greater than 7 days	0.2	0.25	0.25

gastrointestinal (GI) bleeding), thrombocytopenia, coagulation defects, or significant renal function impairment.

Adverse Effects Major adverse effects experienced with the use of indomethacin include bleeding and coagulation problems, renal dysfunction characterized by decreased urinary output and elevated serum creatinine, and GI bleeding. Apnea has been reported following administration of indomethacin. However, a causal relationship to indomethacin therapy has not been established.

Precautions The use of indomethacin may conceal the signs and symptoms of infection. The drug should be stopped if clinical signs and symptoms of liver disease develop. The drug may be very irritating and should be administered carefully to avoid leaking into the tissue (**extravasation**).

Alprostadil-Prostaglandin E1 (Prostin® VR Pediatric) As the name indicates, asprostadil is a prostaglandin.

Indications Alprostadil is indicated to maintain the patency of the ductus arteriosus until corrective surgery can be performed. It is used in neonates with congenital heart defects who depend on the patent ductus for survival.

Dosages Alprostadil is administered by continuous intravenous infusion into a large vein or through an umbilical artery catheter. The infusion should be started at a rate of 0.1 mcg/kg/min until an adequate therapeutic response is seen. The response is an increased PaO_2 for infants with restricted pulmonary blood flow or increased systemic blood pressure and blood pH in infants with restricted systemic blood flow. The rate of infusion should be reduced to as low a level as possible that still maintains an adequate response.

Effects Alprostadil causes vasodilation, inhibits platelet aggregation, and relaxes smooth muscle of the ductus arteriosus. Infants with an initially low PaO_2 value (less than 40 mmHg) appear to have a greater increase in blood oxygenation than those with PaO_2 values greater than 40 mmHg.

Contraindications There are no known contraindications to the use of alprostadil.

Adverse Effects Fever, seizures, flushing, bradycardia, hypotension, apnea, and diarrhea are several of the major adverse effects seen with alprostadil use.

Precautions Alprostadil should be infused for the shortest length of time in the lowest dose possible to produce positive effects. Use cautiously in infants with bleeding tendencies due to the drug's inhibition of platelet aggregation. Alprostadil should not be used in patients with respiratory distress syndrome. Routine or constant monitoring of arterial pressure, blood oxygenation, systemic blood pressure, and blood pH should be performed.

Dopamine HCl (Intropin®) Dopamine is a simple organic chemical in the catecholamine family. It is classified as a monoamine neurotransmitter and hormone.

Indications Dopamine is indicated for the correction of hemodynamic imbalances present in the shock syndrome due to decreased cardiac function in congestive heart failure, trauma, endotoxic septicemia, renal failure, and myocardial infarction.

Dosages Dopamine is administered by continuous intravenous infusion only at a rate of 2 to 20 mcg/kg/min and titrated according to the patient's response.

Effects Dopamine is a catecholamine that is naturally occurring within the body. Its effects are seen both directly on alpha and beta-1 receptors as well as indirectly by releasing norepinephrine throughout the system. Beta-1 effects cause an increase in cardiac output through positive inotropic effects on the myocardium. Dopamine dilates the renal vasculature and causes an increase in GFR, renal blood flow, and sodium excretion. In low doses, cardiac stimulation and renal vascular dilation occur, and in larger doses, the alpha-adrenergic effect of vasoconstriction occurs.

Contraindications Contraindications are **pheochromocytoma** (an adrenal gland tumor) tachyarrhythmias, or ventricular fibrillation.

Adverse Effects The most common adverse effects encountered with the use of dopamine are ectopic heartbeats, tachycardia, hypotension, vasoconstriction, and vomiting.

Precautions Dopamine should be used in conjunction with blood, plasma, and fluid replacement. Routine and/or constant monitoring of blood pressure, pulse pressure, and urine output should be performed. If extravasation occurs, phentolamine (Regitine®) should be administered throughout the area of extravasation.

Dobutamine (Dobutrex®) Dobutamine is a sympathomimetic drug that specifically targets the β_1 receptors in heart muscle.

Indications Dobutamine is indicated for short-term treatment to increase cardiac output due to decreased contractility from organic heart disease or cardiac surgical procedures.

Dosages Dobutamine is administered by continuous intravenous infusion only at a rate of 2.5 to 10 mcg/kg/min and titrated according to the patient's response. The maximum recommended infusion rate is 40 mcg/kg/min.

Effects Dobutamine is a drug chemically related to dopamine with most of its effects exhibited on the beta-1 receptors. Dobutamine has very little effect on the alpha receptors and does not cause the release of norepinephrine, nor does it have any effect on the renal vasculature.

Contraindications Dopamine is contraindicated in patients with idiopathic hypertrophic subaortic stenosis (IHSS).

Adverse Effects There are several dose-related adverse effects, including increased heart rate, increased blood pressure, and increased ventricular ectopic activity. Infusions continuing longer than 72 hours have not been associated with more adverse effects than shorter-duration infusions with the exception that tolerance to the drug has been reported with infusions lasting longer than 3 days.

Precautions Dobutamine should be used in concert with blood, plasma, and fluid replacement. Continuous monitoring of ECG and blood pressure should be performed.

Tolazoline (Priscoline®) Tolazoline is an α-adrenergic antagonist that is used primarily as a vasodilator.

Indications Tolazoline is indicated for the treatment of persistent pulmonary hypertension of the newborn. Treatment should only be started when arterial oxygenation cannot be maintained by oxygen and/or mechanical ventilation.

Dosages Tolazoline is given as an initial dose of 1 mg/kg, followed by an infusion of 1 to 2 mg/kg per hour. The response to the drug usually occurs within 30 minutes of administration.

Effects Tolazoline has a direct effect on blood vasculature, causing vasodilation. It has additional stimulatory effects on the heart and gastrointestinal tract. Tolazoline reduces pulmonary artery pressure by reducing vascular resistance.

Contraindications The only contraindication is a hypersensitivity to the drug.

Adverse Effects Adverse reactions following the administration of tolazoline have been observed; however, their frequency of occurrence is not documented. Adverse effects include hypotension, tachycardia, arrhythmias, nausea, vomiting, diarrhea, pulmonary and gastrointestinal hemorrhage, skin flushing, thrombocytopenia, and edema.

Precautions In the presence of acidosis, the effects of tolazoline on the pulmonary vasculature may be decreased.

Diuretics

The class of drugs termed *diuretics* encompasses a wide variety of agents, including carbonic anhydrase inhibitors, thiazides, loop diuretics, potassium-sparing diuretics, and osmotic diuretics. The use of carbonic anhydrase inhibitors, osmotic diuretics, thiazides, and potassium-sparing diuretics in neonates is very limited. Even though thiazides are the most common diuretic in use today, they are not as effective as the loop diuretics (that is, furosemide) in the neonate due to immature renal tubular function, and a lesser GFR, compared with children and adults.

Acetazolamide (Diamox®)

Indications As a diuretic, acetazolamide is often used in conjunction with furosemide to slow the progression of hydrocephalus in patients who are not candidates for surgery.

Dosages The initial dose is 5 mg/kg every 6 hours, injected slowly intravenously (IV) or orally (PO). The dosage is increased to 25 mg/kg as tolerated.

Effects Acetazolamide works by inhibiting carbonic anhydrase in the renal tubules. The result is sodium and bicarbonate remain in the tubule and an alkaline diuresis occurs. Acetazolamide also decreases the rate of cerebral spinal fluid (CSF) formation and inhibits seizure activity.

Adverse Effects and Precautions Premature infants are at risk of developing metabolic acidosis, which may be severe even in low doses. Hypokalemia is also a possibility.

Bumetanide (Bumex®)

Indications Bumetanide is a diuretic used in patients with congestive heart failure, renal insufficiency, or edema that is refractory to furosemide.

Dosages The dosage of bumetanide is 0.015 to 0.3 mg/kg per dose, given once every 24 hours.

Effects Bumetanide is a loop diuretic and is 40 times more potent than furosemide. It also decreases CSF production by a weak carbonic anhydrase inhibition.

Adverse Effects and Precautions Imbalances in water and electrolytes are frequently seen. In particular, hyponatremia, hypokalemia, and hypochloremic alkalosis are seen. This drug is also potentially ototoxic, but not to the degree of furosemide.

Chlorothiazide (Diuril®)

Indications Chlorothiazide is a diuretic used to treat mild to moderate edema and hypertension. It may be used in conjunction with furosemide or spironolactone. It has been shown to improve pulmonary function in patients with BPD.

Dosages Chlorothiazide is dosed at 10 to 20 mg/kg every 12 hours. It can be given intravenously or orally.

Effects Chlorothiazide's diuretic action is a result of inhibition of sodium reabsorption in the distal nephron. This causes an increase in sodium loss and with it, an increase in water loss.

Adverse Effects and Precautions The most commonly seen adverse effects are hypokalemia and other electrolyte abnormalities. Hyperglycemia and hyperuricemia are also seen.

Furosemide (Lasix®)

Indications Furosemide is indicated for the treatment of fluid overload, symptomatic patent ductus arteriosus, hypertension, and pulmonary interstitial edema.

Dosages Furosemide may be administered orally, intravenously, or intramuscularly. The recommended oral dose is 2 to 6 mg/kg administered every 8 to 12 hours. The recommended intravenous or intramuscular dose is 1 mg/kg initially followed by 2 mg/kg no sooner than 2 hours after the initial dose. An intravenous or intramuscular dose of 1 mg/kg/day to a maximum of 6 mg/kg/day divided every 4 to 12 hours is recommended.

Effects Furosemide inhibits the reabsorption of electrolytes (specifically sodium and chloride) in the proximal and distal tubules and in the loop of Henle. Diuresis from furosemide results in enhanced excretion of multiple electrolytes. Furosemide also has some renal vasodilator effects by decreasing renal vascular resistance and increasing renal blood flow, causing an increase in GFR.

Contraindications Furosemide is contraindicated in patients with **anuria**, a cessation of urine output, or who are hypersensitive to the drug.

Adverse Effects Fluid and electrolyte imbalances are the most common and important adverse effects and should be monitored carefully, especially in the neonate. Electrolyte imbalances (particularly hypokalemia and hypochloremia) may lead to metabolic alkalosis, and potassium supplementation may be necessary in the neonate during furosemide therapy. Other adverse effects include reversible or permanent hearing impairment (usually caused by rapid intravenous administration of too high a dose), dizziness, anorexia, blood **dyscrasias** (abnormal blood or bone marrow condition), and hyperglycemia and glycosuira.

Precautions Observation for signs of hypovolemia and electrolyte imbalances should be carefully monitored. Periodic urine and blood glucose monitoring should be performed.

Spironolactone (Aldactone®)

Indications Spironolactone is used in combination with other diuretics in the treatment of congestive heart failure and BPD.

Dosages Spironolactone is dosed 1 to 3 mg/kg every 24 hours orally.

Effects Spironolactone is a competitive antagonist of mineralocorticoids (aldosterone). It increases the excretion of calcium, magnesium, sodium, and chloride, and decreases the excretion of potassium. The effects are usually not seen before 2 to 3 days after starting therapy.

Adverse Effects and Precautions The most common adverse effects are rashes, vomiting, diarrhea, and headaches. There is also a dose-dependent androgenic effect in females.

Respiratory Drugs

The medications given for the respiratory system are those that cause a relaxation of the bronchial smooth muscles leading to bronchodilation. These drugs are given to the patient aerosolized in a small volume nebulizer or through the intravenous line. We will first examine the aerosolized drugs, and then turn our attention to the bronchodilators administered intravenously.

Aerosolized Drugs

The aerosolized bronchodilators, as with other drugs given to neonates, are not specifically approved for use in neonates, so extreme care and caution must be used when administering these drugs. This category of drugs is divided into four groups: sympathomimetics, parasympatholytics, corticosteroids, and other drugs. We will examine the drugs that fall in each group.

Sympathomimetics Sympathomimetics are also called beta-adrenergics. The name *adrenergic* comes from their ability to act like adrenalin on the beta sites and cause smooth muscle relaxation. At the effector site, which, in this case, is the bronchial smooth muscle cell, the stimulation of the beta site results in the stimulation of adenyl cyclase, which, in turn, catalyzes the formation of cyclic 3′,5′ adenosine monophosphate (cAMP) from adenosine triphosphate (ATP). This series of reactions is illustrated in Figure 14–2. The presence of cAMP causes the smooth muscle to relax,

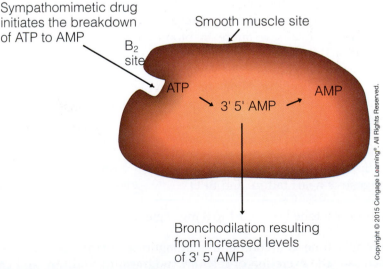

Sympathomimetic drug initiates the breakdown of ATP to AMP

B₂ site

Smooth muscle site

ATP

3′ 5′ AMP

AMP

Bronchodilation resulting from increased levels of 3′ 5′ AMP

FIGURE 14–2. Sympathetic reactions leading to bronchodilation.

leading to bronchodilation. cAMP is inactivated by the enzyme phosphodiesterase into AMP, losing the bronchodilatory effect. Stimulation of the bronchial smooth muscle beta site, whether by the sympathetic system or by a sympathomimetic drug, increases the level of 3', 5' AMP and causes dilation.

All sympathomimetic drugs share the same indication for use, that is, the prevention and treatment of reversible bronchospasm. They also share common adverse reactions and interactions. Adverse reactions include tremors, nervousness, dizziness, insomnia, headache, tachycardia, palpitations, hypertension, nausea, and vomiting. The adverse reactions are often secondary to the inherent stimulation of the beta-1 cardiac sites and may also be due to a slight degree of alpha-site stimulation.

A drug interaction common with all sympathomimetics occurs when they are used in combination with propranolol or other beta-blockers. Beta-blocking drugs may inhibit the bronchodilatory effect of the sympathomimetic drug, and care must be exercised when used together. A common, potentially dangerous effect of sympathomimetics is a paradoxical bronchospasm that may occur following abuse of the drug.

Albuterol

Concentration and Dosage Albuterol (Proventil®, Ventolin®) comes in a 20-mL vial at a concentration of 5 mg/mL, or 0.5% solution. It is also supplied in unit dose, 3 mL of a 0.083% solution, which is 2.5 mg of albuterol, mixed in 2.5 mL normal saline. When given via a small volume nebulizer, the dosage for the patient 13 and older is 0.5 mL of the 0.5% solution, mixed with 2.5 mL of normal saline. This results in a total dosage of 2.5 mg of albuterol per treatment, given 4 times a day. The dosage of aerosolized albuterol given to children of less than 13 years should be examined on an individual basis, with the dosage titrated as needed.

Metaproterenol Sulfate

Concentration and Dosage Metaproterenol (Alupent®), for inhalation comes in a solution with a concentration of 5%. Normal dosage for inhalation is 0.3 mL of a 5% solution diluted with 2.5 mL normal saline. Again, when used with smaller patients, the dosage is titrated according to size and age.

Terbutaline Sulfate

Concentration and Dosage Terbutaline (Brethine®, Bricanyl®, Brethaire®) comes in a concentration of 1 mg/mL, or a 0.1% solution. It is designed to be given subcutaneously at a dosage of 0.01 mg/kg, but can also be aerosolized for inhalation. The dosage for that route has not been established and must be determined by the physician on an individual basis. Terbutaline is also available as a metered dose inhaler (MDI), giving a dose of 0.2 mg/puff. In tablet form, terbutaline comes in 2.5- and 5-mg sizes.

Racemic Epinephrine

Concentration and Dosage Racemic epinephrine (Micronephrine®, Vaponephrine®) is supplied for inhalation as a 2.25% solution. The normal dosage is 0.5 mL of solution, diluted with 2.5–3 mL of normal saline or sterile water. In addition to being used to treat bronchospasm, racemic epinephrine is indicated for use with upper airway edema producing disease, such as croup. The stimulation of the alpha sites, on the laryngeal blood vasculature, results in vasoconstriction, with a reduction of edema and swelling.

Parasympatholytics The action of the parasympathetic system in bronchospasm (Figure 14–3) is opposite that of the sympathetic system. When the parasympathetic system is stimulated, acetylcholine is released at the cholinergic receptor site and stimulates the production of guanyl cyclase. Guanyl cyclase is the enzyme that converts guanosine triphosphate (GTP) to cyclic 3.5 guanosine monophosphate (cGMP). The action of cGMP causes smooth muscle contraction and also enhances the release of mediators from the mast cell.

The action of the parasympatholytic drugs is to block the cholinergic receptor site to acetylcholine, thus stopping the formation of cGMP and reducing the bronchospasm. Drugs that exert this effect are called cholinergic blockers or parasympatholytic drugs. Due to the slow nature of the parasympathetic system, these drugs are of no value during an acute attack, but are used as prophylaxis to bronchospasm.

Atropine

Concentration Atropine comes in ampules in a concentration of 1 mg/0.5 mL, which results in a 0.2% solution. It is also available as 2.5 mg/0.5 mL, resulting in a 0.5% solution.

Dosage The recommended dosage for a child is 0.05 mg/kg given 3 to 4 times per day.

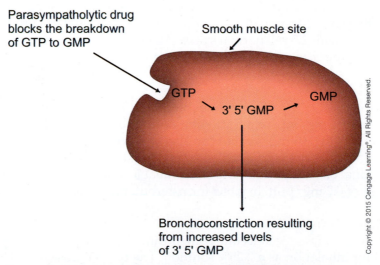

Parasympatholytic drug blocks the breakdown of GTP to GMP

Smooth muscle site

GTP

GMP

3' 5' GMP

Bronchoconstriction resulting from increased levels of 3' 5' GMP

FIGURE 14–3. Parasympathetic reactions that cause bronchoconstriction.

Side Effects Side effects of atropine include dry mouth, blurred vision, and palpitations. Atropine also has a drying effect on secretions. This may pose problems in the patient with thick, viscous secretions.

Ipratropium bromide (Atrovent®) Chemically, ipratropium bromide is a quaternary ammonium derivative of atropine. As such, it is poorly absorbed, is not rapidly removed from the site of deposition, and does not cross the blood-brain barrier, as does atropine. It is, therefore, the drug of choice in the parasympatholytic class. These traits give it a wider therapeutic margin, with fewer side effects.

Dosage The dosage of ipratropium bromide per treatment is in the range of 40–80 µg for adults. Each puff of the MDI gives 18 µg of medication. It is also available as an inhalation solution of 0.02%. This gives 0.5 mg of medication in 2.5 mL. Dosages should be titrated by the physician when used on neonatal and pediatric patients.

Glycopyrrolate (Robinul®) Glycopyrrolate is another quaternary ammonium derivative of atropine. When aerosolized, it provides bronchodiliatory effects similar to atropine with fewer side effects. Experimentally, the drug has been nebulized in 1-mg dosages.[10] However, it was never released for aerosol therapy, and is not available for use.

Tiotropium Bromide Monohydrate (Spiriva®) Tiotropium is a newer anticholinergic with specificity for muscarinic receptors. The patient inhales a dry powder contained within a capsule, from a hand held inhalation device. It is presently only indicated for the long-term treatment of COPD.

Aclidinium Bromide (Tudorza® Pressair®) Aclidinium is another new anticholinergic with a high specificity for the muscarinic receptors. It is administered as a dry powder from a multidose breath-actuated device. It currently has an indication for the long-term treatment of bronchospasm associated with COPD.

Corticosteroids The use of steroids in respiratory disorders is usually reserved for those cases in which other methods have not produced the desired results. This is because of the serious side effects of steroids, namely, suppression of immunologic and inflammatory responses. Patients on chronic steroid therapy may develop adrenal insufficiency and may be more prone to infection.

When aerosolized and delivered to the respiratory tract, steroids appear to reduce the inflammatory response of asthma. This effectively reduces the swelling, edema, bronchoconstriction, and increased outpouring of secretions seen during asthma attacks. It has been shown that steroids do produce short-term improvements in pulmonary function. The long-term effects of steroids on the neonate are unknown.

Aerosolized corticosteroids are delivered via MDI unless otherwise noted. All share the same indications, which are the treatment of bronchopulmonary dysplasis and asthma that does not respond to other conventional treatments. Steroids delivered via MDI share some common adverse reactions, which include hoarseness, dry throat, and mouth and oral *Candida* infections.

Common steroids and their dosages are listed below. Dosages are those prescribed for adults. Neonatal and pediatric dosages must be titrated to the individual patient as prescribed by a physician.

Beclomethasone (Vanceril®, Beclovent®)
Dosage 1 to 2 inhalations of the MDI taken 3 or 4 times per day.

Budesonide (Pulmicort Respules®)
Dosage 0.5 mg once daily or 0.25 mg twice daily, up to 0.5 mg twice daily via a nebulizer.

Flunisolide (Aerobid®)
Dosage 1 to 2 inhalations of the MDI taken 2 times per day.

Dexamethasone (Respihaler®)
Dosage 2 to 3 inhalations of the MDI taken 3 to 4 times per day.

Triamcinolone (Azmacort®)
Dosage 1 to 2 inhalations of the MDI taken 3 to 4 times per day.

Other Drugs for Inhalation
This group of drugs includes those respiratory drugs that do not fit into the above groups.

Pentamidine Isethionate (Nebupent®, Pentam 300®)
Indications Pentamidine is an antibiotic specifically used for the prophylactic treatment of protozoan infections. In particular, pentamidine has been designated for prophylactic treatment of *Pneumocystis jirovecii* pneumonia (PCP) in patients infected with HIV. Pentamidine must be delivered via a special nebulizer.

Dosage The inhalation dosage for primary or secondary prevention of PCP using the Respirgard II® jet nebulizer is 300 mg administered every 4 weeks. Another regimen uses the FISOneb® nebulizer with an initial loading dose of five 60 mg. doses given at 24- to 72-hour intervals over a 2-week period. This is followed by a maintenance dosage of 60 mg every 2 weeks.

Adverse Effects The most commonly seen adverse effects with inhaled pentamidine are coughing and bronchospasm. Both can often be controlled by interrupting the treatment and administering a bronchodilator. Pretreatment with a bronchodilator may also reduce the incidence and severity of coughing and bronchospasm. Coughing has also been controlled by slowing the delivery of the aerosol stream. Other respiratory effects include laryngitis, shortness of breath, chest pain, congestion, and pneumothorax. Occasional adverse effects include rhinitis, hyperventilation, hemoptysis, gagging, cyanosis, and tachypnea.

Hepatic effects include elevated liver function tests, hepatitis, hepatomegaly, and hepatic dysfunction.

Adverse effects seen in the nervous system include neuralgia, confusion, hallucinations, and dizziness. Less often seen are tremors, anxiety, depression, memory loss, seizure, insomnia, loss of taste and smell, and fatigue.

Other adverse effects include hypocalcemia, fever, anaphylactic reactions, shock, conjunctivitis, eye discomfort, blurred vision, and blepharitis.

Exposure Risks and Precautions The U.S. Centers for Disease Control and Prevention have issued an advisement for health care personnel to be aware of possible exposure to tuberculosis in HIV infected patients receiving pentamidine aerosol, due to the coughing that often accompanies it. Patients should be screened and anti-tuberculosis therapy initiated before beginning aerosolized pentamidine therapy.

Because the risk of potential effects of pentamidine on a fetus and pregnancy, as well as the risk of long-term exposure by health care workers is not totally understood, precautions should be taken by those who have contact with these patients. Pregnant and potentially pregnant females are advised that any exposure to pentamidine be avoided. For all others, precautions such as the use of gloves, gowns, goggles, and masks should be followed. The patient receiving treatment should be isolated in a room or chamber and the air inside the room or chamber vented and filtered. Ideally the room or chamber will be negatively pressured to prevent the escape of the drug and exhaled droplets from the room.

Aerosolized Antibiotics The aerosolization of antibiotics directly to the bronchial tree is advocated for treatment of organism colonization in the pulmonary tree. The advantage to this type of delivery is that it targets the specific site of infection and avoids systemic side effects. The aminoglycoside tobramycin, delivered at a dosage of 600 mg every 8 hours, has been successful in treating *pseudomonas*. Another antibiotic, colistin, has also been used in aerosol therapy, as well as gentamyacin.

Intravenous Respiratory Drugs

While a majority of medications used for the respiratory system are delivered via inhalation, this section address those that are given intravenously

Methylxanthines There still exists much controversy in the literature about whether theophylline or caffeine is the preferred respiratory drug of choice in premature infants however, caffeine has certain therapeutic advantages over theophylline. There are several general differences in the newborn system's ability to manage theophylline or caffeine, compared with adults. Theophylline has a greater tissue distribution and also has less protein-binding capacity in infants than in adults. Therefore, lower doses as well as a lower therapeutic range are necessary for infants.

Theophylline is not metabolized in premature and full-term infants via the same mechanism as it is in adults. In infants, theophylline is metabolized to caffeine, and serum concentrations of both theophylline and caffeine can and should be measured. In adults, caffeine is significantly metabolized, and, in contrast, most of the administered dose of caffeine (85%) is excreted unchanged in the urine in newborns.

Caffeine Citrate and Theophylline Intravenous or oral solutions of caffeine citrate are not commercially available, and must be prepared by the pharmacist. Many oral solid and oral liquid dosage forms and strengths of theophylline are available. The intravenous formulation for theophylline is aminophylline (theophylline ethylenediamine), which is 80% theophylline.

Indications Caffeine and theophylline are indicated for the treatment and management of neonatal apnea and for the treatment of acute and chronic bronchospasm.

Dosages for Caffeine Citrate An initial loading dose of 10 mg/kg caffeine followed by a maintenance dose of 2.5 mg/kg administered once a day is recommended. Plasma caffeine levels ranging from 5 to 20 mcg/mL are associated with control of neonatal apnea.

Dosages for Theophylline and Aminophylline For intravenous therapy an initial loading dose of 5 to 6 mg/kg theophylline (6.3–7.5 mg/kg aminophylline) followed by a maintenance dose of 3 to 6 mg/kg/day total dose of theophylline divided every 8 to 12 hours is used. Plasma theophylline levels ranging from 6 to 13 mcg/mL are associated with control of neonatal apnea.

Effects Caffeine and theophylline exhibit their bronchodilatory effects by directly relaxing the smooth muscle of the bronchi and pulmonary blood vessels. The exact mechanism of relaxation that the xanthines produce is unknown; however, two mechanisms of action are currently accepted. The older of the two theories is based on the discovery that the xanthines inhibit the breakdown of cAMP by inhibiting phosphodiesterase. Phosphodiesterease is the enzyme that reduces cAMP to AMP. Therefore, if phosophodiesterase is inhibited, the cyclic AMP remains longer, exerting its effect of bronchodilation.

A newer finding suggests that the xanthines may block the action of adenosine. Adenosine is formed from intracellular AMP and has been shown to cause bronchoconstriction in asthmatics.

Other effects of the xanthines are stimulating the central nervous system, inducing diuresis, increasing gastric acid secretion, and as central respiratory stimulants.

Contraindications Contraindications are hypersensitivity to xanthines and active gastritis or peptic ulcer disease.

Adverse Effects Adverse effects are usually not seen with the xanthine-related products when appropriate serum levels are maintained. When normal serum levels are exceeded, adverse effects (in order of increasing toxicity) include nausea, vomiting, diarrhea, insomnia, irritability, tachycardia, cardiac arrhythmias, seizures, coma and death.

Precautions Because of the effects of caffeine and theophylline on the heart, caution should be exercised in patients with severe cardiac disease, congestive heart failure, and severe hypertension. Routine monitoring of serum theophylline and/or caffeine levels should be performed.

Anticonvulsants

Anticonvulsants are a diverse group of drugs used to control seizures. Recently, they have been gaining popularity in the treatment of bipolar disorder.

Phenobarbital
Indications Phenobarbital is indicated for the treatment of generalized tonic-clonic and cortical focal seizures and also for the acute control of convulsive episodes, including status epilepticus, eclampsia, meningitis, and tetanus. Phenobarbital is also indicated as a sedative for use in pediatric patients. Phenobarbital has been used for the management of narcotic withdrawal in the newborn.

Dosages For the management of acute convulsive episodes, the recommended dose is 15 to 20 mg/kg administered intravenously immediately. The maintenance dose for the treatment of seizures or narcotic withdrawal is 1 to 5 mg/kg/day administered orally, intravenously, or intramuscularly every 8 to 12 hours. The recommended therapeutic serum levels are between 15 and 40 mcg/mL.

Effects Phenobarbital is a drug in the barbiturate class. This class of drugs produces all levels of central nervous system alterations ranging from excitation to depression. Generally, barbiturates depress the sensory cortex causing a depression in motor activity, drowsiness, and sedation. Barbiturates can also cause respiratory depression in large enough doses.

Contraindications Barbiturates are contraindicated in patients with impaired liver function or respiratory distress.

Adverse Effects Barbiturates may cause a variety of adverse effects, including sleep disorders, nervousness, apnea, respiratory depression, vomiting, diarrhea or constipation, skin rashes, and liver damage with chronic use.

Precautions Monitoring of liver and renal functions is recommended. The half-life of phenobarbital in the immediate newborn is very long, because of the immaturity of the newborn liver enzyme metabolizing system. As the age of the infant increases and the liver enzyme system matures, the half-life of phenobarbital decreases rapidly. For these reasons, monitoring of phenobarbital serum levels is highly recommended.

Phenytoin Sodium (Dilantin®)

Indications Phenytoin is indicated for the control of grand mal seizures, for the prevention of seizures during or following surgery, and has been used investigationally (non-FDA approved use) as an antiarrhythmic agent.

Dosages The recommended loading dose for neonates is 15 to 20 mg/kg administered via slow intravenous push in two divided doses separated by 20 minutes. The phenytoin maintenance dose for seizure control is 1 to 3 mg/kg/dose administered every 12 hours. The recommended serum levels for phenytoin are between 5 and 20 mg/mL. Even though oral suspension forms of phenytoin are commercially available, they should not be used in neonates owing to unpredictable absorption from the gastrointestinal tract.

Effects The specific effects of phenytoin are not completely understood; however, it appears that phenytoin inhibits the spread of seizure activity in the motor cortex of the brain via multiple biochemical mechanisms.

Contraindications Phenytoin should not be used in patients with sinus bradycardia, sinoatrial block, and second- or third-degree AV block.

Adverse Effects There are many adverse effects associated with the use of phenytoin and many are related to long-term use of the drug. Major short-term adverse effects include motor twitching, irritability, insomnia, hypotension when rapidly administered intravenously, diarrhea or constipation, hepatitis, jaundice, liver damage, blood dyscrasias, and, occasionally, hyperglycemia.

Precautions It is very important that intravenous doses of phenytoin be administered slowly to avoid some of the adverse effects of the drug. The pH of phenytoin injection is alkaline and irritating to the vein, and doses should be followed with normal saline for injection to flush the catheter. Due to its chemical composition, phenytoin, is incompatible with the majority of IV solutions. For this reason, intravenous administration should be made as close to the catheter injection site as possible to avoid potential incompatibilities with IV solutions. Phenytoin should not be administered intramuscularly due to unpredictable absorption and pain and muscle damage at the injection site.

Felbamate (Felbatol®)

Indications In the pediatric population, felbamate is used to control partial and generalized seizures associated with Lennox-Gastaut syndrome.

Dosage In the child aged 2 to 14 years, felbamate is added at 15 mg/kg/day in 3 or 4 divided doses. If other antiseizure medicines are in use, they are reduced by 20% to control plasma levels. Felbamate is then increased 15 mg/kg/day at weekly intervals to a maximum dosage of 45 mg/kg/day.

Adverse Effects The most commonly seen side effect is a rash. Acne is also occasionally seen.

Valproic Acid (Depakene®, Depakote®)

Indications Valproic acid is indicated for the treatment of simple and complex absence seizures, including petit mal seizures.

Dosage Valproic acid is dosed 15 mg/kg/day initially, and then increased as tolerated weekly 5 to 10 mg/kg/day until the optimal clinical response is achieved. The maximum dosage is 60 mg/kg/day.

Adverse Effects and Precautions The use of this drug carries a risk of hepatotoxicity, especially within the first 6 months of therapy. The risk is highest in patients younger than 2 years of age. To avoid this problem, liver function tests should be performed before starting therapy and at regular intervals thereafter.

Carbamazapine (Tegretol®)

Indications Carbamazapine is used for pediatric patients with epilepsy.

Dosage For the child 6 to 12 years of age, 100 mg BID (twice daily) is given to start with weekly increases of 100 mg/day, up to a maximum of 1,000 mg/day in 3 to 4 divided doses. For the treatment of the child above age 12, the dose is started at 200 mg BID and increased 200 mg/day on a weekly basis up to a maximum of 1200 mg/day given 3 to 4 times per day.

Steroids

The steroid discussed in this section relates to its use outside the realm of respiratory disorders. Its use in the treatment of asthma and BPD is covered in the respiratory drug section of this chapter.

Dexamethasone (Decadron®) Dexamethasone is the primary steroid that is used in neonates. It has less sodium retention activity than most of the other glucocorticoid steroids.

Indications Dexamethasone is indicated for use in neonates for the treatment of tracheal edema, cerebral edema, and bronchopulmonary dysplasia (BPD). Dexamethasone is also indicated in the treatment of various dermatologic conditions, allergic conditions both systemically and topically, bronchial asthma, and inflammatory diseases.

Dosage General neonatal recommendations for dexamethasone therapy are 0.2 to 0.5 mg/kg as an intravenous loading dose, followed by 0.1 to 0.4 mg/kg/day divided every 6 to 8 hours and administered either orally or intravenously. There are several guidelines for dexamethasone dosing in BPD. Each protocol is different in its exact dosing; however, a gradual tapering of the dose over 7 to 21 days has been used and found to be effective.

Effects Glucocorticoids exhibit their effects on virtually all body systems. Their mechanism of action is extremely complex and is involved with all levels of each cell's biochemical activity. This action includes the stabilization of cell membranes, inhibiting macrophage accumulation in inflamed areas, interference with the complement system, promoting gluconeogenesis, and suppressing the release of adrenocorticotropic hormone (ACTH).

Contraindications Intravenously administered glucocorticoids are contraindicated in patients who are hypersensitive to them.

Adverse Effects Some of the adverse effects associated with the short-term use of dexamethasone include hypertension, adrenal suppression, anaphylactic reactions, sodium and fluid retention, suppression of skin test reactions, and masking of the symptoms of infection.

Precautions Dexamethasone therapy should be monitored by observing patients for weight increase, edema, and hypertension.

Sedation and Control of Ventilation

During mechanical ventilation, it may be necessary to sedate the patient to reduce the associated anxiety.

Chloral Hydrate (Noctec®)

Indications Chloral hydrate is indicated when sedation of the patient is desired, to calm agitation, and to aid in sleep.

Dosage Chloral hydrate is given orally or rectally at a dosage of 25 to 50 mg/kg. The oral preparation should be given after feedings or should be diluted to decrease the risk of gastric irritation.

Contraindications Chloral hydrate should not be given in large doses in those patients with severe cardiac disease.

Adverse Effects Chloral hydrate may cause CNS depression, gastric irritation, vasodilation, respiratory depression, cardiac arrhythmias, and myocardial depression. Because chloral hydrate does not provide any analgesic effect, a patient in pain may demonstrate a paradoxical excitement.

Precautions Chloral hydrate should be used with caution on patients with renal and/or hepatic disease. In addition, caution must be employed when used with other CNS depressant drugs, furosemide, and anticoagulants.

Benzodiazepines The benzodiazepines are depressant psychoactive drugs that enhance the effect of gamma-aminobutyric acid (GABA). This leads to sedation and a reduction in anxiety, as well inducing sleep. Benzodiazepines additionally have an amnestic effect. Benzodiazepines are a schedule IV drug under the controlled substance act. There are roughly 15 benzodiazepines marketed in the United States and 20 others marketed in other countries.[11] The use of benzodiazepines in the pediatric and neonatal population is known to cause adverse effects; however, the risk to benefit ratio has yet to be determined.[12]

Diazepam (Valium®)

Indications Diazepam is used to relieve anxiety, for sedation, and as an anticonvulsant. Additionally, diazepam is used in the management of opiate withdrawal.

Dosage Diazepam is given orally, intravenously, or intramuscularly at a dosage of 0.04 to 0.25 mg/kg, every 2 to 4 hours as needed. The maximal total dosage given should not exceed 5 mg/kg.

Contraindications Diazepam should not be used on patients in shock or on patients with narrow-range glaucoma.

Adverse Effects Adverse effects seen with the use of diazepam include hypotension, tachycardia, hypotonia, respiratory depression, elevated respiratory rate, increased risk of hyperbilirubinemia, urinary retention, constipation, and irritation at the site of administration.

Precautions Caution must be used when delivering diazepam with other anticonvulsant drugs due to the additive effect of both drugs. Additionally, diazepam should be used cautiously on patients with renal and hepatic dysfunction.

Midazolam (Versed®)

Indications Midazolam is a short-acting benzodiazepine that has a rapid onset of action. It is used as a sedative/hypnotic to reduce anxiety during invasive procedures, and to induce anesthesia.

Dosage Midazolam is given intravenously (IV) or intramuscularly (IM) at a rate of 0.07 to 0.2 mg/kg over 2 to 5 minutes, repeated as required every 2 to 4 hours.

Adverse Effects and Precautions Respiratory depression with apnea is commonly seen with administration of midazolam and personnel must be prepared to provide artificial ventilation if necessary. Other adverse effects include hypotension and seizures.

Opioids Opioid medications are some of the oldest known for their pain treatment. The therapeutic effect of the opium poppy predates recorded history. Opioids are chemicals that attach to opioid receptors in the CNS and gastrointestinal tract. Their effect in the CNS is to decrease the perception of pain and increase pain tolerance. Side effects include sedation, respiratory depression and constipation. It is recommended whenever an opioid is used that the drug naloxone be available.[13] Naloxone is an opioid antagonist that has no pharmacologic activity. It is used to prevent or reverse the side effects of opioids previously mentioned.[14]

Morphine Sulfate

Indications Morphine sulfate is indicated when analgesia from pain is desired, for sedation, and to induce respiratory depression, which enhances mechanical ventilation.

Dosage Morphine sulfate is given subcutaneously, intramuscularly, or slow intravenous push at a dosage of 0.1 to 0.2 mg/kg, every 4 to 6 hours as needed.

Contraindications Morphine sulfate should not be given when there is a known hypersensitivity to opiates and should not be administered to patients in shock, those with elevated intracranial pressures, or to those having convulsions.

Adverse Effects Administration of morphine sulfate may cause hypotension, bradycardia, histamine release, increased intracranial pressure, respiratory depression, gastrointestinal irritation, muscle rigidity, and a dependence on the drug.

Precautions Oxygen and ventilatory support should be kept at the bedside of patients receiving morphine sulfate. The drug should be used cautiously on those patients with renal and hepatic impairment and on those with cardiac arrhythmias.

Fentanyl Citrate

Indications Fentanyl citrate is used to produce analgesia, sedation, and anesthesia in the patient. It is often used before performing an invasive procedure such as bronchoscopy.

Dosage Fentanyl citrate is given intravenously by slow push at a dosage of 1 to 4 µg/kg, every 2 to 4 hours.

Adverse Effects At dosages greater than 5 µg/kg, respiratory depression may occur unexpectedly. Other adverse reactions include muscle rigidity, seizures, hypotension, and bradycardia. There have been anecdotal case studies of "chest wall rigidity syndrome" and stiff lung (ARDS) associated with fentanyl use; however, they appear to be rare and occur only at high dosages.[15]

Precautions Fentanyl citrate should be used cautiously to avoid tolerance to the drug. The patient may additionally show signs of withdrawal when the drug wears off.

Barbiturates Like the benzodiazepines, barbiturates act on the GABA receptors to produce inhibition of the CNS. They are used to produce a range of therapeutic effects from anti-anxiety and sedation to total anesthesia, however, they have no analgesic effect. As previously mentioned, they are also effective as anticonvulsants. Barbiturates have been shown to lower intracranial pressure, thus providing neuroprotection. Side effects include hypotension, hypoventilation and apnea.

Pentobarbital

Indications Pentobarbital is a short-acting barbiturate used primarily for sedation during procedures.

Dosage 2–2.5 mg/kg/dose given via a slow IV push, or 2–6 mg/kg/dose when given IM. The total dosage should not exceed 100 mg.

Contraindications Sensitivity to barbiturates.

Precautions Because pentobarbital is fast acting, the means to provide ventilatory and respiratory support must be available along with personnel trained in intubation and ventilatory support.

Methohexital (Brevital®)

Indications Methohexital is used primarily as a procedural sedative in the emergency department and intensive care unit. It has been studied as an alternative to etomidate in endotracheal intubation.[16] It is ultra-short-acting with an onset of less than 1 minute and a duration of around 10 minutes. Methohexital has a black box warning which states, "Methohexital should be used in hospital or ambulatory care settings that can provide continuous monitoring of respiratory (e.g., pulse oximetry) and cardiac function. Resuscitative drugs and age- and size-appropriate equipment for bag valve mask ventilation and intubation and personnel trained in their use and skilled in airway management should be readily available. For deeply sedated patients, a designated individual other than the practitioner performing the procedure should be present to continuously monitor the patient."

Dosage The induction dose is 0.75–1 mg/kg/dose via IV with a maintenance dosage of 0.5 mg/kg every 2–3 minutes.

Thiopental (Sodium Pentothal®)

Indications Thiopental is used primarily as an induction agent for endotracheal intubation and to reduce ICP. It has a short onset of action of 30–40 seconds with a half-life of 3–8 hours.

Dosage Induction dosing is 2–5 mg/kg/dose, given via IV.

Paralytics Paralytics are classified as neuromuscular-blocking drugs and are further defined as non-depolarizing blocking agents and depolarizing blocking agents. A majority of the clinically relevant paralytics are non-depolarizing. They act at the neuromuscular junction by blocking acetylcholine to its receptors, leading to a paralysis of skeletal muscle. In contrast, the depolarizing agents cause a persistent depolarization of skeletal muscle. This makes them resistant to further stimulation by acetylcholine. The primary depolarizing agent is succinylcholine. The non-depolarizing agents are used as an adjunct to anesthetics to induce skeletal muscle relaxation and facilitate ventilation. They are also used to control muscle contractions during seizures. Paralytics must always be used with analgesics, anxiolytics, and amnestics. Any of the neuromuscular-blocking drugs can cause a fast and severe rise in body temperature and severe muscle contractions (**malignant hyperthermia**) up to 24 hours after administration. Non-depolarizing agents can be reversed with acetylcholinesterase inhibitors, most commonly neostigmine and edrophonium.

Pancuronium Bromide (Pavulon®)

Dosage Neonates: pancuronium is given intravenously at an initial test dose of 0.02 mg/kg followed by a maintenance dose of 0.03 to 0.09 mg/kg. Children >1 year of age: an initial dose of 0.04 to 0.1 mg/kg is given IV followed by 0.01 mg/kg every 30 to 60 minutes as needed.

Contraindications Pancuronium should not be used on any patient with a preexisting tachycardia.

Adverse Effects Adverse effects of pancuronium include an increase in blood pressure, wheezing, and tachycardia.

Precautions Whenever pancuronium is used, there must be full respiratory support immediately available. Extreme caution should be used when giving the drug to patients with poor renal perfusion or renal disease. Because pancuronium does not provide analgesia, the patient must be monitored for signs of pain and treated with appropriate analgesics.

Succinylcholine Chloride (Anectine®)

Indications Due to its short duration of action, succinylcholine is indicated to induce skeletal muscle relaxation in order to facilitate intubation. It is also used as a muscle relaxant in concert with anesthetic agents.

Dosages The dosage of succinylcholine in children is 1 to 2 mg/kg IV or 2.5 to 4 mg/kg IM.

Contraindications Succinylcholine is contraindicated in those patients who have genetically determined deficiencies of plasma **pseudocholinesterase**, an enzyme in the plasma that metabolizes certain drugs. Additionally, succinylcholine should not be used on patients with myopathies which result in increased serum creatine kinase (CPK, for example) values or those patients with eye injuries.

Adverse Effects Adverse effects include transient bradycardia, tachycardia, hypertension and hypotension, sinus arrest, respiratory depression, and wheezing.

Precautions Whenever succinylcholine is used, full respiratory support must be immediately available. Succinylcholine should be used with extreme caution on patients recovering from severe trauma, electrolyte imbalances, those receiving quinidine or cardiac glycosides, and those with hyperkalemia.

Miscellaneous Agents Certain sedating drugs cannot be classified into any of the typical categories based on their mechanism of action.

Ketamine Ketamine is classified as an NMDA (N-methyl d-aspartate) receptor antagonist. In addition to being an effecting anesthetic, Ketamine also provides analgesia and has amnestic effects. Ketamine is beneficial in that it has a minimal effect on respiratory drive and preserves airway reflexes. It also has bronchodilatory effects, which are helpful in the presence of bronchospasm. Ketamine has a good safety profile in children.[17] There appears to be an idiosyncratic laryngospasm associated with ketamine use.[18] One of the effects of ketamine is that it produces dream-like states, hallucinations and a state known as dissociative anesthesia, which unfortunately, makes it popular as a recreational drug.[19]

Etomidate Etomidate is a short-acting anesthetic administered via IV primarily used as an induction agent for general anesthesia and as a procedural sedative. In adults, it is used in rapid sequence intubation; however, its use in the pediatric population remains to be determined.[18]

Nitrous Oxide Nitrous oxide, also known as laughing gas, is used as an anesthetic and analgesic. It typically gives the patient a feeling of euphoria, which led to the name laughing gas. While used primarily in dentistry, it is also used as an anxiolytic/analgesic during medical procedures.

Propofol Propofol is a sedative that has no analgesic or amnestic properties. Its primary use is in the induction and maintenance of general anesthesia; however, it is gaining in popularity as a procedural sedative. In all uses, an anesthesiologist should be present to monitor the patient and intervene if deep sedation/anesthesia occurs.

Dexmedetomidine Dexmedetomidine is a clonidine-like drug that acts as an agonist of the α_2-adrenergic receptors in certain parts of the brain.[20] A benefit is that it does not induce respiratory depression. More studies are needed to ascertain its usefulness in the pediatric population.[21]

EFFECTS OF MATERNAL DRUG ABUSE ON THE FETUS

The transfer of drugs across the placenta was previously discussed in this chapter. Abusable "street drugs" such as heroin, cocaine, and marijuana have the same potential teratogenic effects as do many prescription and over-the-counter drugs. Drug abuse not only includes the illicit use of street drugs but also the inappropriate and overuse of prescription drugs. Prescription drugs to lessen pain (narcotics) and those to aid in sleep disturbances (sedatives/hypnotics) are frequently prescribed during pregnancy and can lead to abuse, complications during delivery, fetal addiction, and birth defects.

Withdrawal from addictive drugs in the neonate may present itself with many signs and symptoms, many of which may be misinterpreted as meningitis, gastroenteritis, hypocalcemia, or intracranial hemorrhage. The most common withdrawal symptoms include restlessness, irritability, tremors, high-pitched cry, and vomiting. These symptoms will be noticeable within a few hours after birth. Phenobarbital is routinely used to treat the irritability, tremors, or twitching.

Neonatal addiction itself can be initially treated with tincture of opium (10% opium) administered as 1 to 2 drops per pound of body weight and can be increased until the symptoms dissipate. The tincture of opium is then gradually withdrawn over a 7- to 14-day period.

SUMMARY

The use of pharmacologic agents is a challenging science. It is more so in the neonatal patient population because of the wide differences in metabolic rates, sizes, and weights in these patients. The response of a patient to any delivered drug is impossible to predict and two patients of equal age, and size, may respond totally opposite to the same drug given at the same dosage.

The effect of maternal drug use on the fetus has gained much attention in recent history. It is now well known that many drugs can reach 50% to 100% of maternal levels in the fetus. Depending on when the drug is taken, severe teratogenic effects may be seen in the fetus. Drugs taken late in pregnancy may make the baby flaccid and unresponsive when delivered. The best advice to follow is to avoid all medications during pregnancy, unless medically necessary.

Pharmacokinetics is the term used to describe the entire life of a drug, from when it enters the body, how it is distributed throughout the body, and how it exits.

A common type of drugs used on the neonatal and pediatric populations is antibiotics. Antibiotics fall into one of several categories, and each has a specific group of organisms for which it is effective. Proper use of antibiotics requires identification of the pathogen and use of the appropriate drug at the appropriate dosage, for the appropriate time period.

Cardiovascular drugs are used to control and treat cardiac arrhythmias, hypotension, congestive heart failure, pulmonary hypertension, and to close or keep open the ductus arteriosus.

Aerosolized respiratory medications are used in the neonatal and pediatric populations to treat reversible bronchospasm, improve mucus removal, reduce airway inflammation, and to treat or prevent infections. Other medications given intravenously are used to stimulate respirations, especially in neonates suffering from apnea.

Other common medicines used include those to control and prevent seizures, steroids to reduce edema, and sedatives to reduce agitation and anxiety.

POSTTEST

1. Drug transfer across the placenta is affected by which of the following?
    I. concentration difference
    II. lipid solubility of the drug
    III. degree of ionization
    IV. diffusion coefficient
    V. molecular drug weight
        a. II, III
        b. I, III, V
        c. II, III, IV
        d. I, II, III, V

2. Teratogenic drugs generally have their greatest effect during:
    a. ovulation and fertilization
    b. the first trimester
    c. the second trimester
    d. the third trimester

3. A lipid-soluble drug has which of the following characteristics?
    I. readily crosses cell membranes
    II. concentration is higher in tissues than in plasma
    III. high affinity for protein binding
    IV. 10% is bound to albumin
    V. distributed slowly to the heart and kidneys
        a. I, III
        b. I, III, V
        c. I, II, III, V
        d. I, II, III, IV, V

4. Of the following, which is *not* a type of biochemical reaction of drug metabolism in the liver?
    a. excretion
    b. conjugation
    c. reduction
    d. hydrolysis

5. Of the following antibiotics, which is considered to be bacteriostatic?
    a. tetracycline
    b. ciprofloxacin
    c. cefaclor
    d. penicillin

6. For each of the following antibiotic categories, list at least one drug that belongs to that category.
   a. penicillin
   b. cephalosporins
   c. aminoglycosides
   d. macrolides
   e. quinolones
   f. tetracyclines
   g. sulfonamides
   h. antifungals
   i. antivirals

Use the following list to answer questions 7 through 9.
   a. adenosine
   b. epinephrine
   c. digoxin
   d. indomethacin
   e. dopamine

7. Which drug would be most appropriate to treat congestive heart failure?
8. Which drug would be most appropriate to treat supraventricular tachycardia?
9. Which drug would be most appropriate to treat severe hypotension?
10. Acute bronchospasm would best be treated with which of the following drugs?
   a. atropine
   b. ipratropium bromide
   c. albuterol
   d. theophylline
11. Neonatal apnea is treated with which of the following?
   a. caffeine
   b. phenobarbital
   c. cromolyn sodium
   d. ribavirin
12. Which of the following best describe the effects of glucocorticoids?
   I. combat infections
   II. stabilize cell membranes
   III. inhibit macrophage accumulation
   IV. increase the release of adrenocorticotropic hormone
   V. promote gluconeogenesis
       a. I, III, IV
       b. II, III, IV
       c. III, IV, V
       d. II, III, V
13. The drug that inhibits mast cell degranulation is:
   a. theophylline
   b. dexamethasone
   c. atropine
   d. cromolyn sodium

14. Which of the following would be the drug of choice in sedating a neonate following surgery?
    a. pavulon
    b. chloral hydrate
    c. fentanyl
    d. morphine sulfate
15. Restlessness, irritability, tremors, high-pitched cry, and vomiting are all signs of:
    a. respiratory distress
    b. fetal drug withdrawal
    c. fetal drug addiction
    d. maternal heroin abuse

REFERENCES

1. Soranus. *Gynecology.* Baltimore, MD: Johns Hopkins University Press, 1956.
2. Bartlett JG. Clinical practice. Antibiotic-associated diarrhea. *N Engl J Med.* 346(5):334–339, 2002.
3. Bartlett JG, Perl TM. The new Clostridium difficile: what does it mean? *N Engl J Med.* 353(23):2503–2505, 2005.
4. Gruchalla RS, Pirmohamed M. Clinical practice. Antibiotic allergy. *N Engl J Med.* 354(6):601–609, 2006.
5. Neugut AI, Ghatak AT, Miller RL. Anaphylaxis in the United States: an investigation into its epidemiology. *Arch Intern Med.* 161(1):15–21, 2001.
6. Ghislain P-D, Roujeau J-C. Treatment of severe drug reactions: Stevens-Johnson Syndrome, Toxic Epidermal Necrolysis and Hypersensitivity syndrome. *Dermatology Online Journal.* 8(1), 2002.
7. Nandyal RR. Update on group B streptococcal infections: perinatal and neonatal periods. *J Perinat Neonatal. Nurs.* 22(3):230–237, Jul–Sep 2008.
8. Woods, C.J. Streptococcus Group B Infections. http://emedicine.medscape .com/article/229091-overview.
9. Drugs.com; Guifenesin. http://www.drugs.com/guaifenesin.html.
10. Rau JL. *Respiratory Care Pharmacology.* 8th ed. Chicago, IL: Year-Book Medical Publishers Inc., 2011.
11. Drugs of Abuse, 2011 edition. U.S. Dept. of Justice. http://www.justice.gov/dea/pr/multimedia-library/publications/drug_of_abuse.pdf
12. E Ng, et.al. Safety of Benzodiazepines in Newborns. Ann Pharmacother 36(7/8):1150–1155, Jul.-Aug, 2002.
13. Hom J, et al. Pediatric Sedation. http://emedicine.medscape.com/article/804045-overview#aw2aab6b9.
14. Drugs.Com. Naloxone. http://www.drugs.com/pro/naloxone.html.
15. Vaughn RL. Fentanyl chest wall rigidity syndrome--a case report http://www.ncbi.nlm.nih.gov/pmc/articles/PMC2516388/?page=1

16. Diaz-Guzman E, et al. A comparison of methohexital versus etomidate for endo-tracheal intubation of critically ill patients. *AmJ Crit Care.* 19(1):48–54, 2010.

17. emedicine.medscape.com/article/804045-overview#aw2aab6b9.

18. Green SM, et al. Laryngospasm during emergency department ketamine sedation: a case-control study. http://www.ncbi.nlm.nih.gov/pubmed/20944510.

19. Drug Free.org. Ketamine. http://www.drugfree.org/drug-guide/ketamine.

20. Cormack JR, Orme RM, Costello TG. The role of alpha2-agonists in neurosurgery. *J Clin Neurosci.* 12(4):375–378, 2005.

21. Mason KP, et al. Intramuscular dexmedetomidine sedation for pediatric MRI and CT. *AJR Am J Roentgenol.* 197(3):720–725, Sep. 2011.

BIBLIOGRAPHY AND SUGGESTED READINGS

Cottrell GP, Surkin HB. *Pharmacology for Respiratory Care Practitioners.* Philadelphia, PA: WB Saunders Co, 1995.

Daglin JH, Vallerand AH. *Davis's Drug Guide for Nurses.* 13th ed. Philadelphia, PA: FA Davis, 2012.

Merenstein GB, Gardner SL. *Handbook of Neonatal Intensive Care.* 7th ed. St. Louis, MO: Mosby, 2010.

CHAPTER 15

Assessment of Oxygenation and Ventilation

OBJECTIVES

Upon completion of this chapter, the reader should be able to:

1. For each of the following, describe how it is used in the assessment of oxygenation and ventilation:
   a. Respiratory rate
   b. Patient color
   c. Work of breathing
   d. Breath sounds
   e. Tactile fremitus
2. List the indications for obtaining an arterial or capillary blood gas sample in neonatal and pediatric patients.
3. Identify the methods of obtaining blood samples for analysis, and describe why the UAC is the preferred blood sampling site.
4. Identify arterial sampling sites that are pre- and postductal, and describe how a right-to-left shunt through the ductus arteriosus can be detected using blood gas PaO_2, transcutaneous monitors, and/or pulse oximetry.
5. Identify the hazards and contraindications associated with each of the blood gas sampling methods.
6. Define "normal" and "safe" levels of PaO_2, $PaCO_2$, pH, base excess, and HCO_3^-. Describe why values in the midrange are desirable.
7. Compare total blood oxygen to PaO_2.
8. Describe the limitations of PaO_2.
9. Identify and discuss the determinants of $PaCO_2$.
10. Define pH and using the Henderson–Hasselbalch equation, describe the relationship between CO_2 and HCO_3^- in maintaining proper pH.

11. For each of the following, describe how each is calculated and how each is used in the clinical assessment of oxygenation:
    a. Oxygen content
    b. Arteriovenous oxygen content difference
    c. Alveolar to arterial oxygen gradient
    d. Arterial to alveolar oxygen ratio
    e. PaO_2/F_iO_2 ratio
    f. Intrapulmonary shunt
12. Identify two causes for each of the following: respiratory and metabolic acidosis and alkalosis, and describe briefly the compensatory mechanisms for each of these disorders.
13. Describe the role of bicarbonate in buffering blood acids.
14. Define base excess and deficit.
15. Briefly describe the mechanical aspects of a transcutaneous monitor (TCM).
16. Discuss how a transcutaneous monitor (TCM) can be useful even if not reading arterial values.
17. List six factors that could cause a TCM to read lower than the actual PaO_2.
18. Explain the limitations, complications, and hazards of TCMs and how they can be avoided.
19. Describe how a pulse oximeter determines arterial oxygen saturation.
20. Discuss the clinical uses of pulse oximetry.
21. Compare and contrast sidestream and mainstream CO_2 monitors.
22. Describe how increased deadspace ventilation and increased shunt perfusion can cause erroneous capnography readings.
23. List and explain the limitations of capnography.

KEY TERMS

calcaneus	spectrophotometric	stratum corneum
hyperalimentation	infrared analysis	
logarithm		

INTRODUCTION

Clinical assessments of oxygenation and/or ventilation imply specific knowledge of the physical measures that influence the process of moving gasses into and out of the lungs. These are generally "tools" that help guide the respiratory therapist in evaluating, recommending, and/or intervening in the clinical management of diseases and abnormalities affecting the cardiopulmonary system. It cannot be overstated that simple assessments are easily obtainable (or electronically gathered in quick glances at a bedside monitor) and give valuable insight into the pathology of the pediatric patient. These assessments can be informal visual clues (respiratory rate, color [cyanosis], work of breathing [retractions], or evidence of dyspnea), auscultated breath sounds, or specific objective measures (i.e., PaO_2 or $PaCO_2$ [ABG], transcutaneous monitoring (TCM), capnography, oxygen saturation, oxygen content, A-a gradient, a/A ratio, PaO_2/F_iO_2 ratio, or intrapulmonary shunt) that evaluate the efficiency of *the diffusion of pulmonary gasses. The goal of recognizing changes in the measurements of these assessments includes improving the underlying disease, understanding and managing a patient's clinical condition, and effectively correcting the pathophysiology observed in the physical assessments.*

RESPIRATORY RATE

The rate required to stabilize the elimination of metabolically generated carbon dioxide (35–45 mmHg) generally keeps the respiratory rate about 24–30 breaths per minute at rest in pediatric populations. An increased respiratory rate (higher than appropriate for a particular activity) indicates a trend that requires further investigation. Included in any assessment of respiratory rate is the degree of chest rise, appearance of fatigue, or difficulty breathing. Rates greater than 30 breaths per minute often indicate distress and can reach up to 60 to 80 breaths per minute or higher for infants in severe distress requiring immediate treatment and a thorough assessment to investigate for underlying causes.

COLOR

The appearance of the skin or evaluation of the nailbeds can reveal much in the way of oxygen transport. Pale or ashen color is present in hypotensive states or poor peripheral perfusion. Additionally, the presence of cyanosis (bluish coloration) is an indicator of oxygenation that reveals 5% reduced oxyhemoglobin. Comparisons with pink skin tone may not be an accurate assessment of oxygenation because chronic hypoxemia (in specific pathology) encourages polycythemia and can mask deficient oxygenation even if the PaO_2 is low. Evidence of anxiety, cold, or peripheral obstruction may also influence the appearance of cyanosis. Nevertheless, it is a quick assessment that is utilized by a skilled respiratory therapist in conjunction with multiple measures that help assess oxygenation.

WORK OF BREATHING/DYSPNEA

Dyspnea is an uncomfortable awareness of breathing caused by anxiety, pain, or V/Q mismatch in pulmonary disease. This is often manifest by use of accessory muscles aiding inspiration particularly the sternocleidomastiod, trapezius, intercostals, and pectoralis major muscles. Use of these muscle groups assists the diaphragm to increase interthoracic pressure to improve inspiratory volume in the lungs to "blow off" carbon dioxide through increased minute ventilation. Increased work of breathing is often evident by the presence of thoracic retractions (substernal, intercostals, and/or supraclavicular) which paradoxically move the sternum and intercostals spaces inward on inspiration. This is often associated with tachypnea and/or tachycardia in the pediatric patient. Dyspnea may occur suddenly or over an extended period, characterizing increased effort to breathe. As "work of breathing" increases, the pediatric patient may reveal signs consistent with difficulty to move air and anxiety that matched the degree of dyspnea.

BREATH SOUNDS

The evaluation of breathing accompanies any examination or physical assessment of the chest. The presence of air over the lung fields should be indicative of normal gas exchange. The volume and depth of the breathing pattern during auscultation can encourage hyperventilation and the respiratory therapist must guard against dizziness or tingling extremities. Diminished breath sounds can be heard with quiet breaths but they can help predict low PaO_2's (and correspondingly lower SaO_2) and higher $PaCO_2$'s on a blood gas analysis corresponding with abnormal assessments. With poor aeration, crackles, or rhonchi in the airways, a respiratory therapist could speculate the degree of V/Q mismatch in the lungs with the presence of adventitious (abnormal) breath sounds. Further assessment or evidence should be evaluated via chest x-ray for definitive explanation of gaseous transport in the lungs.

TACTILE FREMITIS

Assessment by palpation can often present quick clues to the presence of pulmonary pathology in the pediatric patient. Chest consolidation is evaluated by vibrations and is assessed by placing the hand on the back of the patient and evaluating congestion by the presence of vocal/tactile crepitus.

ARTERIAL BLOOD GAS ANALYSIS

Gaseous diffusion of oxygen and carbon dioxide are measured in a small sample of arterial blood. Additionally, it provides objective measures for pH (acid-base balance), HCO_3, Hb, COHb, MetHb, CaO_2, SaO_2, and P_{50} to evaluate physiologic function of the transport of pulmonary gasses. Most blood gas machines require less than a 0.95 µL sample size to perform the analysis and objectively relate measurements for further clinical interpretation.

Indications

The indications to order an arterial blood gas vary slightly between the neonate and pediatric patient and warrant separate discussions.

Neonatal Patients Premature neonates, in the first hours, days, and weeks of life, can experience dramatic changes in their status very quickly, sometimes even from one minute to the next.

It is very difficult to base therapeutic decisions simply on observation, especially when it comes to changes in oxygenation and ventilation. Some neonates may require blood gas analysis every 10 to 20 minutes; others may only need one every few weeks. The important fact to remember is that each neonate is different and will have different requirements regarding the need for blood gases.

Keep in mind that a small preemie may only have 100 cc of blood in its entire body, and frequent blood gases can deplete that limited supply quickly. A fine line exists between getting too many blood gases and getting too few. If in doubt however, it is better to get too many than not enough. Blood gas values are a critical part of neonatal care, and many decisions affecting the outcome of the neonate are based on blood gas values.

There are certain rules that apply to most neonates that help determine when an arterial blood gas analysis is needed. They are presented here, not necessarily in order of their importance.

1. Any neonate showing signs of respiratory distress such as nasal flaring, retractions, grunting, and cyanosis should have arterial blood drawn for analysis.
2. Any neonate whose clinical course, appearance, vital signs, or condition has changed for no obvious reason should also have an arterial blood gas analysis. It is important not to wait for the blood gas results before reacting to and treating a problem. The patient should be treated first, then an arterial sample obtained. For example, if the respiratory therapist notices that the patient is a dusky blue color or the HR has dropped, the patient should be treated first; after treatment a blood gas can be obtained.
3. It is advisable to obtain an arterial blood gas analysis within 15 to 30 minutes after any change in ventilator or F_iO_2 settings.
4. Once the neonate on a ventilator has stabilized, it is advisable to obtain an arterial blood gas analysis on a regular basis to ensure proper ventilator settings. Regular analysis also helps to document transcutaneous and pulse oximetry readings. The timing of blood gases should be made on an individual basis, as need dictates.

Specific units will have varying criteria for blood gases on long-term ventilator patients.

Pediatric Patients The indications for arterial blood gas analysis on pediatric patients are basically the same as for adults. The primary indication for a blood gas analysis is to objectively assess the oxygenation and ventilation status of the patient. Any patient who shows signs of distress, such as increased respiratory rate, retractions, and cyanosis, should have an arterial blood gas analysis.

In addition, blood gas analysis is indicated on pediatric patients being managed on a mechanical ventilator. Monitoring of PaO_2, $PaCO_2$, and pH allows for optimal settings to be achieved, as well as dictating proper changes in ventilator parameters as needed.

Arterial blood gases are indicated as a follow-up to oxygen therapy or the administration of medications or therapy for the treatment of a pulmonary disorder. Follow-up blood gases indicate if inspired oxygen is adequate and if treatments and medications are effective in reversing concerns.

Considerations in Obtaining Samples in the Neonate

There are two primary sources of arterial blood sampling in the neonate: the umbilical and the radial artery. Other arteries such as the brachial, dorsalis pedis, and posterior tibial arteries are more difficult to puncture and should only be used when the radial site is contraindicated. Capillary blood is another source; however, it is not arterial but rather a mixed sample. It is important to remember that at any time blood or blood products are to be handled, the possibility of contact exists and universal precautions must be observed.

Umbilical Artery Catheter The umbilical artery catheter (UAC) blood gas sample is the preferred method for obtaining arterial blood samples. This is because it causes no pain to the neonate (pain may lead to erroneous values secondary to crying and agitation), and the blood is easily obtained through the catheter. Arterial punctures can be very traumatic to neonates and can drastically change the blood gas values due to the crying and fussing of the patient. It should also be noted that punctures can damage the neonate's fragile skin.

If a right-to-left shunt is suspected through the patent ductus arteriosus (PDA), a right radial arterial sample should be drawn simultaneously with the UAC blood gas to compare the pressure of oxygen in each sample. In normal cardiovascular anatomy, the right radial arterial blood will be preductal, and in the presence of a ductal shunt will reflect a higher oxygen tension than in the postductal location of the UAC (Figure 15–1).

An easier method of detecting a right-to-left ductal shunt is to place a transcutaneous PaO_2 monitor on the upper-right quadrant of the chest and another on the abdomen (Figure 15–2). The higher PaO_2 on the upper-right quadrant, compared to the lower abdominal PaO_2, would reflect the right-to-left ductal shunt. A relative uniformity between PaO_2 at these two sites helps to rule out a right-to-left ductal shunt.

Several problems are associated with the use of the UAC. Most UACs rarely remain in place longer than 3 to 4 weeks in the neonate due to clot formation and problems with infection. A premature neonate may be on a ventilator or require supplemental oxygen for months. In these patients, the loss of the UAC makes the assessment of oxygenation and ventilation more difficult, as capillary samples and external monitors must then be relied upon to assess these functions.

As discussed previously, the arterial blood obtained from the UAC may reflect a low PaO_2 from a ductal shunt. The arterial blood that supplies the head is normally preductal. If the F_iO_2 is increased in response to a low arterial PO_2 (caused by the ductal shunt), the arterial blood supplying the head and eyes may increase to a dangerous level.

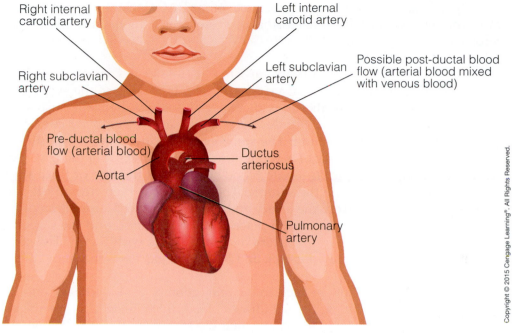

FIGURE 15–1. Normal cardiovascular anatomy.

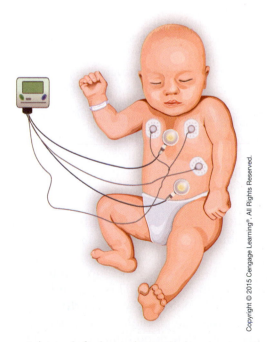

FIGURE 15–2. Detecting a right-to-left shunt through the ductus arteriosus using two transcutaneous monitors. The monitor on the abdomen measures postductal blood, while the monitor on the right-upper chest measures preductal blood.

Complications associated with the use of a UAC include thromboembolism, hypertension, infection, hemorrhage, vessel perforation, and necrotizing enterocolitis.

Procedure for a Blood Draw from an Umbilical Artery Catheter To draw blood from the UAC line, two 3 cc syringes are obtained. One of the syringes is filled approximately two-thirds full with a special neonatal heparin flush solution. A clean gauze pad is placed under the stopcock and the empty 3 cc syringe is placed on the luer lock opening. The stopcock to the incoming IV solution is then turned off and 2.0 to 2.5 cc of blood is slowly withdrawn from the UAC into a "safe set" syringe so as not to waste blood. This clears the line of flush solution, which may contaminate the sample. The stopcock is then turned off one-quarter turn to stop flow from the artery and to prevent IV contamination of the sample. The blood gas syringe is next placed on the luer lock, and the stopcock is opened one-quarter turn to the artery and the sample withdrawn. The stopcock is now turned off to the luer lock and the blood gas syringe removed and capped.

Close attention must now be paid to the reinjection of the blood back into the patient. The syringe containing the withdrawn blood/flush mixture, if not already in-line, can be placed on the luer lock, turning the stopcock off to the IV line. Air bubbles that may be present in the luer are now removed by first flicking the stopcock with a finger and then slowly drawing back 0.25 to 0.5 mL of blood into the syringe, drawing any air out of the stopcock. The blood is now slowly reinjected into the UAC. The line is now flushed using the syringe with the heparin flush solution and following the same steps outlined above.

Radial Artery Catheter An indwelling radial artery catheter can be a useful alternative to a UAC. The main advantage to the radial artery catheter is that the artery is accessible when the UAC has to be pulled out. It is also available in instances where the umbilical artery has lost its accessibility.

Another advantage is that right radial artery samples reflect preductal flow. In the presence of ductal shunting, knowledge of preductal PaO_2 is critical for proper maintenance of F_iO_2 as it reflects the PaO_2 supplying the eyes. An additional advantage is that thrombosis formation, which is often seen when major vessels are used, is less common.

The hazards associated with radial artery catheters include infection, air embolism, arterial occlusion, infiltration of fluids, and nerve damage.

Procedure for a Radial Artery Puncture Compared to the UAC, arterial punctures are fairly difficult to obtain in neonates. This is mainly due to the extremely small size of the neonate's arterial anatomy. When performing an arterial puncture on a neonate, one does not have the advantage of palpating the pulse to help locate the artery, as in adults. It is often done blindly, using only external landmarks to approximate the location of the artery. The distance from the skin to the artery is also deceiving, making it difficult to judge how deep to insert the needle.

One method that may enhance the capability of obtaining a radial sample is to use a transillumination light under the wrist to allow visualization of the artery. Care must be taken to not use a hot light, which may burn the patient.

Another problem with radial punctures is that it is not practical to do an arterial puncture as often as a UAC sample. This is the result of the trauma inflicted on the patient and the inaccuracies in the blood gas that are created from the crying and fussing. In these situations the use of transcutaneous monitors and pulse oximeters is invaluable.

Before performing a radial artery puncture on a neonate, an Allen's Test should be done to ensure collateral circulation. On the neonate, this is accomplished by first manually occluding both the radial and ulnar arteries, then passively squeezing the hand closed, and then opening it while releasing the ulnar artery. A positive test is indicated by diminished blanching (pink appearance) once pressure is released. This indicates sufficient collateral circulation to the hand.

The primary complications found in arterial puncture include infection, bleeding, nerve damage, embolism, and hematoma.

Capillary Samples Arterialized capillary samples are used primarily after the UAC has been removed and the patient requires ongoing blood gas monitoring.

Capillary samples are less hazardous to the patient and are more easily obtained than arterial punctures. Capillary samples are useful in assessing pH and $PaCO_2$, assuming adequate peripheral circulation. Capillary samples are not, however, reliable in the assessment of arterial PO_2.

Without arterial access, arterial oxygenation may be determined by pulse oximetry or transcutaneous monitoring. Another problem with capillary PaO_2 is that there are no defined normal values. On some neonatal patients, a capillary PaO_2 of 35 mmHg might be the equivalent of a 65 mmHg PaO_2, and on another patient the capillary and arterial values might correlate closely. However, one study showed correlated values between heel sticks and arterial values to be close and, therefore, indicated heel sticks to be reliable as an alternative to arterial blood gases.[1]

Indications According to the AARC Clinical Practice Guideline,[2] indications for capillary blood gas sampling are the following: an arterial blood gas analysis is indicated, but arterial access is not available; transcutaneous, pulse oximetry, or capnography readings are abnormal; assessing the patient following initiation, administration, or change in therapy; a change in the patient's status by history or physical exam; and monitoring the severity and progression of a documented disease process.

Contraindications Contraindications as outlined in the AARC Clinical Practice Guideline[2] are that capillary punctures should not be performed at or through the following sites: the posterior curvature of the heel; the heel of any patient who has begun walking and has callus development; the fingers of neonates; previous puncture sites; inflamed, swollen, or edematous tissues; cyanotic or poorly perfused tissues; localized areas of infection; peripheral arteries; and patients less than 24 hours old. Additionally, capillary samples should not be done when there is a need for direct analysis of oxygenation or of arterial blood. Relative contraindications include peripheral vasoconstriction, polycythemia, and hypotension.

The most reliable results from the arterialized capillary sample are obtained if the following steps are done consistently. The heel must be warmed to the same temperature for each puncture, and it must be warmed for the same length of time (5 to 7 minutes). At the end of the appropriate time period, the equipment is readied and the heel is unwrapped and wiped with an appropriate antiseptic pad. The foot is grasped in the nondominant hand and the heel is punctured in the area outlined in Figure 15–3. Puncturing in the outlined area avoids lacerating the posterior tibial artery and additionally averts the accidental puncture of the heel bone (**calcaneus**). The puncture should be made with a neonatal lance to avoid excess trauma to the heel. The blood should flow freely and quickly into the collection tube without needing to squeeze the heel.

Complications Complications of capillary sampling are often related to improper procedure. Puncturing the calcaneus bone may lead to osteomyelitis or bone spurs. Other complications include infection, burns, hematoma, nerve damage, bruising, scarring, tibial artery laceration, pain, bleeding, and inappropriate patient management by relying on capillary PO_2 values.[2]

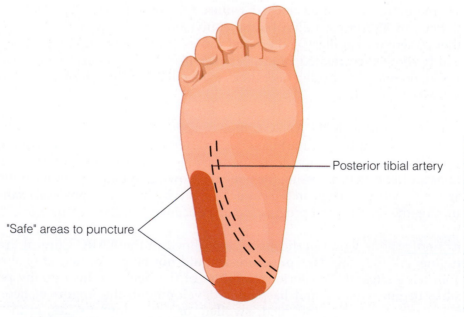

"Safe" areas to puncture

Posterior tibial artery

FIGURE 15–3. The heel is punctured in the outlined area.

Considerations for Obtaining Samples in Pediatric Patients

The pediatric population offers the same arterial sampling sites as the adult, with one exception. It may be possible on smaller pediatric patients up to 9–12 months of age to perform a capillary puncture on the heel of the foot (recognizing that $PaCO_2$ and pH are relatively accurate for acid-base assessment). Less common is a finger stick to quickly assess pH and/or $PaCO_2$.

The safest and most common site for sampling pediatric arterial blood is the radial artery. Arterial blood can also be drawn from the brachial artery and the femoral artery in emergencies. Other sites include the temporal artery and the dorsalis pedis artery if it is palpable. The femoral artery is always the last option; however, it should be considered when blood gas data is critically necessary.

Before performing a puncture on the radial artery, the respiratory therapist should perform an Allen's Test to ensure good collateral circulation through the ulnar artery. A positive test means that there is collateral circulation when the radial artery is occluded. The technique for performing arterial punctures on a pediatric patient is the same as on adult patients.

Indwelling arterial catheters are another method of obtaining arterial samples in the pediatric population. This method, however, is usually reserved for those patients on ventilators, in critical care areas, and others requiring repetitive blood gases and/or continuous blood pressure monitoring.

ARTERIAL BLOOD GAS ASSESSMENT

The assessment of blood gas status relies on an understanding of basic blood gas physiology and normal values. The physiologic concerns apply to both neonatal and pediatric patients. Differences in blood gas interpretation between these two groups are found in the normal (safe) values, which will be identified for each group.

An important point to remember when examining neonatal blood gas values is that there are no normal values. Values change over the first hours and days of life with changes in lung function and cardiac shunts. The neonatal normal values listed here refer to what is considered to be the safe range.

PaO$_2$

Neonatal Safe Range
50 to 70 mmHg
Pediatric Normal Range
80 to 100 mmHg (sea level)
55 to 80 mmHg (5000 ft.)

Basics of PaO$_2$ The arterial PO_2 tells something about oxygenation, but only that of arterial blood. The most important information would be tissue oxygenation, if it were available.

It should be remembered that PaO$_2$ is only one factor in oxygenation of arterial blood, representing the amount of oxygen dissolved in the plasma. According to the law of diffusion, movement through a membrane occurs following a concentration gradient. The larger the gradient, the more movement or diffusion takes place from the alveoli to the plasma in the blood. The diffusion gradient for oxygen at the capillary level is represented by the PaO$_2$ in the blood being on the high end of the gradient and the PaO$_2$ of the tissues being on the low end. We can consider the PaO$_2$ as being the driving pressure for tissue oxygenation, not the total amount of oxygen present.

The PaO$_2$ is the partial pressure of oxygen in the plasma relative to the barometric pressure. As a patient descends to sea level from elevation, the partial pressure generally increases (F$_i$O$_2$ does not change but the altitude decreases exerting more pressure on the body to increase the partial pressure of oxygen into the plasma). In cardiopulmonary disease, PaO$_2$ is a generalized measure of the transport of gas across the alveolar-capillary membrane. At sea level, it is expected to be between 80–100 mmHg. As an assessment, it can be assumed that with a normal oxygen dissociation curve a PaO$_2$ of 60 mmHg equals a saturation of about 90%. As an evaluation of oxygenation, it is only a partial representative of the efficiency of oxygen transport and should be evaluated with other factors that influence oxygen transport. Specifically, it can be influenced by the amount and ability of hemoglobin present to carry oxygen or the degree to which the molecule can be saturated. Low PaO$_2$ in the blood is called hypoxemia and the body's compensatory mechanism to improve oxygen transport is to increase the respiratory rate and/or heart rate.

Total Blood Oxygen and PaO$_2$ The vast majority of oxygen is carried by binding to hemoglobin. How much oxygen is bound to hemoglobin is determined by how much enters the plasma from the alveoli. The higher oxygen level in the plasma (PaO$_2$), leads to a higher driving pressure and causes more oxygen to attach to the hemoglobin. The amount of oxygen bound to hemoglobin is also affected by the position of the oxygen dissociation curve and the presence of pathologic species of hemoglobin such as carboxyhemoglobin and methemoglobin, or fetal hemoglobin.

Limitations of PaO$_2$ in Arterial Samples The PaO$_2$ value only reflects the level when the sample was drawn. At that moment, it may have been at a high, mid, or low point. It is for this reason that mid-range values are the safest when interpreting blood gas data. The patient's clinical status always needs to be considered before making any changes or accepting the validity of a value.

Use of Transcutaneous Monitors and Pulse Oximetry During the acute and recovery phases of RDS and particularly after surfactant replacement, rapid changes in PaO$_2$ may be expected and close monitoring of PaO$_2$ is required. With the advent of transcutaneous monitoring and pulse oximetry, the need for numerous blood gases has diminished. Indeed, the value of the blood gas measurements in these patients is to verify the accuracy of the monitors.

If the PaO$_2$ on the transcutaneous monitor parallels that of the arterial blood, then PaO$_2$ can easily be monitored continuously, allowing the respiratory therapist to make changes as needed to maintain adequate oxygenation.

Pulse oximeters can be reliably used to assess adequate arterial PO_2, as long as the respiratory therapist understands the limitations, explained later in this chapter.

$PaCO_2$

Safe Range
(pediatric and neonatal) 35 to 45 mmHg
Chronic Disease
<60 mmHg

Basics of $PaCO_2$ Carbon dioxide is the byproduct of aerobic metabolism and is excreted as bicarbonate by the kidneys and as CO_2 through the lungs. As with oxygen, the $PaCO_2$ is the partial pressure of carbon dioxide in the plasma. It provides the "driving force" for the carbon dioxide to leave the plasma.

In the blood, 85% of the total carbon dioxide is carried as bicarbonate, 10% is bound to hemoglobin, and 5% is carried as a dissolved gas or carbonic acid.

$PaCO_2$ greater than 45 usually indicates alveolar hypoventilation with respiratory failure being indicated when $PaCO_2$ is greater than 60 mmHg.

$PaCO_2$, then, defines the adequacy of alveolar ventilation, or that part of the tidal volume that is in direct contact with perfused alveolar surfaces.

Determinants of $PaCO_2$ The arterial $PaCO_2$ at any given time is the product of tissue metabolism versus the amount removed by the lungs. As metabolism increases, alveolar ventilation must also increase to remove the excess CO_2 in the blood. Any time there is an imbalance between alveolar ventilation and metabolism, $PaCO_2$ will increase or decrease respectively.

Alveolar ventilation is determined by minute ventilation minus deadspace (V_D). Minute ventilation is the total of all gas moved into the patient's respiratory system in 1 minute. It is calculated by multiplying the respiratory rate and the tidal volume.

V_D is the volume of air moved in and out of the respiratory tract that does not come into direct contact with perfused pulmonary units, that is, alveoli not engaged in gaseous exchange. V_D is composed of gas occupying the nasal, oral, and pharyngeal passages, endotracheal tubes, and the trachea down to the respiratory bronchioles. This includes air that is not physiologically important or is wasted. V_D is also made up of ventilated alveoli that are not being perfused by blood.

With each inspiration, the first gas into the alveoli is from the deadspace, the gas that was left in the airways from the previous exhalation. Only after an inspiration large enough to move the deadspace volume into the alveoli does fresh gas begin to enter the alveoli. Gas exchange will not occur, then, if tidal volume does not exceed deadspace ventilation.

If shallow rapid respirations occur, the V_D may be all that is moved into the alveoli. Even though minute ventilation is high, alveolar ventilation is absent and $PaCO_2$ increases.

This shows that $PaCO_2$ is affected exclusively by alveolar ventilation, not minute ventilation. Alveolar ventilation may be increased by elevations in tidal volume or respiratory rate, as long as the tidal volume is greater than V_D. Tidal volumes that are inadequate or ventilator frequencies that are too low lead to a high $PaCO_2$.

In contrast, a low $PaCO_2$ indicates excessive tidal volumes and/or respiratory rates. In a spontaneously breathing patient, a low $PaCO_2$ is not a stimulus for ventilation and, therefore, indicates the neonate is hyperventilating in response to another drive. Stimulants that can cause hyperventilation include hypoxia, metabolic acidosis, hyperthermia, or a central nervous system disorder (asphyxia, intracranial hemorrhage).

pH

Safe Range
(neonatal and pediatric) 7.35 to 7.45
Acceptable Range
(neonatal and pediatric) 7.30 to 7.50

Basics of pH The pH of the blood is a direct result of the number of hydrogen ions present. Hydrogen ions in the blood are the result of CO_2 reacting with water or derived from lactic acid secondary to anaerobic respiration. The definition of pH is the negative **logarithm** of the hydrogen ion concentration. The logarithm of a number is the *exponent* to which another fixed value, the *base*, must be raised to produce that number. As pH becomes more acidic or alkalotic, the number of hydrogen ions increases or decreases logarithmically.

In the safe range of pH, enzyme systems function optimally and oxygen transport is generally within physiologic ranges. The acceptable range is used for those patients with acute or chronic pulmonary disorders to serve as a guideline for initiation of support or to dictate changes in ventilator settings. A pH that falls below the acceptable range causes pulmonary vasoconstriction and a disruption of vital bodily functions.

Henderson–Hasselbalch Equation To understand pH disorders, one must understand the Henderson–Hasselbalch equation. This equation compares the pH to the bicarbonate ion concentration and $PaCO_2$:

$$pH = 6.1 + \log \frac{HCO_{3^-}\ mEq/L \quad \text{(base)}}{0.03 \times PaCO_2 \quad \text{(acid)}}$$

The $PaCO_2$ is multiplied by 0.03 to convert the partial pressure of carbon dioxide to carbonic acid (H_2CO_3). This weak acid freely donates hydrogen ions in the body. Thus, the higher the $PaCO_2$, the lower the resulting pH.

With a normal blood pH of 7.40, the ratio of bicarbonate ions to dissolved carbonic acid is 20:1. Alterations of blood pH can therefore occur whenever this ratio is altered above or below this ratio. The pH increases whenever the bicarbonate concentration increases or the $PaCO_2$ decreases. Conversely, pH decreases whenever the bicarbonate decreases or the $PaCO_2$ increases.

Whenever these imbalances occur, the body attempts to correct the pH by returning the ratio of bicarbonate to $PaCO_2$ back to normal. This knowledge lays the groundwork for understanding pH disorders and how the body compensates for them.

Primary pH disorders may be the result of respiratory or metabolic disorders, or a combination of both, and may occur with or without compensatory mechanisms. Causes of various pH disorders are outlined in Table 15–1.

OXYGEN CONTENT

Tissue oxygenation is determined by the amount of oxygen transported to the peripheral cells for metabolism. Under normal circumstances, the lungs are capable of delivering about 20 grams% (about 1000 mL/min [DO_2] oxygen delivered to tissues) to the peripheral tissues for aerobic metabolism. This is based on a cardiac output of 5 L/min for adults recognizing that pediatric perfusion is much less. Normal oxygen delivery to pediatric patients is between 550 and 650 mL/min. The tissues extract about 25% (5 grams% expressed as the O_2 Exchange Ratio [O_2ER]) of the oxygen delivered for use to create energy for physiologic functions. Oxygen content is the product of the amount of oxygen bound to hemoglobin added to the amount dissolved in the plasma. It is measured from the following equation:

$$CaO_2 \text{ or } O_2 CT = (Hb \times 1.34 \times SaO_2) + (.003 \times PaO_2)$$

TABLE 15–1

CAUSES OF pH DISORDERS

Respiratory:
Acidosis—generated by the retention of CO_2 in the blood
    Causes—sedation, BPD, meconium aspiration, TTN, maternal sedation or anesthesia, sepsis, intraventricular hemorrhage, metabolic disturbances that affect the respiratory centers (hypoglycemia), abnormalities or trauma to the thorax, diaphragmatic hernia, pneumothorax, and paralysis
Alkalosis—generated by a loss of CO_2 in the blood
    Causes—mismanagement of ventilator rates and volumes, RDS, stimulation of the central nervous system, and hypoxia-induced hyperventilation

Metabolic:
Acidosis—generated by an excess of hydrogen ions, a reduction in the loss of hydrogen ions, or a loss of bicarbonate ions
    Causes—hypoxemia with resulting lactic acidosis, starvation, hyperalimentation, renal tubular acidosis, and diarrhea
Alkalosis—generated by an excessive loss of hydrogen ions or by the addition of bicarbonate to the blood
    Causes—gastric suctioning, vomiting, diuretic use without adequate potassium replacement, IV administration of bicarbonate

Arteriovenous Oxygen Content Difference (C[a-v]O$_2$)

Oxygen content can be measured from a blood gas analysis of the arterial and mixed venous (pulmonary artery sample) blood. Comparisons can be drawn as to the relative oxygen consumption at the tissue level by the oxygen content in mixed venous blood. Under normal conditions, 15 grams% (CvO$_2$) returns to the lungs. The assessment reflects the difference between arterial oxygen and tissue utilization. Values lower than 5 grams% suggests that impairment of cells such that the tissues cannot extract oxygen for metabolism. On the other hand, a value higher than 5 grams% might indicate that perfusion to peripheral tissue is diminished.

A-a Gradient

The pressure difference of alveolar to arterial oxygen tension (P[A-a]O$_2$) reflects the partial pressure change across the alveolar capillary membrane. Under normal circumstances, transfer of gas should reach equilibrium resulting in a gradient difference less than 15 mmHg. Thus, whenever oxygen is necessary to treat hypoxemia the A-a gradient generally widens. Assessment of this parameter gives credibility to the fact that lung pathology that influences gaseous transport of oxygen requires a higher fraction of inspired O$_2$ to normalize oxygen delivery to the tissues.

a/A Ratio

Arterial oxygen relative to the measurement of alveolar oxygen tension assesses the integrity of the lung to diffuse oxygen across the alveolar-capillary membrane. Under normal circumstances at sea level, arterial oxygen (PaO$_2$) is 80–100 mmHg. Values less than 0.80 (80/100) determine a diffusion defect limiting gaseous transfer of oxygen across the alveolar capillary membrane.

PaO$_2$/F$_i$O$_2$ Ratio

The relationship of oxygen tension to the fraction of inspired O$_2$ is an assessment that assists the respiratory therapist to make clinical decisions about lowering PEEP or oxygen level. A value of 200 or greater represents an assessment that allows for reducing expiratory pressure toward normal physiologic levels. For example, a PaO$_2$ of 100/F$_i$O$_2$ of 0.5 is within range to make decisions about reducing PEEP or O$_2$ depending on pathology and clinical progress toward spontaneous breathing.

Intrapulmonary Shunt

An intrapulmonary shunt should be evaluated with the pediatric patient breathing 100% to account for a uniform PaO$_2$ exposing relative and absolute shunts as a cause of hypoxemia. Shunting creates a venous admixture which mixes with re-oxygenated blood and lowers PaO_2 and CaO_2 returning to the left heart. It is measured with the following calculation:

$$Qs/Qt = \frac{CcO_2 - CaO_2}{CcO_2}$$

As an assessment, the shunt relates the percentage of cardiac output returning to the arterial system that had not participated in gaseous transport of oxygen. Between 3 and 5% is normal whereas higher levels alert the respiratory therapist to employ ventilation strategies that help reverse hypoxemia improving oxygen delivery to the tissues.

HCO₃

Normal Range
22 to 26 mEq/L

Basics of Bicarbonate Levels The level of bicarbonate in the blood is controlled by tissue metabolism and the function of the kidneys. There are two components to plasma bicarbonate: the respiratory portion, which is the smaller of the two, and the metabolic portion.

In the bloodstream, hydrogen ions (H^+) combine with bicarbonate ions (HCO_3^-) to form carbonic acid ($H^+ + HCO_3^- = H_2CO_3$). Carbonic acid is then able to dissociate into carbon dioxide and water ($H_2CO_3 = CO_2 + H_2O$). The carbon dioxide is then removed from the blood by the lungs. The bicarbonate component of carbonic acid is said to be the metabolic portion of acid-base balance.

The metabolic portion of bicarbonate is that component that is controlled by the kidneys. The kidneys have the ability to excrete bicarbonate (HCO_3^-) or to retain bicarbonate as needed to maintain the pH.

HCO_3^- is calculated from the pH and $PaCO_2$. It is decreased in metabolic acidosis and respiratory alkalosis and increased in metabolic alkalosis and respiratory acidosis.

A level of 22 to 26 mEq/L shows adequate levels of buffering capacity. As the levels fall, the blood is less able to correct acid states. Conversely, as the levels rise, it signifies that the body has produced too much bicarbonate in relation to acid present, and an alkalotic state presents itself. An increase in CO_2 shifts the equation to the right by generating more H^+ and HCO_3^- and lowering pH. A lowering of CO_2 shifts the equation to the left, thus lowering H^+ concentration and raising pH.

Application of the Henderson–Hasselbalch Equation Understanding the application of the Henderson–Hasselbalch equation is facilitated by likening it to a balance with HCO_3^- on one side and CO_2 on the other side (Figure 15–4A). As illustrated, a normal balance of 20:1 results in a normal pH. As bicarbonate increases or decreases (see Figure 15–4B), the balance is disrupted and metabolic alkalosis or acidosis occurs. As the lungs now alter ventilation, CO_2 is either excreted or retained to counterbalance the effects of the bicarbonate (Figure 15–4C).

When CO_2 increases or decreases, the balance is again offset and acidosis or alkalosis results (Figure 15–4D). The body then responds by either retaining or removing plasma bicarbonate, returning the balance to normal (Figure 15–4E).

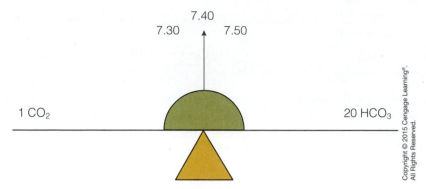

FIGURE 15–4 A. The balance between HCO_3^- and CO_2 results in a normal pH.

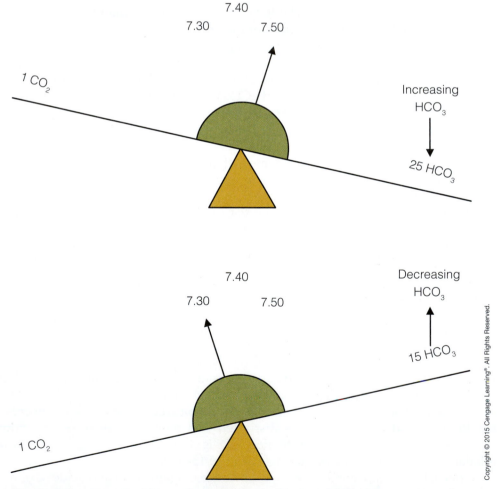

FIGURE 15–4 B. Increasing or decreasing HCO_3^- results in an imbalance, upsetting the pH.

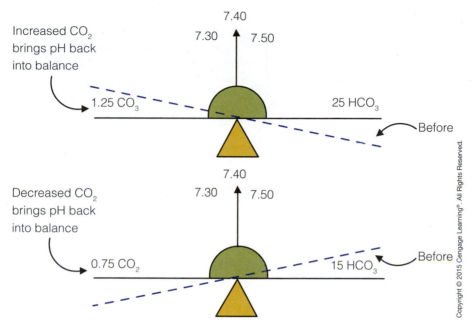

Increased CO_2 brings pH back into balance

7.40
7.30   7.50

1.25 CO_3 25 HCO_3

Before

Decreased CO_2 brings pH back into balance

7.40
7.30   7.50

0.75 CO_2 15 HCO_3

Before

FIGURE 15–4 C. Correction of the pH by retaining or removing CO_2 from the blood.

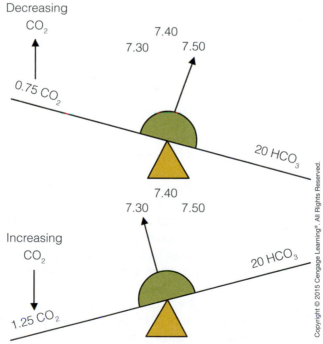

Decreasing CO_2

7.40
7.30   7.50

0.75 CO_2

20 HCO_3

Increasing CO_2

7.40
7.30   7.50

1.25 CO_2

20 HCO_3

FIGURE 15–4 D. As with HCO_3^-, and imbalance of CO_2 causes a change in pH.

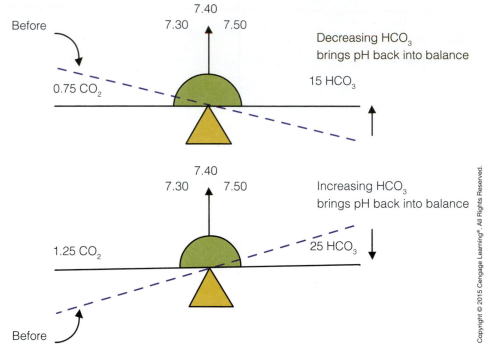

FIGURE 15–4 E. Retaining or removing HCO_3- balances CO_2, normalizing the pH.

Base Excess/Deficit

Normal Range
± 4 mEq/L

Basics of Base Excess Base excess is a reflection of the non-respiratory (metabolic) portion of the acid-base balance and reflects an excess or deficit of plasma bicarbonate. The buffering capacity of the red blood cells also has an effect on the base excess.[2]

Base excess must be viewed considering pH and $PaCO_2$, from which it is calculated, and the patient's clinical course. A base excess above 4 mEq/L indicates too much bicarbonate or too little acid in the blood. A negative value, called a base deficit, or a negative base excess, occurs whenever there is too little base or too much acid.

Base excess can be estimated by multiplying the calculated bicarbonate by 1.2 and then subtracting the normal value (24 mEq) from the product.[2]

Additionally, the bicarbonate binds with the hydrogen ions, forming carbonic acid, which then dissociates into carbon dioxide and water. If alveolar ventilation is not adequate, carbon dioxide levels increase and worsen the acidosis.

RESPIRATORY DISORDERS

In the neonatal and pediatric populations, there are several disorders that have the capability of affecting the blood gas status of the patient.

Respiratory Acidosis

Respiratory acidosis is the result of increased levels of $PaCO_2$ and is caused by alveolar hypoventilation. Possible causes of respiratory acidosis include obstructive lung diseases such as BPD, meconium aspiration, and transient tachypnea of the newborn.

Alveolar hypoventilation could result from the effects of maternal anesthesia before delivery, depressed ventilatory drive from sepsis, intraventricular hemorrhage, and metabolic disturbances that affect the respiratory centers. Abnormalities or trauma to the thorax, including diaphragmatic hernia, pneumothorax, or paralysis, can lead to hypoventilation.

The response of the body to respiratory acidosis is to reduce the excretion of bicarbonate from the kidneys and to excrete H^+ ions. Each increase of 1 mmHg in $PaCO_2$ results in an increase of plasma bicarbonate of 0.1 mEq/L. This then restores the ratio of bicarbonate to $PaCO_2$.

Respiratory Alkalosis

Respiratory alkalosis occurs when the arterial partial pressure of CO_2 is blown off due to alveolar hyperventilation. Respiratory alkalosis is often caused by mismanagement of ventilator rates and volumes.

Respiratory alkalosis is also caused by restrictive lung diseases, such as early RDS, stimulation of the central nervous system, and hypoxia-induced hyperventilation. The body responds to respiratory alkalosis by eliminating excess bicarbonate through the kidneys, restoring the appropriate ratio of bicarbonate to $PaCO_2$. In acute cases of respiratory alkalosis, there is a 0.2 mEq reduction in bicarbonate for every 1 mmHg decrease in $PaCO_2$.

METABOLIC DISORDERS

The body's energy derives from the metabolism of the proteins, fats, and carbohydrates in food. Any abnormality in this process can disrupt metabolism and lead to an interruption of the acid-base status of the patient.

Metabolic Acidosis

Metabolic acidosis is the result of an increased production or reduced loss of hydrogen ions. It is also caused by an abnormal loss of bicarbonate. Metabolic acidosis is commonly due to hypoxia with resulting lactic acidosis. It may also be caused by starvation, **hyperalimentation**, a procedure in which nutrients and vitamins are given to a person in liquid form through a vein, or renal tubular acidosis, from the inability of the premature kidney to excrete acid and reabsorb bicarbonate. Diarrhea may also lead to a loss of bicarbonate and may lead to metabolic acidosis.

The response of the respiratory system to metabolic acidosis is to increase alveolar ventilation and reduce arterial $PaCO_2$. For every mEq reduction in bicarbonate, there is a 1.2 mmHg reduction in $PaCO_2$.

Frequently, the neonate is unable to hyperventilate due to prematurity or the nature of the disease process.

Metabolic Alkalosis

Metabolic alkalosis is the result of an excessive loss of hydrogen ions from the gastrointestinal tract, or the kidneys, or by the addition of bicarbonate to the blood. Hydrogen ions are lost through gastric suctioning, vomiting, or with the overzealous use of diuretics without adequate potassium replacement.

The response of the respiratory system to metabolic alkalosis is a decrease in alveolar ventilation, causing $PaCO_2$ to increase. The response is about 0.6 mmHg increase in $PaCO_2$ for every mEq increase in bicarbonate.

TRANSCUTANEOUS MONITORING

Frequent measurement of arterial blood gases is essential in the treatment and maintenance of oxygenation and ventilation in the diseased neonate. However, traditional methods of assessing arterial blood gas status have inherent shortcomings that make them less than ideal. For example, the small neonate that requires frequent blood gas sampling may have a large portion of its blood volume depleted in a short period. A sample drawn from an umbilical catheter or by puncture, show the status of the patient when the sample was obtained but may be invalid within a few minutes due to the rapid changes that neonates encounter.

The ideal situation would be the ability to constantly monitor arterial blood gas values as they exist in the artery without causing pain or diminishing the blood supply. Although this ideal situation is not available, transcutaneous monitoring offers a welcome alternative.

Functional Design and Mechanics

Transcutaneous monitors (TCMs) evolved from the discovery in the early 1950s that oxygen diffuses through the skin from the capillaries. Modern TCMs use the same electrodes found in blood gas analyzers, except in miniature form.

Heating the area directly beneath the electrode results in three main effects:

- The heat changes the lipid structure of the superficial layer of skin, the **stratum corneum**, allowing a faster diffusion of oxygen through the skin.

- By heating the tissue and blood beneath the electrode, the oxygen dissociation curve is shifted to the right, enhancing the release of oxygen from the red blood cell.
- Finally, the heat causes a local vasodilation of the capillaries and causes an arterialization of the blood.[2]

Heat is provided by a small donut-shaped heater that surrounds the electrode. The temperature is regulated by a thermistor on the sensor that relays the temperature back to the monitor, which then supplies more or less power to the heater as needed. A cutaway view of a modern transcutaneous monitor is shown in Figure 15–5. Technology has now advanced to the point where both oxygen and carbon dioxide can be measured on one sensor, approximately the diameter of a quarter.

In general, transcutaneous PO_2 levels are lower than PaO_2 values. This could be due to the possibility that the TCM is measuring tissue oxygenation.

It is this author's experience that the $PtcCO_2$ tends to correlate more closely to arterial levels. This is possibly due in part to two factors. First, CO_2 diffuses easier than does oxygen, and second, the surface area of the Severinghaus electrode that measures $PaCO_2$ is larger than the Clark electrode.

The result is a monitor or monitors that can be placed on the surface of the patient's skin, which give a continual readout of oxygen and carbon dioxide tensions that are reliable indicators of arterial values.

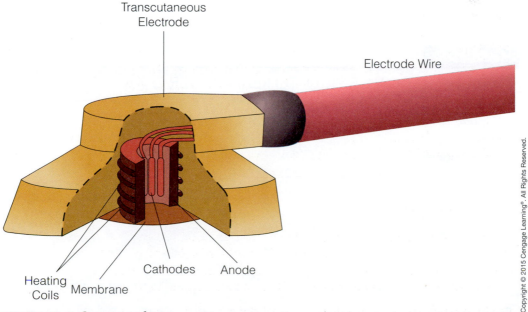

Transcutaneous
Electrode

Electrode Wire

Heating Coils   Membrane   Cathodes   Anode

FIGURE 15–5. Cutaway of a transcutaneous monitor probe.

Clinical Uses

In addition to monitoring the TCM can be used in the clinical setting to help diagnose and follow disease states that otherwise might go underdiagnosed or treated.

Trending An advantage in the use of a TCM is its ability to follow trends. The gradient between $PtCO_2$ and PaO_2 is most stable in noncritical patients. The unfortunate reality is that in critically ill patients, the gradient is highly variable.[3] In other words, the patient in whom we want the highest trending ability may be the one in whom we are least likely to get it. Before relying on the TCM in making critical therapeutic decisions, it must be determined that the monitor is trending adequately.

A patient on a ventilator whose $PaCO_2$ is trending downward can efficiently be weaned following the TCM values. Conversely, a patient with worsening status can be treated more quickly and effectively if the changes in oxygen and carbon dioxide can be continuously monitored. The TCM accomplishes this with minimal discomfort to the patient and, if used appropriately, with no harmful side effects.

The TCM should not be discontinued if it fails to correlate exactly with arterial values. A TCM has only lost its usefulness when its values are significantly different from arterial values and it does not trend in a reproducible way.

Factors that result in the $PtCO_2$ to measure lower than actual arterial PO_2 are those factors that reduce tissue perfusion. These factors, listed in Table 15–2, include shock, severe acidosis, hypothermia, severe cyanotic heart disease, severe anemia, skin edema, hyperoxemia with PaO_2 greater than 100 mmHg, and the use of Tolazoline given for pulmonary hypertension.

Detection of Shunting Blood Another clinical use of the TCM is in its ability to detect right-to-left shunting through the ductus arteriosus. This is done by placing

Table 15–2
FACTORS THAT CAUSE $PtCO_2$ TO READ LOWER THAN ARTERIAL VALUES
Shock
Severe acidosis
Hypothermia
Severe cyanotic heart disease
Severe anemia
Skin edema
PaO_2 greater than 100 mmHg
Tolazoline delivery

one electrode on the right shoulder, which is fed by the preductal right subclavian artery, and placing another electrode on the lower abdomen or leg.

A shunt is indicated when the preductal PaO_2 of the right shoulder is significantly higher than the post-ductal PaO_2 of the abdomen.

Indicator of Skin Perfusion The TCM can also be used as an indicator of skin perfusion.[4] If the monitor tracks the power required to heat the sensor to the preset level, changes in perfusion will show as changes in the amount of power required maintaining the probe temperature.

As perfusion increases, the blood carries the heat away more rapidly, requiring more power to maintain the temperature. Conversely, as perfusion decreases, less power is needed to maintain the temperature. Thus, the power output is a direct indication of perfusion at the electrode site.

Limitations

A task force on transcutaneous oxygen monitors identified seven limitations to their use.

1. $TcPaO_2$ may underestimate the PaO_2 in a hyperoxemic infant.
2. An inappropriate electrode temperature may adversely influence the performance of the monitor.
3. $TcPaO_2$ may underestimate the PaO_2 in infants with a compromised hemodynamic status or when there is excessive pressure on the electrode.
4. The performance of the $TcPaO_2$ may be suboptimal if placed over poorly perfused sites such as distal extremities, pressure points, and bony prominences.
5. $TcPaO_2$ may underestimate PaO_2 in infants with chronic lung disease.
6. The heated electrode may cause skin blistering, especially in very low birth weight infants and those with impaired perfusion.
7. $TcPaO_2$ cannot be used without periodic correlation with arterial blood gas analysis.

Complications and Hazards

Thermal injury is the greatest hazard in the use of TCMs. Recommended temperatures may produce an erythema, or reddening of the skin that can last from several hours to days.

Temperature settings above 44°C may cause thermal injury to the skin. Blistering has been reported when the sensor has been left at one site too long or at too high a temperature. It can also occur if perfusion is diminished.[5] Thermal injury can be avoided by correct temperature selection and appropriate site change intervals every 2 to 3 hours.

The double-gummed disk adhesives used to hold the sensor in place may cause epidermal stripping when removed. When used on the very small preemie, it may be advisable to use a Velcro or Coban wrap to hold the sensor in place. In any case, removal of the sensor should be gentle, avoiding the tendency to pull the sensor off too quickly.

Another potential hazard exists if the respiratory therapist begins to rely on the TCM for total blood gas information. As advanced as technology has become, TCMs cannot be relied on alone in place of arterial blood gases. All TCMs are vulnerable to physiologic changes in skin perfusion that can cause erroneous readings. Whenever a TCM is being used to monitor and change oxygen or ventilator settings, blood gases must be done on a routine basis to verify the accuracy of the TCM.

PULSE OXIMETRY

Another continuing development in noninvasive blood gas monitoring is pulse oximetry. Pulse oximeters utilize light absorption to calculate the saturation of arterial hemoglobin. The pulse oximeter is placed on any location that allows the passage of light. The ideal location is on a toe, finger, or ear, as these areas are fairly thin on the neonate and allow easy passage of light.

Modern pulse oximeters contain both a light source and a photodetector on the probe. The light source uses light-emitting diodes, which transmit both infrared and red light. The pulse oximeter probe is placed on the patient with the light source and photodetector opposite each other, separated by the selected body part. Proper placement is depicted in Figure 15–6. As light passes through the skin it is partially absorbed by the tissues, muscle, bone, etc. These absorb a constant amount of the light, which passes through the body part. Blood pulsing through the arterioles absorbs more light every time a fresh supply of arterial blood passes the site. The result is a variable absorption of light reaching the photodetector.

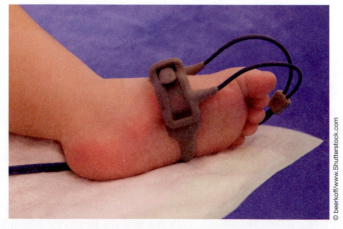

© beerkoff/www.Shutterstock.com

FIGURE 15–6. Proper placement of a pulse oximeter on a patient's foot.

Oxyhemoglobin (O_2Hb) and deoxyhemoglobin (Hb) are distinctly different in their capability to absorb red and infrared light. During systole, as the arterial blood pulsates between the light and photodetector, the pulse oximeter detects the variation in light absorption, and by comparing the ratio of infrared light to red light absorbed, calculates oxygen saturation.

Clinical Uses

Pulse oximeters require no warm-up time and do not need to be calibrated. Probes used on pulse oximeters are available for use on different areas of the body and on different-sized patients. Pulse oximeters have been found to be accurate in critically ill patients whose arterial oxygen saturation exceeds 75%.[3]

For the larger pediatric patient, it may be desirable to use an ear probe or a finger probe specifically designed for that site. For the smaller patient, sensors come built into a small length of flexible plastic, which can be wrapped around a finger, wrist, foot, or toe.

This type of sensor is held in place by small double-gummed adhesives, applied on each end of the sensor. These prevent the movement of the light source and photodetector on the skin surface and may or may not be used, depending on the maturity and health of the patient skin. The entire probe should then be secured to the body part using tape or a Velcro strap limb restraint.

External light sources, especially heat lamps and phototherapy lights, can interfere with the light detector. In these instances, if a limb restraint is not used, a cover should be placed over the sensor. It has also been noted that inaccuracies in measurement are seen in patients with heavy skin pigmentation.[3] Although the risk of skin trauma is small, the pulse oximeter probe site should be changed every 8 hours to prevent skin breakdowns and pressure sores.

A saturation of greater than 90% is usually indicative of normal oxygenation (PaO_2 of 60 mmHg with a normal oxyhemoglobin curve). It is important to remember, however, that the relationship between SaO_2 and PaO_2 is not linear and many factors affect that relationship.[3] The presence of different types of hemoglobin, such as methemoglobin or carboxyhemoglobin, in the blood will cause erroneously high readings on the pulse oximeter. This is because the pulse oximeter does not differentiate between different species of hemoglobin. Again, blood gas analysis should accompany the use of a pulse oximeter on a regular basis to ensure its accuracy.

The use of pulse oximetry has become routine in the emergency department and has been found to detect low saturations on patients who, by clinical evaluation, were not thought to be desaturated.[6] It is of interest to note also that pulse oximetry is being used to evaluate the presence of fetal hypoxia.[7]

Capnography/Capnometry

The introduction of capnography, or capnometry, the measurement of exhaled CO_2, has added one more noninvasive tool to assess the blood gas status of a patient. It has been shown to provide an accurate estimation of $PaCO_2$, even in the presence of severe hypocarbia.[8] It has also proven helpful in confirming ETT position following intubation and during transport.[9] A typical $PetCO_2$ waveform is shown in Figure 15–7.

Basics

Capnography uses **spectrophotometric infrared analysis** of the exhaled gas to determine end-tidal $PaCO_2$ ($PetCO_2$). An infrared spectrometer is an instrument that measures compounds absorption of infrared radiation. Infrared spectroscopy exploits the fact that molecules absorb specific frequencies that are characteristic of their structure. There are two methods available to sample and analyze the end-tidal breath: sidestream and mainstream monitors. The difference in the two methods is in how the sample is collected, not in the analysis itself.

Sidestream Analyzer The sidestream analyzer removes a continuous sample of the exhaled gas through a small tube and carries it to the analysis chamber. Because it is small and lightweight, the sidestream analyzer may be less likely to cause inadvertent extubation. It can also be adapted for use in nonintubated patients.

There are several downsides to the sidestream analyzer. First, the sample must pass through the tubing and water trap before it reaches the sample chamber. This makes it less responsive to high respiratory rates. Additionally, the displayed $PetCO_2$ is delayed from the actual breath. Water or mucus can accumulate in the sample tube and cause erroneous readings. Finally, the amount of gas sampled is important. If too much is drawn out, gas from the ventilator circuit may be entrained and dilute the sample. If used on a small neonate, excessive sampling may reduce the amount of delivered tidal volume.[10]

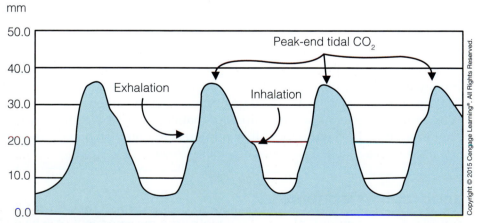

FIGURE 15–7. A normal $PetCO_2$ waveform.

Mainstream Analyzers Mainstream analyzers place the analyzing chamber at the airway. It is heated with a small wire to help prevent condensation in the chamber, reducing errors. An advantage to this type of system is that it gives current $PetCO_2$ readings, unlike the sidestream analyzer. This may make it more useful for patients with a high respiratory rate.

A disadvantage to this type of monitor is that the analyzing chambers are bulky and heavy, making the chance of accidental extubation a hazard. The chamber itself also has a large amount of deadspace, up to 15 mL, that could affect ventilation in the small neonate.

Physiologic Factors

$PetCO_2$ monitoring is valuable provided the respiratory therapist understands the physiology of end-tidal CO_2 production and the factors that can alter it. $PetCO_2$ may be most valuable in the monitoring of trends over time. Changes in patient condition can be quickly observed and treated. Trend evaluation may also make weaning and extubation more exacting to patient conditions. The remainder of this section will describe those factors that are important to understand to properly use the $PetCO_2$ monitor in the clinical setting.

Physiology of CO_2 Production Normal $PaCO_2$ in the healthy patient averages 40 mmHg and reflects the amount of CO_2 dissolved in the plasma of arterial blood. As body cells metabolize energy, they consume oxygen and produce carbon dioxide as a byproduct. From the cell, the CO_2 diffuses into the venous blood to be carried back to the lungs for removal. This addition of CO_2 from the cells raises the $PaCO_2$ of venous blood to about 46 mmHg. The pressure of CO_2 in the alveoli ($PaCO_2$) is lower owing to the inhalation of fresh atmospheric gas, which contains very little CO_2.

Upon reaching the alveoli, the CO_2 in the venous blood diffuses into the alveoli following a pressure gradient. The result is that the CO_2 in both the alveoli and in the blood equilibrate at a value of 40 mmHg. Thus, in the healthy, well-perfused lung, $PetCO_2$ as it has previously been defined. ($PetCO_2$) levels are equal to arterial $PaCO_2$ levels, as depicted in Figure 15–8.

Unfortunately, most patients being monitored for $PetCO_2$ do not possess healthy, well-perfused lungs. The practitioner must understand the physiologic changes that occur in the diseased lung and what the effect will be on $PetCO_2$ to adequately manage the patient using the $PetCO_2$ monitor.

The Effect of Ventilation/Perfusion (V/Q) Imbalances The basis of understanding $PetCO_2$ monitors is that ultimately they reflect changes in pulmonary perfusion. The $PetCO_2$ monitor looks at both lungs as though they were one respiratory unit. This is because exhaled gas at the level of the mouth is a mixture of all of the respiratory units in the lungs.

The healthy patient, with normal ventilation and perfusion, maintains 4 liters of ventilation for every 5 liters of blood flow. This produces a ratio of 4:5 or 0.8 when divided. Thus, for every liter of blood perfusion in the lungs, there is 0.8 liter of gas

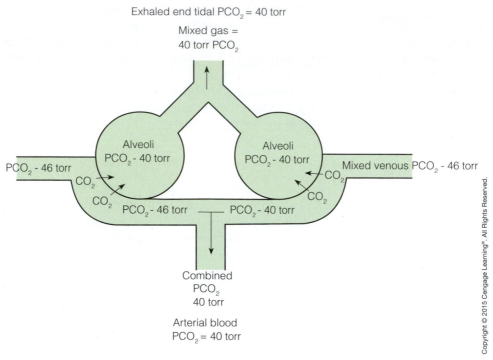

FIGURE 15–8. Well-perfused lungs resulting in a correlation between $PetCO_2$ and $PaCO_2$.

in the alveoli for exchange. We will now examine how changes in the V/Q ratio can alter $PetCO_2$ readings.

Deadspace Ventilation Deadspace ventilation is at one extreme of the V/Q range. This type of abnormality has the greatest effect on the $PetCO_2$ monitor. Deadspace ventilation occurs when the lungs are adequately ventilated, but perfusion is interrupted to a portion of the lung, as depicted in Figure 15–9. In this situation, the gas that enters the nonperfused alveoli does not participate in gas exchange, while the perfused alveoli do. The result is that the gas in the nonperfused alveoli remains with atmospheric partial pressures of CO_2, which is essentially 0 mmHg. The perfused alveoli participate in gas exchange and produce an exhaled gas that has a typical $PaCO_2$ of 40 mmHg.

As these two gases mix in the airways and are exhaled, the resultant mixed gas that exits the patient represents the average $PaCO_2$ of both gases, which is 20 mmHg (40 mmHg from the perfused alveoli, 0 mmHg from the nonperfused alveoli). The arterial blood in this example has a normal $PaCO_2$ of 40 mmHg. This is because the blood perfused good alveoli and participated in gas exchange, resulting in a normal $PaCO_2$. If this patient was monitored with a $PetCO_2$, the monitor would show a value of 20 mmHg, when in reality the arterial $PaCO_2$ is 40 mmHg. Thus, in the presence of increased deadspace ventilation, the $PetCO_2$ will read lower than arterial values.

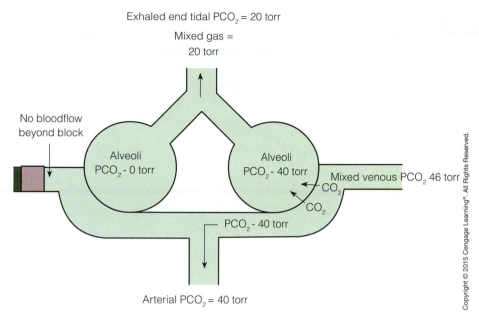

Exhaled end tidal PCO_2 = 20 torr

Mixed gas = 20 torr

No bloodflow beyond block

Alveoli PCO_2 - 0 torr

Alveoli PCO_2 - 40 torr

Mixed venous PCO_2 46 torr

CO_2

CO_2

PCO_2 - 40 torr

Arterial PCO_2 = 40 torr

FIGURE 15–9. Pulmonary embolism leading to deadspace ventilation.

Conditions Increasing Deadspace Ventilation There are several clinical conditions that can lead to an increase in deadspace ventilation, listed in Table 15–3.

Pulmonary embolus, causing an occlusion to blood flow in the lung, is a cause of deadspace ventilation. Depending on the severity of the embolism, the effect of $PetCO_2$ may be minimal with a small pulmonary embolus or dramatic in the case of a large embolus.

Severe hypotension can lead to an underperfusion of the lungs and is another cause of deadspace ventilation. Mechanical ventilation with high airway pressures may overdistend alveoli and compress the nearby pulmonary capillaries, leading to deadspace ventilation. The higher the ventilator pressures, the more the compression and resultant hypoperfusion.

Shunt Perfusion At the other extreme of the V/Q range is shunt perfusion. Shunts occur when blood perfuses areas of nonventilated alveoli. This type of mismatch does not have as drastic effects on the $PetCO_2$ monitor.

The maximal level that $PetCO_2$ can rise to is determined by the $PaCO_2$ of the mixed venous blood. Referring to Figure 15–10, if two arterial blood flows combine, one from an area of no ventilation, the other from an area of normal ventilation, the resultant $PaCO_2$ would be an average of the two, or 43 mmHg. In this example, the $PetCO_2$ would reflect the ventilated alveoli and show a $PaCO_2$ of 40 mmHg when the $PaCO_2$ is 43 mmHg. Only in cases of severe, life-threatening shunting would the $PetCO_2$ be significantly lower than $PaCO_2$.

Table 15–3
CONDITIONS LEADING TO INCREASED DEADSPACE VENTILATION
Pulmonary embolism
Hypotension
High pressures associated with mechanical ventilation

Conditions Causing Shunt Perfusion Clinical situations that result in shunting are listed in Table 15–4 and include atelectasis and obstruction of the airways by foreign objects or mucus.

Limitations to Capnography $PetCO_2$ monitors can only show a change in the patient's condition, not an improvement or subsequent deterioration. Consider the following scenarios, which further examine this limitation of capnography.

An increasing $PetCO_2$ may reflect a decrease in minute ventilation, a marked decrease in cardiac output, or a worsening of the V/Q ratio. All of these are considered

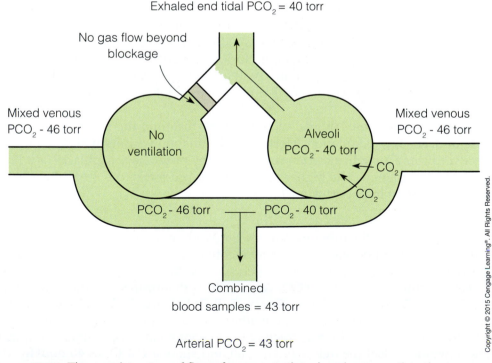

FIGURE 15–10. The combination of flows from a ventilated and nonventilated area.

Table 15–4

CAUSES OF PULMONARY SHUNTS

1. Venoarterial (right-to-left) shunting
   a. Tetralogy of Fallot
   b. Atrial septal defect
   c. Tricuspid atresia

2. Atelectasis

3. Obstruction of the airway

4. Pulmonary consolidation

a worsening of patient condition. Conversely, an increasing PetCO$_2$ may come from an improvement in alveolar deadspace disease, leading to an improvement in gas exchange. This condition would be a reflection of an improvement in patient status.

A decrease in PetCO$_2$ may be due to an improvement in ventilation or in the V/Q ratio, indicating an improvement of patient condition. However, a decreased PetCO$_2$ could also occur as alveolar deadspace increases, thus reflecting a worsening patient condition.

Another limitation of capnography is its inability to provide information on oxygenation. Arterial PO$_2$ may drop to dangerous levels, with little or no change in PetCO$_2$. Oxygenation must be monitored concurrently to get an overall view of respiratory status.

SUMMARY

In order to expertly care for the neonatal and pediatric patient, the respiratory therapist must know how to properly obtain and interpret data concerning the oxygenation, ventilation, and acid-base balance of the patient.

The most compelling method of measuring these parameters is with arterial blood gas analysis. In order to get results that are of value, the blood must be obtained in a manner that does not contaminate the sample, and in which the patient is not traumatized. The most common method of obtaining arterial blood from a neonate is through an umbilical artery catheter (UAC). Because of the possibility of shunting through a patient ductus arteriosus (PDA), and the position of the catheter tip in the descending aorta, blood gas results may be lower than what the upper extremities and head are receiving. Understanding this possibility can help the respiratory therapist make intelligent choices in the face of a low PaO$_2$ from the UAC. Another danger is in the possible dislocation of the catheter with resultant blood loss. In older patients, catheters may be inserted in the radial artery.

Other methods of obtaining blood for analysis are through arterial punctures and capillary samples. Because these inflict pain and usually result in an unhappy child, the results obtained may be skewed. Additionally, it must be remembered that capillary PO_2 does not adequately correspond to arterial PO_2 and should not be used to determine oxygenation status.

Once obtained, it is important for the respiratory therapist to interpret the values correctly. The value for oxygen in the plasma, PaO_2 is often misused. It must be remembered that PaO_2 is only one determinant of oxygenation and that it is only a reflection of the amount of oxygen actually present. Ideally, PaO_2 is used with oxygen saturation measurements to give a more complete view of oxygenation status.

$PaCO_2$ reflects the adequacy of ventilation. If too high, ventilation is not adequate and respiratory acidosis may ensue. If too low, the patient is hyperventilating and respiratory alkalosis may occur.

The pH of the blood is a measurement of the number of hydrogen ions present. The relationship is inverse, with a low pH indicating a high amount of hydrogen ions and vice versa. A low pH is called acidosis, and a high pH is called alkalosis. The pH is affected by both metabolic acids and alkalis and by CO_2.

HCO_3^-, or bicarbonate, is controlled by tissue metabolism and the kidneys and is responsible for maintaining proper pH balance. As more hydrogen ions become available, the bicarbonate quickly combines with them to form carbonic acid. Carbonic acid then dissociates into CO_2 and water, both of which are eliminated from the body. An excess or deficit of bicarbonate is reflected in the base excess/deficit measurement. A base excess above 4 mEq/L indicates too much bicarbonate, while a base deficit reflects too little bicarbonate to buffer the hydrogen ions.

Technology in the past decade has introduced several methods of noninvasive blood gas monitoring. One of the first to be introduced was the transcutaneous monitor (TCM). By measuring PaO_2 and $PaCO_2$ through the skin, constant monitoring can be accomplished and the amount of blood required for analysis reduced. If trending, the TCM can significantly aid in ventilator and oxygen management. Because of the risk of burning, the probe site must be changed every 2 to 3 hours.

Another technological advance is the pulse oximeter. In contrast to the TCM, which measure PO_2, the pulse oximeter measures the amount of oxygen bound to hemoglobin, a potentially more useful measurement. Because it is noninvasive, it can also be used continuously and is very helpful in monitoring for hypoxic spells.

Finally, capnography has been shown to accurately reflect arterial PCO_2. It does this by measuring a sample of the patient's exhaled breath through either a sidestream analyzer or a mainstream analyzer. In order to properly use the data, the factors affecting CO_2 production (such as ventilation/perfusion imbalances, deadspace ventilation, and shunt perfusion) must be understood.

POSTTEST

1. Of the following, which would *not* be an indication for obtaining a blood gas sample?
    a. signs of respiratory distress
    b. change in patient status
    c. departmental policy
    d. significant blood loss
2. Which of the following are common sites used to obtain arterial blood in neonates?
    I. umbilical artery
    II. radial artery
    III. femoral artery
    IV. capillary
    V. carotid artery
        a. I, II, IV
        b. I, III, V
        c. II, IV, V
        d. I, III, III, V
3. In the presence of right-to-left shunting of blood through the ductus arteriosus, arterial blood from the UAC would show:
    a. a low arterial PO_2
    b. a high arterial PO_2
    c. an alkalotic pH
    d. a low arterial $PaCO_2$
4. The complication of necrotizing enterocolitis is most prevalent in which of the following blood gas access sites?
    a. radial artery
    b. umbilical artery
    c. femoral artery
    d. carotid artery
5. Reliable values obtained from capillary samples require which of the following?
    a. heating the heel to at least 45°C
    b. consistency in the technique
    c. adequate squeezing or milking of the heel
    d. puncturing with a beveled needle
6. Which of the following best describes PaO_2?
    a. the total amount of oxygen present in the blood
    b. the amount of oxygen attached to hemoglobin
    c. the pressure of oxygen dissolved in plasma
    d. the best indicator of adequate tissue perfusion

7. Which of the following defines alveolar ventilations?
    a. tidal volume times respiratory rate
    b. minute ventilation minus deadspace ventilation
    c. minute ventilation minus tidal volume
    d. minute ventilation minus respiratory rate
8. As respiratory rate increases at a static tidal volume, which of the following occurs?
    I. $PaCO_2$ decreases
    II. $PaCO_2$ increases
    III. alveolar ventilation increases
    IV. alveolar ventilation decreases
        a. II, III
        b. I, III
        c. I, IV
        d. II, III, IV
9. At a pH of 7.40, which of the following represents the correct balance of bicarbonate to dissolved carbon dioxide?
    a. 1:10
    b. 10:1
    c. 15:1
    d. 20:1
10. In the presence of respiratory acidosis, which of the following is the amount of bicarbonate the body retains for each 1 mmHg increase in $PaCO_2$?
    a. 1.0 mEq/L
    b. 0.1 mEq/L
    c. 0.01 mEq/L
    d. 10 mEq/L
11. Carbonic acid is formed by a combination of:
    a. HCO_3- and CO_2
    b. HCO_3- and H^+ ions
    c. HCO_3- and H_2O
    d. CO_2 and H^+ ions
12. $NaHCO_3-$, if given too rapidly, could lead to:
    a. intraventricular hemorrhage
    b. cardiac arrest
    c. intestinal bleeding
    d. diminished PaO_2
13. The purpose of heating the skin at the attachment site of the TCM is to:
    a. decrease capillary shunting
    b. increase the tissue PaO_2
    c. increase the perfusion to the area
    d. cause the skin to sweat

14. Which of the following factors would cause $PtCO_2$ to measure lower than actual arterial PO_2?
    I. shock
    II. severe acidosis
    III. skin edema
    IV. hyperthermia
    V. severe anemia
        a. I, II, III, V
        b. I, III, IV
        c. III, IV, V
        d. I, II, III, IV, V

15. The greatest hazard associated with transcutaneous monitors is:
    a. erythema
    b. epidermal stripping
    c. hemorrhage
    d. thermal injury

16. Which of the following would cause erroneous pulse oximetry readings?
    a. presence of carboxyhemoglobin
    b. PaO_2 above 100 torr
    c. decreased hemoglobin levels
    d. increased hemoglobin levels

17. A major disadvantage of a mainstream end-tidal CO_2 monitor is:
    a. accidental extubation
    b. occlusion with condensed water
    c. increased risk of pneumothorax
    d. thermal injury

18. The greatest effect on the end-tidal CO_2 monitor is exerted by:
    a. a pneumothorax
    b. shunt perfusion
    c. deadspace ventilation
    d. hyperventilation

19. An increasing $PetCO_2$ may indicate which of the following?
    I. worsening oxygenation
    II. worsening V/Q ratio
    III. improving V/Q ratio
    IV. improvement in alveolar deadspace disease
    V. increasing alveolar deadspace
        a. I, II
        b. II, IV
        c. I, III, V
        d. I, III

REFERENCES

1. Yang KC, et al. The comparison between capillary blood sampling and arterial blood sampling in an NICU. *Acta Paediatr Taiwan*. 43(3):124–126, May–June 2002.
2. AARC Clinical Practice Guideline: capillary blood gas sampling for neonatal and pediatric patients. *Resp Care*. 46(5):506–513, 2001.
3. Durbin CG Jr. Monitoring gas exchange: clinical effectiveness and cost considerations. *Resp Care*. 39:123–137, 1994.
4. Powell CC, et al. Subcutaneous oxygen tension: a useful adjunct in assessment of perfusion status. *Crit Care Med*. 23:867–873, 1995.
5. Avery GB, et al. American Academy of Pediatrics Task Force on transcutaneous oxygen monitors: report of consensus meeting. *Pediatrics*. 83:122–125, 1989.
6. Maneker AJ, et al. Contribution of routine pulse oximetry to evaluation and management of patients with respiratory illness in a pediatric emergency department. *Ann Emerg Med*. 25:36–40, 1995.
7. Luttkus A, et al. Continuous monitoring of fetal oxygen saturation by pulse oximetry. *Obstet Gynecol*. 85:183–186, 1995.
8. Flanagan JKF, et al. Noninvasive monitoring of end-tidal carbon dioxide tension via nasal cannulas in spontaneously breathing children with profound hypocarbia. *Crit Care Med*. 23:1140, 1995.
9. Bhende MS, et al. Evaluation of a portable infrared end-tidal carbon dioxide monitor during pediatric interhopsital transport. *Pediatrics*. 95:875–878, 1995.
10. Walsh BK, et. al. *Perinatal and Pediatric Respiratory Care,* 3rd ed. St. Louis, MO: Saunders/Elsevier, 2010.

BIBLIOGRAPHY AND SUGGESTED READINGS

Kaufman DA. Interpretation of Arterial Blood Gases. American Thoracic Society. http://www.thoracic.org/clinical/critical-care/clinical-education/abgs.php.

MacDonald MG, et al. *Atlas of Procedures in Neonatology.* Philadelphia, PA: Lippincott Williams and Wilkins, 2007.

Mechem CC. Pulse oximetry. UpToDate, Wolters Kluwer. http://www.uptodate.com/contents/pulse-oximetry.

Ortega R, et al. Pulse oximetry. *N Engl J Med*. 364:e33, 2011.

Schwarz AJ. *Blueprints Pocket Pediatric ICU.* Philadelphia, PA: Lippincott Williams and Wilkins, 2007.

WebMD. Arterial Blood Gases. http://www.webmd.com/lung/arterial-blood-gases.

CHAPTER 16

Interpretation of Chest X-Rays

OBJECTIVES

Upon completion of this chapter, the reader should be able to:

1. Explain why x-rays alone cannot be used for a differential diagnosis.
2. Describe the basic mechanics of how an x-ray is taken.
3. List and describe the four densities found on an x-ray.
4. Discuss the diagnostic usefulness and limitations of x-ray.
5. Describe how each of the following are determined when interpreting a chest x-ray:
   a. Patient identification
   b. Orientation of the x-ray
   c. Quality of the x-ray
   d. Patient position
   e. Determination of inspiration or expiration
   f. Proper heart size
   g. Proper position of the umbilical artery and vein catheter
   h. Congestive heart failure and right-to-left shunting
   i. Proper position of the endotracheal tube
6. Describe the cause and appearance of air bronchograms.
7. Describe the appearance of the following neonatal disorders on a chest x-ray:
   a. Respiratory distress syndrome
   b. Atelectasis
   c. Transient tachypnea of the newborn
   d. Pneumonia
   e. Meconium aspiration syndrome
   f. Diaphragmatic hernia
   g. Congenital lobar emphysema
   h. Pneumothorax
   i. Pneumomediastinum
   j. Pneumopericardium
   k. Pulmonary interstitial emphysema (PIE)
   l. Bronchopulmonary dysplasia

8. Describe the radiographic appearance of the following pediatric disorders:
   a. Adult respiratory distress syndrome (ARDS)
   b. Foreign body aspiration
   c. Cystic fibrosis
   d. Asthma
   e. Epiglottitis
   f. Croup

KEY TERMS

air bronchograms	hilum	radiopaque
costophrenic angle	hyperlucency	reticulogranular
decubitus	mAs/kVp	scaphoid
densities	pseudocysts	thymus

INTRODUCTION

An x-ray allows observation of the internal structures of the chest. Utilized as a routine assessment or examination, radiographic evidence of disease processes has revolutionized the assessment and treatment of abnormalities of the cardiopulmonary system. An x-ray can provide meaningful insight into clinical observations or reveal an explanation for the signs or symptoms identified by a clinical examination. It can provide evidence that treatment is working and that support can be weaned away or that a new strategy should be considered. Technology is improving and the images produced are profoundly changing the way respiratory therapists perform their work at the bedside.

BASIC CONCEPTS

X-rays have become an important tool in managing newborns with lung disease because of their ability to give views of the effect of various disease processes on the internal body structures. When interpreting x-rays, it must be kept in mind that the disease itself is not seen. Respiratory therapists may be instrumental in describing physical characteristics to interpret the x-ray by evidence identified as signs of a particular disease. The radiograph represents a visual confirmation of the therapist's suspicions of the presence or absence of a disease process. The physical alterations resulting from a disease are presented on the x-ray film. For example, the air between the chest wall and the lung in a typical pneumothorax is not visible, but the lung tissue being pushed aside and compressed is visible. The space between both, filled with air, is distinct on the x-ray.

Under suspicion of particular pathology, for example in a deteriorating infant with low saturations and falling TCM values or observed asymmetric chest rise, a respiratory therapist may recommend to an attending physician that an x-ray is warranted. In some instances, a physician will be present to interpret the chest x-ray; however, there will be times when the physician is not available and other practitioners may be the first to view the film. In those instances, it is important that the respiratory therapist be able to identify those abnormalities on the x-ray that could be vital in the emergent care of the patient.

X-Ray Projections

A chest x-ray is a two-dimensional black and white picture (with shades of grey) but it has transformed the practice of medicine by allowing a view of the inside of the human body. Its purpose is to confirm pathologic processes related in the history or physical, evaluate the placement of tubes and lines, and observe the progression of disease or effectiveness of therapy. In order to fully visualize an abnormality in the chest of a patient, two x-ray views are required, a frontal (usually a PA view) and lateral view is taken. If the patient is able to stand, the film plate is placed in front of the patient and the x-ray is projected from behind the patient. Because of the x-rays travel from the posterior to the anterior of the patient, this is called a posterior/anterior or PA view. On patients who cannot leave the bed, such as those being ventilated, the film plate is placed under the patient and the x-ray passes from anterior to posterior, creating an anterior/posterior or AP view.

It can usually be expected that a chest film of any newborn or intubated pediatric patient is an AP view, but the respiratory therapist should always make sure which view was obtained. This is because PA and AP views cause the internal structures to appear differently and can cause a misdiagnosis if not understood. As an example, because the heart lies more anterior in the chest, it will appear larger on an AP film than on a PA film, that is, it is either farther away or nearer to the x-ray plate, positioned on the back or chest, respectively.

While the frontal view identifies whether an abnormality is on the right or left side of the chest, the lateral view identifies its position as anterior or posterior in the chest. The lateral view is also used on the neck to identify an enlarged epiglottis characterized by supraglottic swelling.

Mechanics of the X-Ray Device

The basic mechanism of the x-ray is similar to photography. The x-ray is a frequency of light, outside the visible spectrum, that can penetrate most body substances. A film that is sensitive to x-rays is placed on the opposite side of the body from the x-ray "camera." The x-rays are then aimed through the desired part of the body (Figure 16–1). Some of the x-rays pass through and expose the film, while others are blocked from passing through. The film is developed and a transparent picture is obtained.

Densities Seen on an X-Ray

Four **densities** can usually be distinguished on x-ray; air (black), bone (white), fluid (gray), and tissue (grayer) (see Table 16–1).[1] First is an air or gas density. X-rays pass easily through gases, totally exposing or penetrating the x-ray film and turning it black. Second are the fluid densities. Fluids partially absorb the x-rays and allow only a portion of the x-rays to reach the film. The result is a gray shade on the developed

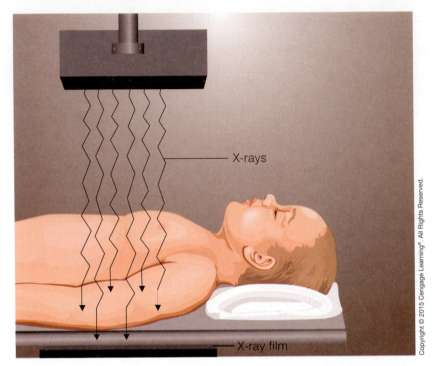

X-rays

X-ray film

FIGURE 16–1. X-rays pass through the body, creating an image on film.

film. Various tissues of the body are largely liquid, and so create a hue very similar to fluids (grayer) on the radiograph. Fluid and tissue are often indistinguishable: however, recognizing the different densities may be helpful. When these patterns appear in anatomic places that one would not expect, this indicates pathology. When such tissue is irregular in its density, the film will be patchy, stippled, or look like ground window glass. Fourth is bone density, which absorbs a large portion of the x-rays. If no x-rays penetrate the film, that area of the x-ray will appear white. The amount of calcium in the bone will determine whether the bone is white or slightly transparent. Well-calcified bone is often white on x-ray, compared to less calcified bone, which appears slightly more transparent.

Table 16–1

DENSITIES FOUND ON X-RAYS

1. Air (black) density—produces the darkest (black) patterns

2. Fluid (gray) density—produces gray patterns

3. Tissue (grayer) density—produces grayer patterns

4. Bone (white) density—produces the lightest (white) patterns

Diagnostic Usefulness and Limitations

It is important to remember that x-rays cannot be used to diagnose lung disease in newborns. The patient's diagnosis is made from physical examination, laboratory data, and clinical signs that correspond to RDS characteristics. Radiographs are then used to confirm the diagnosis based on a thorough evaluation of the data available to the respiratory therapist. X-rays are also used to differentiate between diseases with similar signs and symptoms. They are limited by the fact that artifacts, improper techniques in taking the x-ray, and patient movement may all lead to erroneous interpretation. The person examining the x-ray must be careful to avoid mistaking these factors for disease. For example, excessive distance from the source magnifies the appearance of the structures in the chest. A heart may appear to be enlarged if the distance is greater than 6 feet from the target.

Anatomic Considerations

There are anatomic differences in the chest x-rays of neonates and children, which may cause confusion if not understood. First, the position of the carina—the point at which the trachea splits into the left and right mainstream bronchi—is higher than in adults. In a neonate, it is near the level of the third vertebrae and by age 10 it has descended to the level of the fifth vertebrae.[2]

The **thymus** is a gland located in the mediastinum extending from the lower edge of the thyroid gland in the neck to near the fourth rib. On x-ray, it appears less dense than the heart, but more dense than lung tissue. It is often confused with the heart border and can even appear as an upper lobe atelectasis or pneumonia. Often, it is triangular shaped and is called the "sail sign" when identified on x-ray (Figure 16–2). Its size in relation to the rest of the body is largest at about 2 years of age.

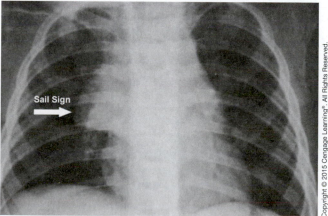

Sail Sign

FIGURE 16–2. Radiography showing the "the sail sign".

METHOD OF INTERPRETATION—A SYSTEMIC APPROACH

Often, when reading or interpreting pathology in an x-ray, attention is drawn to a single overwhelming feature and significant details may be overlooked. To avoid this, the respiratory therapist should use a systematic approach when examining a chest x-ray, outlined in Table 16–2.

Patient Identification and Date

Above all else, check the patient identification stamp, date, and time. For accurate assessment of the patient's current problems, it is important to use the most recent x-ray. This may also alleviate some embarrassment when presenting a dazzling interpretation of the x-ray, just to find out it is the wrong patient or the film is a week old.

Table 16–2

SYSTEMATIC APPROACH TO READING A CHEST RADIOGRAPH

1. Confirm correct patient and date.

2. Correct orientation. Patient's left side should be on your right as you view the radiograph.

3. Check the quality of the radiograph. Check for over- or underexposure.

4. Confirm proper patient position (rotation).

5. Determine whether the radiograph is in the inspiratory or expiratory phase.

6. Examine the ribs

7. Examine the diaphragm.

8. Examine the abdomen.

9. Inspect the cardiac silhouette.

10. Examine the area of the lung at the hilum.

11. Inspect the respiratory tract:
    a. Trachea
    b. Position of the endotracheal tube
    c. Mainstream bronchus
    d. Lung fields
    e. Pleural surface

Orientation

Next orient the x-ray so that the patient's right side is on the respiratory therapist's left. This feature is often marked by the x-ray technician, but you should always check the anatomy yourself. Determining the infant's position at the time of the x-ray will help in orientation. Look for landmarks such as heart leads, a transcutaneous monitor, and chest tube sites. The heart should be centered but slightly to the left. If a stomach bubble is present, it should be on your right as you look at the film. Also, make certain that the film is not reversed or upside down. Many normal infants have mistakenly been diagnosed as having a diaphragmatic hernia, when the only problem was an upside-down film.

X-Ray Quality

Next check the quality of the x-ray. Determine if it is over-, under-, or normally exposed. Spaces between the vertebrae are visible and distinct when a proper exposure has been made. If the spaces between the vertebrae are not visible, too little energy was used and the film is underexposed. Too much energy overexposes the film, making the intervertebral spaces excessively dark. An x-ray that is over- or underexposed will be very difficult to interpret. The lung fields in an overexposed chest x-ray may look well aerated when in reality they are very underaerated. Conversely, the lung fields in an underexposed chest x-ray may appear vastly underaerated when in fact they are well aerated.

It is good practice to post the **mAs/kVp** which help control the density and contrast the duration of exposure, and the energy used that resulted in a good exposure at the patient's bedside or on the incubator. This will help in consistently getting good exposures.

Patient Position

Next check the position of the infant on the film. The infant should be relatively straight on the film, and not rotated to either side. Identify the position of the spinal processes of the thoracic vertebrae with respect to the clavicles and the sternal notch, that is, the spine should center between the clavicular attachments at the sternum. Rotation will alter the heart size and cover areas it may be necessary to see. The clavicles should be examined for symmetry in relation to the spinal column. When the infant is straight, the clavicles and spine should form a "T," with both clavicles symmetrical and at right angles to the spine, as shown in Figure 16–3. The peripheral ribs should turn downward, and not be flat or turning upward. A rotated chest x-ray may give you the impression of an enlarged heart or shifted trachea.

Determination of Inspiration and Expiration

The next step is to determine if the film was exposed during inspiration or expiration. On an inspiratory x-ray the diaphragm should be at or below the ninth rib, as shown

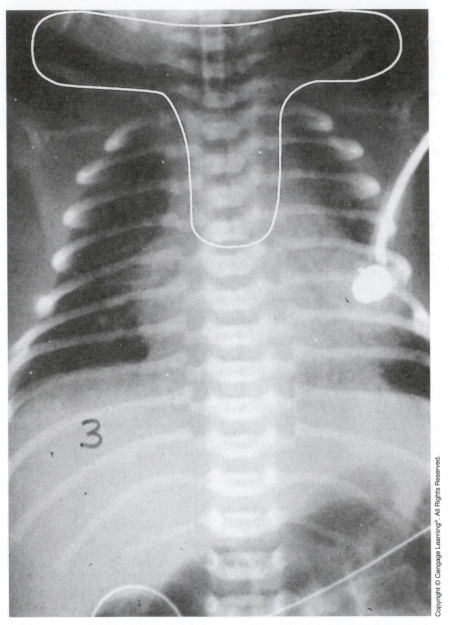

FIGURE 16–3. Chest x-ray showing the "T" formed by clavicles and vertebrae.

in Figure 16–4. Overdistention or hyperaeration will be near or below the 10th rib. A radiograph taken during expiration will show the diaphragm at the sixth or seventh rib. Hyperaeration will cause the ribs to appear flattened or the chest to be "bell" shaped. At this point take the time to examine the ribs for any deformities or fractures.

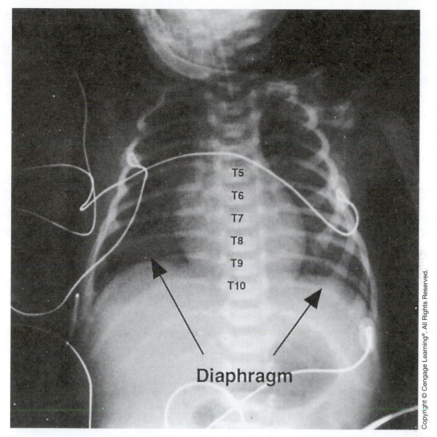

FIGURE 16–4. Position of the diaphragm during inspiration.

Examination of the Ribs

The ribs are examined for any sign of abnormality or fracture. One common method used to evaluate the ribs is to start the examination at the posterior portions of the ribs first, then proceed to the anterior portions. The rib examination is finished by examining the lateral aspects of each rib. Any time an abnormality is seen, that rib should be followed in its entirety.

Rib fractures will appear as a break in the smooth outline of the rib. A lucent fracture line may also be seen. Keep in mind however, that a rib fracture may not be visible on a CXR. In children, multiple bilateral rib fractures in various stages of healing may be associated with abuse.

Examination of the Diaphragm

Now examine the shape of the diaphragm. It should be dome-shaped on both sides, with the right diaphragm usually being one rib higher than the left. This is caused by the liver pushing the diaphragm upward. If the diaphragm does not meet this description, there may be a water density in the lung adjacent to the diaphragm. Next, observe the **costophrenic angles** on either side of the thorax. These angles are formed by the posterior curve of the diaphragm as it arches downward toward the spine. They should be sharp and well-defined points at the outer edges of the film. Fluid in the pleural space may cause "blunting" of these angles. Air trapping and hyperaeration will cause the diaphragms to appear flat anteriorly to posterior on a lateral view or extend beyond the 10th rib on the x-ray.

Examination of the Abdomen

Chest x-rays do not often include a great deal of the abdomen, but the respiratory therapist should learn to examine the portion of the abdomen that is present. The presence of a stomach bubble helps to orient the film to the left. A large air bubble in the stomach and excessive air in the bowel (Figure 16–5) are indicative of gastric

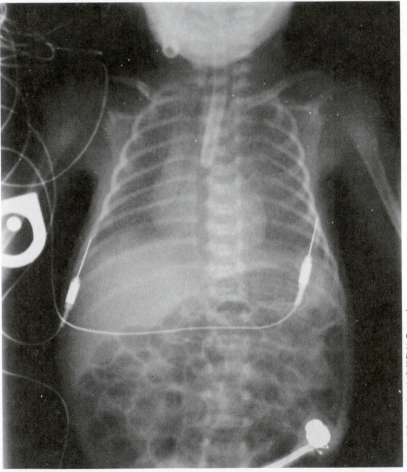

FIGURE 16–5. Excessive gastric air resulting from an esophageal intubation.

distention. Excessive distention in the stomach can decrease the ventilation of the infant by pressing upward against the diaphragm.

Examining the upper right side of the abdomen, the posterior edge of the liver is seen as the lowest visible edge. The liver appears as gray-to-white shade on the film because it is a fairly thick tissue. The liver should not be more than 1 to 1.5 cm below the rib cage. A liver that is below that level may be an indication of blood engorgement resulting from right-sided heart failure.

If enough of the abdomen is showing, check the position of the umbilical artery or vein catheter. The tip of the umbilical artery catheter (UAC) should lie between the seventh and eighth thoracic vertebrae (T7–T8) or between the third and fourth lumbar vertebrae (L3–L4), as shown in Figure 16–6. One study found a higher incidence of leg blanching and cyanosis in infants with the UAC tip at L3–L4. Finding the appropriate vertebrae can be done by locating the 12th thoracic vertebra (T12). T12 is the vertebra to which the last floating rib is attached. The next vertebra down is the first lumbar vertebra. Counting upward, T7 and T8 can be located. Placing the tip at T7–T8 positions the tip above the celiac arteries. Positioning the tip of the UAC between L3 and L4 places it above the division of the aorta into the legs and below the inferior mesenteric artery. These two positions prevent direct instillation

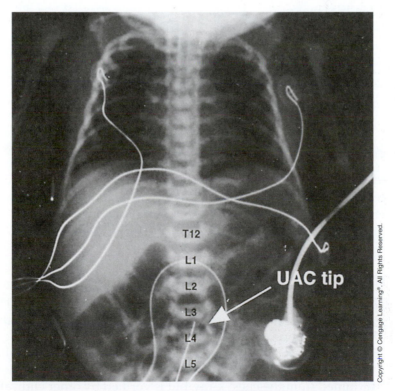

FIGURE 16–6. The tip of the UAC in proper position between L3 and L4.

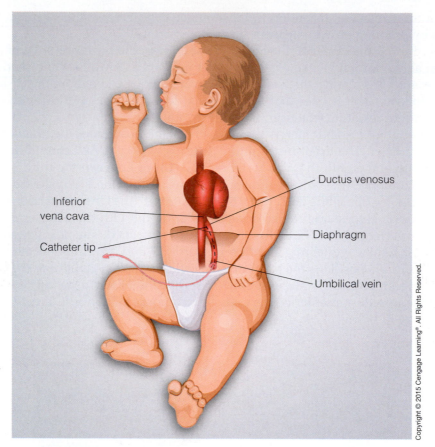

FIGURE 16–7. Proper position of the UAC.

of fluids and drugs into the celiac or mesenteric arteries. The L3–L4 position may also help prevent hypoperfusion to the kidneys when blood is withdrawn from the catheter. The UAC is positioned in the interior vena cava, just above the diaphragm, as illustrated in Figure 16–7.

Examination of the Cardiac Silhouette

The silhouette of the heart and thymus should now be examined. The cardiac silhouette (Figure 16–8) is extremely variable in size and should be less than 60% of the thoracic width (from one costophrenic angle to the other). A cardiac silhouette larger than 60% implies an enlarged heart, although the silhouette includes other structures in the mediastinum, including the thymus. A diagnosis of cardiomegaly is not solely determined from the chest x-ray, but is verified by other clinical signs and symptoms the patient demonstrates.

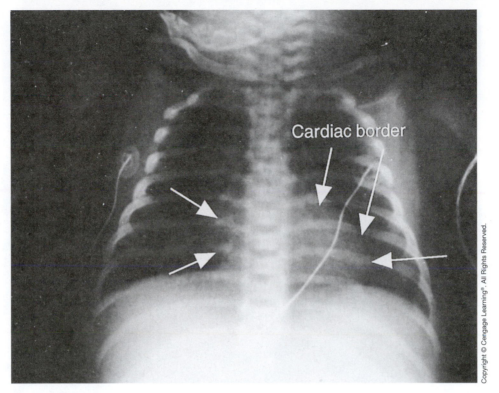

Cardiac border

FIGURE 16–8. The cardiac silhouette as seen on the chest x-ray.

Examination of the Hilum

Now examine the hilum area of the chest. The **hilum**, outlined in Figure 16–9, is the area where the trachea splits and enters both lungs. Of special concern in this area is the amount of vascularity that is visible. The blood vasculature appears as gray–white streaks fanning out from the center of the cardiac silhouette. Excess vascularity is seen in congestive heart failure and certain congenital heart malformations. Undervascularity is seen in right-to-left shunting, resulting in decreased pulmonary blood flow.

Examination of the Respiratory Tract

Leaving the lungs to the last prevents focus on gross pathology in other structures that may otherwise be missed. Now focus attention on the respiratory tract.

Trachea First, examine the trachea, beginning at the larynx and following it to the carina. The trachea often deviates slightly to the right, but should be located near the center of the spinal column. A trachea that is deviated significantly may indicate the presence of atelectasis, pneumothorax, or tension pneumothorax. In the instance of atelectasis, the trachea will be deviated toward the affected side, whereas a pneumothorax under pressure will deviate the trachea away from the affected side.

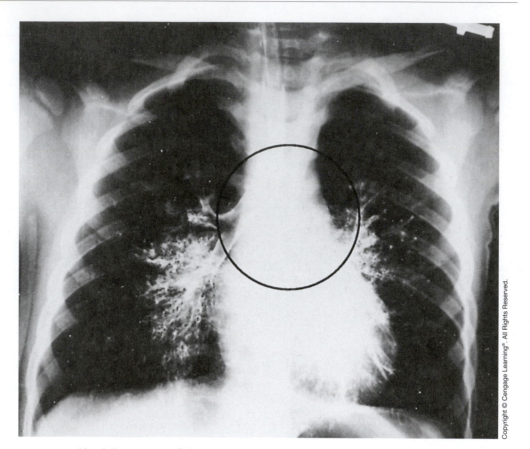

FIGURE 16–9. The hilum area of the lungs. The bronchus are highlighted by the inhalation of radiopaque gas.

Endotracheal Tube If the patient is intubated, check the location of the tip of the endotracheal tube. It should have a **radiopaque** (white) stripe on the tip, which makes it easily seen on the x-ray. The tip of the tube should be halfway between the carina and the clavicles, as shown in Figure 16–10. If the tube is in too far and near the carina, the chance of the tube entering the right mainstem bronchus is greatly increased. Conversely, if the tube tip is near the clavicles, the chance of accidental extubation increases. The position of the tube tip may vary with the position of the patient's head. If the infant's chin is down at the time the x-ray is being taken, the tip of the ET tube may be higher in the trachea. When the chin is elevated, the tube may be pushed farther down the trachea.

Mainstem Bronchus Now follow the trachea past the carina to the mainstem bronchi. The right bronchus may appear as an extension of the trachea, whereas the left angles off at almost a 90-degree angle. It is unusual to see the bronchi beyond the hilum of the lung because the air-filled lungs do not provide a contrast to the air-filled airways. However, if the lung tissue increases in density, such as in pneumonia,

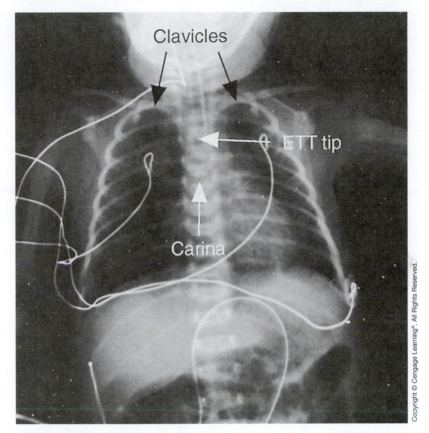

FIGURE 16–10. Proper position of the endotracheal tube is determined by the tip being above the carina and below the clavicles as shown.

atelectasis, or in aspiration, it may be possible to see the bronchi outlined into the lung periphery, as seen in Figure 16–11.

This is caused by two factors. First, as the lung consolidates, it begins appearing whiter on the x-ray film. The air-filled bronchus, passing through the lung, is contrasted against the lung and becomes increasingly more visible on the x-ray.

Second, in the presence of atelectasis the bronchi may dilate, making them more visible against the whiter lung fields, that is, visible black airways surrounded by white lung parenchyma. These visible bronchi are called **air bronchograms**.

Lung Fields Next examine the lung fields. Generally speaking, the lung tissue should be expanded with air, if taken during inspiration, and thus appear dark (black) on the x-ray (Figure16–12). Lungs that appear whiter in appearance are either underexpanded or are involved in some type of disease process that is making them atelectatic. The appearance of the lungs with different disease entities is examined in the following section. It is at this point that the respiratory therapist should evaluate the lungs in light of the following descriptions.

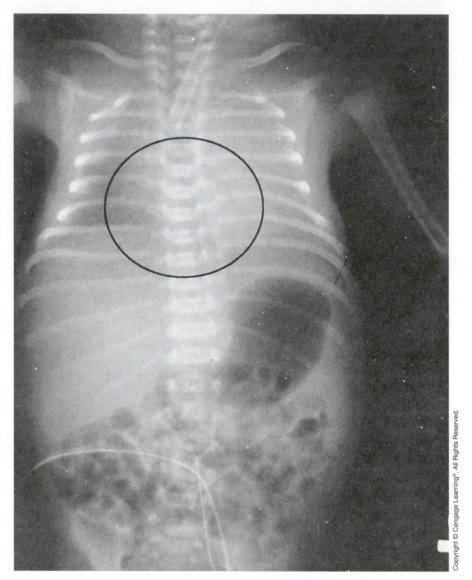

FIGURE 16–11. Air bronchograms as seen in the circled area.

Pleural Surface The surface of the pleura should next be examined. This is best done at the interface of the peripheral lungs and the chest wall at a point between the ribs. Lung markings should extend to the outermost pleural border. Pneumothoraces are often detected only by the absence of lung markings in a section of the thorax. Chest tubes, if present, should be checked to make sure they are positioned to evacuate the free air in the thorax.

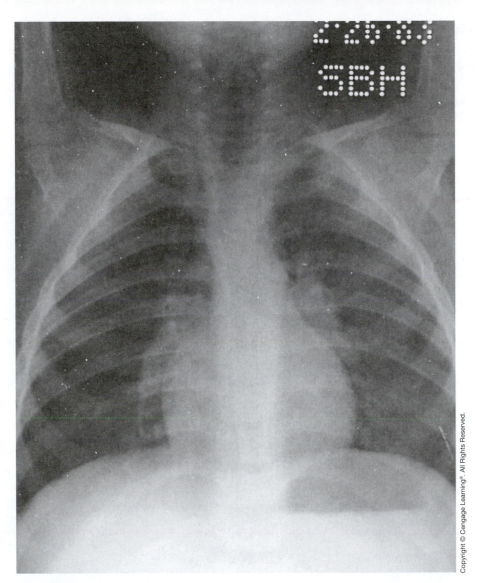

FIGURE 16–12. Normally aerated lung fields.

RADIOGRAPHIC FINDINGS IN NEONATAL LUNG PATHOLOGY

A routine examination of the chest often includes a quick picture as a baseline to compare complicating pathology in the care of the neonate. By examining the underlying pathology and associated treatment, the respiratory therapist can asses and evaluate whether a particular strategy is effective by an improving x-ray.

Respiratory Distress Syndrome (RDS)

RDS is the most common lung disease found in premature infants. Radiographic findings in RDS are quite characteristic. Fine **reticulogranular** patterns, alveoli with increased tissue and fluid densities surrounding small areas (interstitial space) of aerated alveoli, are found in both lung fields. This is commonly called a ground glass or a frosted glass appearance (Figure 16–13).

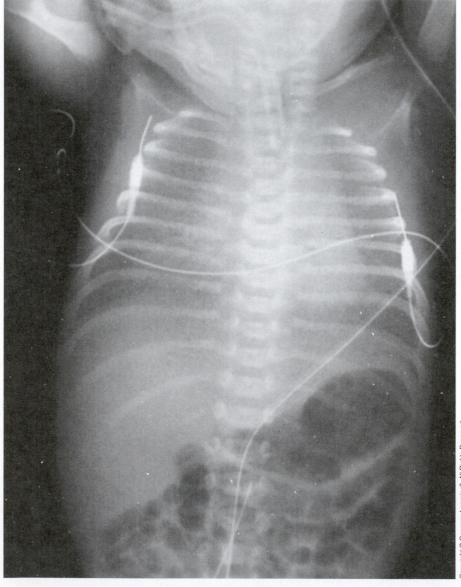

FIGURE 16–13. The "ground glass" appearance of RDS.

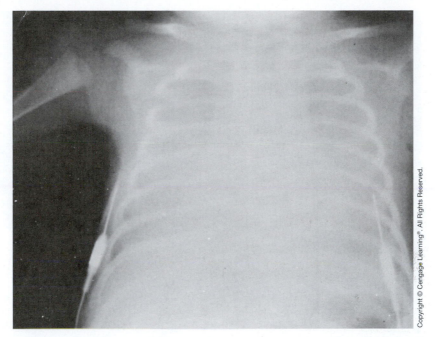

FIGURE 16–14. Total "white out" of the lungs.

Both lungs appear as opaque white density, reflecting the lack of lung aeration and expansion. Air bronchograms are prominently seen, particularly at the lung bases. Pleural fluid is absent, helping to differentiate the disease from an infectious process. Pleural fluid can be present in RDS, however, if the infant has been overloaded with IV fluid following birth.

The bilateral opaque appearance continues until the lungs begin to recover. If the disease worsens, the lungs can become completely white on the x-ray film. This is called, fittingly, a white-out, shown in Figure 16–14. White-outs are due to an almost total absence of aeration, with massive atelectasis and collapsed lung segments. As the disease improves, lung clearing occurs over a period of a few days indicated by lobar aeration outlined in black. Clearing usually starts with the apical and peripheral areas first, followed by the central and basal lung areas.

Atelectasis

Atelectasis is a consolidation of part or all of a lung due to a collapse of the alveoli. Radiographic atelectasis is shown in Figure 16–15. This loss of volume may be due to surfactant deficiency, as in RDS, bronchial obstruction, or scar formation. Bronchial obstruction may result from mucous plugging or from an aspirated object in small children.

The signs of atelectasis include an elevated diaphragm on the affected side and a mediastinal shift toward the atelectatic area. There may also be a decrease in the spaces between the ribs, and possibly a hyperinflation of the adjacent lung lobes or of the opposite lung.

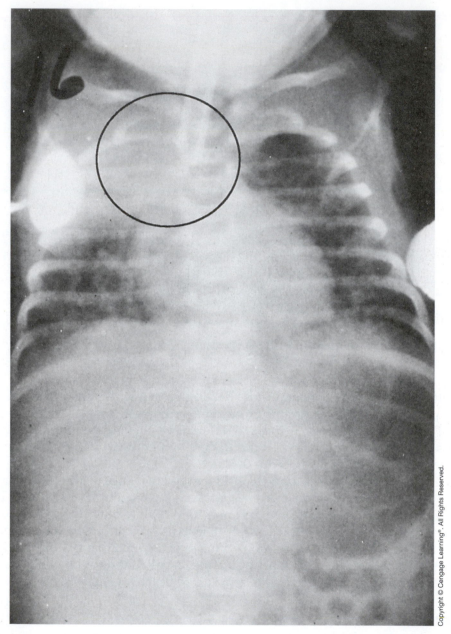

FIGURE 16–15. Areas of atelectasis seen within the circled areas.

Transient Tachypnea of the Newborn (TTN)

TTN is a common cause of respiratory distress in newborns, especially those born via cesarean delivery. Covered earlier in more depth in Chapter 7, TTN is thought to be partially caused by retention of fetal lung fluids from nonvaginal births.

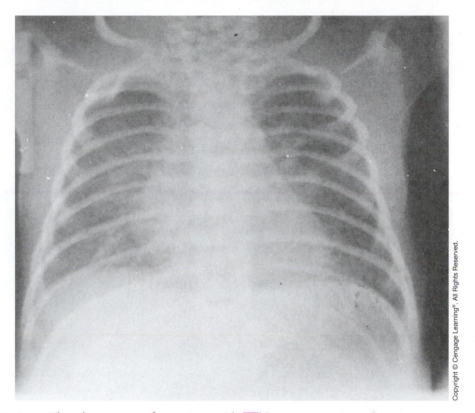

FIGURE 16–16. The chest x-ray of a patient with TTN.

Radiographically, if seen within the first few hours of life, TTN may closely resemble hyaline membrane disease (Figure 16–16). A possible difference is that the lungs are hyperaerated rather than hypoaerated.

It is common to see small amounts of pleural fluid and symmetrical, stringy infiltrates in the hilar region, which may be due to engorged veins and lymphatic vessels. An important point in distinguishing TTN from other causes of respiratory distress is that the infiltrates clear rapidly, often within 24 hours.

Neonatal Pneumonia

Contamination of the infant most commonly occurs just before, during, or after birth. Colonization of organisms on the infant's skin, gastrointestinal tract, or respiratory system may occur following premature rupture of membranes, dystocia, or the use of contaminated equipment or hands on the infant. With pneumonias, the radiologic pattern may be variable. Neonatal pneumonia is very difficult to determine on the chest x-ray because fluid and atelectatic lung tissue is generally indistinguishable.

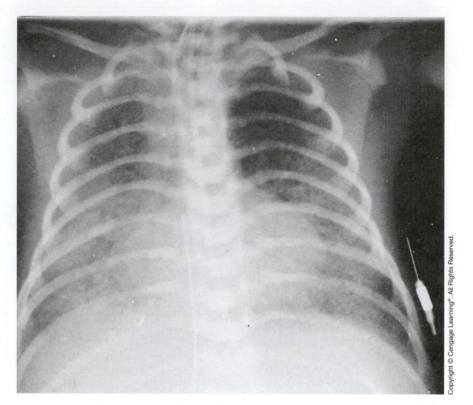

FIGURE 16–17. Neonatal pneumonia as seen on x-ray.

Lung markings are described as being diffuse, which may also describe many other lung diseases. A chest x-ray of pneumonia is depicted in Figure 16–17. The presence of excessive pleural fluid helps establish the diagnosis of pneumonia. Consolidation of a lobe or segment, often seen in older patients, is very rare in neonates.

Often, pneumonia is diagnosed in a normal right-lower lobe. This is because of a prominence of vessels and airways on the x-ray at that location, giving the appearance of consolidation. In contrast, pneumonia in the lower-left lobe may be difficult to see behind the cardiac shadow. Diaphragmatic boarders may help to distinguish the heart shadow from the lung boarder. A comparison of heart shadow densities from top to bottom and right to left may reveal increased density in the lower-left region, indicating lower lobe pneumonia.

Group B hemolytic streptococci has recently become a common source of neonatal infection. The fetus may become infected while still in utero and present at birth with systemic symptoms of the disease. These symptoms may be indistinguishable from RDS in that the neonate may grunt, flare the nostrils, and have substernal and intercostal retractions. The chest x-ray may also appear as a complete white-out and be mistaken for RDS, especially in the preterm neonate.

Meconium Aspiration Syndrome (MAS)

The chest x-ray of an MAS patient may be normal, in mild cases, or very abnormal, in severe cases. Severe MAS shows bilateral infiltrates and evidence of air trapping. Air trapping predisposes the lungs to pulmonary interstitial emphysema (PIE), pneumomediastinum, and pneumothorax. Blockage of the airway by meconium often leads to atelectasis distal to the occlusion. Additionally, there may be signs of inflammation and edema caused by the chemical irritation of the meconium. Pleural effusions, indicated by a loss (blunting) of the costophrenic angle by fluid (the angle between the diaphragm and the lateral chest wall) may also be present.

Diaphragmatic Hernia

Diaphragmatic hernias may occur at birth or in utero. Diaphragmatic hernias that occur in utero cause severe damage to the lung by hampering its growth and development. Roughly 80% to 85% of diaphragmatic hernias occur on the left side. X-ray findings in congenital diaphragmatic hernia show the presence of the stomach and bowel loops in the left thoracic cavity (Figure 16–18).

Diagnosis is simplified when the stomach and intestines contain air. Air-filled intestines are easily identified when located in the thorax. The abdominal cavity will also be noticeably void of a stomach bubble or intestinal markings.

There is usually a severe deviation of the mediastinal structures and its contents away from the side of the hernia. If a gastric tube is present, the tip is commonly seen ending in the thorax instead of the abdomen. A diaphragmatic hernia is almost always accompanied by severe respiratory distress and a flat or sunken abdomen (**scaphoid**). X-ray findings are then used to verify the diagnosis.

Congenital Lobar Emphysema

X-ray findings in this disorder show a single lobe, commonly an upper lobe or the right middle lobe, becoming overdistended and emphysematous. The remaining lobes of the lung become atelectatic and collapsed. Depression of the diaphragm and displacement of the mediastinum to the opposite side is also seen. In later stages of the disease, atelectasis occurs in the opposite lung.

Pneumothorax

Radiographically, a pneumothorax is identified when the lung is displaced away from the chest wall by a dark (black) band of air (Figure 16–19). The dark air space will have no lung markings, and, frequently, the border of the lung is seen as a sharp white line, medial to the air sack. In the presence of a tension pneumothorax, the diaphragm on the affected side will be depressed, and the intercostal spaces will be widened. The mediastinum is also displaced away from the pneumothorax.

It is sometimes possible to mistake a skinfold for a pneumothorax. Although skinfolds may appear as the border of the lung, the space surrounding the line will have lung markings, which is inconsistent with a pneumothorax. The skinfold may

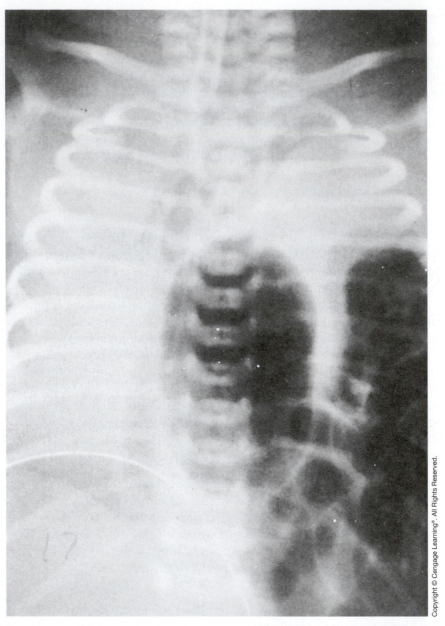

FIGURE 16–18. Congenital diaphragmatic hernia. Note the stomach bubble and bowel loops in the left thorax.

also be seen beyond the confines of the pleural cavity and into the soft tissues of the chest wall.

Patient symptoms are invaluable in diagnosing a pneumothorax. Lack of distress or other symptoms helps to rule out a pneumothorax when x-ray findings are inconclusive.

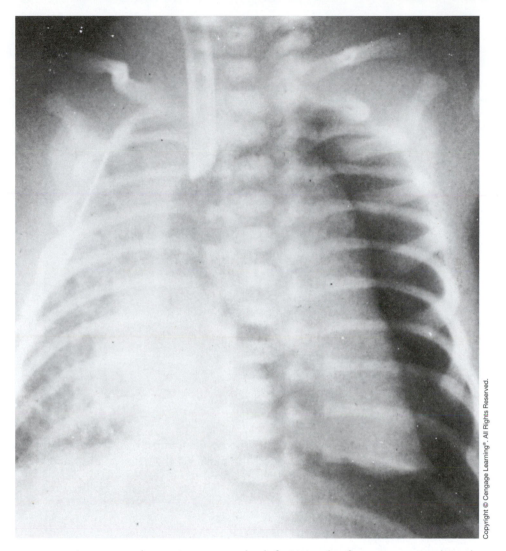

FIGURE 16–19. A pneumothorax is seen on the left. Note the free air surrounding the left lung.

Pneumomediastinum

A pneumomediastinum is detected radiographically by the presence of air (black) in the mediastinum, outlining the thymus and the lateral aspects of the heart (Figure 16–20). This outlining of the thymus has been called "bat wing" and "angel wing," because of its appearance as a wing. On a lateral view, the thymus is lifted, giving it the appearance of a sail. Collections of mediastinal air around the lung hilum are often confusing. They may be seen in areas of the lung not thought of as being the mediastinum. These collections, called **pseudocysts**, are often mistaken for other abnormalities, but are actually mediastinal air.

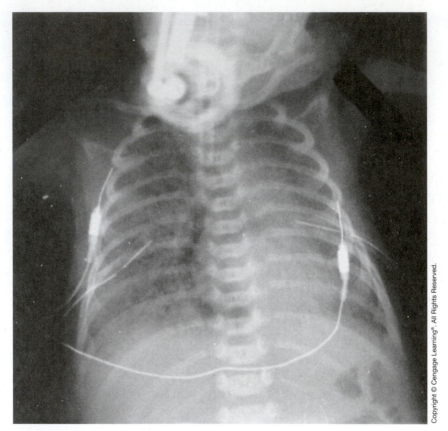

FIGURE 16–20. A radiograph showing a pneumomediastinum. Note the outlining of the lateral edge of the heart. The free air does not surround the apex of the heart.

Pneumopericardium

The accumulation of air within the pericardial sac is called a pneumopericardium. On x-ray, the air completely surrounds the heart (Figure 16–21), in contrast to a pneumomediastinum, which only surrounds the lateral sides of the heart. The air pocket around the heart may appear as a halo. The amount of air present is of concern, because larger accumulations of air may tamponade the heart, reducing cardiac output and leading to shock.

Pulmonary Interstitial Emphysema

Pulmonary interstitial emphysema (PIE) is caused by air leaking from a lung rupture and migrating throughout the lung parenchyma. The radiographic appearance is unique to this disease. The interstitial air compresses the alveoli and bronchioles, leading to atelectasis and collapse. On x-ray, the lungs have small dark streaks and cysts, surrounded by the white of the lung tissue. Figure 16–22 shows a radiograph

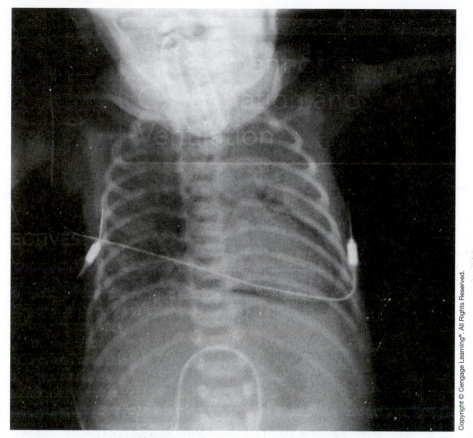

FIGURE 16–21. A radiograph showing a pneumopericardium. Notice the free air completely surrounds the heart.

of PIE. Some have described its appearance as looking like black paint flicked onto a white background. It is also described as having a sponge-like appearance, or looking like ground hamburger with air in it.

PIE may affect one lung, but is most likely found in both lungs. PIE may show areas of air accumulations, as in a pneumothorax, or a cystic formation.

Bronchopulmonary Dysplasia

Bronchopulmonary dysplasia (BPD) is recognized when infant lungs show the presence of hyperaeration in association with alternating areas of dark cystic areas and strand-like densities. Radiologic characteristics of BPD have been classified into four stages.

- Stage I (mild BPD): Stage I has an appearance similar to that of RDS and occurs within 2 to 4 days following delivery (Figure 16–23A).

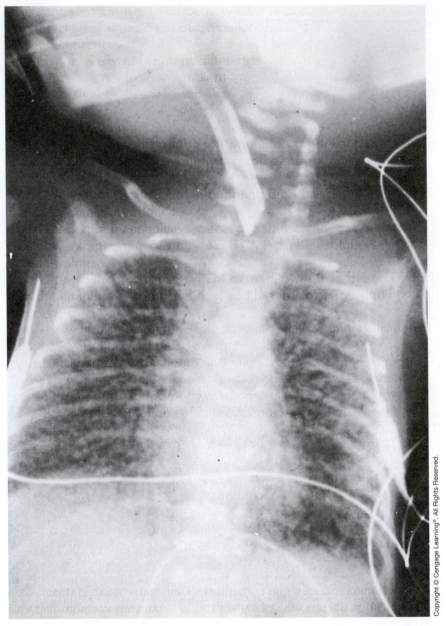

FIGURE 16–22. The small cystic areas throughout the lung fields are consistent with PIE.

- Stage II (moderate BPD): The RDS appearance now changes to coarse, irregularly shaped densities that are often grouped together and contain very small cystic areas. The coarse infiltrates are often dense enough to obscure the cardiac markings. These areas are caused by interstitial edema, as well as alveolar septal edema, with subsequent atelectasis. The cystic areas represent early emphysematous changes. Stage II generally occurs 4 to 10 days following delivery.

- Stage III (severe BPD): The small cysts now become arranged in generalized patterns. Dense cystic patches that appear are evidence of the progressive, emphysematous changes. In this stage, extensive repair is taking place in the alveolar walls. Fibrotic areas show up as irregular white streaks throughout the lungs. The size and number of irregular areas increases as the days pass. There may also be some areas of lung hyperexpansion. This stage occurs around 10 to 20 days following delivery (Figure 16–23B).
- Stage IV (chronic, advanced BPD): During this stage, lung hyperexpansion is less severe, as are the streaky opacities found between the large cystic areas. The lung field has a "bubbly" appearance caused by the continued enlargement of the cysts. Signs of chronic air trapping, with low set, flattened diaphragms and hyperaeration, are usually present. The patient with stage IV BPD has continued oxygen requirements that may persist for months. Occasionally, the infant requires mechanical ventilation for long periods, while the lungs slowly heal during stage IV.

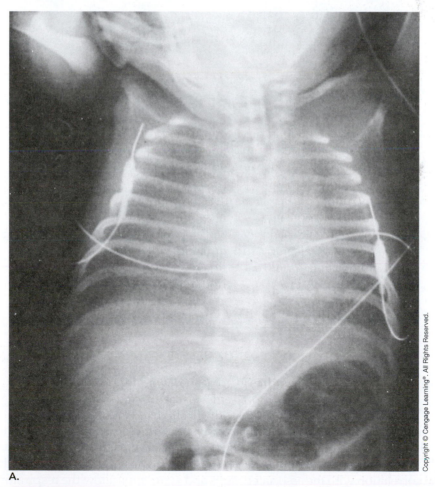

A.

FIGURE 16–23A. Stage 1 BPD.

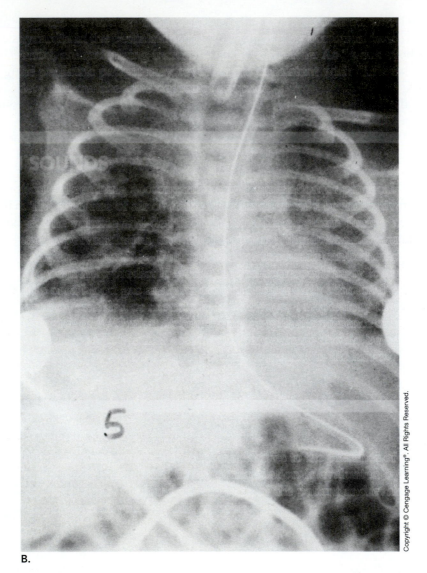

B.

FIGURE 16–23B. Stage 3 BPD.

RADIOGRAPHIC FINDINGS IN PEDIATRIC LUNG PATHOLOGY

The pediatric patient has a larger proportion of pathologies to evaluate and consider than a typical neonate. X-rays may help identify airway obstructions, croup, or bronchiolitis, as well as infections or inflammation of the lung or other abnormalities in the chest. Clinical correlation with the associated signs and symptoms allow the respiratory therapist to interpret the findings of a chest x-ray with a diagnosis for a specific pathology.

Adult Respiratory Distress Syndrome (ARDS)

Depending on when the chest x-ray is obtained in the course of ARDS, the respiratory therapist may see a variety of pathologic findings on the chest x-ray. The progression of ARDS involves an accumulation of lung pathologies, which result in acute widespread damage to the lung parenchyma.

Initially, the x-ray of the chest shows diffuse, fluffy infiltrates due to the accumulation of fluid and debris in and around the alveoli from leaky pulmonary vessels. Perpetuated by hypoxemia, acidosis, and necrosis, fluid leak leads to inflammation and scaring of the tissue which accentuates atelectasis. These infiltrates then give way to patchy, nodular densities as the disease progresses. As the lungs become fibrotic, the lungs take on a stringy interstitial pattern with diffuse areas of consolidation. The lung fields often become "whited out" secondary to diminished aeration as progressive atelectasis in the damaged, fluid-filled lungs.

Foreign Body Aspiration

The aspiration of a foreign body into the pulmonary tree is commonly seen in the pediatric population. Frequently, the aspirated object is not visible on the radiograph, making it necessary to look for signs of air trapping and atelectasis, which may be present distal to the offending object. If the object is causing a complete blockage of a major airway, air volumes in the areas distal to the blockage are often greatly diminished due to atelectasis.

A partial blockage of the airway leads to a ball-valve effect, in which gas passes the obstruction on inspiration but becomes trapped on exhalation as the airway collapses on the object. This results in areas of **hyperlucency** on the radiograph in those areas distal to the blockage. Of most value in this situation is an expiratory film, which more clearly shows areas of air trapping. An expiratory film may be obtained on younger patients by placing the patient in a **decubitus** position, where the lung on the downside is compressed into exhalation.

Cystic Fibrosis

The chest x-ray of the patient with cystic fibrosis may be normal in the early stages of the disease. As the disease progresses with increased mucous production in the lungs (and other body systems) by involvement of goblet cells, submucosal or bronchial glands, and thickening of the peribronchial areas (producing mucous plugging) hyperaeration begin to be apparent. As the disease progresses, the chest radiograph shows areas of consolidation, cystic changes, and fibrosis of the lungs affecting gaseous exchange.

Asthma

The chest x-ray of an asthmatic patient appears normal with no signs of lung pathology in the absence of an acute attack. Although during an acute asthmatic attack (or in status asthmaticus), the classic lung radiograph is that of hyperinflation with a slight depression of the diaphragm and an overall hyperlucency of both lung fields. Additionally, bulging at the intercostals margins may be present. It must be noted, however, that even in the presence of an acute asthmatic attack, the lung fields may show little radiographic change.[3] In these cases, clinical and physical signs may be more diagnostic than the chest x-ray.

Epiglottitis

Epiglottitis may be seen radiographically on a lateral neck x-ray (Figure 16–24). Epiglottic swelling (supraglottic) of three to four times normal is seen at the base of the tongue and appears as if someone left a thumb print, thus the term "thumb sign," which is used to describe the swollen epiglottis. There is also involvement of the hypopharynx with swelling and thickening of the tissue.

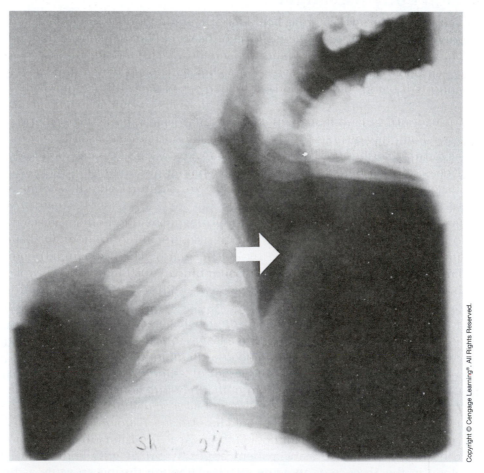

FIGURE 16–24. Lateral neck x-ray showing epiglottitis. The arrow shows the swollen epiglottis, which appears as a thumb print.

Croup

Croup may be diagnosed radiographically with an anteroposterior view of the neck. The area of the swelling in the subglottic region is seen as an "hourglass" or "steeple" (Figure 16–25). Because these findings are also seen with subglottic stenosis, severe symptoms in patients younger than 6 months may require bronchoscopy to provide a differential diagnosis.

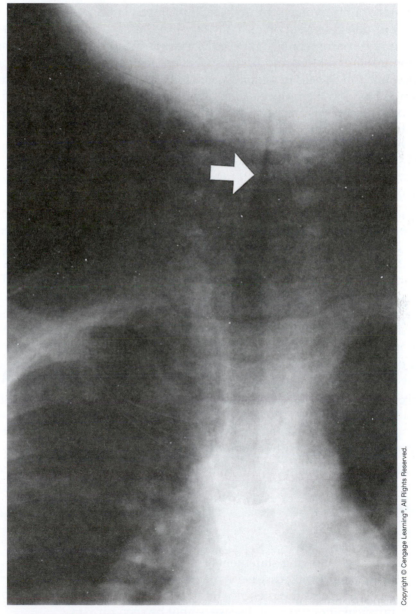

FIGURE 16–25. AP x-ray showing croup. The arrow points to the "steeple" shape of the airway resulting from subglottic swelling.

SUMMARY

X-rays of the chest are one of the most commonly ordered tests in the neonatal and pediatric group of patients. An x-ray gives an internal view of the effect that a disease process is having on the organ systems. While not used alone for diagnosis, a chest x-ray is invaluable at verifying the presence of a process and monitoring its progression or improvement from therapeutic intervention.

The four densities seen on an x-ray (air, fluid, tissue, and bone) form the details of the internal environment. Air spaces are seen as the darkest areas and bone is seen as the lightest areas. Fluid and tissue spaces are seen as areas of gray in between.

Anatomic differences in neonates and children can hinder proper interpretation if not understood in the proper context. For example, the carina is higher in the thorax in younger patients and may prove deceptive if the respiratory therapist is used to looking for the carina lower in the chest. Additionally, the thymus gland adds an extra shadow to the chest x-ray of young patients, which may be mistaken for an enlarged heart or for lung pathology.

When reading a chest x-ray, it is important to follow a systematic approach. Begin by checking the name and date of the x-ray. Next, orient the x-ray on the viewbox so the patient's right side is on your left. The quality of the x-ray is next evaluated for proper exposure. The position of the patient on the x-ray is then examined to ensure that no, or minimal, rotation has occurred.

Next, determine the extent of expiration or inspiration by counting and examining the characteristics of the ribs, and by evaluating the diaphragm and abdomen. Moving back to the thorax, the respiratory therapist next examines the cardiac silhouette, the hilum, and respiratory tract. Placement of the endotracheal tube is evaluated on intubated patients, with the tip ideally placed between the carina and the clavicles.

Before the x-ray is obtained, the differential diagnosis has often been narrowed to two or three processes. The radiographic findings are then used to confirm or rule out the diagnoses. X-ray findings of commonly seen lung pathologies are particularly characteristic for specific disease and knowledge of those findings is vital in identifying the disease process and its progression. The respiratory therapist is encouraged to examine as many x-rays as possible, both normal and abnormal, and to discuss the findings with others. By this mechanism, reading x-rays becomes almost second nature.

POSTTEST

1. Which of the following statements is true?
   a. Diagnosis of lung disease is made by x-ray alone.
   b. X-ray confirms the presence or absence of a disease process.
   c. Physical alterations of disease cannot be seen on x-ray.
   d. X-rays should only be done on neonates in an emergency.

2. Of the following, which are densities seen on x-ray?
    I. gas
    II. skin
    III. fluid
    IV. cartilage
    V. bone
        a. II, III, IV
        b. I, III, IV
        c. I, III, IV, V
        d. I, III, V

3. Which of the following may limit the interpretation of a chest x-ray?
    I. artifact
    II. patient movement
    III. old film
    IV. improper technique
    V. the presence of bony material
        a. I, II, IV
        b. I, II, IV
        c. I, II, V
        d. II, IV

4. As you examine a chest x-ray, you note that the spaces between the vertebrae are visible and distinct. This film is:
    a. overexposed
    b. underexposed
    c. exposed correctly
    d. backwards

5. Flattened diaphragms seen on a chest x-ray indicate:
    a. meconium aspiration
    b. hypoaeration
    c. air trapping
    d. hyperventilation

6. The neonatal cardiac silhouette is considered normal size if it is less than what percentage of the thoracic width?
    a. 60%
    b. 50%
    c. 40%
    d. 30%

7. Undervascularization of the hilar region would indicate:
    a. heart failure
    b. right-to-left shunt
    c. RDS
    d. central vasospasm

8. As you examine a patient's chest x-ray, you note the tip of the endotracheal tube to be near the carina. You would:
   a. pull the tube back slightly
   b. push the tube in slightly
   c. leave the tube in its present position
   d. rotate the tube 90 degrees

9. Examination of a chest x-ray reveals a slightly elevated left diaphragm, with a slight mediastinal shift toward the left. The left lower lobe appears whiter than the upper lobes with a slight hyperinflation of the right lower lobe. What is the probable diagnosis?
   a. atelectasis in the left lower lobe
   b. atelectasis in the right lower lobe
   c. left lung pneumothorax
   d. right lung pneumothorax

10. A newborn infant presents from delivery with severe respiratory distress. On examination, the abdomen is scaphoid. The radiograph shows a severe mediastinal shift to the right. The likely diagnosis is:
    a. diaphragmatic hernia
    b. pneumothorax
    c. pneumoperitoneum
    d. pneumonia

11. On examination of a chest radiograph, you note an air pocket on the right lateral heart border. This indicates (a) possible:
    a. pneumomediastinum
    b. pneumopericardium
    c. pneumothorax
    d. congenital lobar emphysema

12. Dense cystic patches arranged in generalized patterns that gradually increase in size and number describes which stage of BPD?
    a. stage 2
    b. stage 3
    c. stage 4
    d. stage 5

13. A decubitus film is best used to diagnose which of the following?
    a. croup
    b. epiglottitis
    c. foreign body aspiration
    d. cystic fibrosis

14. Which of the following is (are) true regarding the chest radiograph of an asthma patient?
    I.   hyperinflation is common during an acute attack
    II. air trapping is chronically seen
    III. the chest x-ray may be normal
    IV. the lungs may appear hyperlucent during an attack
        a. I, III, IV
        b. I, II, III
        c. II, IV
        d. I, III

REFERENCES

1. Wilkins S, Dexter JR, Heuer A. *Clinical Assessment in Respiratory Care*. 6th ed. St. Louis, MO: Elsevier/Mosby, p. 166, 2010.
2. Karlson KH, Seibert JJ. Radiographic assessment techniques. In: Barnhart SL, Czervinske MP. *Perinatal and Pediatric Respiratory Care*. 3rd ed. Philadelphia, PA: WB Saunders Co., 2010.
3. Burton GG, Hodgkins J, Ward J. *Respiratory Care: A Guide to Clinical Practice*. 4th ed. Philadelphia, PA: JB Lippincott Co., 1997.

BIBLIOGRAPHY AND SUGGESTED READINGS

Bierman CW, Pearlman DS, Shapiro GG, Busse WW. *Allergy, Asthma, and Immunology from Infancy to Adulthood*. 3rd ed. Philadelphia, PA: WB Saunders Co., 1995.

Chapman S. *Essential Pediatric Radiology*. Philadelphia, PA: WB Saunders Co., 2000.

Chernik V, Boat TF. *Kendig's Disorders of the Respiratory Tract in Children*. 8th ed. Philadelphia, PA: WB Saunders Co., 2012.

Cloherty JP, Stark AR (eds). *Manual of Neonatal Care*. 7th ed. Philadelphia, PA: Lippincott, 2011.

Dantzker DR, MacIntyre NR, Bukow ED. *Comprehensive Respiratory Care*. Philadelphia, PA: WB Saunders Co., 1995.

Flores MT. Understanding neonatal chest x-rays part I: what to look for. *Neonatal Network*. 12:9–17, 1993.

Glanze WD (ed.). *Mosby's Medical, Nursing, and Allied Health Dictionary*. 6th ed. St. Louis, MO: CV Mosby Co., 2005.

Goodman LR. *Felson's Principles of Chest Roentgenology*. 3rd ed. Philadelphia, PA: WB Saunders Co., 2006.

Hicks GH. *Cardiopulmonary Anatomy and Physiology*. Philadelphia, PA: WB Saunders Co., 2000.

MacDonald MG, et al. *Avery's Neonatology Pathophysiology and Management of the Newborn* . 6th ed. Philadelphia, PA: JB Lippincott Co., 2005.

Merenstein GB, Gardner SL. *Handbook of Neonatal Intensive Care*. 7th ed. St. Louis, MO: CV Mosby Co., 2010.

Management of Ventilation and Oxygenation

Whenever I feel blue, I start breathing again.
—*L. Frank Baum*

CHAPTER 17

Concepts of Mechanical Ventilation

OBJECTIVES

Upon completion of this chapter, the reader should be able to:

1. Describe the primary goal of mechanical ventilation and the skills required to reverse respiratory failure.
2. Define each of the following terms. Include a description of how each is determined and the ventilator parameters that determine each one.
   a. Peak inspiratory pressure (PIP)
   b. Positive end-expiratory pressure (PEEP)
   c. Frequency or rate
   d. Inspiratory time (IT)
   e. Mean airway pressure (MAP)
   f. Tidal volume (Vt)
   g. Minute ventilation (VE)
   h. Deadspace (V_D)
   i. Alveolar ventilation
   j. Opening pressure
   k. Driving pressure
   l. Functional residual capacity (FRC)
   m. Diffusion time
   n. Flow rate
3. Discuss the relationships that exist between ventilator parameters, using Figure 17–12 as a guide.
4. Define compliance and describe how lung compliance is measured.
5. Compare and contrast static and dynamic lung compliance.
6. State the normal range of lung compliance values in the neonate.
7. Describe the determinants of pulmonary compliance.
8. Discuss the compliance of the thorax and how it is developed.
9. Describe the relationship between the lungs and thorax that determines the overall compliance.

10. Compare and contrast the three positions on the lung compliance curve. Describe conditions that create each position.
11. Identify and discuss several lung disorders that alter lung compliance.
12. List the four factors that create resistance and identify the factor that is responsible for airway resistance changes.
13. State range of airway resistance in the normal newborn and how it is measured.
14. List and describe three factors that increase resistance in the neonatal airway and how each can be countered.
15. Define a time constant. Discuss the significance of three time constants and expiratory time.
16. When given compliance and resistance values, calculate a minimal expiratory time needed.
17. Describe how changes in resistance and compliance change time constants.

KEY TERMS

compliance	elastic	static attraction
diffusion time	opening pressure	unstressed volume
driving pressure	resistance	viscosity

INTRODUCTION

This chapter will cover the goals of mechanical ventilation as well as definitions and inter-relationships that exist among ventilator settings. Patient lung dynamics and mechanical ventilator interface will also be discussed.

GOALS OF MECHANICAL VENTILATION

The goal of mechanical ventilation is to reduce the work of breathing by providing adequate alveolar gas exchange with minimal damage to lung tissue (barotrauma) and/or interference with the circulatory system. This can only be achieved with a thorough understanding of the physiology and pathophysiology of diseases a newborn or pediatric patient is likely to encounter.

To gain this understanding, a respiratory therapist must possess a thorough knowledge of basic concepts of mechanical ventilation, the many options (a repertoire of ventilation strategies), modes, and settings that are available to function adequately at the bedside. With such wide flexibility, the respiratory therapist must be sensitive to the potential physiologic damage and changes that may occur with each setting change.

The respiratory therapist must also have the ability to interpret blood gas results and radiologic findings, which are assessed frequently throughout the course of the disease. The goals of mechanical ventilation are listed in Table 17–1.

Table 17–1

GOALS OF MECHANICAL VENTILATION

Normalization and Maintenance of Blood Gases and Acid-Base Balance

- PaO_2—Maintain arterial PO_2 above hypoxic levels (< 50 mmHg with supplemental oxygen) and below hyperoxic levels (especially in neonates).
- PCO_2—Reverse hypercapnic states through adequate alveolar ventilation.
- pH—Maintain blood pH within homeostatic range by managing the balance between $PaCO_2$ and HCO_3^-.

Prevention of Iatrogenic Complications

- Barotrauma—Careful regulation of rate and pressures.
- Infection—Follow sterile technique whenever the airway is suctioned and limit breaks in the circuit, which may allow bacteria to be introduced into the airway
- Sedation—Pharmacologic sedation and analgesia as needed to reduce anxiety and pain.

Support of the Patient's Respiratory Needs

- Decrease work of breathing—Mechanical ventilation should provide the support required by the patient to decrease work of breathing and achieve acceptable blood gases without placing the patient at risk for barotrauma.
- Apnea—Mechanical ventilation is indicated in neonates with apnea due to prematurity, secondary to intraventricular hemorrhage (IVH) or secondary to drug depression.

DEFINITIONS

In order to appropriately manipulate mechanical ventilator settings to achieve desired outcomes, it is necessary to understand each setting, the affect it has on the patient, the affect it has on other settings and how the patient's lung and airway dynamics respond and alter the effects of each setting. The following definitions will assist in this understanding.

Peak Inspiratory Pressure

Most common conventional neonatal ventilators use pressure-limiting modes in order to protect the newborn's lungs from barotrauma. In pressure-limited modes, a mechanical positive pressure breath will be terminated once a preset peak inspiratory pressure (PIP) has been reached, illustrated in Figure 17–1. PIP is a limit variable that will not allow the delivered breath to result in a pressure greater than the set PIP.

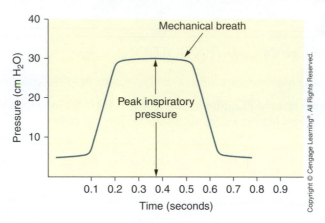

FIGURE 17–1. Peak inspiratory pressure as seen on a pressure waveform.

The level of PIP is one determinant of the delivered tidal volume and is changed as needed to alter ventilation. Initially, PIP is set at a level that achieves good chest excursion and provides an adequate predicted tidal volume based on the patients weight in kilograms. The tidal volume achieved in pressure-limited ventilation is variable, depending on lung compliance and airway resistance. Patients with poor lung compliance require higher PIP levels than those with good compliance to achieve the same tidal volume. A suggested starting point for PIP is between 16 and 20 cm H_2O.[1] Once the desired tidal volume is achieved as a result of the set PIP, rate should be adjusted to maintain appropriate minute ventilation.

If PIP is reached too soon, limiting the resulting tidal volume, it may be due to airway obstruction, a kink in the endotracheal tube, bronchospasm, or decreased lung compliance. If the ventilator is unable to reach the set PIP before the breath is cycled into exhalation, it may be due to a leak, such as an endotracheal tube cuff leak or a ventilator circuit leak. Failure to reach PIP may also be due to an insufficient inspiratory flow rate, preventing the ventilator from reaching the set PIP in the pre-determined inspiratory time.

Positive End-Expiratory Pressure (PEEP)

PEEP, depicted in Figure 17–2, is a positive pressure maintained in the patient's airway and throughout the closed ventilator circuit during the expiratory phase of ventilation. PEEP is considered a baseline variable, which means at the end of exhalation the airway pressure will return to this level prior to the trigger of the next breath. The maintenance of pressure during expiration prevents alveolar collapse in the patient with RDS or other conditions of decreased lung compliance, thus increasing the functional residual capacity and decreasing the need to overcome critical opening pressure with each positive pressure breath. PEEP also improves oxygenation. PEEP levels are usually kept between 4 and 6 cm H_2O.[1] Higher levels of PEEP may lead to increased mean airway pressure, resulting increased intrathroacic pressure and the possible reduction of cardiac output. If higher levels of PEEP are necessary

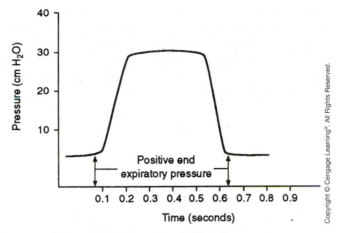

FIGURE 17–2. Positive end-expiratory pressure (PEEP) seen on a pressure waveform.

to increase oxygenation or to overcome critical opening pressure in noncompliant lungs, hemodynamic status must also be considered.

If PEEP is increased in pressure-limited modes, the resulting tidal volume will be reduced. In order to maintain the same minute ventilation in this instance, it is necessary to either increase PIP to maintain the same tidal volume, thus maintaining the minute ventilation, or increase respiratory rate to maintain the same minute ventilation.

Frequency

The frequency of ventilation, or rate, shown in Figure 17–3, is the number of inspirations that occur in 1 minute. Frequency or rate is considered a trigger variable determined by the cycle time of each breath. With the determination of adequate PIP

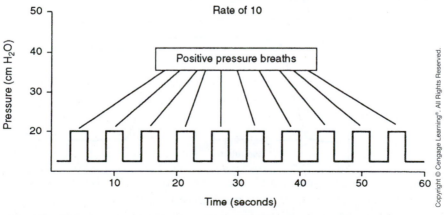

FIGURE 17–3. The frequency or rate of ventilation is equal to the number of positive pressure breaths delivered per minute.

and PEEP levels, the rate is set to achieve minute ventilation that will maintain the desired $PaCO_2$. The initial breath rate varies but should be started at 20 to 40 bpm.[1,2] Preterm neonates may require rates as high as 60 bpm.

Modern conventional neonatal ventilators have the capacity of providing rates of up to 150 bpm. However, when rates this high are indicated high-frequency oscillatory or jet ventilation should be considered. This strategy is recommended for patients with extremely noncompliant lungs in an attempt to maintain adequate minute ventilation, to preserve lung integrity and to prevent barotrauma associated with increased PIP and MAP. High-frequency ventilation is discussed in Chapter 20.

Inspiratory Time

Inspiratory time (IT), depicted in Figure 17–4, is set by the operator and is a cycle variable that will cycle the breath into exhalation once the preset IT is achieved. The combination of IT and rate determines the I:E (inspiration to expiration) ratio. The IT further determines the amount of time the inspired gas is in contact with the alveoli. As ventilator rates increase, it becomes necessary to decrease the IT to prevent air trapping and to allow for sufficient exhalation of the delivered breath. The clinical use of IT and the determination of I:E ratios are discussed in Chapter 18.

Mean Airway Pressure (MAP)

MAP (Figure 17–5) is the average pressure exerted on the airway and lungs from the beginning of inspiration until the beginning of the next inspiration. Most ventilators calculate MAP by electronic ventilator monitors that measure all pressure variables over a time period and then determine the average airway pressure during each complete breath cycle. MAP can also be approximated by using the formula in Table 17–2.

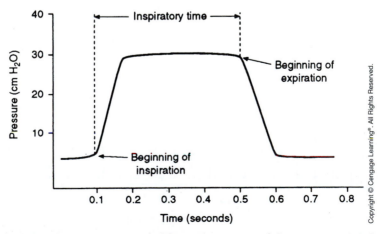

FIGURE 17–4. Inspiratory time, measured from the onset of the inspiratory phase to the onset of the expiratory phase.

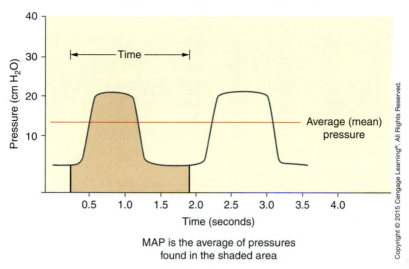

MAP is the average of pressures
found in the shaded area

FIGURE 17–5. Mean airway pressure (MAP) is the average pressure in the airway over a time period. It is calculated by measuring all of the pressure variables during the time period and averaging the overall pressure.

MAP is the most powerful influence on oxygenation and must be carefully monitored because high levels of MAP lead to decreased cardiac output, pulmonary hypoperfusion, and increased risk of barotrauma. MAP is affected by PIP, PEEP, IT, and rate. Because MAP takes into account these factors that affect ventilation, it is the best indicator of balance between adequate ventilation and excessive pressures. MAP levels above 12 cm H_2O have been shown to contribute to barotrauma.[2]

Table 17–2

CALCULATION OF MEAN AIRWAY PRESSURE

MAP = (PIP) × (inspiratory time/total breath duration) + (PEEP) × (expiratory time/total breath duration)

For example, current ventilator settings:

PIP, 23 cm H_2O; PEEP, 5 cm H_2O; I:time, 0.51 second; E:time, 1.53 seconds; total breath duration, 2.04 seconds.

Inserting the above setting into the formula, we get:

$$23 \times (0.51/2.04) + 5 \times (1.53/2.04)$$
$$(23 \times 0.25) + (5 \times 0.75)$$
$$5.75 + 3.75$$
$$MAP = 9.5 \text{ cm } H_2O$$

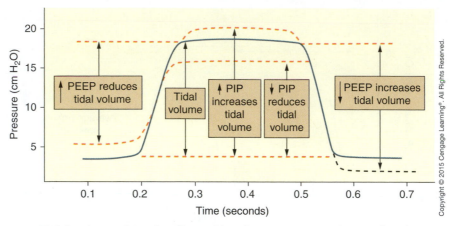

FIGURE 17–6. Tidal volume directly affected by changing PIP and PEEP levels.

Tidal Volume (V$_T$)

The amount of gas inhaled in a single breath is called the tidal volume. During mechanical ventilation, the tidal volume is the volume of gas that enters the patient's lungs during the inspiratory phase. Adequate tidal volume can be determined when appropriate chest expansion is observed and equal bilateral breath sounds are heard during auscultation of the inspiratory phase.

The two ventilator parameters that most directly affect tidal volume in pressure control ventilation are PIP and PEEP. Referring to Figure 17–6, the delivered tidal volume is directly related to the vertical distance from the baseline pressure to the PIP level. As PIP is increased, the distance between baseline and PIP increases, thus increasing tidal volume. If the baseline pressure, which is the PEEP level, is decreased or increased, the distance is again changed, and tidal volume changes.

Minute Ventilation (VE)

Minute ventilation is equal to the tidal volume multiplied by the respiratory rate. Therefore, in pressure control ventilation a change in either the PIP or PEEP, which alter tidal volume, or a change in frequency will alter minute ventilation.

Minute ventilation is broken down into alveolar ventilation, the portion actually participating in gas exchange and deadspace ventilation, the portion not participating in gas exchange.

Deadspace and Alveolar Ventilation

Deadspace is any gas that does not participate in gas exchange. Deadspace is divided into two categories: anatomic deadspace and alveolar deadspace.

Anatomic deadspace is the volume of tidal gas that fills the airways at the end of inspiration. It comprises the airways beginning at the nose and ending at the terminal bronchioles, as shown in Figure 17–7A. Anatomic deadspace in a neonate is roughly 2 to 2.2 mL/kg. Alveolar deadspace, depicted in Figure 17–7B, is that portion of the tidal gas that fills unperfused alveoli. Alveolar deadspace, in contrast to anatomic deadspace, is impossible to determine and can vary tremendously from hour to hour in the same patient.

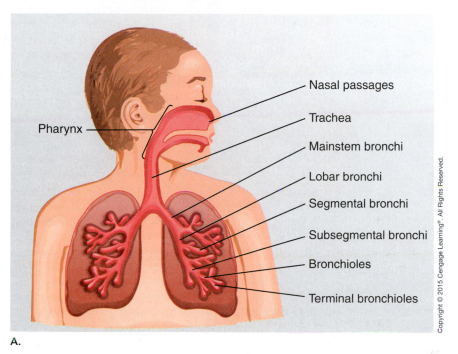

Nasal passages

Trachea

Pharynx

Mainstem bronchi

Lobar bronchi

Segmental bronchi

Subsegmental bronchi

Bronchioles

Terminal bronchioles

A.

FIGURE 17–7A. Anatomic deadspace comprises the nose to the terminal bronchioles.

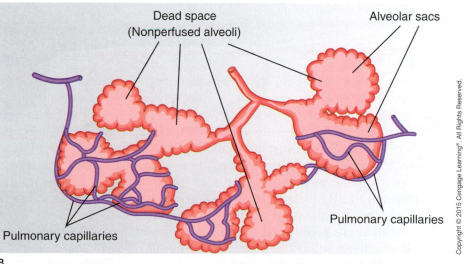

Dead space (Nonperfused alveoli)

Alveolar sacs

Pulmonary capillaries

Pulmonary capillaries

B.

FIGURE 17–7B. Alveolar deadspace encompasses all nonperfused alveoli.

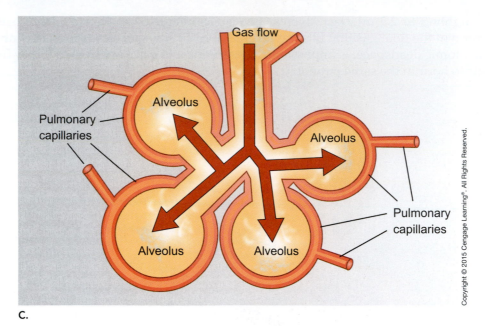

C.

FIGURE 17–7C. Alveolar ventilation is the result of all alveoli participating in gas exchange with the blood.

The total of anatomic and alveolar deadspace is called physiologic deadspace (V_D). When V_D is compared to tidal volume (V_T), the ratio (V_D:V_T) reflects the portion of the tidal breath that is not participating in gas exchange. This portion is called wasted ventilation. The amount of physiologic deadspace varies from patient to patient.

Alveolar ventilation, shown in Figure 17–7C, is the portion of tidal gas actually participating in gas exchange. Anatomically, it comprises the respiratory bronchioles to the alveoli.

Opening Pressure

To open and expand an alveolus, a certain amount of pressure must be applied to the alveoli. This pressure must overcome the surface tension that is causing the alveoli to pull inward. Surface tension is increased when there is a lack of surfactant, requiring a higher pressure to open the alveoli. To ventilate the lungs, the combined surface tensions of all the alveoli must be overcome. The pressure that must be applied to the airways to overcome the combined tensions is the critical **opening pressure**.

When applying positive pressure ventilation to neonatal lungs, it is important to maintain sufficient PEEP to keep the airways from complete collapse at the end of exhalation. This prevents the need of excessive pressures to overcome critical opening pressure with every breath and reduces lung tissue damage. Once the lung is recruited and stabilized with PEEP, it is much easier to ventilate and requires lower airway pressure to achieve volume delivery.

Opening pressure and alveolar recruitment can be assessed when crackles are heard in the lungs during inspiration. Often this sound is heard at the end of inspiration as the volume of air being delivered reaches the alveolar sacs. As the wet alveoli are opened, the pulling apart of the alveolar walls creates the crackles.

Driving Pressure

The **driving pressure**, created by the ventilator, is the difference between the baseline pressure, or PEEP (if the baseline is above 0 cm H_2O), and the PIP. If we are using a PIP of 20 cm H_2O with a PEEP of 4 cm H_2O, the driving pressure is 16 cm H_2O.

In theory, when mechanically ventilating a neonate, the driving pressure must be equal to the opening pressure to open and ventilate the alveoli. For example, if the opening pressure is determined to be 20 cm H_2O and we desire a PEEP of 4 cm H_2O, a PIP of 24 cm H_2O would have to be used to achieve a driving pressure that is equal to opening pressure. In this instance, if the PIP were set at 20 cm H_2O, the driving pressure would only be 16 cm H_2O, and in theory, the alveoli would not be adequately ventilated.

Clinically, in addition to assisting with oxygenation, PEEP is used to stabilize the alveoli and reduce the surface tension. The opening pressure is thus reduced and lower driving pressure is needed to ventilate the lungs.

Functional Residual Capacity (FRC)

The FRC is the amount of gas remaining in the lungs at the end of a passive exhalation. In the presence of RDS, the lack of surfactant and subsequent collapse of the alveoli reduces the FRC (Figure 17–8A). As alveoli get smaller during exhalation, surface tension increases and higher pressure is required to reopen them.

PEEP helps prevent the collapse of the alveoli following exhalation and allows the FRC to stabilize or possibly increase (Figure 17–8B). The surface tension in the alveoli is reduced as FRC increases, resulting in less pressure being required to open the alveoli during inspiration. Therefore, the application of PEEP to the airways increases FRC and consequently increases lung compliance, decreasing opening pressures.

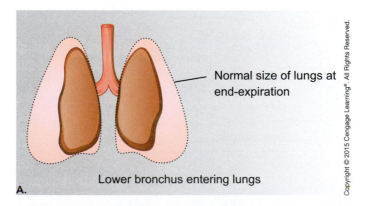

Normal size of lungs at end-expiration

Lower bronchus entering lungs

A.

FIGURE 17–8A. Atelectatic lungs causing a decreased FRC at end-expiration.

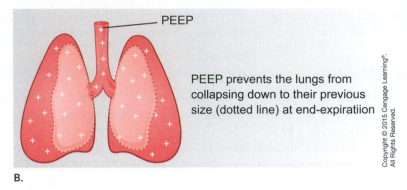

PEEP

PEEP prevents the lungs from collapsing down to their previous size (dotted line) at end-expiratiion

B.

FIGURE 17–8B. FRC is increased as PEEP is added to the airways.

Diffusion Time

Alveolar ventilation is also affected by the length of time that the gas is in contact with the alveoli, or the **diffusion time**. The longer the inflating gas is in contact with the alveoli, the more gas can diffuse to and from the blood. The diffusion time is controlled by the inspiratory time and peak flow.

Referring to Figure 17–9, the diffusion time is represented by the area under the volume curve. Increasing inspiratory time increases the duration of the volume curve and thus increases the amount of time the gas is in contact with the alveoli. Increasing or decreasing peak flow changes the speed at which the gas enters the alveoli. At a constant inspiratory time, increasing the peak flow allows the gas to inflate the alveoli sooner. With a quicker opening of the alveoli, inspired gas is in contact with diffusing surface area for a longer portion of the inspiratory time. Obviously, a change in peak flow has less of an effect on the diffusion time than does inspiratory time.

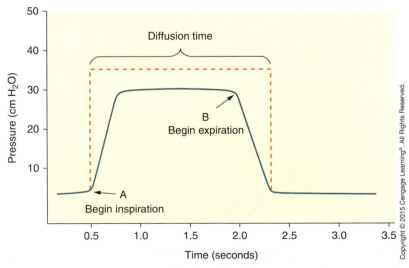

FIGURE 17–9. A representation of the diffusion time, determined from the time the breath begins (point A) until pressure returns to baseline (point B).

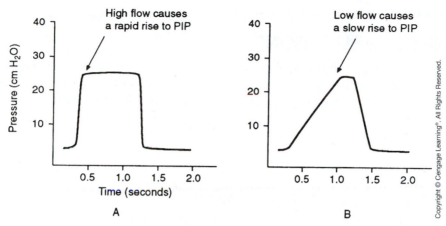

FIGURE 17–10. Pressure patterns at high flows (wave A) and low flows (wave B).

Flow Rate

The flow rate used determines the wave pattern of the ventilator breath. Figure 17–10 shows the wave patterns that are achieved at high flow rates (wave A) and at low flow rates (wave B).

As illustrated, flow rate should be set high enough to achieve the desired pressure level before inspiratory time is reached. If the flow rate is set too low, the inspiratory time may be reached before PIP is attained, thus limiting the delivered breath. This will also decrease contact time between the delivered gas and alveoli (Figure 17–11). A flow rate that is too high causes turbulent airflow, resulting in increased airway resistance, decreased uniform gas delivery and decreased tidal volume delivered to the patient due to prematurely reaching the set PIP.

Any adjustment made to the flow will alter the delivered breath; therefore, the practitioner must monitor the patient carefully whenever flow is changed to ensure airway resistance hasn't increased and predicted tidal volumes haven't decreased.

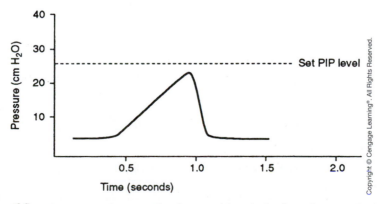

FIGURE 17–11. If flow is set too low, expiration may begin before the set PIP level is reached.

CLINICAL APPLICATIONS

An understanding of the clinical applications of the above-mentioned concepts will help the respiratory therapist appropriately care for the ventilator patient. Changes in ventilator parameters may be indicated by altered clinical signs, changes in the chest x-ray, or laboratory data. Any change in ventilator parameters will change another parameter to some degree. The exception to this is the F_iO_2. Changes in F_iO_2 do not change other parameters per se, but may necessitate other changes to be made. The interwoven relationship of all ventilator parameters is shown in Figure 17–12.

Referring to Figure 17–12, follow the changes when two common ventilator parameters are altered. A change in PIP will change both compression pressure and tidal volume, leading to a change in minute ventilation and an alteration of alveolar ventilation. The alteration of alveolar ventilation leads to changes in $PaCO_2$, which changes pH. The changes in PaO_2 due to alterations in alveolar ventilation exist but are small in comparison to the changes that occur in $PaCO_2$ and pH.

A change in the PEEP level also changes driving pressure and tidal volume leading to the same alterations mentioned with PIP changes. Additionally, changes in

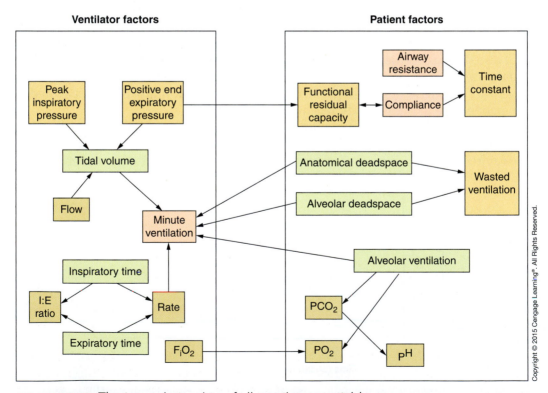

FIGURE 17–12. The interrelationship of all ventilatory variables.

PEEP may impact the FRC, which can then alter compliance. A change in compliance might require altering PIP, resulting in possible alterations of time constant, expiratory time, and the I:E ratio.

If this discussion appears confusing, then it has served its purpose. The point is to demonstrate that all ventilator parameters influence one another to some degree. Ventilator management is no easy task and requires an understanding of these complicated interrelationships.

PRESSURE–VOLUME RELATIONSHIPS (COMPLIANCE)

The relationships that exist between pressure and volume in the lungs play a significant role in strategic manipulation of the mechanical ventilator in order to achieve a desired result. This section reviews these relationships.

Basics

The airways, lungs, and chest wall, like other body organs and structures, are elastic structures. An **elastic** structure, by definition, has the ability to resist deformation when a force is exerted against it, and thus produces a recoil force.

According to Hooke's law of elasticity, when an elastic substance is stretched, tension develops that is proportional to the degree of deformation that is produced. Thus, the more it is stretched, the more force it produces to recoil to its original size and shape.

To measure the elasticity of a hollow, spherical organ, such as the lung, it would be difficult to stretch the tissue and measure its recoil force. Instead, recoil is measured by applying a known pressure to the lung and the change in volume that occurs is measured. This relationship between a given change in volume and the pressure difference required to achieve that volume change is called **compliance** and directly reflects the ability of the lungs to stretch.

Static and Dynamic Compliance

Static compliance defined as the change in volume for any given applied pressure. It is measured when there is no airflow through the lung at the end of inhalation through an inspiratory hold maneuver. This hold eliminates the effects of airway resistance from the measurement. A plateau pressure is measured during the 0.5 second inspiratory hold. Tidal volume is then divided by the difference between plateau pressure and PEEP. Static compliance only reflects the elastic properties of the lungs.

Compliance measured during an active breath is called dynamic compliance. It is calculated by dividing tidal volume by the difference between PIP at the end of inspiration and PEEP. Dynamic compliance better reflects the elastic recoil of the lungs.

Normal Compliance

Lung compliance is measured in mL of volume change per cm H_2O of pressure applied to the trachea. Normal compliance in a newborn is approximately 2.5 to 5 mL/cm H_2O and can decrease to as low as 0.5 mL/cm H_2O/kg with RDS.

Compliance Curves

The amount of pressure required to increase the volume in the lungs is directly related to the number of elastic elements that are present in the lung tissue. The more elastic elements, the more pressure required to stretch them and the lower the compliance.

A graphic representation of the three possible compliance curves of the lung is shown in Figure 17–13. Curve A shows the curve in a stiff, noncompliant lung, curve B is the normal lung compliance curve, and curve C shows a very compliant lung.

Determinants of Pulmonary Compliance

The two main determinants of lung compliance are alveolar surface forces and elastic elements in the lung tissue. Alveolar surface forces are the direct result of surface tension in the alveoli created by the interface between the moist alveoli and the gas in them. (See Chapter 1 for a review of surface tension and surface forces.)

The degree to which surface tension affects lung compliance is illustrated in Figure 17–14. This graph shows a compliance curve of a normal lung when the air–liquid interface of the alveoli is removed by filling and then ventilating the lungs with normal saline, compared to the same lung when ventilated with air. Notice that

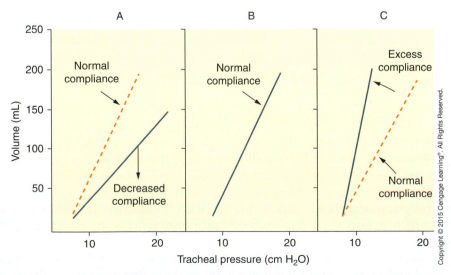

FIGURE 17–13. Various compliance curves of the lungs. Curve A represents a stiff lung, Curve B represents a normal lung, and Curve C represents an excessively compliant lung.

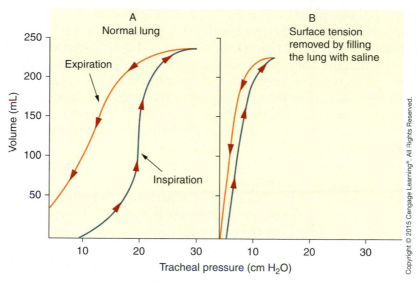

FIGURE 17–14. The relationship between surface tension and lung compliance. Compliance dramatically increases when surface tension is removed (graph B).

the saline-filled lung is far more compliant than the air-filled lung. This difference is the result of alveolar surface tension.

In the healthy lung, these alveolar surface forces are counteracted by the presence of surfactant, which chemically reduces the surface tension of the alveoli. Elastic elements in lung tissue remain fairly constant in the healthy lung, but in disease states these elastic elements may increase and contribute to a decrease in compliance.

Compliance of the Thoracic Cage

The thorax, like the lungs, is an elastic structure. It differs from the lung in that it recoils inward or outward, whereas the lung only recoils inward. The direction of thoracic recoil depends on the volume in the thorax.

If all the organs were removed from the chest and the chest were reclosed, the ribs would be at a neutral point, neither recoiling nor expanding. At this point, the pressure inside the thorax is the same as outside the thorax. This is referred to as the **unstressed volume**. If we were to add volume to the thorax, the ribs would begin to pull inward as they are stretched beyond their unstressed level. This inward pull of the ribs increases the pressure inside the thorax. If volume is now removed from the thorax below the unstressed volume, the ribs attempt to recoil outward, which would decrease the pressure inside the thorax.

Relationship between the Lungs and the Thoracic Cage

To ventilate the lungs adequately, both lung forces and chest wall forces must be overcome. A thin layer of fluid found between the visceral pleura surrounding the lungs and the parietal pleura lining the chest wall maintains the intimate relationship between the lungs and the chest wall. This thin layer of fluid creates a **static attraction** between the external surface of the lung and the internal lining of the lung. The net result is that the compliance of the chest wall and of the lungs, although two separate entities, become one compliance when ventilating the lungs.

FRC is determined when the inward pull of the lungs is balanced with the outward pull of the thorax and the unstressed volume in the chest is reached. At this point, the pressure in the thorax, and thus the lungs, is equal to atmospheric pressure. To inflate the lungs, the pressure inside the thorax must drop below atmospheric pressure, as occurs in spontaneous breathing, or atmospheric pressure must rise above thoracic pressure, as in mechanical ventilation.

As volume increases in the thorax, the elastic forces of both the lungs and the chest recoil inward, increasing the pressure in the thorax and allowing passive exhalation to occur. The gas then exits the thorax to the point that the unstressed volume is once again reached.

Therefore, if the compliance of the lung decreases, the inward pull of the lung exceeds the outward recoil of the ribs and a new unstressed volume is reached, which is less than the previous volume; thus the FRC has decreased.

Compliance Curve of the Lungs

The relationship between volume and pressure is graphically represented in Figure 17–15. The "S"-shaped curve represents the compliance of the lung with pressure on the horizontal and volume on the vertical axis.

Point B in Figure 17–16 shows the location on the curve of the lung with a normal FRC. Notice that it is located on the steep portion of the compliance curve, indicating a high compliance. In other words, small changes in pressure produce large changes in volume.

With diseases such as RDS, as the alveoli lose surfactant, increased surface tension causes an increasing collapse of the alveoli and the FRC decreases. In this lung, the compliance is low. This is represented as point A in Figure 17–17. On the flat

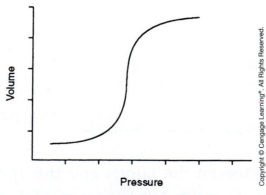

FIGURE 17–15. The volume–pressure curve of the lung.

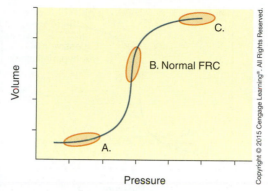

FIGURE 17–16. The location of a lung with a normal FRC on the volume–pressure curve. Small changes in pressure cause large changes in volume.

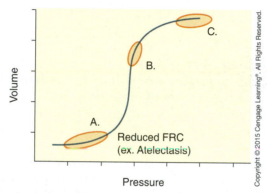

FIGURE 17–17. The loss of FRC places the lung at the low end of the volume–pressure curve. Large pressure changes result in only small changes in volume.

portion of the curve, increases in pressure produce only small changes in volume, indicating a very stiff noncompliant lung.

With the addition of PEEP, the alveoli are held open at the end of exhalation, causing an increase in FRC and moving the lungs back to point B on the compliance curve.

When the lungs are over expanded, FRC increases above normal and the elastic elements in the lung interstitium are stretched. The compliance becomes lower as the lung loses its ability to stretch further. The lungs are now at another flat portion of the compliance curve, represented by point C in Figure 17–18. Again, in this circumstance, changes in pressure produce only small changes in volume.

The hazard when ventilating at this portion of the curve is a tearing or rupture of the lung interstitium because the lung cannot stretch any more in response to pressure increases. A high FRC (point C) can be caused by air trapping or from excessive levels of PEEP.

Successful ventilation techniques require the use of appropriate PEEP levels to keep the lung on the steep portion of the compliance curve.

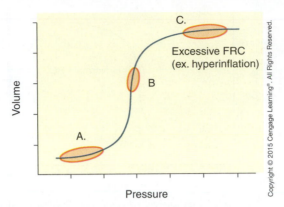

FIGURE 17–18. An increase in FRC causes the lung to be at the high end of the volume–pressure curve. Large pressure changes result in only small changes in volume.

Clinical Applications

Any time mechanical ventilation is initiated on a patient, an understanding of lung compliance is vital. Diseases that increase surface forces in the alveoli (RDS) decrease compliance and increase the amount of pressure required to ventilate the lungs. As the alveoli shrink in size, the FRC is reduced. Higher pressure is now needed to inflate the alveoli. The addition of PEEP increases the FRC and allows the use of lower pressures for ventilation.

Certain fibrotic diseases may cause an increase in the amount of elastic elements in the lung, thus altering compliance. Paralyzation of the chest wall reduces thoracic compliance and requires increased inspiratory pressures to overcome the increased stiffness.

With the need for increased pressure to open the alveoli, there is an increased risk of barotrauma. High pressure also further decreases cardiac output by decreasing venous return to the right heart. Pulmonary vascular resistance increases as ventilatory pressures rise, resulting in diminished blood flow to the lungs and increased V/Q mismatch.

An important goal when ventilating the lungs is to maintain the lung on the steep portion of the compliance curve resulting in lowering inspiratory pressures and decreasing the chance of barotrauma and other mentioned effects on the cardiopulmonary systems.

PRESSURE–FLOW RELATIONSHIPS (RESISTANCE)

There are several factors that impact airway resistance. Understanding these factors and their relationship to pressure and flow will assist in making appropriate clinical decisions that can decrease the patient's work of breathing and potentially improve the patient's outcome.

Basics

There are several factors that determine the level of flow through a tube. They are: 1) the difference between the inlet and the outlet pressures, which is the driving pressure, 2) the radius of the tube, 3) the length of the tube, and 4) the **viscosity** or thickness of the gas or fluid, illustrated in Figure 17–19. This is the basic expression of Poiseuille's law. The pressure difference between the inlet and the outlet determines the rate of flow, with a greater pressure difference resulting in a greater flow and vice versa. The other three factors offer a **resistance** to that flow.

When dealing with the airways, the length of the airway and the viscosity of the gas remain relatively constant, so the only factor that changes resistance to airflow is a change in the radius of the airway. This is important to remember when selecting an endotracheal tube for a patient in order to secure an artificial airway and provide assisted ventilation.

Measurement of Airway Resistance

Resistance is measured as the ratio between the driving pressure, measured in cm H_2O, and the amount of flow in liters per second. The basic definition of airway resistance is the driving pressure needed to move gases through the airways at a constant flow rate.

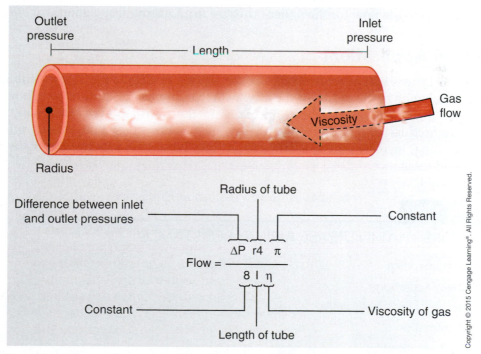

FIGURE 17–19. Poiseuille's law determining flow through a tube. Flow is proportional to the viscosity of the gas and the length of the tube. Flow is inversely proportional to the fourth power of the radius of the tube.

In the lung, the driving pressure is the difference between the pressure at the mouth (inlet pressure) and the alveoli (outlet pressure). We can then calculate resistance by measuring the driving pressure and dividing it by the flow of gas. The measurement of airway resistance is usually accomplished during pulmonary function studies. The normal airway resistance in a spontaneously breathing neonate is between 20 and 30 cm $H_2O/L/sec$.

Other Causes of Increased Resistance

There are other factors that may lead to increased airway resistance that are not associated with the normal anatomy of the airway. Neonates have an increased level of interstitial fluid in the lungs, which reduces the radius of the airway.

The presence of an endotracheal tube (ETT) and the associated ventilator tubing also increases airway resistance. The resistance offered by an ETT is directly related to its length and inversely related to its diameter. Turbulent flow is present in a 2.5 mm ID ETT at flow rates exceeding 3 Lpm and at flows exceeding 7.5 Lpm in a 3.0 ETT. Subsequent changes in flow above these levels cause disproportionate increases in resistance, secondary to the increased turbulent flow. Although suggested inspiratory flow rates for neonates on mechanical ventilation range from 6 to 10 Lpm depending on gestational age, respiratory rate and inspiratory demand, much of this flow is not delivered to the airway but rather used to drive the ventilator and to provide flow for the patient to draw from during inspiration.

Clinical Applications

Of all the factors that affect resistance in the airway, by far the most powerful influence is a change in the radius of the airway. According to Poiseuille's law, for every decrease in the radius, resistance increases to the fourth power. Therefore, anything that reduces the radius of the airway, such as bronchospasm, mucus, edema, and swelling, increases the resistance to airflow. Table 17–3 lists possible causes of increased resistance.

Table 17–3
FACTORS THAT INCREASE AIRWAY RESISTANCE
1. Bronchospasm
2. Airway secretions
3. Edema of the airway walls
4. Inflammation
5. Artificial airway
a. Endotracheal tube
b. Tracheostomy tube

Treatment is aimed at increasing the airway diameter and reducing the resistance to air flow. This is done with bronchodilators to relieve bronchospasm, vigorous chest physiotherapy and suctioning to mobilize and remove airway secretions, diuretics to reduce edema, and antibiotics and anti-inflammatories to reduce inflammation.

Airway resistance that exists due to the placement of an endotracheal tube can be reduced by shortening the tube and only allowing 4 cm of the tube extends beyond the lips. The shorter the tube, the less resistance it will offer. Shortening the length of the ETT will also decrease deadspace ventilation. When intubating a patient, it is desirable to use an endotracheal tube with the largest diameter possible, further reducing airway resistance.

To avoid extremes in turbulent airflow that increase airway resistance, attempts should be made to keep ventilator flow rates at or below those levels at which turbulence increases. The clinical implications of turbulent airflow are less pressure being delivered to the alveoli with a resultant reduction in tidal volume. This is prevalent more so when high rates and short inspiratory times are being used.

Additionally, the airway resistance offered by the ETT is greater than that of the upper airways, and spontaneous ventilation by the neonate through the ETT may require more work than the neonate is able to handle. The neonatal patient should be extubated when ventilator settings are weaned to a low rate and PIP. They should not be required to breathe spontaneously on CPAP through an ETT for any length of time due to the work of breathing necessary to overcome the resistance of the ETT.

TIME CONSTANTS (Kt)

Time constants reflect the amount of time required for alveolar and proximal airway pressures to equilibrate. In other words, time constants are the amount of time required for the lungs to inhale or exhale. Our focus in this section will be on expiratory time constants.

Calculating Time Constants

The two forces that determine the time required for exhalation are the elastic recoil of the lung and chest wall (compliance) and the opposition to airflow (resistance). The formula for calculating one time constant is to multiply compliance by resistance. Compliance must be changed to L/cm H_2O before calculating the time constant.

The compliance and resistance of the respiratory system as a whole is used to calculate time constants. This is done realizing that we are using an average, when some alveoli having longer time constants and some shorter. An understanding of time constants will help the caregiver choose the safest and most effective ventilator settings for each patient.

Table 17–4	

CALCULATION OF TIME CONSTANTS

Kt = compliance (L/cm H_2O) × resistance

Kt = 0.006 × 25

Kt = 0.15 sec

0.15 × 3 (amount of time to exhale 95% of the VT) = 0.45 sec needed for exhalation

One time constant equals the time required for the alveoli to discharge 63% of the tidal volume. Three time constants are required before 95% of the tidal volume is emptied.

An example of calculating time constants, using a lung compliance of 0.006 L/cm H_2O and a resistance of 25 cm H_2O/L/sec, is demonstrated in Table 17–4. In this instance, one time constant equals 0.15 second. This patient would therefore require a minimum of 0.45 second (3 × 0.15 sec) to exhale 95% of the tidal volume and avoid air trapping.

Clinical Applications

All possible combinations of resistance and compliance changes, and the effect on time constants, are demonstrated in Table 17–5. We will briefly discuss three common clinical situations that demonstrate these relationships.

If airway resistance remains constant, a decrease in lung compliance results in a decreased time constant. This means that less time is needed for exhalation and the patient can tolerate shorter expiratory times. Shorter expiratory times allow for faster ventilatory rates without the risk of air trapping. This combination is often present in RDS, where the decreased amount of surfactant affects the alveolar compliance, but not airway resistance.

If airway resistance increases along with a decrease in compliance, as would occur if bronchospasm accompanied RDS, the time constant would increase and expiratory times would need to be lengthened to prevent air trapping.

A possible clinical situation in which this could be dangerous is in a patient being mechanically ventilated at a high rate of RDS. If bronchospasm occurred, the time constant would increase and air trapping would result. To avoid air trapping, the expiratory time would need to be increased to allow the lungs time to empty. The administration of a bronchodilator may reduce the bronchospasm, reducing airway resistance and returning the time constants to previous levels.

It should be apparent that the clinical disease state of the infant is continuously changing and must be closely monitored and anticipated so that appropriate ventilator changes can be made.

Table 17–5

EFFECTS OF COMPLIANCE AND RESISTANCE CHANGES ON KT

Changes	Effect on Kt
Compliance unchanged	
Increased airway resistance	Longer duration
Decreased airway resistance	Shorter duration
Airway resistance unchanged	
Improved compliance	Longer duration
Worsening compliance	Shorter duration
Improved compliance	
Increased airway resistance	Longer duration
Decreased airway resistance	No change
Worsened compliance	
Increased airway resistance	No change
Decreased airway resistance	Shorter duration
Increased airway resistance	
Improved compliance	Longer duration
Worsening compliance	No change
Decreased airway resistance	
Improved compliance	No change
Worsening compliance	Shorter duration

Another possible clinical situation surrounds the administration of surfactant. This example involves a preterm neonate, with RDS being ventilated at high pressures and frequency, receiving a dose of surfactant. The surfactant reduces the alveolar surface tension, increasing compliance. As the compliance improves, time constants also increase. The respiratory therapist must be aware of these changes and slow the rate of ventilation to allow adequate expiratory time in the presence of longer time constants. It should also be noted that the administration of surfactant requires close monitoring and weaning of PIP in order to maintain estimated tidal volumes. Increased lung compliance will result in increased tidal volumes that may exceed the desired volumes for the patient and may result in barotrauma.

Procedures such as suctioning and reintubation with a larger endotracheal tube cause a decrease in resistance and decreased time constants. An understanding of these concepts will allow the respiratory therapist to maintain the ideal patient/ventilator system.

SUMMARY

In order to appropriately manage a mechanically ventilated patient, the respiratory therapist must understand the basic concepts involved in mechanical ventilation. Before committing a patient to a ventilator, the goals of the treatment must be understood. The overriding goal is to provide adequate alveolar gas exchange while decreasing work of breathing and causing minimal damage to the lungs and minimal interference with the circulation.

Understanding mechanical ventilation begins with an understanding of terminology. The peak inspiratory pressure (PIP) a limit variable and is the maximum pressure reached during the inspiratory phase. Positive end-expiratory pressure (PEEP) is a baseline variable and is the level of positive pressure applied to the airway during the expiratory phase. Frequency, or rate, is a trigger variable and is the number of inspiratory breaths delivered by the ventilator in one minute. The inspiratory time (IT) is a cycle variable and is the amount of time, usually measured in seconds or tenths of a second, that the inspiratory breath lasts.

A slightly more difficult concept to grasp is that of mean airway pressure (MAP), which is the average pressure being applied to the airway throughout the inspiratory and expiratory cycle, or the complete cycle time. There are many variables that determine MAP, such as rate, PIP, PEEP, and IT. In general, it is prudent to maintain MAP as low as possible in order to protect lung tissue from damage and still meet the ventilatory requirements of the patient.

Tidal volume is the amount of gas, measured in milliliters or liters, given to the patient during inspiration. When the tidal volume is multiplied by the rate of ventilation, the result is the minute volume, or the total amount of gas delivered to the patient in one minute. Deadspace is defined as those portions of the respiratory tract that do not participate in gas exchange. Deadspace is either anatomic or alveolar. Anatomic deadspace involves airways that do not engage in gas exchange, basically from the terminal bronchioles upward. Alveolar deadspace includes alveoli that fill with gas, but are not perfused with blood. The combination of the two is called physiologic deadspace. Alveolar ventilation, therefore, is equal to the tidal volume, minus the physiologic deadspace.

The amount of pressure needed to open and expand the alveoli is called opening pressure. It may be determined when crackles are heard during inspiration. The driving pressure of the ventilator is equal to the total amount of pressure rise during an inspiration, or PIP minus PEEP. Ideally, the driving pressure should be equal to or above the opening pressure in order to ventilate the alveoli. In the presence of PEEP compliance is improved, opening pressure is reduced and less driving pressure is needed to provide ventilation.

The functional residual capacity (FRC), is the amount of gas remaining in the lungs at the end of inspiration. In the presence of surfactant deficiency, the FRC drops and compliance worsens. The addition of PEEP brings the FRC back to its appropriate level and improves lung compliance. The amount of time that the inspiratory gas is in contact with the alveoli is called diffusion time. The longer the contact time, the more gas is able to diffuse between the alveoli and the blood. Finally, the flow rate determines how quickly gas is delivered during inspiration. It can be likened to a water faucet in which the wider it is opened, the faster the flow escaping. Likewise, the more an inspiratory flow valve is opened, the faster the gas will flow through the circuit and into the patient.

Terminology, as it relates to the structures of the pulmonary tree, is also important to understand. Compliance reflects the ability of the lungs to expand at any given pressure. In states of high compliance, the lung expands easily at low pressures. Conversely, in states of low compliances, high pressures are required to make the lungs expand. Compliance is determined by alveolar surface forces and by the elastic elements of the lungs. Low compliance is the result of increased alveolar surface forces, an increase in the elastic elements, or a combination of both. The compliance curve of the lung is useful to understand the role of FRC and its effect on lung compliance. As FRC increase above normal, the lung tissue is stretched beyond its normal length. As pressure is applied to the lungs, they can expand only a small amount and thus compliance is low. When FRC is below normal, the alveoli shrink due to their surface forces. Now as pressure is applied, a greater amount is required to overcome the surface forces. Again, compliance is low. At its normal volume, neither the lung tissues are stretched exceedingly, nor are the alveoli shrunk abnormally, and compliance is within its normal range. At that point, ventilation can be accomplished without having to resort to excessive pressures, which could damage the lungs and impede circulation.

As gas flows through the airways, its movement is resisted by several factors including the size and length of the airway. Of the factors affecting gas flow in the airways, all remain constant except for the size, or diameter. Therefore, the major factor in determining resistance to airflow is the changing diameter of the airways. As the diameter decreases, such as with bronchospasm, airway resistance increases. The opposite is true when airway diameter increases.

The final term covered is time constant which is the amount of time required for alveolar and proximal pressures to equilibrate. Lung compliance and airway resistance determine time constants. This is an important concept to understand when providing mechanical ventilation to a neonate. For example, if a patient has a long time constant secondary to increased airway resistance, a longer period of time will be required for exhalation to occur. If the expiratory time is too short, the next breath will be delivered before exhalation is complete, leaving inspired gas in the alveoli. The results could be air trapping and possibly air leaks.

POSTTEST

1. Which of the following is the goal of mechanical ventilation?
   a. the reversal of acute lung disorders
   b. maintain a patent airway in the presence of lung disease
   c. treatment and diagnosis of acute and chronic lung disorders
   d. decrease work of breathing and provide adequate alveolar ventilationwith minimal lung damage

2. Which of the following is the best definition of peak inspiratory pressure?
   a. the maximum pressure exerted against the patient's airway during inspiration
   b. a positive pressure maintained in the airway during expiration
   c. the pressure required to open the lungs to 75% of capacity
   d. the pressure generated by the ventilator before a tidal volume delivery
3. Of the following, which best describes wasted ventilation?
   a. alveolar deadspace
   b. physiologic deadspace
   c. the ratio of physiologic deadspace to tidal volume
   d. the amount of tidal gas that leaks around the endotracheal tube
4. Of the following, which alter the duration of ventilation?
   I. rate
   II. flow
   III. PIP
   IV. PEEP
   V. I:T
   a. II, V
   b. I, III, IV
   c. II, III, V
   d. I, II, III, IV, V
5. Assuming an alveolar opening pressure of 24 cm H_2O, which of the following combinations of PIP and PEEP would achieve the desired compression pressure?
   a. PIP-24, PEEP-4
   b. PIP-20, PEEP-5
   c. PIP-28, PEEP-4
   d. PIP-26, PEEP-5
6. Normal lung compliance in a newborn is:
   a. 2.5 to 5 mL/cm H_2O
   b. 7 to 10 mL/cm H_2O
   c. 10 to 15 mL/cm H_2O
   d. 25 to 30 mL/cm H_2O
7. Of the following, which are determinants of pulmonary compliance?
   I. elastic elements
   II. alveolar surface forces
   III. plateau pressure
   IV. airway resistance
   V. dynamic ventilatory pressures
   a. II, IV
   b. I, III, IV
   c. I, II
   d. III, IV, V

8. As volume is extracted from the thorax at its unstressed volume, the ribs:
    a. pull inward
    b. spread apart
    c. recoil outward
    d. pull closer together

9. With overexpansion of the lungs caused by air trapping, lung compliance is:
    a. normal
    b. high
    c. reduced
    d. inverse to the level of airflow

10. RDS lowers lung compliance by:
    a. increasing pulmonary blood flow
    b. increasing airway resistance
    c. increasing air trapping
    d. increasing alveolar surface forces

11. Which of the following is the main factor that determines airway resistance?
    a. airway radius
    b. airway length
    c. outlet pressure
    d. viscosity of the gas

12. The normal airway resistance in a spontaneously breathing neonate is:
    a. 10 to 20 cm $H_2O/L/sec$
    b. 20 to 30 cm $H_2O/L/sec$
    c. 20 to 30 mm $Hg/cc/sec$
    d. 30 to 40 mm $Hg/cc/sec$

13. Endotracheal tube resistance can be reduced by:
    a. lengthening the tube
    b. increasing gas flow
    c. shortening the tube
    d. decreasing tidal volume

14. In the presence of which of the following scenarios could shorter inspiratory times and faster rates be used without the risk of air trapping?
    a. RDS with bronchospasm
    b. administration of surfactant to an RDS patient
    c. improving RDS
    d. RDS

15. With a compliance of 3.6 mL/cm H_2O and an airway resistance of 42 cm $H_2O/L/sec$, what would be an appropriate expiratory time?
    a. 0.46 sec
    b. 0.28 sec
    c. 0.16 sec
    d. 0.15 sec

REFERENCES

1. Merenstein GB, Gardner SL. *Handbook of Neonatal Intensive Care.* 7th ed. St. Louis, MO: CV Mosby Co., 2011.
2. Koff PB, et al. *Neonatal and Pediatric Respiratory Care.* 2nd ed. St. Louis, MO: CV Mosby Co., 1993.

BIBLIOGRAPHY AND SUGGESTED READINGS

Chang DW. *Clinical Application of Mechanical Ventilation.* 4th ed. Albany, NY: Delmar, Cengage Learning, 2013.

Goldsmith JP, Karotkin EH. *Assisted Ventilation of the Neonate.* 5th ed. Philadelphia, PA: WB Saunders Co., 2010.

Levin D, Morriss F, et al. *Essentials of Pediatric Intensive Care.* 2nd ed. St. Louis, MO: Quality Medical Publishing, Inc., 1997.

MacIntyre NR, Branson RD. *Mechanical Ventilation.* 2nd ed. Philadelphia, PA: WB Saunders Co., 2008.

Pilbeam SP. *Mechanical Ventilation.* 4th ed. St. Louis, MO: Mosby, 2006.

OBJECTIVES

Upon completion of this chapter, the reader should be able to:

1. List and describe several indications for mechanical ventilatory support of the neonate and child.
2. Compare and contrast partial ventilatory support and full ventilatory support.
3. Describe how the following initial ventilator parameters are determined: ventilator mode, peak inspiratory pressure, set rate, sensitivity, PEEP, F_iO_2, inspiratory flow rate, inspiratory time, I:E ratio, and/or tidal volume.
4. Describe volume-control versus pressure-controlled ventilation.
5. Describe how changes are made in ventilator settings based on arterial blood gases and clinical assessment and evaluation.
6. Discuss several hazards/complications of mechanical ventilation.
7. Discuss weaning procedures and extubation strategies to remove the neonatal and pediatric patient from mechanical ventilation.
8. Discuss indications/considerations for early extubation of the neonatal and pediatric patient.

KEY TERMS

conditional variable
control variable
full ventilatory support
mode of ventilation
pallor

partial ventilatory
  support
pressure-controlled
  ventilation

rebound effect
volume-controlled
  ventilation

INTRODUCTION

Intubation, with subsequent mechanical ventilation, is a common lifesaving intervention in the NICU and pediatric intensive care units. The length of stay in the units can be for days, weeks, and even months. Given the length of time the patient is on the ventilator, it is essential that the respiratory therapist has a good understanding of those techniques used to optimize the interaction between the ventilator and patient, and minimize complications.

INDICATIONS FOR VENTILATORY SUPPORT OF THE NEONATE AND CHILD

In the neonatal or pediatric intensive care unit, a thorough clinical evaluation and rapid patient assessment of the signs and symptoms of impending respiratory failure are key to a successful resuscitation. The immediate indication for mechanical ventilation is respiratory failure. This is commonly subdivided into three classifications: hypoxemic respiratory failure, hypercapnic respiratory failure, and mixed respiratory failure.

Hypoxemic Respiratory Failure

Hypoxemic respiratory failure is commonly manifested by a PaO_2 $\leq$50 mmHg on a F_iO_2 of $\geq$60% (PaO_2/F_iO_2 ratio < 300 observed in acute lung injury) despite the use of continuous positive airway pressure (CPAP), or a decreasing PaO_2 (or SpO_2 <90–92%) despite an increase in F_iO_2. Frequently, these patients will have an accompanying hypocapnia ($PaCO_2$ $\leq$30 mmHg) and respiratory alkalemia (pH $\geq$7.5), as they attempt to compensate for hypoxemia by increasing spontaneous minute ventilation. Clinical features include agitation, cyanosis, tachycardia, or bradycardia (late), tachypnea (>70–80 breaths/min in neonates; >50 breaths/min in children). Classic signs of distress in neonates also include nasal flaring, grunting, and marked thoracic retractions (substernal, sternal, intercostal, supraclavicular, and suprasternal).

Hypercapnic Respiratory Failure

Hypercapnic respiratory failure is commonly manifested by a $PaCO_2$ $\geq$60 mmHg, accompanied by acidemia (pH $\leq$7.25). The infant may appear apneic, listless, and cyanotic. Bradycardia or tachycardia may be present depending on the presence of asphexia (primary or secondary apnea) in the newborn, that is, decelerations recognized in fetal heart monitoring and prolonged periods of bradycardia as asphexia progresses. The end result is hypoxic-ischemic encephalopathy.

Mixed Respiratory Failure

Mixed respiratory failure is manifested by both hypoxemia and hypercapnia. Marked acidemia will be present as well. Table 18–1 indicates the clinical conditions that may necessitate mechanical ventilation of the neonate and child.

Table 18–1

CAUSES OF DEPRESSED RESPIRATORY DRIVE

Drug overdose

Acute spinal cord injury

Head trauma

Neurologic dysfunction

Sleep disorders

Metabolic alkalosis

CAUSES OF EXCESSIVE VENTILATORY WORKLOAD

Acute airflow obstruction

Deadspace ventilation

Congenital heart disease

Cardiovascular decompensation

Shock

Increased metabolic rate

Drugs

Decreased compliance

CAUSES OF VENTILATORY PUMP FAILURE

Chest trauma

Premature birth

Electrolyte imbalance

Geriatric patients

Other Considerations

It is generally accepted that mechanical ventilation is indicated when one or more reversible problems (ventilation, acidemia, and oxygenation) exist. However, not all problems in neonates or children are reversible and there is an ethical dilemma about whether to withhold or withdraw life support from some children. Diagnoses in which the decision is made to withhold life support include birth weight less than 800 g, severe intracranial hemorrhage, periventricular leukomalacia, severe necrotizing enterocolitis, hypoxic-ischemic encephalopathy, intractable respiratory failure, and major congenital anomalies or chromosomal abnormalities. In the presence of one or more of these problems, the pediatrician, neonatologist, and parents may choose to forgo therapy because it may be futile, the abnormality may lead only to lifelong impairment, or the treatment may cause great social, cultural, and/or economic suffering.[1,2]

MODES OF MECHANICAL VENTILATION

A **mode of ventilation** is described as the combination of control, phase, and conditional variables.[3] The **control variable** is that which does not change when compliance or resistance changes. In **volume-controlled ventilation**, if compliance or resistance changes in the lung, volume does not change; pressure changes. In **pressure-controlled ventilation**, when compliance or resistance changes, pressure remains constant. This means that when compliance decreases or resistance increases, tidal volume necessarily decreases. The phase variables are trigger, limit, cycle, and baseline. A trigger variable refers to how a breath is initiated (i.e., how the breath is triggered, by time, pressure, or flow). The patient's inspiratory effort may be time, pressure, flow, or volume triggered. Breaths that are begun only when dictated by an inspiratory timer are time triggered. The limit variable is that which is reached before the end of inspiration and may include time, pressure, volume, or flow. The cycle variable is that which ends inspiration. Cycle variables also include time, pressure, volume, or flow. The baseline variable defines expiration, which is usually measured only by pressure. **Conditional variables** describe the conditions that must exist for initiating a sigh breath, or a mandatory breath during synchronized intermittent mandatory ventilation (SIMV). A given mode may be classified in one of two categories, partial or full ventilatory support.

PARTIAL VENTILATORY SUPPORT (PVS)

Partial ventilatory support includes those modes indicated for patients who are capable of maintaining all or part of their minute ventilation spontaneously. Included are CPAP, pressure support ventilation (PSV), intermittent mandatory ventilation (IMV) at low mandatory rates, and synchronized intermittent mandatory ventilation (SIMV) at low mandatory rates. CPAP and IMV are the primary modes used for neonates. CPAP, SIMV, and PSV, among others, are used in the mechanical ventilation of children.

Continuous Positive Airway Pressure (CPAP)

CPAP is the application of a continuous positive distending pressure to the airways while the patient is spontaneously breathing. It is a technique that is used on infants and children suffering from respiratory distress syndrome in an attempt to prevent the need for continuous mechanical ventilation. It accomplishes this by increasing the functional residual capacity (FRC), increasing compliance, decreasing total airway resistance, and decreasing respiratory rate, which are the desired outcomes of nasal CPAP.[3]

In RDS, one of the last organs to mature in utero is the respiratory system. Alveolar surfactant quantity produced by alveolar type II cells and properly functioning gas exchange are insufficient due to prematurity to maintain alveolar geometry, thus causing surface tension to increase. The increased surface tension of the alveoli causes an ever-decreasing FRC. With each breath, the patient must overcome the higher surface tension, and the work of breathing correspondingly increases. The administration of a continuous positive pressure to the airway physically holds the alveoli and airways open during exhalation and increases FRC, as shown in Figure 18–1. With an increase in FRC, lung compliance improves, easing the work of breathing, and PaO_2 increases while usually allowing a decrease in the F_IO_2 and its accompanying toxic side effects. CPAP may be administered to the neonate or infant through an endotracheal tube in the trachea. Alternative airways used on neonates include a trimmed endotracheal tube in the posterior oral pharynx adjacent to the uvula, or nasal prongs. To use the trimmed tube technique, an appropriately sized endotracheal tube is inserted into a nare and advanced until it is palpated adjacent to the uvula. Once there, it is trimmed outside the nare to decrease dead space, then taped in place above the upper lip. The endotracheal tube-ventilator circuit adapter is replaced and fitted to the ventilator circuit.

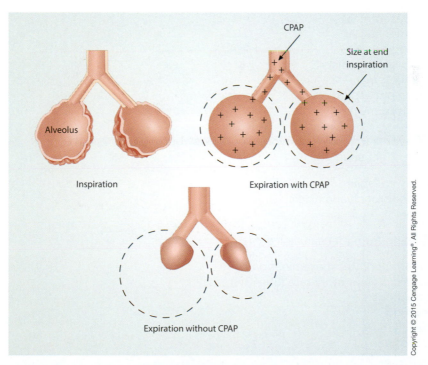

FIGURE 18–1. The presence of positive pressure during the expiratory phase prevents alveolar collapse when surfactant is not present.

The nasal prongs are attached to the ventilator circuit at the endotracheal tube adapter. The prongs are fitted into the nares and secured with tape to the infant's face.

CPAP is administered to a child through the endotracheal tube. A mask is not advised, because the child may aspirate air, leading to gastric distention, vomiting, and aspiration of gastric contents. The child may fear the mask, exhibit anxiety, and frequently dislodge it unless sedated.

Indications CPAP is useful for the treatment of conditions resulting in airway or alveolar instability. Five general indications for CPAP exist, as shown in Table 18–2. The first indication is any disease or condition that causes a decrease in the FRC. Causes of a decreased FRC include: infectious processes such as pneumonia; a loss of lung volume as seen with atelectasis, pulmonary edema, or thoracotomy; an inability for gas to reach the alveoli as occurs in meconium aspiration, or severe airway blockage with mucus; conditions that lower lung surfactant such as RDS; and other conditions, including RDS type II (transient tachypnea) and left-to-right shunting present with certain cardiac defects.

Table 18–2

INDICATIONS FOR CPAP

A. *Decreased FRC*
   Pneumonia
   Atelectasis
   Pulmonary edema
   Thoracotomy
   Meconium aspiration
   Increased mucus
   RDS
   RDS type II (transient tachypnea of the newborn)
   Left-to-right shunting

B. *Airway collapse*
   Tracheobronchial malacia
   Apnea

C. *Weaning from mechanical ventilation*

D. *Abnormal physical examination*
   Increased respiratory rate (30–40%)
   Retractions
   Grunting
   Nasal flaring
   Cyanosis

E. *Abnormal arterial blood gases*
   $PaO_2 < 50$ mmHg at an F_iO_2 of 60% (with adequate ventilation)

The second indication includes those processes that cause airway collapse. One of the primary causes of airway collapse is tracheobronchial malacia, in which the cartilage of the trachea is abnormal and does not offer the necessary rigidity to prevent collapse during inspiration and expiration. This is sometimes observed in congenital anomalies such as heart defects or in long-term intubations. Airway collapse can also lead to apnea, making CPAP helpful in treating apnea.

A third indication for CPAP is to assist in weaning the patient from mechanical ventilation. A study by Tapia and associates, however, failed to demonstrate any difference in extubation outcome whether CPAP was used or not.[4]

The fourth and fifth indications may be seen in the above conditions, but are not exclusive to them and are listed separately. An abnormal physical examination that shows a 30% to 40% increase in respiratory rate, retractions, grunting, flaring, or cyanosis is the fourth indication. The fifth involves blood gas (oxygenation) abnormality. Assuming ventilation is adequate, the inability to maintain the PaO_2 greater than 50 mmHg at an F_iO_2 of 60% is an indication for CPAP.[5]

CPAP is most effective when it is instituted early in the progression of the disease. Initial pressures should start at between 4 and 5 cm H_2O. The pressure is increased in increments of 2 cm H_2O, as needed, to achieve the desired PaO_2 and SpO_2 level, up to a CPAP of 10 cm H_2O.[3] CPAP is considered successful if the F_iO_2 is stabilized at ≤60% with a PaO_2 ≥50 mmHg or SpO_2 >90%, a decreased work of breathing, decreased retractions, nasal flaring, or grunting, improved aeration on the chest radiograph, and subjectively improved patient comfort.

Nasal CPAP is considered to have failed when the PaO_2 remains below 50 mmHg despite an F_iO_2 of 80% to 100% on CPAP pressures of 10 to 12 cm H_2O. A $PaCO_2$ ≥60 mmHg with a pH less than 7.25 specially occurring with marked retractions on CPAP, metabolic acidosis that does not respond to treatment, or frequent apneic episodes while on CPAP are all indications that CPAP has failed. In this instance, intermittent mandatory ventilation is initiated.

Classification of Breaths and Waveforms CPAP breaths are classified as pressure controlled, pressure triggered, pressure limited, and pressure cycled. The baseline variable is pressure. All breaths are spontaneous. That is, all breaths are initiated by patient effort and all breaths end owing to the patient's compliance and resistance characteristics. A representative pressure waveform is shown in Figure 18–2.

Hazards The principal hazard of CPAP therapy is that associated with high pressures (barotrauma). In the presence of excessive pressures, pulmonary blood flow is diminished secondary to the compression of pulmonary vessels. Cardiac output may also be reduced owing to the decrease in venous return to the heart. For these reasons, CPAP is not useful in the patient with persistent pulmonary hypertension and other diseases where the problem is not one of alveolar instability.

Additional hazards include renal effects such as a decrease in glomerular filtration rate, sodium excretion, and reduced urine output. CPAP also elevates intracranial pressure, increasing the incidence of cerebral hemorrhage. Further hazards include pneumothorax, nasal obstruction, gastric distention, and necrosis or erosion of the nasal septum. Nasal deformities from the use of nasal prongs has also been recognized.[6]

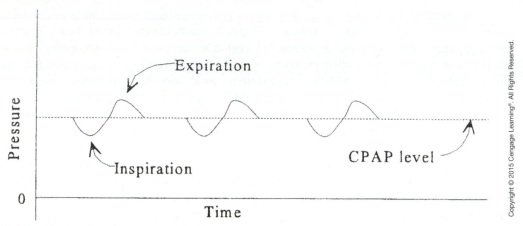

FIGURE 18–2. Pressure wave form for continuous positive airway pressure. All breaths are spontaneous, pressure triggered, limited, and cycled.

Contraindications CPAP should not be used in the presence of upper airway abnormalities such as choanal atresia, cleft palate, or tracheoesophageal fistula, because it could be ineffective or dangerous. CPAP increases intrapulmonary pressure; therefore, it should not be used in cases of untreated air leaks such as pneumothorax, pneumomediastinum, pneumopericardium, and pulmonary interstitial emphysema. The increase in intrathoracic pressure may also further worsen cardiovascular instability and should not be used in those patients. Secondly, because the patient must maintain spontaneous ventilation, CPAP should not be used on the severely apneic patient who experiences episodes of desaturation or bradycardia. Any patient who cannot maintain an adequate spontaneous tidal volume and, therefore, have hypercapnic respiratory failure should not be treated with CPAP. Neonates with untreated congenital diaphragmatic hernia should not be treated with CPAP. One study raised the possibility of bronchiolitis being a contraindication for CPAP.[7]

Weaning from CPAP As soon as the patient begins to show signs of clinical improvement, the F_iO_2 is decreased in 5% decrements until the F_iO_2 reaches 40% to 60%. At that point, the CPAP is lowered in decrements of 2–5 cm H_2O, as tolerated and as indicated by the blood gas status. Continuous monitoring of blood gases with a transcutaneous monitor and/or a pulse oximeter is recommended during the weaning phase. CPAP is lowered until it reaches 2 to 3 cm H_2O, at which point the CPAP device can be safely removed and the patient placed in an oxyhood at the preexisting F_iO_2, which is then weaned as tolerated.

Pressure Support Ventilation (PSV)

PSV is a mode of ventilation that supplements spontaneous patient inspiratory effort with a clinician-selected pressure level. PSV is indicated for any patient in whom a greater tidal volume (5–8 mL/kg) and decreased spontaneous ventilatory rate are desired during spontaneous breaths in the SIMV or CPAP modes. It is also used to overcome the resistance of the airways and ventilator circuit, or may be used to deliver a specified tidal volume (i.e., 10 mL/kg for FVS). Tidal volume is proportional to the PSV level and compliance, but inversely proportional to resistance.

BiPAP™ is the same as PSV with PEEP. It was popularized for patients with hypoventilation syndromes, to augment spontaneous ventilation, or to initiate weaning trials. Ventilators that incorporate this mode have settings for inspiratory positive airway pressure (IPAP) and expiratory positive airway pressure (EPAP). The pressure difference between EPAP and IPAP determines tidal volume. Breaths may be flow or pressure triggered, or the mode control may be set so time-triggered breaths can be delivered for patients with central apnea disorders.

A modification of PSV found on the Siemens Servo 300 ventilator, volume support (VS), is "compliance-sensitive." In VS, the user selects a tidal volume and the ventilator delivers successively higher pressures until the inspiratory tidal volume sensing mechanism senses the delivery of the desired tidal volume.[8] In the event of a decrease in compliance or increase in resistance, the ventilator automatically increases the PSV pressure until the desired tidal volume is restored. The ventilator automatically and continuously makes these adjustments. Waveforms are the same as in PSV. The correlate mode for patients who need time-triggered mandatory breaths is pressure-regulated volume control (PRVC).[9]

Hazards of PSV It is important to realize that in PSV, there are no mandatory breaths, so the patient must have a reliable, spontaneous ventilatory pattern. If the patient becomes apneic, the ventilator must provide an alarm and/or may switch automatically to a mode of ventilation that provides mandatory breaths.

PSV Waveforms Once a patient makes an inspiratory effort, the ventilator inflates the lungs until the pressure reaches the user-specified PSV level and holds it there until the gas flow tapers to approximately 25% of the peak flow, owing to the patient's airway resistance. PSV breaths are pressure controlled, flow, pressure, or volume triggered (not time triggered, except in the case of PRVC), flow limited, and flow or time cycled. The baseline variable is pressure, because PSV may be used with PEEP (Figures 18–3A and B).

Weaning from PSV To wean the patient from pressure support, the support pressure is gradually decreased, while ensuring that tidal volume is being maintained without an increase in ventilatory rate. This is thought to occur as muscle strength increases maintaining sufficient tidal volume over declining pressure support levels. Once the PSV level is 5 cm H_2O and the mandatory rate is discontinued, the patient should be thoroughly assessed for extubation.

Intermittent Mandatory Ventilation

Intermittent mandatory ventilation (IMV) is a mode of ventilation that provides mandatory breaths (a clinician-specified rate), which allows the patient to breathe spontaneously during the periods between mandatory breaths. The rate of mandatory breaths can be adjusted from 1 to 150 breaths/minute on several of

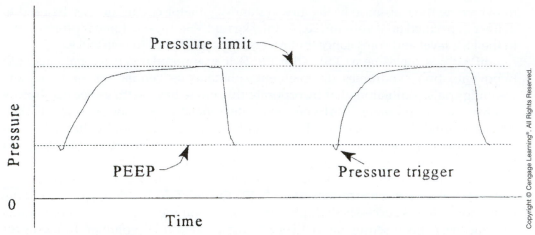

FIGURE 18–3A. Pressure waveform of pressure-support ventilation. All breaths are pressure or flow triggered from the baseline, which is often elevated, pressure limited, and flow cycled. Tidal volume depends on set pressure, resistance, and compliance.

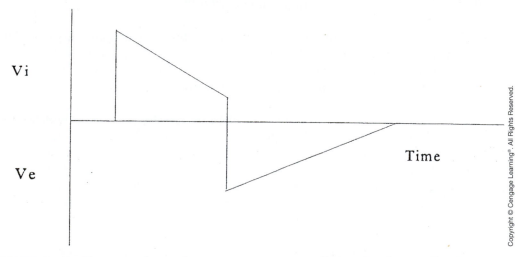

FIGURE 18–3B. Flow waveform of pressure-support ventilation. Inspiratory flow is above the baseline. Flow begins to taper in response to the patient's compliance and resistance. Inspiration ends at approximately 25% of peak flow. Vi = inspiratory flow; Ve = expiratory flow.

the neonatal ventilators, so the time available for spontaneous breathing can vary widely, depending on the patient's ventilatory status. For IMV to be referred to as a mode of PVS, the mandatory rate must be low (<30 breaths/min in the neonate) to allow for effective spontaneous ventilation. The spontaneous breaths that occur during IMV are best described as CPAP breaths because the baseline pressure is nearly always above ambient. Neonatal ventilators provide a continuous flow of mixed gas from which the infant breathes spontaneously.

To initiate the IMV mode, the therapist need only turn the mode knob from CPAP to IMV/CPAP, which then powers the drive mechanism to begin delivering mandatory breaths.

IMV is indicated when CPAP proves ineffective, or in any instance of hypercapnic ventilatory failure is apparent. Signs of the failure of CPAP include progressive hypoxemia, apnea, increased retractions, worsening tachypnea, tachycardia or bradycardia, and cyanosis. If the $PaCO_2$ rises above 60 mmHg and pH decreases below 7.25, the patient's ventilatory demand has outpaced their ventilatory capacity and hypercapnic respiratory failure is evident. The set IMV rate depends on the patient's carbon dioxide production. The greater the carbon dioxide produced, the greater the $PaCO_2$, which means that to normalize the $PaCO_2$, the IMV rate will need to be increased. As the IMV rate is increased, this mode is more appropriately classified as a mode of full ventilatory support. There is no arbitrary mandatory rate at which FVS is commenced; however, it is usually begun at 30 to 40 breaths/minute. If the infant appears to have little or no ventilatory effort while being mechanically ventilated, FVS is assumed.

IMV Waveforms Because IMV combines two breath types, each has its own classification characteristics. The mandatory breaths are pressure controlled, time triggered, pressure limited, and time cycled. The baseline variable is pressure. The spontaneous breaths are classified as described above in CPAP. The pressure waveform for IMV is shown in Figure 18–4.

Hazards of IMV Because IMV increases the mean airway pressure more than CPAP, the hazards previously described may become more evident as peak, plateau, and mean airway pressures increase. A more complete discussion of the hazards

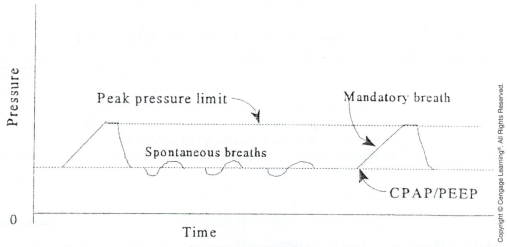

FIGURE 18–4. Pressure waveform of IMV/CPAP. Mandatory breaths are time triggered, pressure limited, and time cycled. Spontaneous breaths are pressure triggered, limited, and cycled.

of mechanical ventilation follows. Only that extent of peak pressure necessary to observe adequate chest expansion and to auscultate adequate breath sounds should be used. Otherwise, barotrauma and a decrease in cardiac output may occur.

Contraindications to IMV IMV is only contraindicated when it is not necessary. If the infant is maintaining adequate blood gases and an acceptable ventilatory pattern within normal parameters, IMV is unnecessary.

Synchronized Intermittent Mandatory Ventilation (SIMV)

SIMV differs from IMV in that in SIMV, the mandatory breaths are synchronized with the patient's inspiratory effort. In IMV, the ventilator delivers the mandatory breaths arbitrarily, according to the set total cycle time. In SIMV, the ventilator imposes a flexible "window" of time during which patient effort may trigger a mandatory breath. If the mandatory breath is not patient triggered, the window closes, and a time-triggered mandatory breath is given to maintain the mandatory rate. Ventilators that provide SIMV allow patient triggering by pressure, flow, or volume, which opens a demand valve to provide the volume for the patient's spontaneous breathing. SIMV has two advantages over IMV. First, breath stacking is avoided. Breath stacking occurs when the ventilator gives a mandatory breath arbitrarily during a patient's spontaneous breath, leading to discomfort, excessive tidal volume, and possibly, barotrauma. Second, because the patient breathes from the ventilator's demand flow system in SIMV, monitoring is considerably easier and more accurate because a continuous flow is unnecessary.

SIMV has been used as both a weaning mode and for continuous ventilation. The difference is in whether or not weaning is implemented and the magnitude of the mandatory rate. SIMV used for FVS will have a mandatory rate high enough so the patient has very little opportunity to take a spontaneous breath without causing iatrogenic hyperventilation, unless that is desired, as in a closed head injury.

Because there are several breath types during SIMV, each breath type is individually classified. Mandatory breaths may be volume or pressure controlled. Volume-controlled breaths are usually time, pressure, or flow triggered. They are flow limited and time cycled, and the baseline is pressure. Pressure-controlled breaths are time, pressure, or flow triggered. Most of the newer neonatal ventilators provide a volume- or flow-triggering mechanism to provide SIMV as well as pressure-, volume-, or flow-triggered continuous mandatory ventilation . They are pressure limited and flow or time cycled, and the baseline is pressure. Spontaneous breaths are as described above in CPAP or PSV (Figure 18–5).

FULL VENTILATORY SUPPORT

Modes of **full ventilatory support** provide all of the required minute ventilation for a particular patient. They include synchronized intermittent mandatory ventilation (SIMV) at normal rates and continuous mandatory ventilation (CMV).

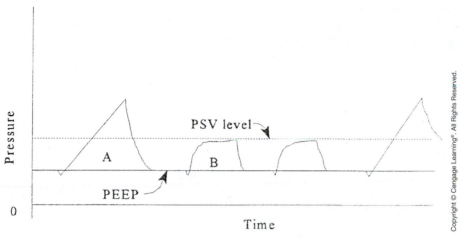

FIGURE 18–5. Pressure waveform of SIMV–PSV. Breath A is a synchronized, pressure-triggered mandatory breath. Breath B is a pressure-triggered, pressure-supported breath.

Continuous Mandatory Ventilation

Continuous mandatory ventilation (CMV) is indicated when all of the minute ventilation must be supplied by mandatory breaths. Each breath, regardless of trigger variable, has the same tidal volume or peak pressure depending on patient compliance). Time-triggered CMV is applied to patients who have been paralyzed traumatically or pharmacologically. Pressure- or flow-triggered CMV may be used to rest the muscles of ventilation in those patients who have muscle fatigue. The mode once known as assist/control is now classified as time- and pressure-triggered CMV. It is less commonly applied now than in past decades, with the advent of newer modes (i.e., SIMV–PSV) for patients who are able to partially support ventilation.

Breaths during CMV may be pressure or volume controlled. Volume-controlled breaths (VC-CMV) may be time, pressure, or flow triggered, flow limited, and time cycled. The clinician sets the mandatory rate and tidal volume (Figure 18–6).

Pressure-controlled breaths (pressure-controlled ventilation, PCV, PC-CMV) may be time, pressure, or flow triggered, pressure limited, and flow or time cycled. The clinician sets the mandatory rate and peak pressure.

Indications for PCV PCV is indicated for patients (children and adults) with acute respiratory distress syndrome (ARDS) that results in a plateau pressure ≥35 cm H_2O or a peak pressure ≥40 cm H_2O while on volume ventilation. Sedation and paralysis may be indicated if the patient is unable to tolerate this ventilatory pattern.

Pressure-Controlled Inverse Ratio Ventilation

CMV is usually administered with an inspiratory-to-expiratory time ratio of less than 1:2 (1:3–1:4). A variation of CMV wherein I:E ratio is adjusted to ≥1:1 is inverse ratio ventilation (IRV). IRV may be pressure or volume controlled (PC-IRV or VC-IRV), and usually requires that the patient be sedated and pharmacologically paralyzed,

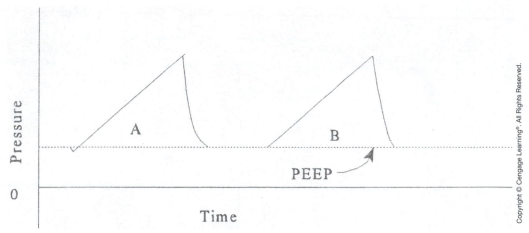

FIGURE 18-6. Pressure waveform of continuous mandatory ventilation (CMV). Breath A is pressure triggered. Breath B is time triggered. Because these pressure waveforms are linear, it is implied that the flow waveform is square, so these breaths are flow limited.

because it is an uncomfortable ventilatory pattern. I:E ratio may be adjusted up to 4:1. IRV is indicated for those patients who fail to oxygenate despite high F_iO_2 and PEEP. Patient management becomes more difficult in IRV because mean airway pressure rises precipitously. As mean airway pressure rises, there is a greater tendency for venous return, cardiac output, and blood pressure to decrease. IRV should not be used unless the patient care team is familiar with its use and the management of decreased cardiac output recognized. Respiratory therapists should be thoroughly familiar with monitoring inadvertent PEEP during ventilation.

Other Less Commonly Used Modes

Research is continually examining novel modes of ventilatory support to reduce the side effects associated with positive pressure ventilation. Some of these modes are experimental and may one day replace the traditional methods of ventilating a patient.

Airway Pressure Release Ventilation In airway pressure release ventilation (APRV), the patient is placed on a physiologic level of CPAP above baseline to restore his or her FRC. The patient is allowed to breathe spontaneously through the circuit at the upper level of CPAP. Ventilation occurs when the exhalation valve opens, allowing the pressure to fall to ambient, resulting in a patient exhalation. CPAP is restored the moment exhalation ceases. Mandatory breaths in APRV are pressure controlled, time triggered, pressure limited, and time cycled. Spontaneous breaths are pressure triggered, pressure limited, and pressure cycled. Breaths may be mandatory or spontaneous, depending on the patient's spontaneous effort.

Mandatory Minute Ventilation and Augmented Minute Ventilation Both of these modes are similar in that they measure the patient's spontaneous breathing effort and provide assistance to the patient if he or she is unable to reach a predetermined minute volume. This is usually done by measuring the exhaled volume and comparing it to the desired minute volume. If the patient does not reach the desired volume, the machine provides assisted breaths, allowing the targeted volume to be achieved. This mode is used mainly during weaning to prevent patient exhaustion during spontaneous breathing.

SETTING INITIAL VENTILATOR PARAMETERS

While patients' medical situations vary tremendously, it is important to have a starting point for each ventilator variable that serves in most cases as an appropriate beginning level.

Mode

Once it is determined that the patient is in respiratory failure, the mode is often the first setting made on the ventilator. Remembering that the ventilator is a device that can supplement oxygenation and/or ventilation in parallel, modes can be selected that provide either or both, depending on the patient's needs. Modes that increase mean airway pressure (i.e., CPAP) are employed for hypoxemic respiratory failure. Modes that increase minute ventilation (i.e., SIMV, CMV) are employed for hypercapnic respiratory failure. On many newer ventilators, the mode setting guides the clinician to setting the other parameters. The clinician then determines the values for the parameters necessary to implement the chosen mode.

First, the choice is made between modes of partial versus full ventilatory support. If a patient is in hypoxemic respiratory failure, CPAP is usually the mode of choice. In this case, the patient relies on his own spontaneous ventilation to maintain the $PaCO_2$. When using CPAP, one sets the flow (on neonatal ventilators), F_iO_2, and expiratory pressure (CPAP). If the patient is in hypercapnic respiratory failure, IMV, SIMV, or CMV is chosen to increase the patient's minute ventilation. This requires setting a sensitivity, flow, mandatory/set rate, and tidal volume/inspiratory time. A specified F_iO_2 and end-expiratory pressure are chosen to maintain an adequate PaO_2. In combined respiratory failure, IMV or SIMV with CPAP/PEEP or CMV with PEEP is chosen to support both ventilation and oxygenation.

Neonates who are in hypoxemic respiratory failure yet breathe spontaneously are first supported with continuous positive airway pressure (CPAP), described below. Should work of breathing increase and blood gases demonstrate hypercapnic respiratory failure as well, pressure-controlled ventilation in the form of intermittent mandatory ventilation is initiated to accompany the previously established CPAP. A decision tree representing guidelines for modes of ventilation for neonates is presented in Figure 18–7.

Pediatric patients are usually ventilated similar to that of adults, with a lower tidal volume (or pressure) and higher ventilatory rates. A decision tree of guidelines for establishing ventilation for children is illustrated in Figure 18–8. These are only guidelines. The modes and techniques used will vary with severity of illness and the experience of the care team.

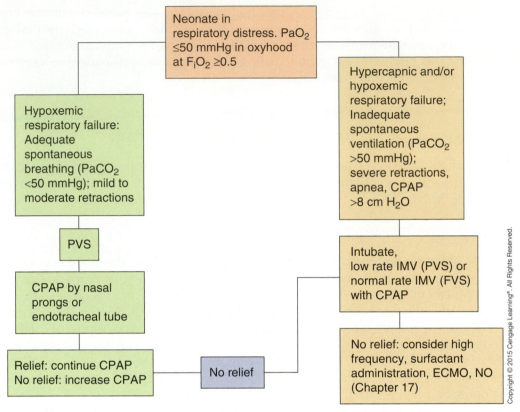

FIGURE 18–7. Decision tree for modes of ventilation in neonates. After classifying the type of respiratory failure, partial versus full ventilatory support is chosen. In hypoxemic respiratory failure, CPAP is initiated and continued, provided that the PaO_2 normalizes. If the PaO_2 remains inadequate, IMV at a low (PVS) or nornal (FVS) rate may be necessary with additional CPAP to provide oxygenation and ventilation. If the PaO_2 remains low, more aggressive therapy may be required.

Peak Inspiratory Pressure

In pressure-controlled ventilation (PC-IMV/SIMV, PC-CMV), the peak pressure is preset by the clinician. The inspiratory pressure is limited by a pop-off valve or by limiting the pressure applied to the expiratory valve and allowing excess pressure to vent through the expiratory side of the ventilator circuit. This pressure limit does not stop inspiration; it limits the inspiratory pressure. Once the inspiratory pressure limit is reached, flow is vented out of the pop-off valve or out the expiratory valve and flow to the patient ceases. The result is an inspiratory hold, where the volume in the lungs remains static until expiration occurs. This inspiratory hold promotes distribution of ventilation and increases mean airway pressure.

To set the PIP for a neonate, PIP is usually maintained at the pressure used during resuscitation, usually at 15 to 20 cm H_2O.[10] The PIP is then changed slowly,

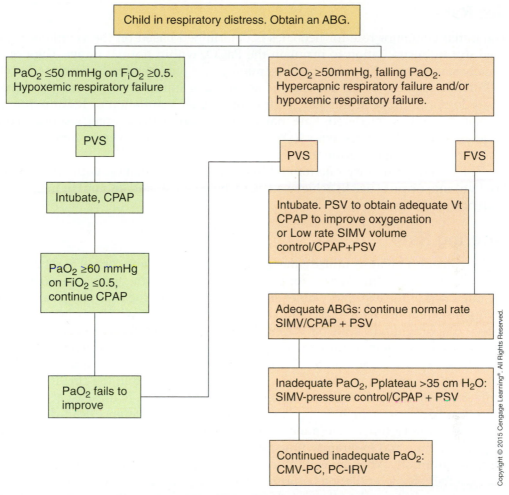

FIGURE 18–8. Decision tree for initial mode of ventilation in children. After classifying the type of respiratory failure, partial versus full ventilatory support is chosen. In hypoxemic respiratory failure, the child is intubated and CPAP is initiated and continued, provided that the PaO_2 normalizes. If the PaO_2 remains inadequate, SIMV may be necessary with additional CPAP to provide oxygenation. If hypercapnic respiratory failure is present, SIMV is necessary in either full or partial ventilatory support as dictated by the $PaCO_2$ and the child's response to the initial mechanical minute ventilation. If PaO_2 remains low and pressure is high, pressure-controlled ventilation is initiated. IRV is necessary only if PaO_2 remains low despite optimal PEEP and a high F_iO_2.

if needed, until there is appropriate bilateral chest expansion, bilateral aeration on auscultation, and an normocapnic arterial $PaCO_2$.

For children, peak inspiratory pressure for PC-SIMV or PC-CMV is generally set to obtain a plateau pressure of ≥ 30 cm H_2O. This should result in a tidal volume of about 6 to 8 mL/kg.

Set Rate

The initial ventilator rate for neonates is determined based on the ventilatory rate used during resuscitation to maintain the $PaCO_2$ within normal limits. The rate is usually set between 30 and 40 breaths/minute, but may need to be increased up to 150 breaths/minute in the presence of severe lung injury. In the event that blood gases do not improve at this rate, high-frequency jet ventilation or high-frequency oscillation can be considered. Rate may be decreased as the neonate's spontaneous effort increases. Neonates with RDS have been shown to tolerate high set rates without developing hyperinflation.[11]

The initial ventilatory rate for children is set in combination with an adequate tidal volume or pressure to achieve a $PaCO_2$ between 40 and 48 mmHg in children with normal lungs.[12]

Altering Rate

Most neonatal ventilators utilize either a rate or expiratory time control to set the IMV rate. When the determined time for exhalation has ended, the timing mechanism of the rate knob or the expiratory timer signals the closure of the expiratory valve. This occurs mechanically with a solenoid valve or a flow of gas, which pushes against a rubber diaphragm and seals off the expiratory side of the circuit. Other ventilators compress a diaphragm against an orifice at the end of the circuit, which occludes the end of the expiratory side of the circuit. With the occlusion of the expiratory side of the circuit, the continuous flow of gas increases pressure within the circuit and flow is diverted into the endotracheal tube and the patient's lungs. In most aspects the rate control and expiratory timer are similar, but one important difference bears discussion.

An expiratory timer determines a set expiratory time that remains fixed. Both inspiratory time and expiratory time must be set by the operator with appropriate I:E ratios in mind. When an expiratory timer is used, a change in inspiratory time changes the rate of ventilation because the total cycle time changes as well.

A rate control, on the other hand, automatically changes the expiratory time to maintain the desired rate, despite changes in inspiratory time. Figure 18–9 demonstrates this concept.

For example, if an expiratory time of 1.0 second was set using an expiratory timer, with an inspiratory time of 0.5 second, the resultant rate would be 40 breaths/minute. This is determined by adding inspiratory and expiratory times and dividing into 60 (1.0 + 0.5 = 1.5 sec; 60/1.5 sec = 40 breaths/min). If inspiratory time is changed to 0.75 second, without changing the expiratory time, the rate would decrease to 34 breaths/minute (1.0 + 0.5 = 1.75 sec; 60/1.75 sec = 34.3 breaths/min). A rate control, in the second scenario, would automatically decrease expiratory time to 0.75 second to maintain the set rate of 40 breaths/minute.

Sensitivity

Once a patient is placed on a mechanical ventilator, one goal should be to reduce the work of breathing. This can be accomplished by triggering mechanical breaths with as little effort as possible. The ventilator must be set to be sensitive to the patient's

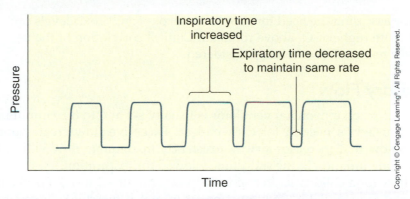

FIGURE 18–9. The expiratory time is automatically adjusted by the rate timer whenever inspiratory time is changed. This results in the rate being maintained at the same level.

spontaneous inspiratory efforts. This is the trigger variable, which may be set to a pressure, flow, or volume. In pressure triggering, the sensitivity is set to -1 to -2 cm H_2O. In flow triggering the sensitivity is set to 0.15 to 1 L/minute. In volume triggering, the sensitivity is set to up to 3.0 mL. The sensitivity method is dependent on the ventilator being used. Regardless, the sensitivity must not be set such that the ventilator triggers without patient effort (autocycle). Nor should the sensitivity be set to make inspiratory efforts too difficult. This artificially increases the work of breathing, and may lead to respiratory muscle fatigue and ventilatory failure. Whereas the main goal for mechanical ventilation is to reduce the work of breathing, a thorough patient assessment using visual clues, and monitoring capabilities is a key component to recognize an appropriate setting and the desired outcome.

Positive End-Expiratory Pressure (PEEP) or CPAP

The PEEP is generally initiated at between 3 and 5 cm H_2O. PEEP is varied as needed to achieve optimal oxygenation and maintenance of adequate FRC. Management of PEEP to obtain optimal oxygenation is described below.

Fraction of Inspired Oxygen (F_iO_2)

The required F_iO_2 is determined during the resuscitation, as the amount needed to keep the baby pink. If a transcutaneous monitor or pulse oximeter is in place, F_iO_2 is varied to keep the PaO_2 and SpO_2 within normal limits. In children, the F_iO_2 is set depending on the preventilation arterial blood gases. In the event the child is cyanotic, has cardiovascular instability, or is severely hypoxemic, a F_iO_2 of 100% is set. Otherwise, a F_iO_2 that maintains the PaO_2 greater than 60 mmHg or SpO_2 greater than 90% is set. Some research advocates lower F_iO_2 (room air) producing positive resuscitation outcomes reducing injury from hyperoxia.[13] However, clinical judgment as to the possibility of free-radical injury versus short-term stabilization must be carefully considered during the resuscitation period. Neonatal resuscitation (2011) guidelines recommend targeted preductal SpO_2 of between 60% and 65% at one minute administering oxygen throughout the range of 21% to 100% via blender by assessing the need for supplemental oxygen.[14] Toxic levels can quickly be achieved with higher F_iO_2 above room air. Clinical correlation of the use of supplemental oxygen must be carefully considered.

Inspiratory Flow

The initial flow on a neonatal ventilator is usually set at 6 to 8 L/minute. The flow is then adjusted as needed for each patient. Excessive flow creates unnecessary turbulent flow that increases airway resistance. Inadequate flow will not provide adequate lung inflation in the short time allowed for inspiration.

The flow for a child is set to maintain an I:E ratio of 1:2 to 1:4. For the child who is triggering the ventilator, flow must be set to match the child's inspiratory effort. Otherwise, an increased work of breathing results. A flow of 25 to 30 L/minute should deliver the set tidal volume within the recommended 1.0 to 1.5 second inspiratory time.

Inspiratory Time

For neonatal ventilation, the inspiratory time is determined by an inspiratory time control and is set by the operator. The inspiratory time control begins timing the breath at the instant the expiratory time control signals the closure of the expiration valve. When the predetermined inspiratory time has elapsed, the inspiratory time control opens the expiration valve and exhalation occurs passively from the patient's lungs.

The inspiratory time must be set to consider the desired set rate, the maintenance of a desired inspiration-to-expiration ratio (I:E), and lung condition. In RDS, the lungs are noncompliant. Therefore, a longer inspiration time may be needed to inflate the lungs. Expiratory time constants are decreased, and less time is needed for expiration. In diseases that are characterized by air trapping, expiratory time constants are longer, and therefore less time is needed for inspiration.

The inspiratory time for ventilation of children is often the result of the desired tidal volume and inspiratory flow, and should result in an I:E ratio that comfortably meets the patient's inspiratory needs. For example, if the child's tidal volume is 0.35 L and the inspiratory flow is set to 25 L/minute, the inspiratory time is 0.83 second (Vt/flow = Ti; 0.35 L/0.42 L/sec = 0.83 sec). The extent to which the patient is comfortable with this flow is determined by noting a constant increase in pressure during inspiration, observing chest rise, and by asking if the patient is comfortable (if possible).

I:E Ratio

The I:E ratio is not ordinarily set, but rather is derived once a pattern of ventilation is established. Once the I:E ratio is derived, it may be changed by manipulation of any of its components. Calculation of the I:E ratio is shown in Table 18–3.

Close attention to I:E ratio is required as the rate is increased. At the maximum rate of 150 breaths/minute, the inspiratory time would have to be decreased to 0.2 second to allow a 1:1 ratio (60 sec/150 breaths/min = 0.4 sec; 0.4 sec/2 = 0.2 sec inspiratory time). In diseases with a severe reduction in compliance, 0.2 second may be enough time for expiration, but in the presence of normal compliance or air trapping, 0.2 second would not allow adequate time for exhalation.

Table 18–3

CALCULATION OF THE I:E RATIO

What is the I:E ratio, given the following data?
f = 50 breaths/min, Ti = 0.4 sec

1. Determine total cycle time.
   60/f = 60 sec/50 breaths/sec = 1.2 sec/breath

2. Determine the Te by subtracting the Ti from the TCT.
   Te = TCT − Ti
   Te = 1.2 − 0.4 = 0.8 sec

3. Determine the expiratory fraction of the I:E by dividing the expiratory time by the inspiratory time.
   Te/Ti = expiratory portion
   0.8/0.4 = 2

4. The I:E ratio is the ratio of 1 to the expiratory fraction.
   I:E ratio = 1:2

The proper setting of rate (or expiratory time) and inspiratory time requires not only an understanding of proper I:E ratios, but also an in-depth understanding of the disease process that is being treated.

Tidal Volume

When ventilating neonates with pressure-controlled ventilation, the tidal volume is the result of the change in airway pressure between the peak and end-expiratory pressures, the lung-chest wall compliance, and the airway resistance. The desired tidal volume varies by birth weight from the very-low-birth-weight infant at 4 to 6 mL/kg, to the term infant at 6 to 8 mL/kg.

Children are usually volume ventilated. Tidal volume for children should be initially set to no more than 8 mL/kg.

In recent years, ventilators have become more flexible in their tidal volume delivery (i.e., Siemens® Servo 300, Bird® VIP, or Dräger® Babylog), so that they can be used for neonates, children, and adults by alerting the ventilator's software to the range of patient size being ventilated. The term "seamless" is used to describe this flexibility. Once this is accomplished, the ventilator may be adjusted to meet the needs of the patient, rather than having to switch ventilators. The ventilatory needs of the pediatric patient—decreased lung compliance, small tidal volumes, high respiratory rates, high airway resistance requiring low flow rates, small dead space volumes, and the need for low compressible volumes in the ventilator circuit—are easily accommodated by the newer ventilators.

Suggested initial ventilator parameter settings are summarized in Table 18–4.

Table 18–4

INITIAL VENTILATORY PARAMETERS

Neonates		Children
PIP	15 to 20 cm H_2O	Keep Pplat <35 cm H_2O
PEEP	3 to 5 cm H_2O	5 cm H_2O
F_iO_2	Set to keep patient pink, or SpO_2 90–92%	1.0 or to maintain SpO_2 >93%
Rate	30–40 breaths/min	To maintain $PaCO_2$ 40–48 mmHg
Flow	6–8 L/min	25–30 L/min
Inspiratory time		1.0–1.5 sec
Low-birth-weight infants 0.25–0.5 sec Term infants 0.5–0.6 sec		
I:E ratio 1:1.5–1:2		>1:2; maintain patient comfort
V_T		6–8 mL/kg
Term 8 mL/kg Low-birth-weight 6 mL/kg Very-low-birth-weight 4–6 mL/kg		

VOLUME VERSUS PRESSURE-CONTROLLED VENTILATION

Pressure-limited, time-cycled ventilation is the primary method of ventilating neonates. When using this method, the peak pressure is set so that it is achieved before the inspiratory time has elapsed. This traditional method has been effective for years, with excellent results, so there has not been a major concern about tidal volumes in neonates. Newer neonatal ventilators monitor the breath-to-breath tidal volume and minute ventilation so respiratory therapists can affect tidal volume, if desired, to keep it within the recommended ranges for a given patient size. Mandatory breaths remain time cycled and pressure limited, but when changes are made to obtain a range of exhaled tidal volumes, those breaths become "volume targeted." While we continue to pressure ventilate, we are concurrently observing and making adjustments to target a range of tidal volume, as suggested in Table 18–4.

Children who weigh less than 10 kg are usually ventilated as described above. Once a child's weight exceeds 10 kg, volume or pressure control is chosen, depending on lung condition. In children with normal lungs (i.e., postoperative ventilation, neuromuscular disease), volume-controlled ventilation with a tidal volume of

6–8 mL/kg and a rate to achieve a $PaCO_2$ within normal limits is instituted. However, in children with noncompliant lungs, pressure-controlled ventilation is instituted, as it is in adults with acute respiratory distress syndrome. The advantages and disadvantages of volume and pressure ventilation are outlined in Table 18–5.

Achieving Volume Targeted Ventilation with a Pressure-Controlled Ventilator

The easiest method to achieve volume-targeted ventilation with a pressure-controlled ventilator is to change the peak pressure limit until the desired range of tidal or minute volume is achieved. For example, a 1000 g low-birth-weight infant might benefit from a targeted volume of between 4 and 6 mL. Subsequent daily weight following surfactant delivery could help the respiratory therapist calculate an appropriate volume taking into consideration patient compliance and adjusting the peak inspiratory pressure (PIP) to reach the desired volume. Assessments to correlate patient tolerance and outcomes that match ventilator goals are continuous and ongoing as the patient improves/deteriorates. If the target ventilation cannot be achieved by increasing the peak pressure, the inspiratory time or inspiratory flow may also need to be increased.

Table 18–5

ADVANTAGES AND DISADVANTAGES OF VOLUME- AND PRESSURE-CONTROLLED VENTILATION IN THE NEONATAL AND PEDIATRIC POPULATION

Volume-Controlled Ventilation		Pressure-Controlled Ventilation	
Advantages	**Disadvantages**	**Advantages**	**Disadvantages**
Delivers a set tidal volume despite changes in compliance or resistance	Potential for volutrauma	Lower mean airway pressure	Inconsistent minute ventilation
	Leaking around cuffless endotracheal tubes	Avoids volutrauma	Changes in tidal volume with changes in compliance and resistance
Consistent minute ventilation	High mean airway pressure		
Better control of $PaCO_2$			

Another method of volume targeting involves increasing the peak pressure limit above that which can be reached during the set inspiratory time. Then, tidal volume can be increased by increasing the inspiratory time or flow rate. Tidal volume may be decreased by decreasing the inspiratory time or flow rate. Care must be taken to ensure that the I:E ratio does not exceed normal limits. Tidal volume then becomes the product of inspiratory time and inspiratory flow, as shown in Table 18–6.

Recognizing a Decreased Compliance or Increased Resistance

Signs of a decrease in compliance include an increase in auscultated crackles caused by alveolar collapse, a decrease in chest wall excursion, a decreased slope of the pressure-volume loop and a decrease in monitored tidal volume. An increase in airway resistance is indicated by an increase in secretions by the presence of wheezing. The respiratory therapist may need to make appropriate changes to the ventilator (i.e., increase the peak pressure) while investigating and correcting the causes of decreased compliance or increased resistance.

Initiation of Pressure-Controlled Ventilation

Initial parameters are usually set according to the disease process and clinical evaluation of the patient who weighs less than 10 kg and who is ventilated with

---

Table 18–6

CALCULATING TIDAL VOLUME USING A PRESSURE-CONTROLLED VENTILATOR

An infant weighs 2.3 kg and is being ventilated at 20 cm H_2O above PEEP of 5 cm H_2O (PIP = 25 cm H_2O). Are the inspiratory flow and time appropriate for delivery of a 6 to 8 mL/kg V_T?

The tidal volume is calculated by multiplying the inspiratory time by the flow rate as follows:
Inspiratory time = 0.4 sec
Flow rate = 6 L/min (flow must be converted to mL)
6 L/min = 6000 mL/min or 100 mL/sec
Tidal volume = 0.4 sec × 100 mL/sec = 40 mL

Volume lost due to tubing compliance:
Pressure = 20 cm H_2O × tubing compliance of 1.5 mL/cm H_2O = 30 mL lost volume
Measured V_T is 40–30 mL lost volume = 10 mL
Desired V_T is 16 mL; if flow is increased to 7 L/min (117 mL/min), delivered V_T should be 46.8 mL; subtracting 30 mL lost volume = 16.8 mL (7.3 mL/kg), which is within the desired range.

pressure-limited, time-cycled ventilator. Peak inspiratory pressure is set to that which obtains good chest excursion and good lung aeration as heard on auscultation.

The mandatory rate is set considering the time constants present in the lung. Noncompliant lungs and those in which resistance is low have a shorter *time constant* than do lungs with normal compliance and can, therefore, sustain shorter expiratory times and faster rates. In contrast, compliant lungs and those with increased resistance have longer time constants and require longer expiratory times and slower rates. The inspiratory time is set to maintain an I:E ratio of 1:2 with the selected frequency. Flow should be set to allow the peak inspiratory pressure to be reached before the end of inspiratory time.

Initiation of Volume-Controlled Ventilation

Under most circumstances, pediatric patients should be ventilated at a tidal volume of up to 8 mL/kg. It is also necessary to use a noncompliant circuit when using volume-controlled breaths on pediatric patients to minimize volume loss due to tubing compliance.

The compliance of the ventilator circuit can be calculated and used to determine the actual delivered tidal volume. Tubing compliance is calculated by delivering a known volume (usually less than 300 mL) into the circuit with the patient connection occluded. The pressure generated is measured from the manometer and is divided into the volume, resulting in the compliance of the circuit. The set tidal volume can be set to deliver the desired tidal volume and the additional tubing loss volume in order to ventilate the patient with the proper volume. The method of calculating corrected tidal volume is shown in Table 18–7.

Table 18–7

DETERMINATION OF CORRECTED TIDAL VOLUME

A patient weighing 35 pounds is to be mechanically ventilated.

Step 1: Determine the weight in kg:
35 lb/2.23 lb/kg = 15.69 kg. This will be rounded to 16 kg.

Step 2: Determine the desired tidal volume by multiplying the patient's weight in kg by 8.0 mL/kg:
16 kg × 8.0 = 128 mL desired tidal volume

Step 3: Determine volume loss due to tubing compliance:
(PIP − PEEP) × circuit compliance = volume lost due to tubing compliance
(23 cm H_2O − 5 cm H_2O) × 2 mL/cm H_2O = 36 mL

continues on the next page

Table 18–7

continued from the previous page

A patient weighing 35 pounds is to be mechanically ventilated.

Step 4:   Determine actual tidal volume:

set V_T − lost volume = actual V_T

130 mL − 36 mL = 94 mL (5.8 mL/Kg)

Step 5:   Increase the set V_T by the value of the lost volume to arrive at the corrected tidal volume.

130 mL + 40 mL = 170 mL (10.6 mL/kg)

The addition of tidal volume may increase the PIP and therefore compressible volume, which may necessitate a further increase in tidal volume.

CHANGING VENTILATOR PARAMETERS IN VOLUME AND PRESSURE VENTILATION

When making changes on the ventilator, one must remember how each parameter affects the blood gas values. Ventilation, reflected by the $PaCO_2$, is affected by changes in the minute ventilation; that is, the ventilatory rate × tidal volume. The tidal volume in pressure-controlled ventilation is determined by the difference in pressure between the PIP and PEEP (the ΔP), resistance, and compliance. $PaCO_2$ is also affected by inspiratory time, because the longer the alveoli are inflated, the more diffusion takes place between the blood and alveoli.

PaO_2 is a function of the F_iO_2 and the end expiratory pressure. It is also affected by the mean airway pressure. Calculation of the mean airway pressure was discussed in Chapter 17. The end-expiratory pressure is the most important parameter determining mean airway pressure, because the relationship between mean airway pressure and end-expiratory pressure is 1:1.

Changing PaCO₂

The $PaCO_2$ is changed by manipulating the ΔP or set rate. Once the PIP is set, as described above, it is usually held constant, unless the patient's compliance or resistance changes. In the event of a decrease in compliance or increase in resistance, PIP may need to be increased in 2 cm H_2O increments to maintain tidal volume and good breath sounds. In the event that compliance increases or resistance decreases, PIP may need to be decreased to avoid overdistension and baro/volutrauma. If the clinician is satisfied with the PIP but the $PaCO_2$ is high, the set rate is increased, usually in increments of 2 to 5 breaths/minute until a satisfactory $PaCO_2$ is obtained. Likewise, if the $PaCO_2$ is low, the rate may be decreased until a satisfactory $PaCO_2$ is obtained. Flow also affects $PaCO_2$. Because pressure-controlled ventilation in neonates is time cycled, the tidal volume is determined by the product of the inspiratory time and the inspiratory flow. Should the pressure limit be reached before the end of the inspiratory time, flow will continue to be delivered until the end of the inspiratory time, thus affecting tidal volume. Pressure or flow waveform graphics may assist the clinician in determining the presence of this phenomenon.[15] Should the inspiratory time be too long, it may be decreased so as to limit the duration of a plateau pressure (which also increases the mean airway pressure). In RDS accompanied by high peak or plateau pressures, it may be desirable to allow the $PaCO_2$ to rise above 50 mmHg, as long as the pH does not decrease below 7.25. This technique, permissive hypercapnia, allows a reduction in tidal volume, and assists in avoiding baro/volutrauma.

In summary, the set rate is the primary parameter used to alter the minute ventilation, and therefore, $PaCO_2$. Other parameters to consider are PIP, flow, and inspiratory time.

In volume-controlled ventilation, $PaCO_2$ is also affected by minute ventilation. The tidal volume (or inspiratory time) is set directly and peak pressure is a function of resistance and compliance. As previously mentioned, the tidal volume is set in the 6–8 mL/kg range for children. Once that is established, it is not usually changed. A factor that may influence the need to increase tidal volume would be persistent atelectasis or air hunger, despite an optimally adjusted sensitivity and flow. The major factor that would contribute to the need to decrease tidal volume would be the desire to institute permissive hypercapnia in ARDS or acute lung injury.

Once the clinician is satisfied with the tidal volume, the remaining factor determining minute ventilation and, therefore, $PaCO_2$ is the mandatory rate, which is increased if the $PaCO_2$ rises and decreased if $PaCO_2$ is low. Rate is usually changed in 1 to 3 breaths/minute increments. The higher the rate is, the greater the increment. For example, if the rate is set at 20 breaths/minute, affecting a 20% change in minute ventilation would require a change of 4 breaths/minute. If the rate is set at 8 breaths/minute, affecting a 20% change in minute ventilation would require a change of 1 to 2 breaths/minute.

An additional factor affecting minute ventilation is the extent of spontaneous ventilation during CPAP or PSV breaths (supplemental minute ventilation based on the patients effort). If tidal volume during CPAP (without PSV) is ≥5 mL/kg, then this fraction of the minute ventilation is contributing to a normal $PaCO_2$. If these tidal volumes are less than 5 mL/kg, this fraction of the minute ventilation is contributing to dead space, and the $PaCO_2$ may increase. It is for this reason that PSV is useful. Initiation of between 5 and 8 cm H_2O PSV will usually increase the spontaneous tidal volume to ≥5 mL/kg and decrease the spontaneous ventilatory rate, both contributing to normalizing the $PaCO_2$.

Changing PaO_2

The PaO_2 is changed by manipulating the F_iO_2, end-expiratory pressure (PEEP/CPAP), and subsequently, the mean airway pressure. The decision to use the F_iO_2 or the end-expiratory pressure depends on the cause of hypoxemia. In case of V̇/Q̇ inequality (pneumonia, bronchiolitis), hypoxemia generally responds to an increase in F_iO_2.

In the case of capillary shunting (RDS, ARDS, ALI), the PaO_2 responds to an increase in end-expiratory pressure, not an increase in PaO_2. This is referred to as refractory hypoxemia. In refractory hypoxemia, alveoli are collapsed, fluid-filled, or smaller than normal (requiring higher distending pressure to reach critical opening pressure in the alveoli), resulting in a decrease in alveolar surface area and reduced functional residual capacity. Therefore, an increase in F_iO_2 alone will have little effect on the PaO_2.

An increase in PEEP is usually indicated if the PaO_2 is inadequate despite a PEEP of 3 to 5 cm H_2O and F_iO_2 of ≥50%. PEEP may be increased in 2 to 3 cm H_2O increments until the PaO_2 increases appreciably. This indicates alveolar surface area recruitment and restoration of the functional residual capacity.

In neonates, a PEEP of 12 to 15 cm H_2O is rarely exceeded. There are two reasons for this. One is that, owing to the cuffless endotracheal tube, additional PEEP would be lost. Second is the decrease in cardiac output and pulmonary barotrauma that may occur as a result of high PEEP. If a PEEP of 12 to 15 cm H_2O fails to provide adequate oxygenation, high-frequency ventilation, nitric oxide, or extracorporeal membrane oxygenation are considered, as appropriate for the etiology of hypoxemia.

Excessive PEEP is also avoided in children for the same reasons. Higher PEEP may be used in children who have a cuffed artificial airway. The highest PEEP that should be used is referred to as optimum PEEP. This is defined as the PEEP that results in a PaO_2 greater than 60 mmHg that does not result in cardiac output depression. Some method of cardiac output measurement, such as thermal dilution or a continuous flow-directed pulmonary artery catheter is necessary when using this method. Another method of obtaining the best PEEP level is to measure the static lung–thorax compliance (static compliance, lung–thorax compliance = exhaled tidal volume/Pplateau-PEEP) at the initial PEEP level. The Pplateau is the end-inspiratory pause pressure. The PEEP is increased in 3 to 5 cm H_2O increments. After each increase in PEEP, the lung–thorax compliance is calculated. The best PEEP is that pressure where lung–thorax compliance is greatest. If PEEP is adjusted above this level, intrathoracic pressure increases, lung–thorax compliance will decrease, cardiac output may decrease, and the child will be susceptible to other forms of barotrauma.

Under most circumstances, hypoxemia will respond to less than 10 cm H_2O of PEEP, at which time the F_iO_2 may be decreased slowly in decrements of 5% to between 30% and 40% F_iO_2. Weaning of PEEP may occur when the F_iO_2 has been decreased to a safe value (generally less than 30%–40%) and the patient is hemodynamically stable. PEEP is decreased 2 to 3 cm H_2O, no more than every 6 hours. After a decrease in PEEP, the PaO_2, SaO_2, or SpO_2 are observed for acute deterioration. If the saturation decreases below 90% or PaO_2 decreases below 60 mmHg, the previous PEEP level should be restored and the patient monitored for acceptable oxygenation. Generally, if F_iO_2 is above 60%, PEEP can be used to increase PaO_2. Below 60%, PEEP can be reduced to minimize hemodynamic compromise.

Mean airway pressure is increased by increasing PEEP, PIP, set rate, or inspiratory time, or by decreasing expiratory time (increasing the I:E ratio). Changing the mean airway pressure other than by increasing PEEP is considered a secondary method of changing the PaO_2. It is the mechanism whereby PaO_2 is improved when using inverse ratio ventilation.

In extreme cases, where a F_iO_2 of 100% is insufficient to maintain oxygenation, several alternatives may improve the oxygenation status. The hypoxemia may be due to blood shunting away from the lungs through the PDA. In this case, a decrease in the MAP by lowering the PIP, PEEP, rate, or inspiratory time may allow more blood to perfuse the lungs by lowering the pulmonary vascular hypertension and thus increase oxygenation.

Ventilator Changes Using Clinical Information

The respiratory therapist may rely on the patient's clinical signs to make appropriate ventilator changes. The adequacy of minute ventilation is best determined by auscultation of breath sounds and the observance of chest excursion. With each mandatory breath, there should be air movement heard in both lung fields, indicating sufficient aeration. In addition, the chest should rise and expand with each mandatory breath. The determination of suitable chest excursion is subjective and changes from patient to patient. The size of the patient and the nature of the lung disease alter the amount of chest excursion. In most circumstances, however, a rise in the chest during inspiration is a sign of adequate lung expansion.

Changes in lung mechanics may be estimated by auscultating changes in the breath sounds and observing chest excursion. In the presence of worsening compliance, breath sounds diminish, fine crackles may be auscultated, and chest excursion may decrease. The slope of the pressure–volume loop may decrease indicating a reduced compliance. An increased resistance may be noted by the observation or auscultation of secretions in the airway and/or the auscultation of wheezing. An increase in airway resistance will also increase the PIP (in pressure control ventilation). Once the cause is determined, therapeutic measures are implemented. In the meantime, minute ventilation or F_iO_2 may need to be increased until the problems are reversed.

In contrast, an improvement in breath sounds and chest excursion from baseline indicates an improvement in compliance or resistance. In this example, tidal volume or rate can be weaned to avoid hyperventilation and/or barotrauma.

HAZARDS OF MECHANICAL VENTILATION AND HOW TO AVOID THEM

The hazards of mechanical ventilation (Table 18–8) can be categorized into the various parameters that constitute total ventilation. The hazards are basically the same for neonates and children, with exceptions noted as needed.

Hazards of Oxygen, CPAP, and PEEP

Hazards of high oxygen concentrations include oxygen toxicity (one factor in the development of bronchopulmonary dysplasia, BPD) and possible absorption atelectasis. Oxygen toxicity may enhance the appearance of hyaline membranes and

Table 18–8

HAZARDS OF MECHANICAL VENTILATION

Oxygen
Oxygen toxicity
Hyaline membrane formation
BPD
ROP

PEEP and CPAP
Excessive pressures
    a. Hypoventilation from excessive FRC
    b. Decreased cardiac output
    c. Barotrauma

Peak Inspiratory Pressure
Barotrauma
    a. Pneumothorax
    b. Pneumomediastinum
    c. Pneumopericardium
    d. Pulmonary interstitial emphysema

BPD
Hyperinflation
    a. Hyperventilation
    b. Respiratory alkalosis
    c. Hemodynamic depression

Respiratory Rate
Respiratory alkalosis
Air leaks
Decreased ventilation-to-perfusion ratios
Increased intrapleural pressure
Decreased pulmonary perfusion
Diminished cardiac output

General Hazards
Infection

Hypoxic-Ischemic Injuries
Intracranial hemorrhage in the neonate
Gastric distention
Complications of endotracheal intubation

cause or worsen ARDS in the pediatric patient, making the lung less compliant. Retinopathy of prematurity (ROP) is caused by an excessive PaO_2. For that reason, only a F_iO_2 necessary to maintain a PaO_2 within normal limits for a given patient is appropriate. A $F_iO_2 \geq 50\%$ is hazardous, and every effort must be made to decrease it, including the application of PEEP/CPAP and increased mean airway pressure (i.e., inverse ratio ventilation) taking care to minimize barotrauma or impair circulation. Misapplied levels of CPAP and PEEP can lead to hypoventilation with resulting respiratory acidosis, decreased cardiac output from a decreased venous return, and air leak syndromes (pneumothorax, pneumomediastinum, pneumopericardium). PEEP/CPAP is increased until the F_iO_2 can be decreased to less than 50%, contingent on a stable cardiovascular status (normal cardiac output and SvO_2).

Hazards of Peak Inspiratory Pressure (PIP)

Complications of excessive PIP include barotrauma leading to air leak syndromes and BPD, and respiratory alkalosis from alveolar hyperventilation. In the pediatric patient, PIP is the direct result of the tidal volume and lung compliance, with higher volumes and stiffer lungs causing higher pressures to be generated. The transmission of PIP to the surrounding vasculature varies depending on the disease state. In the normally compliant lung there is a maximal transmission of pressures to the environment; therefore, the degree of hemodynamic compromise is directly related to the level of PIP and PEEP. Lungs with decreased compliance, as in ARDS, allow for a lesser transmission of pressures, and so the effect on the hemodynamics is not as great until higher pressures are reached.

In pressure-controlled ventilation, PIP should be set such that plateau pressure does not exceed 35 cm H_2O. For neonates, PIP is increased only to the point where there are adequate breath sounds and chest excursion. In volume ventilation, tidal volume should not exceed 8 mL/kg. In ARDS, tidal volume should not exceed 6 to 8 mL/kg. Should PIP exceed 40 cm H_2O, pressure ventilation should be instituted.

Hazards of Frequency/I:E

Respiratory alkalosis is a possible hazard of an unnecessarily high rate or short expiratory time. Inappropriately high I:E ratios lead to air leaks from air trapping, inadvertent PEEP, decreased ventilation-to-perfusion ratios, increased intrapleural pressure leading to decreased pulmonary perfusion, and diminished cardiac output.

The mandatory rate should be maintained to keep the $PaCO_2$ within normal physiologic limits. I:E should be maintained 1:2 or greater to allow for sufficient expiratory time.

General Hazards

General hazards of mechanical ventilation include infection, hypoxic-ischemic injuries, intracranial hemorrhage in the neonate, gastric distention, and complications of endotracheal intubation.

Infection is avoided by careful attention to standard precautions and changing of ventilator circuits no more than every 48 hours or as the circuit requires. Hypoxic injuries may be avoided by ensuring oxygenation during suctioning. Gastric distention is avoided by placing a gastric tube. The hazards of endotracheal intubation are avoided by paying careful attention to aseptic technique during intubation, insertion of the proper size endotracheal tube, and properly securing it once in place.

WEANING AND EXTUBATION

Appropriate management of the patient-ventilator system usually results in a patient who weans rapidly from ventilation and is ready to be extubated in a reasonable amount of time. The goal of removing the patient from ventilatory support should have been in place since the time of intubation and commitment to the ventilator. Weaning or gradual withdrawal of ventilatory support should, therefore, have been in progress since the initiation of support. This section defines weaning as the final process of discontinuing the ventilator and removal of the artificial airway.

When making the decision whether to wean and extubate, two factors must be considered: 1) the ability of the patient to spontaneously maintain adequate gas exchange, and 2) the ability of the patient to maintain the airway and clear secretions. Each of these factors must be approached separately and decisions involving weaning and extubation must be made with these factors in mind.

The success of weaning and extubation depends on many elements. Foremost is that there has been significant progress toward the resolution of the original disease or condition that required mechanical ventilation in the first place. Perhaps the most difficult element is customizing the weaning process on each individual patient. This means that the patient must be closely monitored, and adjustments made as the patient's condition dictates. Too often, we follow a rigid set of guidelines that may not suit a particular patient.

In the older child, it may be necessary to psychologically prepare the patient for weaning and extubation. Following a prolonged time on mechanical ventilation (sometimes months), the patient may have become both physiologically and psychologically dependent on the ventilator. Failure to realize these important aspects will result in failure and the necessity of prolonged mechanical ventilation.

NEONATAL PATIENT

Upon stabilization and improvement of the infant's condition, the ventilator parameters are slowly weaned to allow the neonate to assume responsibility for ventilation.

Clinical Indications For Weaning

Signs that the neonate is ready to be weaned include blood gas values within normal physiologic limits, the presence of adequate spontaneous respirations, and increased muscle tone and activity that allow weaning of supplemental F_iO_2.

Weaning Ventilator Parameters

The decision as to which parameter to wean is based on the patient's condition and the level of support provided by each parameter. The F_iO_2 should be weaned to ≤40% in 20% to 50% increments before starting to wean other parameters. The purpose of weaning is lost if high F_iO_2 is needed to provide adequate oxygenation ($PtcO_2$ 60–80 mmHg or SpO_2 90–92% on F_iO_2 ≤40%) as PIP and rate are lowered. Once the F_iO_2 is ≤0.4, PEEP is decreased in 1 to 2 cm H_2O increments to 3 to 4 cm H_2O before considering extubation.

When adequate arterial oxygenation is ensured, PIP can then be slowly weaned, usually in increments of 1 to 2 cm H_2O to 15 to 18 cm H_2O.

Following reduction of PIP, rate can be lowered in increments of 1 to 5 to allow the patient to assume ventilation. On those patients who have required high set rates, rate may be decreased faster, as previously discussed.

Gas exchange, often by arterial blood gas analysis, must be monitored after each ventilator change to assess the response of the patient. Provided there is good correlation between ABGs and noninvasive monitors of gas exchange, the transcutaneous monitor and/or pulse oximeter make weaning a much easier process and greatly decrease the number of blood gas samples needed.

Duration of Weaning

The speed at which weaning takes place is dictated by the patient's response to therapeutic treatment. Generally, the longer the patient has been on the ventilator, the slower the weaning process. Careful attention to the speed of weaning will help prevent a **rebound effect**, which is a negative reaction to a weaned parameter that requires not only a reinstitution of the parameter but often reinstitution to a level higher than was set before the weaning.

The disease state also dictates the speed at which weaning takes place. In RDS, the lungs often begin stabilizing 48 to 72 hours after birth, resulting in improvement in lung compliance. In these patients, PIP, rate, and F_iO_2 are weaned as tolerated to prevent barotrauma and effects of hyperoxia.

As lung compliance improves, the transmission of excessive pressure, and the depression of hemodynamics that follows, is averted by appropriate weaning of pressures. Indeed, complications often arise if weaning is not conducted rapidly enough. That is, as compliance improves, pneumothorax results in pressures maintained for excessive periods.

Not all neonates respond to the weaning of parameters. Patients with BPD, PDA, and neurologic damage may require long periods of ventilatory support and do not respond well to weaning attempts. This is indicated by the dependence on any of the ventilatory parameters, with a rapid decline in blood gas levels when those parameters are weaned.

Clinical Indications of a Failure to Wean

Tachycardia, bradycardia, pallor, retractions, hypercapnia, and cyanosis during weaning indicate a failure to wean. The ventilator parameters used before the weaning attempt should be restored and the cause of weaning failure investigated and treated.

Extubation

When the PIP is weaned to 15 to 18 cm H_2O, the PEEP to 3 to 5 cm H_2O, the rate to less than 10, and an F_iO_2 of 30% to 40%, the patient can be extubated. Feedings should be withheld for several hours before extubation to reduce the risk of aspiration. Before extubation, tracheobronchial hygiene should be ensured to remove as much mucus as possible. A leak should be audible at the end of a mandatory breath to help assess the absence of airway edema. In the presence of edema (no leak), a racemic epinephrine aerosol is administered.

The patient is prepared for extubation by hyperoxygenating and then carefully removing the tape and holder that are securing the endotracheal tube. Following successful completion of the above preparations, the manual resuscitator is used to deliver several breaths. During one of these breaths, the endotracheal tube is withdrawn. Following removal of the endotracheal tube, oral secretions are removed using a suction device.

Respiratory Care Following Extubation

Following extubation, blood gas values and patient status are closely monitored to ensure safe adaptation off the ventilator. Oxygenation is maintained by the use of an oxyhood, nasal CPAP, or nasal cannula, as dictated by the PaO_2 or SpO_2. One study supports the use of nasopharyngeal SIMV postextubation in a sample of 22 very-low-birth-weight infants.[16] The incidence of postextubation respiratory failure was significantly lower in the SIMV group than in the nasal CPAP group, thus preventing reintubation. Stridor caused by inflammation and edema from the endotracheal tube can be treated with nebulized racemic epinephrine. Chest physiotherapy is performed as indicated to assist with removal of secretions.

PEDIATRIC PATIENT

Weaning

As with the neonate, plans should be made for weaning and extubation as soon as the patient is placed on the ventilator. Weaning then begins when the patient has met the following criteria: 1) The disease process is stabilized and past the acute phase, 2) the cardiovascular system is stable, 3) gas exchange is stable without the need for high pressures or F_iO_2, and 4) the patient is alert with minimal sedation.

Successful weaning requires good communication with and psychological preparation of the patient. The patient must understand what is happening and that he or she has the choice to rest when necessary. When it is determined that the patient is ready to be weaned, the F_iO_2 is lowered to ≤40% and PEEP to ≤5 cm H_2O. The set rate is then weaned slowly to allow the patient to assume the work of breathing. Depending on the duration of mechanical ventilation, this may take a short or long period of time.

It is important to closely monitor and assess the patient during weaning to ensure that the patient does not become anxious or exhausted. A patient who shows signs of tiring or anxiety should be rested on the ventilation by increasing the set rate for a period of time before resuming weaning.

Failure to Wean

Several cardiorespiratory problems contribute to a failure to wean. These factors and possible solutions are shown in Table 18–9.

The mandatory rate is decreased to 3 to 5 breaths/minute. The PEEP is decreased to 3 to 5 cm H_2O during this time. PSV is decreased to 5 cm H_2O, or may be discontinued if the patient is able to completely support minute ventilation with adequate tidal volume. At this point, the patient is placed on CPAP and observed to determine satisfactory aeration. An ABG is frequently obtained to determine tolerance of CPAP/PSV.

In a study of 213 children, ages 32 to 64 months, several respiratory variables were found to predict weaning success or failure. Subjects in this study were ventilated from less than 3 days to in excess of 7 days.[17]

This study represents the scarce evidence in this area. Extubation failure was defined as the need to be reintubated within 48 hours of extubation. Several of the parameters that are useful in predicting successful extubation in adults, such as ventilatory rate, maximum inspiratory pressure, the rapid-shallow breathing index, and the compliance-rate-oxygenation-pressure (CROP) index, were also examined and found to be not predictive in the pediatric population.

Several parameters were predictive of successful extubation. There was a low risk of extubation failure if the spontaneous tidal volume indexed for body weight (mL/kg) was ≥6.5 mL/kg, F_iO_2 <30%, mean airway pressure <5.0 cm H_2O, oxygen index (OI = mean airway pressure × (F_iO_2/PaO_2) × 100) ≤1.4, fraction of minute ventilation by the ventilator (FrVe%) ≤20%, peak inspiratory pressure on the ventilator of ≤25 cm H_2O, dynamic compliance (Vt/PIP − PEEP) ≥0.9 mL/kg/cm H_2O, and mean inspiratory flow of ≥14 mL/kg/sec. Because these parameters are easily measured at the bedside, respiratory therapists using these data may be more confident of a successful extubation in children.

Table 18–9

FACTORS ASSOCIATED WITH FAILURE TO WEAN AND POTENTIAL SOLUTIONS

Factor	Solutions
Increased work of breathing	Ensure appropriate PSV Increase artificial airway diameter Ensure optimal bronchodilation Tracheobronchial hygiene Ensure ventilator synchrony
Atelectasis/secretions	Ensure adequate hydration Tracheobronchial hygiene Chest physiotherapy Frequent position changes
Agitation/dyspnea	Reassure the patient Check ABGs for acute deterioration Antianxiety agents Relieve excessive work of breathing
Respiratory muscle weakness	Slow wean using PSV Check electrolytes Ensure optimal position Ensure proper nutrition Respiratory muscle rest on ventilator

Extubation

Once it is concluded that the patient may be ready for extubation, a leak test is performed. The oral pharynx is suctioned and the endotracheal tube cuff is deflated. The presence and quantity of a leak past the cuff is assessed during a mandatory breath. If there is no leak, laryngeal edema is assumed. This must be treated with racemic epinephrine and/or intravenous steroid administration before extubation is attempted. Otherwise, the airway may spasm following extubation, precipitating respiratory failure and reintubation, which may be traumatic. Extubation is only performed if a leak is present.

The patient is prepared for extubation by first hyperoxygenating and then thoroughly suctioning the endotracheal tube, followed by reoxygenation. The tape or other securing device is loosened from the face and tube. If present, the endotracheal cuff is deflated in preparation for removing the tube. The patient is given a positive pressure breath with a manual resuscitator, and at peak pressure the tube is removed from the trachea.

Following extubation, oxygen is administered to maintain SpO_2 greater than 92%. The patient is observed closely for signs of edema or subglottic stenosis. Aerosolized racemic epinephrine or dexamethasone may be given as needed to reduce postextubation edema. Incentive spirometry is often performed following extubation to prevent atelectasis.

SUMMARY

This chapter discusses the use of conventional modes of ventilation of the neonate and child. It begins with a discussion of the forms of ventilatory failure (hypoxemic, hypercapnic, and mixed) and examples given for each. Modes of ventilation are discussed as they are classified into either partial or full ventilatory support. Partial ventilatory support occurs when the patient is responsible for all or part of his or her minute ventilation. Full ventilatory support occurs when the ventilator is responsible for all of the minute ventilation. The use of full versus partial ventilatory support is based on the patient's physiologic status and ability to support his or her own minute ventilation. The rationale for these modes is discussed and each mode is graphically depicted. The concepts of control, phase, and conditional variables are discussed.

Once the decision is made to utilize full or partial ventilatory support, and a particular mode is chosen, initial values for the parameters of ventilation are selected. These parameters include peak inspiratory pressure, tidal volume, set rate, sensitivity, PEEP, F_iO_2, inspiratory flow, inspiratory time, and I:E ratio. The need to set any of these parameters rests with which mode of ventilation has been selected. Once the patient has been established on mechanical ventilation, decisions are made about how to vary the parameter values to accomplish the goals of mechanical ventilation—reduce the work of breathing, adequate ventilation and oxygenation. Usually, this is done by obtaining and analyzing arterial blood gases and by clinical observation of the patient's synchrony with and toleration of ventilation. Changes in oxygenation and ventilation are accomplished by manipulating the controls of the ventilator until adequate arterial blood gases are achieved and there is patient–ventilator synchrony. Once the original indication for mechanical ventilation has been treated, consideration of how to liberate or wean the patient is made. The fraction of minute ventilation supplied by the ventilator and the F_iO_2 and PEEP are decreased. The spontaneous parameters of ventilation and oxygenation as they pertain to neonates and children are discussed, as are the considerations involved in the extubation and postextubation therapy of these patients.

POSTTEST

1. CPAP increases FRC by:
    a. physically holding the alveoli open during exhalation
    b. increasing inspiratory time and decreasing expiratory time
    c. reducing time constants
    d. increasing PaO_2 and decreasing $PacO_2$

2. Of the following, which is the most common device used to apply CPAP to the neonate?
   a. headbox
   b. face chamber
   c. nasal mask
   d. nasal prongs

3. Which of the following would indicate a failure of CPAP?
   I. PaO_2 less than 50 mmHg with an FiO_2 of 80% to 100% and CPAP of 10 to 12 cm H_2O
   II. $PaCO_2$ greater than 55 mmHg
   III. marked retractions
   IV. frequent apnea spells
   V. reduced FiO_2 needs
      a. I, II, V
      b. II, III, IV
      c. I, III, IV
      d. I, II, III

4. Determination of adequate levels of PIP is initially determined by:
   a. chest excursion, breath sounds, and PaO_2
   b. patient weight and gestational age
   c. FiO_2 requirements
   d. flow and inspiratory time to be used

5. Changing which of the following ventilator parameters would *not* alter minute ventilation?
   a. PIP
   b. expiratory time
   c. rate
   d. PEEP

6. Which of the following parameters has the greatest influence on mean airway pressure?
   a. PIP
   b. PEEP
   c. flow rate
   d. inspiratory time

7. The respiratory care practitioner receives blood gas results on a ventilated infant. The $PaCO_2$ is 48 mmHg and previously it was 43 mmHg. A proper ventilator change would be:
   a. decrease the rate by 5 BPM and the PIP by 3 cm H_2O
   b. increase the rate by 5 BPM or the PIP by 2 cm H_2O
   c. increase the inspiratory time and flow
   d. decrease the flow rate and the F_iO_2

8. The main advantage in using volume-cycled ventilation with neonates is:
   a. reduced barotrauma
   b. improvement in lung compliance
   c. reduction in airway resistance
   d. delivery of a consistent tidal volume

9. A 6-year-old female patient weighing 40 pounds is being ventilated at a tidal volume of 280 mL and a rate of 20 breaths/minute. The PIP is 38 cm H_2O with a PEEP of 4 cm H_2O. The compliance of the circuit tubing is measured at 2.5 mL/cm H_2O. Which of the following accurately describes this patient's corrected tidal volume?
   a. 9.5 mL/kg
   b. 10.8 mL/kg
   c. 12 mL/kg
   d. 13.4 mL/kg

10. Which of the following modes of ventilation should not be used on a spontaneously breathing patient?
    a. IMV
    b. APRV
    c. Inverse ratio ventilation
    d. SIMV

11. Which of the following is not considered a hazard of mechanical ventilation?
    a. barotrauma
    b. infection
    c. intracranial hemorrhage
    d. diaphragmatic paralysis

12. The first parameter weaned from a mechanically ventilated infant should be:
    a. F_iO_2
    b. rate
    c. PIP
    d. flow

13. Which of the following are clinical signs of a failure to wean?
    I. increased chest excursion
    II. bradycardia
    III. retractions
    IV. tachycardia
    V. pallor
       a. I, III, IV
       b. II, III, IV, V
       c. III, IV, V
       d. I, III, V

14. Which of the following are predictive of a low risk of the need for reintubation in the pediatric patient?
    I. spontaneous tidal volume of 3.2 mL/kg
    II. F_iO_2 of 45%
    III. mean airway pressure of 4.0 cm H_2O
    IV. PIP of 20 cm H_2O
    V. V_T/Ti of 16 mL/kg/sec
       a. I, II, III only
       b. II, III, IV only
       c. III, IV, V only
       d. I, III, V only

15. What arterial blood gas change is most likely to be observed when the mean airway pressure is increased?
    a. increased PaO_2
    b. increased $PaCO_2$
    c. decreased $PaCO_2$
    d. decreased PaO_2
16. What mode of ventilation should be instituted if the physician requests an increase in the spontaneous tidal volume during SIMV?
    a. APRV
    b. MMV
    c. PSV
    d. IRV
17. The respiratory therapist observes a PaO_2 of 52 mmHg on an infant despite nasal CPAP of 8 cm H_2O and 60% oxygen. What is the therapist's most appropriate action?
    a. increase the CPAP pressure to 12 cm H_2O
    b. increase the F_iO_2 to 80%
    c. intubation and ventilation in the IMV/CPAP mode
    d. replace the CPAP with an oxyhood at an F_iO_2 of 80%
18. What is the most accurate classification of neonatal mechanical ventilation?
    a. volume controlled, flow limited, time cycled
    b. pressure controlled, pressure limited, flow cycled
    c. volume controlled, flow limited, volume cycled
    d. pressure controlled, pressure limited, time cycled
19. How is hypercapnic respiratory failure identified?
    a. a decreased pH
    b. an increased $PaCO_2$
    c. a decreased PaO_2
    d. a decreased bicarbonate
20. How is tidal volume increased during pressure-controlled ventilation?
    a. increase the PEEP
    b. increase the ΔP
    c. increase the PEEP and ΔP by the same value
    d. increase the expiratory time

REFERENCES

1. Partridge JC, Wall SN. Analgesia for dying infants whose life support is withdrawn or withheld. *Pediatrics*. 99(1):76–79, 1997.
2. Partridge JC, Wall SN. Death in the intensive care nursery: physician practice of withdrawing and withholding life support. *Pediatrics*. 99(1):64–70, 1997.
3. Chatburn RL. Classification of mechanical ventilators. *Respiratory Care*. 37:1026–1044, 1992.

4. Tapia JL, et al. Does continuous positive airway pressure (CPAP) during weaning from intermittent mandatory ventilation in very low birthweight infants have risks or benefits? *Ped Pulmon.* 19:269, 1995.

5. American Association for Respiratory Care. Application of continuous positive airway pressure (CPAP) to neonates via nasal prongs or nasopharyngeal tube. *Respir Care.* 39(8):817–23, 1994.

6. Loftus BC, et al. Neonatal nasal deformities secondary to nasal continuous positive airway pressure. *Laryngoscope.* 104(8pt1):1019–22, 1994.

7. Smith PG, El-Khatib MF, Carlo WA. PEEP does not improve pulmonary mechanics in infants with bronchiolitis. *Am Rev Respir. Dis.* 147:1295–1298, 1993.

8. Siemens-Elema Life Support Division. *Servo ventilator 300 operating manual,* v 7.1. Art. No. 6027416E313E. 84–85, 1994.

9. Siemens-Elema Life Support Division. *Servo ventilator 300 operating manual,* v 7.1. Art. No. 6027416E313E. 82–83, 1994.

10. Bloom RS, Cropley C. *Textbook of neonatal resuscitation.* Dallas: American Heart Association/American Academy of Pediatrics, 1994.

11. Kano S. et. al. Fast versus slow ventilation for neonates. *Am Rev Respir Dis.* 148:578, 1993.

12. Wilson BG. Mechanical ventilation of the infant and child. In: Aloan CA, and Hill TV (eds.). *Respiratory care of the newborn and child,* 2nd ed. Philadelphia, PA: Lippincott, 327, 1997.

13. Corff KE, McCann DL. Room air resuscitation versus oxygen resuscitation in the delivery room. *Journal of Perinatal & Neonatal Nursing.* 19(4): 379–390, 2005.

14. American Heart Association, American Academy of Pediatrics. *Neonatal Resuscitation Textbook.* 6th ed., 2011.

15. Waugh JB, Deshpande VM, Harwood RJ. *Rapid interpretation of ventilator waveforms.* Upper Saddle River, NJ: Prentice Hall, 1999:1997.

16. Freidlich P, et al. A randomized trial of nasopharyngeal-synchronized intermittent mandatory ventilation versus nasopharyngeal continuous positive airway pressure in very low birth weight infants after extubation. *J Perinatol.* 19(6 pt 1):413–418, 1999.

17. Kahn N, Brown A, Venkataraman ST. Predictors of extubation success and failure in mechanically ventilated infants and children. *Crit Care Med.* 24(9): 1568–1579, 1996.

BIBLIOGRAPHY AND SUGGESTED READINGS

Bellettato, M. et.al. "Assisted Ventilation of the Newborn" 2012. Medscape. http://emedicine.medscape.com/article/979268-overview

Klingenberg, M. et.al. "A Practical guide to Neonatal Volume Guarantee Ventilation" J Perinatol. 2011;31(9):575-585

Claure, N. and Bancalari, E. "New modes of mechanical ventilation in the preterm newborn: evidence of benefit" Arch Dis Child Fetal Neonatal Ed. Nov 2007; 92(6): F508–F512

Goldsmith, J. and Karotkin, E. "Assisted Ventilation of the Neonate, 5th ed." 2010. Amsterdam Saunders/Elsevier

Donn, SM and Sinha, SK. "Invasive and Noninvasive Neonatal Mechanical Ventilation" Respiratory Care. 2003: 48(4)

CHAPTER 19

Common Infant and Pediatric Ventilators

OBJECTIVES

Upon completion of this chapter, the reader should be able to:

1. Identify and discuss, for each of the following ventilators, modes, capabilities and monitoring options:
   a. Bio-Med CV-2i+
   b. Carefusion 3100A
   c. Carefusion AVEA
   d. Drager Babylog 8000 plus
   e. Drager EvitaXL
   f. Hamilton Galileo
   g. Maquet Servo-i
   h. Newport HT70 Plus
   i. Puritan Bennett 840
   j. Sechrist Millennium

KEY TERMS

acute lung injury (ALI)
adaptive support ventilation (ASV)
airway pressure release ventilation (APRV)
assist/control (A/C)
assisted spontaneous breathing (ASB)
automode
bias flow
biphasic
DuoPAP

independent lung ventilation (ILV)
mandatory minute ventilation (MMV)
neutrally adjusted ventilator assist (NAVA)
open lung tool (OLT)
pressure regulated volume control (PRVC)
proportional pressure support (PPS)
rapid shallow breathing index (RSBI)

synchronized intermittent mandatory ventilation (SIMV)
synchronized intermittent positive pressure ventilation (SIPPV)
time cycled pressure limited (TCPL)
volume control plus (VC+)
volume guarantee (VG)

INTRODUCTION

Today's mechanical ventilators have developed beyond the days of just a few basic modes. It is not uncommon for ventilator manufacturers to have modes they have developed that are specific to their equipment. Although some may have similar principles in how the breath is delivered, the modes may have different names. Ventilator manufacturers are continuously developing new strategies through evidence-based research that provide safer ventilation and allow for more specific monitoring and careful manipulation of the patient ventilator interface. This chapter will introduce several of the more common ventilators that may be used in an infant or pediatric patient population. This list is not all-inclusive but it provides a broad grouping of infant and pediatric ventilators on the market today.

Each section will provide an overview of specific ventilator modes, capabilities, and monitoring. For further information and prior to using any ventilators in this chapter on a patient, it is recommended that the reader refer to the ventilator manufacturer for training on the device and read the most current evidence based research related to its use on patients.

BIO-MED CROSSVENT 2i+

The Bio-Med Crossvent 2i+ was created to be an ICU and a transport infant/pediatric ventilator.[1] This small simple ventilator has up to a 6-hour battery life, which makes it a viable transport ventilator. A compressor, a blended gas or 100% oxygen can power this ventilator.

Modes

Modes available on this ventilator include Assist-Control, SIMV, Pressure Support, CPAP, and Pressure-Limited Constant Flow.

Capabilities

Table 19–1 outlines specific capabilities of the Bio-Med Crossvent 2i+:

Monitoring

The Bio-Med Crossvent 2i+ uses brightly lit and easy to read monitoring screens. There are two alarm menus with this ventilator. The Alarm 1 menu allows for setting high and low alarms for peak pressure, respiratory rate, exhaled tidal volume, and exhaled minute volume. The Alarm 2 menu allows for setting high and low limits for PEEP pressure, mean airway pressure, and oxygen levels. Auto-set is a function that allows the respiratory therapist to quickly set the alarms at the push of one button. If running on battery power, the alarm will sound when the battery is running low.

Table 19–1	
CAPABILITIES OF THE BIO-MED CROSSVENT 2i+	
Breath Rate (Assist Control)	5–150 bpm
Breath Rate (CMV)	1–150 bpm
Tidal Volume	5–750 mL
Inspiratory Time	0.1–3.0 sec
I/E Ratio	3:1–1:99
Flow Rate	1–15 lpm
Peak Pressure	0–80 cm H2O
PEEP Pressure	0–20 cm H2O
Flow Trigger	1–20 (scale)
Pressure Support	0–50 cm H2O
SIMV Rate	0.6–50 bpm
O_2 Sensor	21–100%
Exhaled Tidal Volume	5–1300 mL

Source: Bio-Med Devices. (n.d.) Product brochure, *Crossvent 2i+*. http://www.biomeddevices .com /index.html?bmdcv2i.html&3

CAREFUSION 3100A

The CareFusion 3100A is a high-frequency oscillatory ventilator that is designed specifically for neonatal and pediatric patients.[2] This ventilator is based upon the understanding that lung recruitment through continuous distending pressure and gentle oscillatory ventilation supports the lung and provides ventilation and oxygenation through very small high-frequency pressure and volume movements. The frequency is delivered in Hz (1 Hz = 60 oscillations). Therefore, it is possible to deliver 180–900 oscillations per minute. Currently, the 3100A is the only FDA approved high-frequency ventilator approved for early intervention in the treatment of neonates in respiratory failure.

Modes

The only mode of ventilation offered on the CareFusion 3100A is high-frequency oscillation. Ventilation and oxygenation is achieved by distending with mean airway pressure. As low as 1 to 3 mL tidal volumes are then applied to the lung through piston driven oscillation, which is active on both inspiration and exhalation.

Capabilities

Table 19–2 outlines specific capabilities of the 3100A High-Frequency Oscillator.

Table 19–2	
CAPABILITIES OF 3100A HIGH-FREQUENCY OSCILLATOR	
Bias flow	0 to 40 L/min
Mean airway pressure	mPaw 3 to 45 cm H2O
Max mean pressure limit	10 to 45 cm H2O
Amplitude (Delta-P)	> 90 cm H2O
Frequency	3 to 15 Hz
Percent inspiratory time	30% to 50%
Piston centering adjust	Applies electrical counterforce to piston coil to maintain piston centering

Source: Carefusion. (2010). *Product brochure, 3100A High-Frequency Oscillatory Ventilator.* http://www.carefusion.com/medical-products/respiratory/ventilation/HFOV /sensormedics-3100a-high-frequency-oscillatory-ventilator.aspx.

Monitoring

Monitoring in the 3100A is somewhat different from that of conventional ventilation. The display monitors mean airway pressure, amplitude (Delta-P), percent of inspiratory time, frequency (Hz), piston displacement, and **bias flow**. The alarms available on the 3100A include high and low mean airway pressure, low battery, low gas source, power failure, oscillator stopped, 45-second alarm silence, and oscillator overheated. There is no alarm for a patient disconnect; therefore it is important to monitor the patient for proper ETT placement and via physical assessment of chest wiggle, oxygen saturation, auscultation, and possibly chest x-ray.

CAREFUSION AVEA VENTILATOR

The CareFusion AVEA ventilator is able to provide invasive and noninvasive ventilator support from neonates to adults.[3] Additionally, it is capable of providing volumetric capnography and transpulmonary pressure monitoring.

Modes

Modes of ventilation available on the CareFusion AVEA include **assist/control (A/C)**, SIMV, CPAP/PS, NPPV and Nasal CPAP/IMV. The respiratory therapist is able to select among several breath types on this ventilator such as **airway pressure release ventilation (APRV/Biphasic)**, volume, pressure, **time cycled pressure limited (TCPL)**, **pressure regulated volume control (PRVC)**, and **volume guarantee (VG)**.

APRV/Biphasic ventilation uses a pressure control mode of ventilation with an inverse inspiratory to expiratory ratio. P_{high} is set as a continuous positive airway pressure (CPAP) with an intermittent release of pressure to P_{low}. This mode may be indicated on patients with **acute lung injury (ALI)** or adult respiratory distress syndrome (ARDS), significant atelectasis or refractory hypoxemia due to alveoli collapse. This mode allows patients to maintain continuous spontaneous breathing while supporting lung recruitment. Caution should be observed when using this mode on patients with hemodynamic instability or patients with high expiratory resistance, such as in chronic obstructive pulmonary disease (COPD) or asthma.

Volume control type breaths are determined by a set tidal volume; thus, the pressure necessary to deliver the breath may vary depending on the patient's lung compliance. If the patient has decreased lung compliance, the pressure necessary to deliver the set volume will be increased. Only the peak airway pressure alarm will limit this breath; thus, care should be taken when selecting volume control ventilation by setting appropriate peak pressure alarms.

Pressure control type breaths are determined by a set peak inspiratory pressure (PIP), thus the volume delivered may vary depending on the patient's lung compliance. If a patient has decreased lung compliance, a smaller volume will result from the set pressure delivered to the lung in comparison to a patient with increased lung compliance. Therefore, care should be taken when setting high tidal volume alarms. As compliance improves, volumes will increase. The high tidal volume alarm is necessary to dump excessive volume and alert the respiratory therapist so adjustments in the PIP can be made. Likewise, low tidal volume alarms should be carefully set. As the patient's compliance decreases, this alarm will alert the respiratory therapist that the set PIP is not sufficient to reach target volumes.

Most approaches to mechanically ventilating infants include time cycled pressure limited (TCPL) breaths. As with pressure ventilation listed above, the PIP is set and the volume that results from the delivered pressure is variable depending on compliance. TCPL implies that time is what terminates inspiration, cycling it into exhalation. In TCPL ventilation, the respiratory therapist sets an inspiratory time. It is important in TCPL to ensure that flow is sufficient to reach the set PIP before the termination of inspiration. If flow is insufficient, the PIP will not be reached in the set inspiratory time.

Pressure regulated volume control (PRVC) is a dual mode of ventilation that requires a set tidal volume, minute volume, and respiratory rate. The ventilator can detect the level of pressure necessary to deliver the set volume, and it can adjust to provide the least amount of pressure to achieve the set volume. Unlike volume control breaths, PRVC may minimize the effects of excessive pressure delivered to the airway, which can cause barotraumas, volutrauma, and adverse hemodynamic issues. An upper pressure limit is set in order to limit excessive peak pressures when the set volume is delivered. If the upper pressure limit is reached, a lower tidal volume will be delivered and an alarm will sound. This type of breathing is not indicated in patients with a spontaneous respiratory drive.

Table 19–3

CAPABILITIES OF THE AVEA VENTILATOR

Rate	1 to 150 bpm (neonatal, pediatric)
Tidal volume	2.0 mL to 2.5 L
Inspiratory pressure	0 to 80 cm H_2O (neonatal), 0 to 90 cm H_2O (adult, pediatric)
Peak flow	0.4 to 150 L/min
Inspiratory time	0.15 to 5.0 sec
Pressure support ventilation (PSV)	0 to 80 cm H_2O (neonatal), 0 to 90 cm H_2O (adult, pediatric)
PEEP	0 to 50 cm H_2O
Flow trigger	0.1 to 20 L/min
%O_2	21% to 100%
Pressure high1 (in APRV mode)	0 to 90 cm H_2O
Time high1 (in APRV mode)	0.2 to 30 sec
Time low1 (in APRV mode)	0.2 to 30 sec
Pressure low1 (in APRV mode)	0 to 45 cm H_2O

Source: Carefusion (2011). Product brochure, *AVEA Ventilator*. http://www.carefusion.com/pdf/Respiratory/Ventilation/AVEA_Standard_spec_sheet_RC0107-02.pdf.

Volume guarantee (VG) is a dual mode of ventilation. A PIP is set as is a minimum tidal volume. The breath delivered is a pressure control breath, but if the minimum volume is not reached, the breath delivery type may switch to a volume breath in order to deliver the minimum volume set.

Capabilities

Table 19–3 outlines specific capabilities of the AVEA ventilator.

Monitoring

Monitoring the patient ventilator interface on the CareFusion AVEA is done in a variety of ways. A number of alarms are available that allow the respiratory therapist the ability to closely monitor all aspects of the patient's breathing and response to the ventilator. Several flow, volume, pressure, and capnography waveforms are available for additional patient interface assessment and monitoring.

Advanced settings and monitoring options are available on the AVEA. Please see the CareFusion AVEA product specifications brochure for additional details.

DRAGER BABYLOG 8000 PLUS

The Drager Babylog 8000 plus is a TCPL ventilator with continuous flow designed to support preterm neonates to pediatric patients.[4] This ventilator also offers BabyFlow nasal CPAP and high-frequency ventilation (HFV)

Modes

There are several modes available on the BabyLog 8000 plus, some of which are unique to this ventilator. Intermittent Positive Pressure Ventilation and Intermittent Mandatory Ventilation (IPPV/IMV), CPAP, **Synchronized Intermittent Positive Pressure Ventilation (SIPPV)**, **Synchronized Intermittent Mandatory Ventilation (SIMV)**, and Pressure Support Ventilation (PSV) are all modes available on this ventilator. Additional functions include Volume Guarantee (VG), High-Frequency Ventilation (HFV), and Variable Inspiratory and Variable Expiratory flow (VIVE), which can be added to several of the modes listed above.

IPPV/IMV is a TCPL ventilation mode for patients without spontaneous breathing. It can be combined with HFV or VIVE.

SIPPV is synchronized with the patient's spontaneous breathing and the patient is in control of the frequency. If the patient experiences apneic periods, the default ventilation will be determined by the set inspiratory and expiratory time. SIPPV can be combined with VG and VIVE.

PSV is synchronized with the patient's spontaneous effort and assists in augmenting the inspired tidal volume. This mode can be combined with VIVE and SIMV with VG.

CPAP is intended for patients who are able to maintain their own spontaneous rate and tidal volume. It provided continuous flow and adjusts the baseline to the PEEP/CPAP level. This mode can be combined with VIVE and HFV.

VG can be combined with SIPPV, SIMV and PSV in order to achieve a consistent tidal volume.

HFV combines high frequency pulses and a mean airway pressure. The CPAP/PEEP level becomes the set mean airway pressure and the pulses move above and below the CPAP/PEEP level. This is intended to reduce the stress on patient's lungs.

VIVE allows for adjustment of inspiratory and expiratory flow. Inspiratory flow is effective during ventilation strokes and the expiratory flow is effective during spontaneous breathing. Increasing expiratory flow may provide increased flow for spontaneous breathing and may assist in flushing deadspace volume from the patient Y-piece.

Capabilities

Table 19–4 outlines specific capabilities of the Babylog 8000 plus ventilator.

Table 19–4

CAPABILITIES OF THE BABYLOG 8000 PLUS VENTILATOR

Inspiratory oxygen concentration	21 to 100%
Peak inspiratory pressure	10 to 80 mbar
PEEP/CPAP	0 to 25 mbar
Maximal frequency	200 bpm
Inspiratory time	0.1 to 2 sec
Expiratory time	0.2 to 30 sec
Inspiratory flow	1 to 30 L/min
Base flow (VIVE)	1 to 30 L/min

Source: Drager Medical. (n.d.). Babylog 8000 Plus: Intensive care ventilator for neonates, instructions for use. http://www.kilimed.com/user_manual/babylog8000 _en.pdf.

Monitoring

Patient monitoring on the Babylog 8000 plus include integrated flow and volume monitoring at the Y-piece, lung function monitoring of compliance, resistance and time constant, oxygen delivery, and peak and mean pressures as well as a graphic trending and a logbook of the last 100 alarms.

For more specific information on ventilator modes or specific control details, please refer to the Drager Babylog 8000 Plus product brochure and instructions for use.

DRAGER EVITA XL

The Evita XL is a ventilator with broad applications.[5] It is able to provide invasive and noninvasive support to patients ranging from neonates to adults. The noninvasive application allows for the Evita XL to provide all modes of ventilation noninvasively through the use of a dynamic leak compensation system. This device also incorporates SmartCare/PS weaning system and **mandatory minute ventilation (MMV)** function to ensure all patients receive the set minute volume despite fluctuating spontaneous breathing levels.

Modes

Modes available on the Evita XL include several mentioned previously in this chapter, such as IPPV, SIMV, A/C, CPAP, and APRV. Additional modes available on this device include mandatory minute ventilation (MMV), biphasic positive airway pressure (BIPAP), **independent lung ventilation (ILV)**, and **proportional pressure support (PPS)**.

MMV allows the patient to breathe spontaneously however a set minute volume must be achieved. If the set minute volume is not achieved, mandatory ventilation strokes will make up the difference, bringing the patient's minute volume up to the set volume. **Assisted spontaneous breathing (ASB)** can be added to this mode, which will assist in augmenting the patient's spontaneous breaths allowing the patient to more easily reach the set minute volume.

BIPAP or BIPAP/ASB is pressure-controlled ventilation that allows for spontaneous breathing and adjustable pressure support. The controlled portion of ventilation is set with a PIP and frequency. Frequency can be reduced during the weaning process. When the frequency is reduced to 0 the device will automatically change to CPAP or CPAP/ASB.

ILV allows two Evita units to be connected and operate in synchrony to independently ventilate the patient's lungs. This is done through an analogue interface. The master device will control the operation. The slave device will follow the control of the master device.

PPS is an optional setting that is intended for differentiated proportional support of spontaneous breathing with pathological compliance and/or resistance.

Capabilities

Table 19–5 outlines specific capabilities of the Evita XL ventilator.

Table 19–5

CAPABILITIES OF THE EVITA XL VENTILATOR

Ventilation frequency (f)	0 to 100/min, 0 to 150/min (Neonatal)
Inspiration time (T insp)	0.1 to 10 sec
Tidal volume (VT)	0.02 to 0.3 L (Pediatric) 0.003 to 0.1 L (Neonatal)
Inspiratory flow	6 to 30 L/min (Pediatric and Neonatal)
Inspiratory pressure	0 to 95 mbar/cm H_2O
PEEP/intermittent PEEP	0 to 50 mbar/cm H_2O
Pressure assist ASB/Psupp	0 to 95 mbar/cm H_2O
Rise time for inspiratory pressure	0 to 2 sec
O_2 concentration	21 to 100%
Multi-sense Trigger Criteria	Internal automatic pressure trigger, Flow, Volume (Flow adjustable 0.3 to 15 L/min)

Source: Drager Medical. (n.d.). Evita XL: Intensive care ventilator, instructions for use. http://www.adhb.govt.nz/achicu/Documents/Evita%20XL.pdf.

Monitoring

Patient monitoring on the Evita XL include a variety of flow, pressure, and volume monitoring capabilities, capnography, lung compliance and resistance measurements, oxygen delivery, deadspace measurements, weaning parameters, and peak and mean pressures, as well as a graphic trending.

For more specific information on ventilator modes or specific control details, please refer to the Evita XL product brochure and instructions for use.

HAMILTON GALILEO

The Galileo ventilator provides a variety of features for supporting patient's ventilator needs including invasive and noninvasive support.[6] It also offers adaptive support ventilation (ASV), which is a feature unique to the brand, and **DuoPAP**, which is a biphasic mode of ventilation.

Modes

Modes available on the Galileo include several mentioned previously in this chapter, such as A/C, SIMV, APRV and SPONT (CPAP). Additional modes available on this device include ASV and DuoPAP.

Adaptive support ventilation (ASV) uses pressure control and pressure support to maintain a set minute ventilation. The goal of this mode is to use the lowest settings necessary to provide the patient a comfortable work of breathing. This mode will adapt to the patient's demand by increasing or decreasing support. The ventilator functions off of the patient's ideal body weight in order to determine the appropriate minute ventilation based on 100 mL/min/kg. If the patient is apneic or if there is a delay in respiratory effort, the ventilator will assume an appropriate respiratory rate, tidal volume and pressure limit in order to deliver mandatory respirations. As the patient increases spontaneous effort, the ventilator will decrease the mandatory breaths delivered.

Duo Positive Airway Pressure (DuoPAP) is very similar to APRV or other biphasic modes of ventilation in that the support alternates between two preset positive pressure levels. The patient can breathe spontaneously at either pressure level. Spontaneous breaths are also synchronized as the pressures shift from low pressure to high pressure.

Capabilities

Table 19–6 outlines specific capabilities of the Galileo ventilator

Monitoring

Patient monitoring on the Galileo includes a variety of flow, airway pressure, auxiliary pressure and volume monitoring capabilities, lung compliance

Table 19–6	

CAPABILITIES OF THE GALILEO VENTILATOR

CMV rate	5 to 120 b/min
SIMV rate	1 to 60 b/min
Tidal volume	10 to 2000 mL
PEEP/CPAP	0 to 50 cm H_2O
Oxygen	21 to 100%
I:E ratio	1:9 to 4:1
Inspiratory time	10% to 80% of cycle time (0.1 to 3 sec)
Pause time	0% to 70% of cycle time (0 to 8 sec)
Peak flow	1 to 180 L/min
Pressure trigger	0.5 to 10 cm H_2O below PEEP/CPAP
Flow trigger	0.5 to 15 L/min
Base flow	4 to 30 L/min, depending on flow trigger setting
Pressure control	5 to 100 cm H_2O
Pressure support	0 to 100 cm H_2O
Pressure ramp	25 to 200 msec
Expiratory trigger sensitivity	10% to 40% of inspiratory peak flow
% minute volume (ASV)	10% to 350%
Bodyweight (ASV)	10 to 200 kg

Source: Hamilton Medical AG. (2000). *Hamilton Galileo Ventilator*. http://www.ventworld.com/equipment/ProdBooth.asp?ProdId=173.

and resistance measurements, oxygen delivery, imposed work of breathing, **rapid shallow breathing index (RSBI),** deadspace measurements, weaning parameters, and peak and mean pressures as well as a waveforms and graphic trending.

For more specific information on ventilator modes or specific control details, please refer to the Galileo product brochure and instructions for use.

MAQUET SERVO-i

The Servo-i ventilator has the capability to provide ventilator support for patients from infant to adult.[7] This ventilator can be used at the bedside, for transport and in the MRI room, depending on ventilator options selected. The Servo-i also has capabilities of providing noninvasive support.

Modes

Modes of ventilation available on the Servo-i include A/C, SIMV, PS, CPAP, and PRVC. Additional optional modes of support unique to the Servo-i include **Neutrally Adjusted Ventilatory Assist (NAVA)**, **Open Lung Tool (OLT)**, and Automode.

NAVA uses monitoring of the electrical activity of the diaphragm (EDI) to determine asynchrony of ventilation support and patient effort. NAVA allows for better control of ventilation synchrony and patient effort.

The OLT is a tool that trends breath-by-breath ventilation parameters, including dynamic compliance. This option can be valuable in assessing alveolar recruitment and lung-protective strategies.

Automode allows for a smooth transition from controlled ventilation to supported ventilation when the patient begins to spontaneously trigger breaths.

Capabilities

Table 19–7 outlines specific capabilities of the Servo-i ventilator

Monitoring

Patient monitoring on the Servo-i includes a variety of flow, airway pressure, and volume monitoring capabilities, lung compliance and resistance measurements, leakage fractions, end tidal CO_2 and CO_2 minute elimination, oxygen delivery, work of breathing pattern, shallow breathing index (SBI), weaning parameters, and peak and mean pressures as well as a waveforms and graphic trending.

For more specific information on ventilator modes or specific control details, please refer to the Servo-i product brochure and instructions for use.

Table 19–7

CAPABILITIES OF THE SERVO-I VENTILATOR

Inspiratory tidal volume	2–350 mL
Inspiratory minute volume	0.3–20 L/min
Apnea, time to alarm	2–45 sec
Automode Trigger timeout	3–15 sec
PC/PS above PEEP	0–(80 – PEEP) cm H_2O
PC/PS above PEEP in NIV	0–(32 – PEEP) cm H_2O
PEEP	0–50 cm H_2O
PEEP in NIV	2–20 cm H_2O
CPAP pressure	2–20 cm H_2O
CMV frequency	4–150 breaths/min
SIMV frequency	1–60 breaths/min

Breath cycle time, SIMV	0.5–15 sec
P High	(PEEP + 1) – 50
T High	0.2–10 sec
T PEEP	0.2–10 sec
PS above P High	0–(80 – P High)
O_2 concentration	21–100%
I:E ratio	1:10–4:1
T Insp	0.1–5 sec
NAVA level	0–30 cm $H_2O/\mu V$
Edi trigger sensitivity	0.1–2.0 μV
NIV Back-up T Insp	0.3–1 sec
T Pause	0–1.5 sec
T Pause	0–30% of breath cycle time
Flow trigger sensitivity level	0–100% fraction of bias flow
Press. trigg sensitivity	−20–0 cm H_2O
Insp. rise time	0–20% of breath cycle time
Insp. rise time	0–0.2 sec
Insp. cycle off	1%–70% of peak flow
Insp. cycle off in NIV	10%–70% of peak flow
Nebulizer time	5–30 min

Source: Maquet. (2011). Data sheet: Ventilation Servo-i Infant. http://www.maquet.com /assets/ documents/product-information/SERVO-i-Infant/SERVO-i-Infant-Data-Sheet-EN-US.pdf.

NEWPORT HT70 PLUS

The Newport HT70 Plus is a multifunctional ventilator that can be used for home care, transport, hospital and long-term care.[8] This portable ventilator provides support for patients from 5 kg to adult. The monitor is geared to provide simple navigation with touch screen controls. The Newport HT70 Plus has a built-in generator and a battery that provides up to 10 hours of use.

Modes

The Newport HT70 Plus is capable of pressure and volume ventilation via A/C, SIMV, and Spontaneous modes with the ability to add PS to spontaneous breaths in SIMV and Spontaneous modes. Each of these modes is also able to run noninvasively.

Capabilities

Table 19–8 outlines specific capabilities of the Newport HT70 Plus ventilator

Table 19–8

CAPABILITIES OF THE NEWPORT HT70 PLUS VENTILATOR

VT (Tidal Volume)	50 to 2,200 mL
RR (Respiratory Rate)	1 to 99 b /min
i Time (Inspiratory Time)	0.1 to 3.0 sec
PEEP/CPAP	0 to 30 cm H_2O/0 to 30 mbar
PS (Pressure Support)	0 to 60 cm H_2O/0 to 60 mbar*
Flow	6 to 100 L/min
I:E Ratio	1:99 to 3:1
PC (Pressure Control)	5 to 60 cm H_2O/5 to 60 mbar
Ptrig (Sensitivity)	−9.9 to 0 cm H_2O/−9.9 to 0 mbar
Flow Trigger	0.0 to 10.0 L/min, Off
Manual Inflation	3 sec maximum
O_2 (oxygen)	21 to 100%
Bias Flow	NIV off: 7 L/min w/PEEP NIV on: 3 to 30 L/min w/PEEP
PS Max i time	0.1 to 3.0 sec
PS % Exp. Threshold	5% to 85%
Slope Rise	1 to 10
Flow Wave Pattern	Square or descending

Source: Covidien. (2013). Newport HT70 Plus Ventilator. http://www.covidien.com/rms/pages.aspx?page=Product/NewportHT70Plus.

Monitoring

Patient monitoring on the Newport HT70 Plus includes a variety of flow, airway pressure and volume monitoring capabilities and alarms. It also provides internal battery dual battery system with a battery use time estimator and an oxygen cylinder monitor. Waveform graphics, trending and recorded events are viewable on specialty screens. There is also an option that allows for capturing and downloading events and trends.

For more specific information on ventilator modes or specific control details, please refer to the Servo-i product brochure and instructions for use.

PURITAN BENNETT 840

The Puritan Bennett 840 ventilator provides diverse ventilator support for patients ranging from 300 grams to 150 kgs. The NeoMode software allows this ventilator to deliver tidal volumes as small as 2 mL. Leak compensation reduces the impact of leaks on intubated patients and those supported in noninvasive modes.

Modes

The Puritan Bennett 840 ventilator modes include A/C, SIMV, SPONT, and Bi-Level ventilation.[9] Mandatory breath types used with these modes include volume control (VC), pressure control (PC), **volume control plus (VC+)**, pressure support (PS), and volume support (VS). All of these modes and breath types have been discussed previously in this chapter with the exception of VC+ and VS.

In VC+, the respiratory therapist will set an inspiratory time and a target tidal volume. A test breath is delivered to the patient. The delivered breath incorporates a decelerating flow and a plateau in order to determine lung compliance. The ventilator will adjust subsequent breaths depending on whether they were greater or smaller than the target volume. The goal of this breath type is to appropriately set flow to meet the needs of the patient without using excess flow. Patients can breathe spontaneously throughout the inspiratory phase of the breath.

Capabilities

Table 19–9 outlines specific capabilities of the Puritan Bennett 840 Neonatal ventilator.

Monitoring

Patient monitoring on the Puritan Bennett 840 includes a variety of flow, airway pressure, and volume monitoring capabilities and alarms on a dual-view touch

Table 19–9

CAPABILITIES OF THE PURITAN BENNETT 840 NEONATAL VENTILATOR

Tidal volume (vt)	2 to 315 mL with neoMode software
Respiratory rate (f)	1 to 150 /min with neoMode
Peak inspiratory flow (vMaX)	1 to 30 l/min with neoMode
Flow pattern	square or descending ramp
Plateau time (tpl)	0.0 to 2.0 seconds
Inspiratory pressure (pi)	5 to 90 cm H_2O
Inspiratory time (ti)	0.2 to 8.0 seconds
I:E ratio	$\leq$ 1:299–4.00:1
Expiratory time (te)	$\geq$ 0.2 second
Trigger type	Pressure or flow
Flow sensitivity (vsens)	0.1 to 10 l/min with neoMode
O_2%	21 to 100%
PEEP	0 to 45 cm H_2O

Source: Covidien. (2013). Puritan Bennett 840 Neonatal Ventilator. http://www.covidien.com / RMS/pages.aspx?page=Product/Puritan-Bennett-PB840-Ventilator &tab=Resources.

screen. A variety of waveform graphics are easily viewable. Trending with up to 58 parameters and recorded events for up to 72 hours is a possibility with an optional trending package. There is also an option that allows for capturing and downloading events and trends.

For more specific information on ventilator modes or specific control details, please refer to the Puritan Bennett 840 product brochure and instructions for use.

SECHRIST MILLENNIUM

The Sechrist Millennium ventilator is specifically designed to support infant and pediatric patients.[10, 11] This ventilator provides simple and reliable modes of ventilation combined with a unique pressure sensing technology called SmartSync, which is a pressure-sensing device that allows for sensitive synchrony between a patient's natural breathing cycle and breath support. The controls are intuitive and easy to operate. The Sechrist Millennium is available as a countertop ventilator or on a rolling stand.

Modes

The Sechrist Millennium ventilator is capable of providing A/C, SIMV/IMV, CPAP, CPAP with backup ventilation, and Standby.

Capabilities

Table 19–10 outlines specific capabilities of the Sechrist Millennium ventilator

Table 19–10	
CAPABILITIES OF THE SECHRIST MILLENNIUM VENTILATOR	
Inspiratory time	0.1 to 3.0 sec
I:E Ratio	Normal Range 1:1.0 to 1:1.10 (sens. off) 1:1.0 to 1:99 (sens on) Inverse range 1:0.1 to 4.0:1
Respiratory Rate	2 to 150 reaths/min
Expiratory Pressure	0 to 20 cm H_2O
Inspiratory Pressure	5 to 70 cm H_2O
Flow	2–32 Lpm; flush 40 Lpm
Waveform	Tapered to square

Source: Sechrist Products. (n.d.). Millennium: Infant and Pediatric Ventilation. http://www.sechristusa.com/pdf/millennium_brochure_rev2.pdf.

Monitoring

Patient monitoring on the Sechrist Millennium includes a variety of flow, airway pressure and volume monitoring capabilities and alarms. Breath status can be visualized in graphic display. A fiber optic data output link allows for data transmission to a secondary computer site.

For more specific information on ventilator modes or specific control details, please refer to the Sechrist Millennium product brochure and instructions for use.

SUMMARY

As technology develops, new ventilators have been developed incorporating modes of ventilation that have greatly improved the ability to ventilate and oxygenate with less risk of injury or side effects to the patient. The advent of microtechnology has allowed neonatal ventilators to enter the realm of synchronization, which may reduce the risk of barotrauma and "fighting" the ventilator. Technological advances have allowed ventilator manufacturers to finely tune supportive modes and monitoring capabilities. These advances provide the respiratory therapist with invaluable information that aids in making critical adjustments to the support being provided to the patient.

New ventilators enter the market with new ventilatory modes and advances, requiring a sound understanding of basic ventilatory techniques by the respiratory therapist. Before working with any ventilator, the respiratory therapist must become familiar with all aspects of the ventilator before applying it to a patient.

The advancement of technology has brought about the ability to closely and accurately measure and display airway pressures, inspiratory and expiratory times, and flow patterns. This allows the well-trained and experienced practitioner to finely tune the ventilator settings to meet the specific needs of the patient. Additionally, these advancements and continued evidence based research have reduced risk of barotrauma and other side effects as long as the ventilator is appropriately managed.

POSTTEST

1. Which of the following ventilators was specifically developed to provide high frequency oscillatory ventilation?
   a. Hamilton Galileo
   b. Newport HT70 Plus
   c. Carefusion 3100A
   d. Sechrist Millennium

2. Which of the following ventilators provides an option for neutrally adjusted ventilator assist (NAVA)?
   a. Drager EvitaXL
   b. Maquet Servo-i
   c. Bio-Med CV-2i+
   d. Puritan Bennett 840
3. In high-frequency ventilation, another term that refers to amplitude is:
   a. Peak pressure
   b. Delta P
   c. Inspiratory time
   d. Pressure control
4. Which of the following ventilators provides an option to combining two ventilators to work in synchrony for independent lung ventilation (ILV)?
   a. Drager EvitaXL
   b. Hamilton Galileo
   c. Carefusion AVEA
   d. Drager Babylog 8000 plus
5. What is the range of Hertz (Hz) that can be set on the Carefusion 3100A?
   a. 1–8 Hz
   b. 7–20 Hz
   c. 4–10 Hz
   d. 3–15 Hz
6. Which of the following is NOT a biphasic mode of ventilation?
   a. DuoPAP
   b. APRV
   c. SIPPV
   d. All are biphasic modes of ventilation.
7. Volume guarantee (VG) can be described as a mode where:
   a. The set tidal volume is guaranteed to be delivered despite the patient's compliance.
   b. PIP is set to achieve a minimum tidal volume but if the volume is not reached, the breath type may switch to a volume breath in order to deliver a minimum volume.
   c. PIP is set to achieve a minimum tidal volume but if the volume is not reached, the PIP is increased automatically in order to reach the minimum volume to be delivered.
   d. Flow and i-time are altered automatically in order to deliver a guaranteed tidal volume.
8. Which of the following statements are true about adaptive support ventilation (ASV)?
   a. The goal is to use the lowest settings necessary to provide the patient a comfortable work of breathing.
   b. Pressure control and pressure support are used to maintain preset minute ventilation.
   c. ASV will adapt to the patient's demand by increasing or decreasing support.
   d. All of the above are true statements.

REFERENCES

1. Bio-Med Devices. (n.d.) Product brochure, *Crossvent 2i+*. http://www
   .biomeddevices.com/index.html?bmdcv2i.html&3.
2. Carefusion. (2010). Product brochure, *3100A High-Frequency Oscillatory
   Ventilator*. http://www.carefusion.com/medical-products/respiratory/
   ventilation/HFOV/sensormedics-3100a-high-frequency-oscillatory-
   ventilator.aspx.
3. Carefusion. (2011). Product brochure, *AVEA Ventilator*. http://www.carefusion
   .com /pdf/Respiratory/Ventilation/AVEA_Standard_spec_sheet_RC0107-02.
   pdf.
4. Drager Medical. (n.d.). Babylog 8000 Plus: Intensive care ventilator for
   neonates, instructions for use. http://www.kilimed.com/user_manual/
   babylog8000 _en.pdf.
5. Drager Medical. (n.d.). Evita XL: Intensive care ventilator, instructions for use.
   http://www.adhb.govt.nz/achicu/Documents/Evita%20XL.pdf.
6. Hamilton Medical AG. (2000). Hamilton Galileo Ventilator. http://www
   .ventworld .com/equipment/ProdBooth.asp?ProdId=173
7. Maquet. (2011). Data sheet: Ventilation Servo-i Infant. http://www.maquet.
   com /assets/documents/product-information/SERVO-i-Infant/SERVO-i-
   Infant-Data-Sheet-EN-US.pdf.
8. Covidien. (2013). Newport HT70 Plus Ventilator. http://www.covidien.com/
   rms/pages.aspx?page=Product/NewportHT70Plus.
9. Covidien. (2013). Puritan Bennett 840 Neonatal Ventilator. http://www
   .covidien.com /RMS/pages.aspx?page=Product/Puritan-Bennett-PB840-
   Ventilator &tab=Resources.
10. Sechrist Products. (2010). Millennium – The Infant/Pediatric Ventilator.
    http://www.sechristusa.com/millennium-ventilator.html.
11. Sechrist Products. (n.d.). Millennium: Infant and Pediatric Ventilation. http://
    www.sechristusa.com/pdf/millennium_brochure_rev2.pdf.

BIBLIOGRAPHY AND SUGGESTED READINGS

Corning HS. (n.d.). New Vent Modes: VS, PRVC, PC+PS and Automode. RC Edu-
    cational Consulting Services, Inc. http://www.rcecs.com/MyCE/PDFDocs/
    course/V7077.pdf.
Kherallah M. (n.d.). *Advanced Modes of Mechanical Ventilation*. http://www.me
    criticalcare.net/downloads/lectures/AdvancedVentilatoryModes.pdf.
Medical University of South Carolina Division of Neonatology. (2006). Ventilator
    terminology and classification of mechanical ventilation. http://www
    .musckids.org/pediatrics/fellowship/neonatal/tools/Classification_of_
    Mechanical_Ventilation.pdf.

CHAPTER 20

Special Procedures and Nonconventional Ventilatory Techniques

OBJECTIVES

Upon completion of this chapter, the reader should be able to:

1. Describe each of the following, as they relate to surfactant replacement therapy.
   a. Patient history
   b. Indications
   c. Administration techniques
   d. Outcomes
2. Identify the major advantage of HFV.
3. Describe, for each of the three types of HFV, the following:
   a. Rates of ventilation
   b. Indications
   c. Clinical uses
   d. Hazards
4. Explain why a conventional ventilator is used in conjunction with HFJV and HFO.
5. Discuss the two theories of gas flow characteristics that are associated with HFJV and HFO.
6. Describe the mechanisms of action of inhaled nitric oxide and its role in treatment of the newborn and pediatric patient in respiratory failure.
7. Describe the basic components of inhaled nitric oxide delivery.
8. Discuss the safety of inhaled nitric oxide and possible adverse effects of its use.
9. Discuss the use of heliox for pediatric patients with airflow obstruction.
10. Describe each of the following as they relate to ECLS:
    a. History
    b. Venoarterial vs. venovenuous bypass
    c. Components of the ECLS circuit
    d. Use of mechanical ventilation during ECLS

11. Identify methods used for selecting patients for ECLS and recognize those for which ECLS is contraindicated.
12. Describe how ECLS is initiated, the indications for termination, and the complications associated with its use.
13. Discuss each of the following, as they relate to negative pressure ventilation:
    a. History
    b. Methods of delivery
    c. Current uses
    d. Advantages and disadvantages
14. Briefly describe the history and use of partial liquid ventilation.

KEY TERMS

air leak syndrome	methemoglobinemia	venoarterial
amplitude	necrotizing	venovenous
dipalmitoyl	tracheobronchitis	
phosphatidylcholine	phospholipid	
(DPPC)	thrombocytopenia	

INTRODUCTION

In addition to conventional methods of treating the critically ill newborn or pediatric patient, adjunct therapy may involve nontraditional methods of resuscitation and ventilation. These special procedures include surfactant replacement therapy (SRT), high-frequency ventilation (HFV), special medical gas administration, extracorporeal life support (ECLS), partial liquid ventilation (PLV), and negative pressure ventilation. Although considered nontraditional, these special procedures are playing a role (where clinically appropriate) in neonatal and pediatric care in the critical care unit and are becoming increasingly routine.

SURFACTANT REPLACEMENT THERAPY

It has long been understood that primary dysfunction in RDS is abnormal alveolar surface forces resulting from capillary leak and a lack of surfactant. It therefore became an item of major interest in the scientific community to develop a surfactant that could be administered to an infant, to replace that which was viewed as a deficiency in physiologic function. Naturally occurring surfactant is composed of several **phospholipids** and lipids, and four or more specific apoproteins. It appears as though each component may have its own distinct characteristics with regard to production, secretion, and removal.[1] These factors have made it difficult to produce an ideal replacement surfactant.

Approximately 90% of surfactant is phospholipid, with phosphatidylcholine (PC) comprising 85% of the total. Roughly 60% of the PC is **dipalmitoyl phosphatidylcholine (DPPC)**. It is the DPPC that allows surfactant to lower surface tension.[2] The remaining phospholipids are phosphatidylglycerol (PG) and phosphatidylinositol (PI). Cholesterol is the predominant neutral lipid in surfactant. The four proteins found in surfactant, given the names of surfactant proteins A, B, C, and D (SP-A, etc.), make up 5% to 10% of the total. Although small in quantity, their presence is essential for proper activity of pulmonary surfactant.[2]

Early studies were discouraging because researchers could not find the right combination of components that formed a useful surfactant. Dosages and method of delivery also inhibited the usefulness of surfactant replacement.

Early surfactants were made with DPPC and were nebulized into the trachea. This type of surfactant alone and method of delivery did not produce the desired results. Continued research and later studies of surfactant and its biochemical and biophysical properties illustrated the important role of the other proteins and lipids. New surfactants were developed that included the additional lipids and proteins. Delivery was changed from nebulization to direct instillation of the surfactant into the patient's trachea at higher dosages than had previously been used.

Indications

There are two primary protocols for the administration of surfactant during the neonatal period. Prophylactic administration of surfactant is indicated for those infants who are at a high risk of developing RDS. Included are those infants born before 32 weeks, those who weigh less than 1300 grams, those with an L/S ratio less than 2:1, or those with an absence of PG in the amniotic fluid. Under this protocol, the infant receives the surfactant as quickly as possible, following delivery. Therapeutic administration (also called rescue) is not given until the patient develops signs of RDS. Indications include those infants who require ventilatory assistance due to an increased work of breathing (grunting, nasal flaring, retractions), increasing oxygen requirements, and having chest x-ray evidence of RDS.[3] SRT has also been effective in other causes of respiratory failure in the newborn, such as pneumonia and meconium aspiration syndrome.[4]

The indications for surfactant use for the pediatric patient in respiratory failure are not as well established. Unlike RDS in preterm infants where surfactant is not produced by mature pathways, the role that surfactant deficiency or inactivation during pathologic processes in the child with acute lung injury remains unclear. SRT for the child with acute hypoxemic respiratory failure may therefore be indicated when current therapy, which includes mechanical ventilator support and treatment of the underlying cause, has failed to yield positive results. Although SRT may not reverse the lung injury, it has been shown to improve lung volumes by stabilizing alveoli and increasing compliance and oxygenation.[5]

Types of Surfactant

Currently, most surfactants fall into two categories: those obtained from mammalian lungs and those that are synthetically produced. Mammalian preparations typically contain all surfactant proteins, but the proportions of their active ingredients are different. Varying the amount of cholesterol, free fatty acids and total phospholipids has been shown to vary the biophysical activity of these surfactant preparations.[6] Additionally, the absorption of lung surfactant is largely controlled by surfactant proteins. Synthetically produced preparations that are protein free contain detergent-like substances that act as spreading agents to enhance disbursement and, thus, absorption by alveolar structures. The difference in relative components of lipids and proteins in exogenous surfactants varies the amount of surface activity from each commercially marketed surfactant.[7] (Refer to Table 20–1.)

Outcomes

There are several reported adverse reactions associated with dosing procedures during SRT. The most common are usually transient with full recovery. Adverse effects can include bradycardia, oxygen desaturation, and ETT reflux. The infant must be monitored during the dosing procedure and appropriate action taken should any of these adverse effects occur. Because SRT can significantly affect oxygenation and lung compliance, the infant must be closely monitored after administration. Improvement in oxygenation may require reduction in the oxygen concentration (sometimes reduced from 100% F_iO_2 to room air over 30 minutes to one hour), and improvement in lung compliance may require a reduction in ventilator pressures.[8]

On the positive side, SRT has been shown to reduce the severity of RDS, pulmonary air leaks, and the subsequent development of BPD.[6] When used in conjunction with other special procedures such as high-frequency oscillatory ventilation[9] and inhaled nitric oxide,[10] SRT has resulted in significant clinical improvement. SRT in the pediatric population has been shown to improve pulmonary dynamic compliance and stabilize gas exchange[11] and reduce the length of ventilatory support and lead to earlier PICU discharge.[12]

Table 20–1

COMPARISON OF EXOGENOUS SURFACTANTS

	Exosurf	Survanta	Infasurf	Curosurf
Source	Synthetic	Calf lung	Calf lung	Pig lung
Proteins	—	SP-B, C	SP-B, C	SP-B, C
Phospholipids	13 mg/mL	25 mg/mL	35 mg/mL	80 mg/mL
Dosage/birth weight	5 mL/kg	4 mL/kg	3 mL/kg	2.5 mL/kg

Since coming of age, SRT has dramatically decreased mortality and morbidity rates in RDS[3] and has become the standard of care for neonates with RDS.

HIGH-FREQUENCY VENTILATION (HFV)

The normally held understanding of ventilation is that the tidal volume must exceed the amount of physiologic dead space for alveolar ventilation to occur. Conventional ventilation utilizes this principle by inflating the patient's lungs with a tidal volume that exceeds dead space and inflates the alveoli for gaseous exchange. Expiration then occurs by the passive recoil of the thorax and lung.

HFV is a technique of ventilation that delivers small tidal volumes at very high respiratory rates with PEEP used for alveolar expansion. According to the FDA, HFV is any form of mechanical ventilation that delivers respiratory rates that are greater than 150 per minute. High-frequency rates are expressed in hertz (Hz), where 1 Hz is equal to 60 cycles per minute or one cycle per second. Amplitude refers to peak-to-peak pressures or the difference between peak inspiratory pressure (PIP) and positive end-expiratory pressure (PEEP). Oxygenation is primarily controlled by adjusting the mean airway pressure, whereas carbon dioxide removal is a result of the amplitude pressure.

Conventional ventilation that depends on the bulk movement of gas in and out of the lungs may require high pressures and volumes in order to achieve adequate oxygenation and ventilation. These high pressures and volumes have been known to contribute to barotrauma and the development of BPD in neonates. Early studies involving HFV showed that adequate ventilation occurred even when tidal volumes far below dead space were used.[13]

The major advantage of delivering small tidal volumes is that it can be done at relatively low pressures, greatly reducing the risk of barotrauma.

Indications

The indications for any type of HFV in the neonatal population are primarily linked to respiratory failure that does not respond to conventional methods of mechanical ventilation. These infants usually have further complications such as pulmonary air leaks or persistent pulmonary hypertension that would be exacerbated by positive pressure ventilation.[14] High-frequency oscillatory ventilation (HFOV) has been shown to be a safe and effective rescue technique in treating patients who have failed conventional ventilation,[15] in newborns with congenital diaphragmatic hernia,[16] and in neonates with RDS or air leak syndrome.[17]

The benefits of HFV for the pediatric population are becoming more apparent. A study by Arnold (1994) demonstrated that HFOV offered rapid and sustained improvements in oxygenation without adverse effects on ventilation in patients with diffuse alveolar disease or air leak syndrome.[18] Other studies have reported decreased mortality in pediatric patients with ARDS as a result of HFV.[19]

Hazards

As with any method of mechanical ventilation, there are problems associated with HFV as well. HFV has been known to cause gas trapping, hyperinflation, obstruction of the airway with secretions, hypotension, and **necrotizing tracheobronchitis**.[20, 21] Furthermore, chest assessment of patients on HFV is difficult. Assessment for adequate ventilation is based on chest wall vibration (wiggle) rather than chest rise and fall. A decrease in chest wall vibration with an increased $PaCO_2$ without a decrease in PaO_2 may indicate an obstruction or malposition of the ETT. Decreased lung compliance and pneumothoraces are observed by a decrease in chest wall vibration, increase in $PaCO_2$ and a decrease in PaO_2. The infant should be assessed for signs of pallor, cyanosis, bradycardia, hypotension, and increased respiratory effort, all of which indicate a worsening of status.

Types of High-Frequency Ventilators

High-frequency ventilators deliver rates between 150 and 3000 bpm. The major types of HFV are categorized by the frequency of ventilation and the method with which the tidal volume is delivered. The four categories examined here are high-frequency positive pressure ventilation (HFPPV), high-flow jet ventilation (HFJV), high-frequency flow interruption (HFFI), and high-frequency oscillatory ventilation (HFOV) (Table 20–2).

High-Frequency Positive Pressure Ventilation High-Frequency Positive Pressure Ventilation (HFPPV) is simply conventional ventilatory breaths delivered at rates between 60 and 150 bpm (1 to 2.5 Hz). The delivery of tidal volume during HFPPV occurs via convective air movement, in which tidal volume exceeds dead space. Studies have shown a reduction in $PaCO_2$ and in F_iO_2 when HFPPV was used. These studies additionally showed a lower rate of pneumothoraces in the neonates ventilated with HFPPV when compared to those receiving conventional ventilation.[14] Other studies have shown that fighting the ventilator by the neonate may be eliminated at ventilatory rates of 100 to 120 bpm.

Table 20–2	
CLASSIFICATION OF HIGH-FREQUENCY VENTILATION	
Mode	**Frequency**
HFPPV	1–2.5 Hz
HFJV	4–11 Hz
HFFI	15 Hz
HFOV	8–30 Hz

High-Frequency Flow Interruption High-frequency flow interruption (HFFI) can deliver frequencies as high as 15 Hz. In this type of HFV a control mechanism, usually a rotating ball with a gas pathway, interrupts a high-pressure gas source in order to deliver rapid rates. As with HFPPV and HFJV, exhalation occurs passively.

High-Frequency Jet Ventilation High-frequency jet ventilators (HFJV) generally operate in the range of 4 to 11 Hz. The high-frequency jet ventilator delivers a high-pressure pulse of gas to the patient airway. This is done through a special adaptor attached to the endotracheal tube, or through a specially designed endotracheal tube that allows the pulsed gas to exit inside the endotracheal tube, depicted in Figure 20–1.

HFJV is used in tandem with conventional ventilators. The purpose of the conventional ventilator is threefold. First, it provides occasional sighs, which help stimulate the production of surfactant and prevent microatelectasis. Second, the conventional ventilator provides PEEP to the patient airway. Third, it makes a continuous flow of gas available at the endotracheal tube for entrainment by the jet ventilation.[20]

High-Frequency Oscillatory Ventilation High-frequency oscillatory ventilation (HFOV) utilizes the highest of rates, usually in the range of 8 to 30 Hz. The oscillatory waves that deliver the gas to the lungs are produced by either an electromagnetically

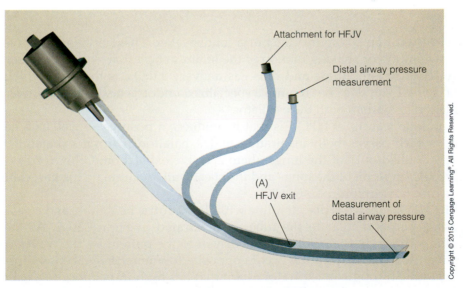

FIGURE 20–1. Endotracheal tube adapted for use with high-frequency jet ventilation. The pulsed jet flow exits into the endotracheal tube at point A.

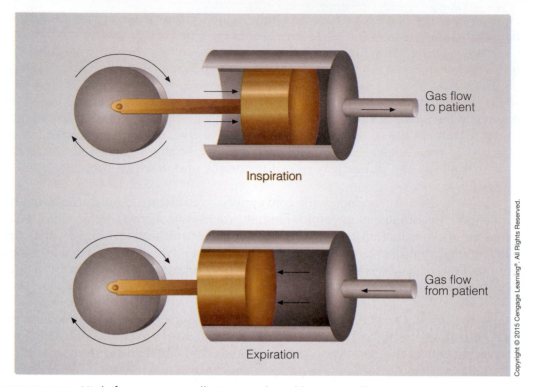

Inspiration

Gas flow
to patient

Gas flow
from patient

Expiration

FIGURE 20–2. High-frequency oscillation produced by an oscillating piston.

driven piston pump (Figure 20–2) or a loudspeaker. These oscillatory waves produce a vibration or shaking motion of the infant's chest that should be observed to verify adequate amplitude and thus gas delivery. HFOV is the most widely used method of HFV. It does not require a specialized endotracheal tube or conventional ventilation in tandem with the oscillator.

A unique feature of HFOV is that it produces a positive as well as a negative stroke, which assists both inspiration and exhalation. During exhalation gas is actively "pulled-out" of the lungs; there is active exhalation. Other forms of HFV simply rely on recoil of the lungs and the chest wall to eliminate the gas; exhalation in this case is, therefore, passive.

The HFOV device is placed inline with the endotracheal tube, and a gas source is passed perpendicular to the tube, as illustrated in Figure 20–3. As the fresh gas enters the endotracheal tube, it is driven to the patient by the waves coming from the oscillator. Expiration occurs opposite to where the gas enters the endotracheal tube through an expiratory limb that has high impedance to oscillations, but low impedance when there is a steady flow of gas. Marked swings in pressure between inspiration and expiration to reopen alveoli do not occur during HFOV because the alveoli remain open continuously usually assessed by the mean airway pressure.

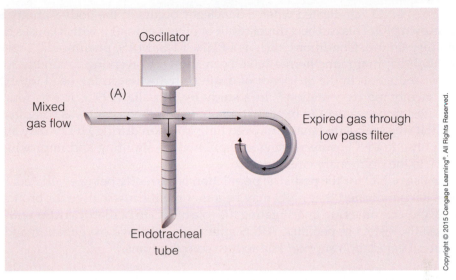

FIGURE 20–3. Mixed gas passes into the endotracheal tube through a side port (A).

SPECIALTY MEDICAL GASES

In addition to oxygen, the administration of other medical gases such as nitric oxide and helium are becoming more popular in respiratory care. Nitric oxide has shown great promise in the treatment of neonates with pulmonary hypertension, while helium has proven its value in severe airway obstructions.

Inhaled Nitric Oxide (i-NO)

Nitric oxide (NO) is a colorless gas that is produced in endothelial cells of the body. In 1987, Palmer and colleagues discovered that NO diffuses from the endothelium into smooth muscle cells that form the vascular walls and is responsible for vascular dilation.[23] NO relaxes vascular smooth muscle by activating guanylate cyclase and increasing the levels of cyclic guanosine 3', 5'-monophosphate (cGMP), which causes vasodilation. Frostell and coworkers (1991) gave experimental proof that when inhaled, NO mimics the effect of naturally released NO and selectively produces pulmonary vasodilation.[24] The pharmacological effect is an increase in oxygenation tension due to dilation of pulmonary vessels in better ventilated areas of the lung.[25]

NO for inhalation is supplied as a gaseous blend of 0.8% NO and 99.2% nitrogen (N_2). The recommended dose of i-NO is upwards of 20 ppm (parts per million) in conjunction with oxygen delivery. Administration of i-NO through a system, such as the INOvent Delivery System provides consistent concentrations of NO throughout the respiration cycle with continuous monitoring of NO, nitrogen dioxide (NO_2), and oxygen concentrations.[26]

Indications i-NO is indicated when a deficiency occurs in the body's ability to produce its own NO. This can be a direct result of illness or injury, which causes hypoxic respiratory failure. Conditions such as PPHN, RDS, MAS, pneumonia, sepsis, and congenital diaphragmatic hernia have been shown to respond favorably to i-NO, by either reduction in the incidence of death or reduction in the need for extracorporeal membrane oxygenation.[27] In a study by Kinsella (1997), it was found that the greatest improvement in oxygenation occurred when i-NO was combined with HFOV.[28] It was speculated that improved lung inflation during HFOV may augment the response to i-NO by decreasing intrapulmonary shunting and improving I-NO delivery to the pulmonary circulation.[28]

The use of NO for the pediatric population is currently being evaluated. Several studies have indicated that i-NO may be a therapeutic alternative for bronchodilation.[19, 29] Other studies are investigating the role of NO in pediatric ARDS with promising results.[30] i-NO in pediatric ARDS appears to improve oxygenation and lower mechanical ventilation support and reduce complications.[29]

Outcomes Positive outcomes require that the patient be monitored for **methemoglobinemia** and NO_2. Methemoglobinemia results when NO comes into contact with blood and binds with the hemoglobin to form nitrosylhemoglobin (NOHb). The presence of oxygen causes nitrosylhemoglobin to become oxidized, forming methemoglobin and NO_2. Once the NO_2 is excreted in the urine, methemoglobin is enzymatically reduced to hemoglobin again. NO_2 levels should not exceed 5 ppm by Occupational Safety and Health Administration (OSHA) standards. Clinically, the goal is to maintain NO_2 levels below 2 ppm during NO administration[31]. This requires accurate and continuous monitoring of NO_2 production. Without accurate monitoring of delivered i-NO and NO_2 production, the patient may develop pulmonary edema, injury, and death.[32]

Care must be taken in the withdrawal of i-NO. A sudden withdrawal of i-NO may cause a rebound effect, resulting in pulmonary hypertension and hypoxemia.[33] Recommended guidelines are that, first, the lowest effective i-NO dose, often less than 10 ppm, be used. Withdrawal should not be considered until the patient shows marked clinical improvement; the patient should be hemodynamically stable on an F_iO_2 less than 40% with a PEEP of 5 cm H_2O or less. If the patient meets these criteria the next recommended step is to increase the F_iO_2 to 60% to 70% before withdrawal of i-NO, and prepare to support the patient hemodynamically if necessary. i-NO withdrawal has been well tolerated when these guidelines are followed.[33]

Heliox Therapy

Helium (He) and oxygen (O_2) mixtures have been used therapeutically since as early as the 1930s. Because of helium's known low density and its being inert, it makes it an ideal gas to mix with oxygen to reduce both turbulence in airflow and resistive pressure in the airways. The therapeutic result is reduction in airway resistance and respiratory muscle work. Delivery of O_2 as well as medicated aerosols can, thus, be enhanced when He is used in place of nitrogen.

Indications The primary indication for heliox therapy is during any clinical situation where airway obstruction prevents or significantly impedes the delivery of gas flow throughout the airways. Clinically, this can be seen during severe bronchospasm or upper airway obstruction due to infection or foreign body aspiration. This may include infants and children with severe asthma, laryngotracheobronchitis, or postextubation stridor.

Heliox can be delivered in 60:40 to 75:25 blends of He and O_2, depending on the patient's F_iO_2 needs. However, as the amount of O_2 increases in the mixture, above 30%, the less the benefit in reducing airway resistance.[34] Heliox can be delivered by a nonrebreather face mask to nonintubated patients or directly to a mechanical ventilator in cases requiring intubation and ventilatory support. Heliox can also be used to power pneumatic nebulizers when aerosolized medication delivery is indicated.

Outcomes Patients treated with heliox therapy during severe asthma showed improvement in $PaCO_2$, pH, increased peak expiratory flow rates, and reduction in the work of breathing. Intubated and mechanically ventilated patients with severe bronchospasm showed reduction in peak inspiratory pressures and $PaCO_2$. All patients on heliox therapy should be monitored for oxygenation either by pulse oximetry or arterial blood gas analysis.

EXTRACORPOREAL LIFE SUPPORT (ECLS)

Oxygenation of blood outside the body, through a membrane oxygenator, was first developed for use in open heart surgery in the 1950s. The technology continued to improve and modifications allowed the long-term use of the technique in the 1960s.[13]

The first use of the extracorporeal membrane oxygenator on an infant was described in 1971.[35] This paved the way for science to perfect and refine the technique used today in many institutions across the country.

Because of the potential risks associated with ELCS, selection is based on strict criteria and only those infants who are at an 80% or greater risk of mortality should be treated with ECLS. Several authors have proposed the use of the alveolar-arterial oxygen difference $P(A\text{-}a)O_2$ or the oxygen index (OI), determined by multiplying the F_iO_2 and the mean airway pressure and dividing by PaO_2 to select infants for inclusion to ECLS. As assessments of the ability of the lungs to transfer oxygen across the alveolar-capillary membrane, these measurements assist in determining eligibility for support. Furthermore, it is recommended that infants at a gestational age less than 35 weeks and those with preexisting intraventricular hemorrhage (IVH) be excluded. ECLS candidates are also excluded in some institutions if they have been managed with conventional mechanical ventilation (CMV) for as little as 7 days. Bower and Petit (1994) report success of these long-term CMV infants diagnosed with bronchopulmonary dysplasia (BPD).[17] (See Table 20–3.)

Mechanisms of Bypass

There are two types of ECLS procedures: venoarterial and venovenous.

Table 20–3

RECOMMENDED CRITERIA FOR ECLS

Include infants with:
  A-a difference: >620 torr for 6–12 hours
  Oxygen Index: >40 for 1–6 hours

Exclude infants with:
  Gestational Age: <35 weeks
  Preexisting Conditions: Intraventricular hemorrhage
                          Conventional ventilaton >7 days

Venoarterial In the **venoarterial** route, blood is drawn from the right atrium via the internal jugular vein. The oxygenated blood is returned to the aortic arch via the right common carotid artery, as shown in Figure 20–4. Venoarterial ECLS not only oxygenates the blood, but also supports the cardiac function of the patient by ensuring systemic circulation.

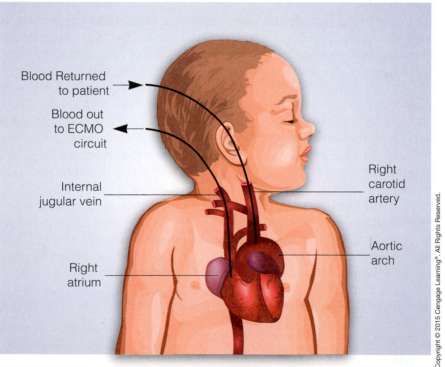

Blood Returned to patient

Blood out to ECMO circuit

Internal jugular vein

Right atrium

Right carotid artery

Aortic arch

FIGURE 20–4. Placement of ECLS catheter when the venoarterial route is used.

Venovenous In the **venovenous** route, blood is removed from the right atrium via a catheter inserted in the right internal jugular vein. The oxygenated blood is returned to the right atrium through a catheter inserted via the femoral vein. This method oxygenates the blood, but does not support cardiac output.

ECLS Circuit The ECLS circuit utilizes a modified heart-lung bypass machine consisting of a venous-blood drainage reservoir, a blood pump, the membrane oxygenator where the exchange of O_2 and CO_2 takes place, and a heat exchanger to maintain body temperature. Figure 20–5 depicts a typical ECLS circuit.

Complications

Complications of ECLS are both technical and physiologic. Common physiologic complications of ECLS are those related to bleeding, secondary to the high level of heparin required for anticoagulation.[36]

Cardiovascular complications arise from both low and high circulating volumes leading to hypo- and hypertension in the infant. Anemia, leukopenia, and **thrombocytopenia** are all possible hematologic complications caused by the consumption of blood components by the membrane oxygenator.[13] Due to the invasive nature of ECLS with tubes and catheters, there is also an increased risk of infection.

Technical complications that may arise during ECLS include failure of the pump, rupture of the tubing, failure of the membrane, and difficulties with the cannuls.[37]

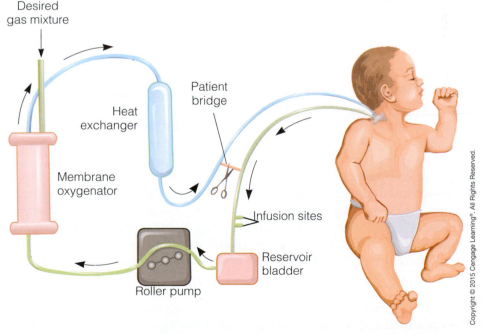

FIGURE 20–5. A typical ECLS circuit.

Outcomes The use of ECLS has added an important tool in the care of patients who previously had no hope. As of October 1994, 9663 neonates had been treated with ECLS with an overall survival rate of 81%, while 845 pediatric patients were treated with a survival rate of 51%.[17] The survival rate appears to be related to the severity of lung disease and to the occurrence of ECLS complications, not the length of time on ECLS.[38]

Due to the invasive nature of the procedure and severity of disease, the outcome of surviving patients may involve serious, long-term problems. Problems such as cerebral palsy, visual and hearing loss, seizures, and severe cognitive disabilities were seen in a higher percentage of ECLS patients than those treated conventionally.[39] Impairment of renal function and marked fluid retention appear to be unique complications when the venovenous route of ECLS is used.[40]

The need for ECLS has declined in patients managed with SRT and HFOV. Furthermore, the use of I-NO may also reduce the use of ECLS in patients with PPHN. Despite this decline, ECLS remains an important life support option for a very select group of critically ill infants.

PARTIAL LIQUID VENTILATION

An exciting technology in the area of neonatal ventilation is partial liquid ventilation (PLV). Although not a new concept, the ability to successfully utilize this technology has only recently been developed. The concept behind liquid ventilation is to obliterate the air/liquid interface at the alveoli and thus substantially lower surface tension. Mechanical inflation could then occur at pressures low enough to not damage lung tissues.

Many substances have been used through the years. In the first experiments, saline was used. It proved, however, to be a poor carrier of oxygen and was too viscous and dense when compared to gas. Other substances, such as oils and silicone, which have a high capacity to carry gases, proved to be toxic to the lungs. Perfluorochemical (PFC) liquids are the first substances that have been shown to support respiration while remaining relatively nontoxic to the lungs.

PFCs have a very high solubility for oxygen and carbon dioxide, and minimize pulmonary surface tension. They are inert, odorless, clear liquids derived from common organic compounds.[41]

PLV with perfluorocarbon liquid occurs by using the liquid to recruit atelectatic lung tissue and reduce surface tension in the alveolar lining. During exhalation the liquid acts as a reservoir of oxygen, preventing alveolar collapse and intrapulmonary shunting. With the next inspiration, tidal volume gas removes carbon dioxide from the liquid and replenishes it with a new supply of dissolved oxygen.

Uses

PLV has potential application for use in several diseases that traditionally have been difficult to treat. Included are RDS, aspiration syndromes, persistent pulmonary hypertension of the newborn, and pneumonia.[41] PLV has been shown to improve pulmonary gas exchange, lung compliance, and reduce lung injury.[42] PLV has been shown to be compatible with surfactant administration, and may even be superior to surfactant.[43]

Clinical trials with perflubron (LiquiVent) in infants with RDS have shown a decrease in mortality rates as well as physiologic improvements in gas exchange and lung compliance.

While the potential of a favorable impact on the treatment of neonates is nearer, more research is still necessary before PLV takes its place among current treatment modalities.

NEGATIVE PRESSURE VENTILATION (NPV)

Although not technically a "new" concept in ventilation, NPV continues to draw interest as a method of ventilation. NPV utilized the application of negative pressure to the external thorax, causing the thorax to expand. The negative pressure generated within the thorax then causes air to enter the lungs (Figure 20–6). Because it mimics normal spontaneous breathing patterns, cardiopulmonary complications that result from positive pressure are not seen.

The concept of NPV was the primary factor that led to the development of the Drinker iron lung in 1928. Researchers have subsequently scaled the iron lung down

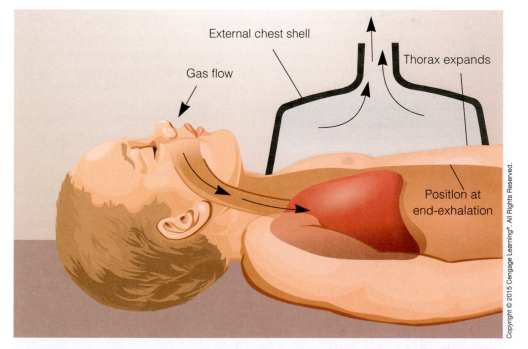

FIGURE 20–6. Negative pressure exerted on the external thorax causes the thorax to expand, allowing gas to enter the lungs.

to allow the technique to be used on infants. Even with some initial success, NPV was never accepted as an alternative to PPV, possibly due to the inconvenience created by limited access to the infant as well as limited success on the infant with severe IRDS.

Current Use

Current research is focusing on an application of NPV that involves the use of high-frequency technology. In one such technology, termed transthoracic oscillation, a chest shell is placed on the infant and pressure is generated external to the thorax at high frequencies. This external pressure causes a forced exhalation, with inhalation occurring passively from chest recoil. A study using this technology showed an improvement in gas exchange and a significant reduction in respiratory rate.[44]

The major advantage to the use of NPV is that ventilation can be accomplished with little risk of barotrauma and the complications of invasive positive pressure ventilation.[45] Additionally, the cardiac system is not compromised as it is during positive pressure ventilation. Disadvantages include poor access to the patient, pressure sores at contact points, and air leaks.

SUMMARY

The advent of new, nonconventional ventilatory techniques and procedures in neonatal and pediatric care has changed the way these patients are treated in a dramatic way. Nothing has had quite as profound an effect in the treatment of ventilator failure as surfactant replacement therapy. While the need for replacement has been understood for many years, only fairly recently has the ability to produce useful surfactants and a method to deliver them, been developed. It is well understood that prematurity predisposes a newborn's lungs to surfactant deficiency, leading to decreased compliance and RDS. Surfactant replacement therapy appears to reduce the severity of RDS and its consequences. Continuing research will undoubtedly uncover further uses for surfactant allowing successful use in all patients.

High-frequency ventilation has been investigated for many years. Early researchers noted that hummingbirds breathe in synchrony with their wing beats, in excess of 2000 times per minute. Observation of a dog on a hot day reveals panting breaths that may approach 200 breaths per minute. The traditional idea of ventilation is that the inhaled tidal volume must be greater than the dead space. It is obvious that at respiratory rates of several hundred to thousands of breaths per minute, the tidal volume is not exceeding dead space. Although the exact mechanism of gas movement with high-frequency ventilation is not fully understood, it appears as though a continuous flow of gas is created. This allows gas exchange to take place continuously and at lower pressures than those required with conventional ventilation.

The four types of high-frequency ventilation are: high-frequency positive pressure ventilation (HFPPV), high-frequency flow interruption (HFFI), high-frequency jet ventilation (HFJV), and high-frequency oscillation (HFO). Each mode delivers its breaths by a different modality. Additionally, each mode operates within a certain frequency: HFPPV between 60 and 150 bpm, HFJV between 250 and 640 bpm, and HFOV between 500 and 2000 bpm.

Another nonconventional therapy that has gained renewed interest in recent years, is extracorporeal life support (ECLS). With ECLS, blood is removed from the patient, passed through a membrane oxygenator, and returned to the patient. Routes of blood removal and return are either venoarterial, in which the blood is removed from the right atrium and returned to the aortic arch, or venovenous, in which the blood is removed and returned to the right atrium. Because of its invasive nature, it is only used on those patients at an 80% or greater risk of mortality. Methods used to determine candidates include the A-a gradient and the oxygen index.

Specialty medical gases have gained popularity in the care of the infant and pediatric patient in recent years. Nitric oxides use as a potent pulmonary vasodilator has proven to be successful in the treatment of PPHN and illness that cause pulmonary hypertension. Heliox has shown success when used in the treatment of severe airway obstruction such as asthma, upper airway, and postintubation inflammation.

Partial liquid ventilation is an exciting new ventilatory technique that has the potential of ventilating at low pressures. The liquids, perfluorochemicals, have been shown to be relatively nontoxic to the lungs, and able to support respiration. As the liquid enters the alveoli, surface tension is obliterated by removing the air-gas interface. Thoracic expansion can then take place with minimal pressure.

Finally, the use of negative pressure ventilation has given rise to less invasive ventilation of the infant and pediatric patient, minimizing the complications of invasive conventional mechanical ventilation.

POSTTEST

1. Rescue surfactant is given:
    a. as quickly as possible following delivery
    b. to any patient less than 32 weeks' gestation
    c. before the onset of RDS symptoms
    d. after the onset of RDS symptoms
2. Artificial surfactant is best administered:
    a. directly instilled into the endotracheal tube
    b. nebulized into the endotracheal tube
    c. through a peripheral IV site
    d. adding it to the ventilator circuitry
3. The major advantage to HFV is:
    a. improved oxygenation
    b. improved ventilation
    c. reduced barotrauma
    d. reduced cost

4. The convective movement of a tidal volume that is larger than dead space is achieved with:
   a. HFPPV
   b. HFJV
   c. HFOV
   d. HFV

5. All of the following are hazards of HFV except:
   a. air trapping
   b. hypertension
   c. hyperinflation
   d. necrotizing tracheobronchitis

6. While managing a patient receiving HFOV the respiratory care practitioner notices that the PaO_2 is decreased. This can be corrected by all of the following except:
   a. increasing the PEEP
   b. increasing the frequency
   c. increasing the amplitude
   d. increasing the PIP

7. Which of the following HFV methods requires the use of an adapted ETT?
   a. HFFI
   b. HFPPV
   c. HFJV
   d. HFOV

8. Which of the following describes the venoarterial route of ECLS?
   a. Blood is taken from the subclavian vein and returned to the subclavian artery.
   b. Blood is taken from the femoral vein and returned to the femoral artery.
   c. Blood is taken from the right atrium and returned to the aortic arch.
   d. Blood is taken from the pulmonary vein and returned to the pulmonary artery.

9. Two criteria used to determine potential ECLS patients are:
   a. patient age and weight
   b. level of $PaCO_2$ and pH
   c. level of hypoxemia and ventilatory support
   d. A-a gradient and the oxygen index

10. The most common complication of ECLS is:
    a. infection
    b. bleeding
    c. barotrauma
    d. machine failure

11. An advantage to the use of negative pressure ventilation is:
    a. better access to the patient
    b. less cost to the patient
    c. allows the use of lower F_iO_2
    d. reduced cardiopulmonary complications

12. Which of the following is not true regarding partial liquid ventilation?
    a. It reduces infection.
    b. Improves pulmonary gas exchange.
    c. Improves lung compliance.
    d. Reduces lung injury.

REFERENCES

1. Jobe AH, Ikegami M. Surfactant metabolism. *Clin Perinat.* 20(4):65–73, 1993.
2. Holm BA, Waring, AJ. "Designer surfactants: the next generation in surfactant replacement." *Clin Perinat.* 20(4):813–29, 1993.
3. AARC Clinical practice guideline: surfactant replacement therapy. *Resp Care.* 39(8):824–829, 1994.
4. Jobe A, Ikegami M. The future of surfactant replacement therapy. *Neonatal Resp Dis.* 7(4):2–10, 1997.
5. Willson D, et al. Calf's lung surfactant extract in acute hypoxemic respiratory failure in children. *Crit Care Med.* 24(8):1316–1322, 1996
6. Bloom B, et al. Comparison of Infasurf (calf lung surfacant extract) to Survanta (beractant) in the treatment and prevention of respiratory distress syndrome. *Pediatrics.* 100(1):31–38, 1997.
7. Forest Pharmaceuticals.
8. GlaxoWellcome.
9. Jackson JC, et al. Reduction in lung injury after combined surfactant and high-frequency ventilation. *Am J Resp Crit Care Med.* 150(2):534–9, 1994.
10. Colburn S, et al. Nitric oxide and surfactant replacement in pediatric ARDS. *RT J Resp Care Pract.* 13(4):84–87, 2000.
11. Perez-Benavides F, et al. Adult respiratory distress syndrome and artificial surfactant replacement in the pediatric patient. *Pediatr Emerg Care.* 11(3): 153–155, 1994.
12. Willson, 1996
13. Carlo WA, Chatburn RL. *Neonatal Respiratory Care,* 2nd ed. Chicago, IL: Year Book Medical Publishers Inc., 1988.
14. Boynton BR. High-frequency ventilation in newborn infants. *Resp Care.* 31(6):480–487, 1986.
15. Clark RH, et al. Prospective, randomized comparison of high-frequency oscillation and conventional ventilation in candidates for extracorporeal membrane oxygenation. *J Pediatr.* 124(3):447–54, 1994.
16. Miguet D, et al. Preoperative stabilization using high-frequency oscillatory ventilation in the management of congenital diaphragmatic hernia. *Crit Care Med.* 22(9 suppl):s77–s82, 1994.
17. Bower L, Betit P. Extracorporeal life support and high frequency oscillatory ventilation: alternatives for the neonate in severe respiratory failure. *Resp Care.* 40(1):61–73, 1994.

18. Arnold, J.H. et al. "Prospective, randomized comparison of high-frequency oscillatory ventilation and conventional mechanical ventilation in pediatric respiratory failure" Crit Care Med. 1994 Oct;22(10):1530–9.

19. Rowan, CM et al. "Preemptive use of high-frequency oscillatory ventilation in pediatric burn patients" J Burn Care Res. 2013 Mar-Apr;34(2):237–42.

20. Gordin P. High-frequency jet ventilation for severe respiratory failure. *Pediatr Nurs.* 15(6):625–629, 1989.

21. Richardson C. Hyaline membrane disease: future treatment modalities. *J Perinat Neonat Nurs.* 2(1):78–88, 1988.

23. Palmer RMJ, et al. Nitric oxide release accounts for biological activity of endothelium derived relaxing factor. *Nature.* 327:524–526, 1987.

24. Frostell CG, et al. Inhaled nitric oxide: A selective pulmonary vasodilator reversing hypoxic pulmonary vasoconstriction. *Circulation.* 83:2038–2047, 1991.

25. Okamoto, K. et al. "Efficacy of Inhaled Nitric Oxide in Children With ARDS" Chest 114:827–833, 1998.

26. http://inomax.com/inomax-delivery-systems.

27. Committee on Fetus and Newborn. "Use of Inhaled Nitric Oxide" PEDIATRICS Vol. 106 No. 2 August 1, 2000 pp. 344–345.

28. Kinsella, J.P. et al. "Early Inhaled Nitric Oxide Therapy in Premature Newborns with Respiratory Failure" N Engl J Med 2006; 355:354–364.

29. Pfeffer, K.D. et al. "The effect of inhaled nitric oxide in pediatric asthma" AmJRespCritCareMed Vol. 153, No. 2 (1996), pp. 747–51.

30. Thompson J, et al. Pediatric application of inhaled nitric oxide. *Resp. Care.* 44(2):177–182, 1999.

31. Okamoto K, et al. Efficacy of inhaled nitric oxide in children with ARDS. *Chest.* 114(3):827–833, 1998.

32. Roberts J. Inhaled nitric oxide for hypoxemic respiratory failure of the newborn. *Resp. Care.* 44(2):169–173, 1999.

33. Hess D. Adverse effects and toxicity of inhaled nitric oxide. *Resp. Care.* 44(3):315–328, 1999.

34. Manthous C, et al. Heliox in the treatment of airflow obstruction: a critical review of the literature. *Resp Care.* 42(11):1034–1042, 1997.

35. Zwishchengerger JB, et al. The role of extracorporeal membrane oxygenation in the management of respiratory failure in the newborn. *Resp. Care.* 31(6):491–495, 1986.

36. Wilson B. Extracorporeal and intracorporeal techniques for the treatment of severe respiratory failure. *Resp. Care.* 41(4):306–317, 1996.

37. Donn SM. ECMO indications and complications. *Hosp Practice.* 25(6):143–146,1990.

38. Green TP, et al. Probability of survival after prolonged extracorporeal membrane oxygenation in pediatric patients with acute respiratory failure. *Crit Care Med.* 23(6):1132, 1995.

39. Robertson CM, et al. Neurodevelopmental outcome after neonatal extracorporeal membrane oxygenation. *Can Med Assoc.* 152(12):1981–1988, 1995.

40. Roy BJ, et al. Venovenous extracorporeal membrane oxygenation affects renal function. *Pediatrics.* 95(4):573, 1995.
41. Greenspan JS. Liquid ventilation: a developing technology. *Neonatal Network.* 12(4):23–28, 1993.
43. Hirschl RB, et al. Liquid ventilation improves pulmonary function, gas exchange, and lung injury in a model of respiratory failure. *Ann Surg.* 221(1):79–88, 1995.
43. Leach CL, et al. Partial liquid ventilation in premature lambs with respiratory distress syndrome: Efficacy and compatibility with exogenous surfactant. *J Pediatr.* 126(3):412–420, 1995.
44. Hardinge FM, et al. Effects of short term high frequency negative pressure ventilation on gas exchange using the Hayet oscillator in normal subjects. *Thorax.* 50(1):44–49, 1995.
45. Klonin H, et al. Negative pressure ventilation via chest cuirass to decrease ventilator-associated complications in infants with acute respiratory failure: a case series. *Respiratory Care.* 45(5):486–493, 2000.

BIBLIOGRAPHY AND SUGGESTED READINGS

Clark RH. High-frequency ventilation in acute pediatric respiratory failure (editorial) *Chest.* 105(3):98, 1994.

Fuhrman B et al. Partial liquid ventilation and the challenges of randomized, controlled trials in acute respiratory distress syndrome. *Resp Care.* 43(12): 1086–1091, 1998.

Gross GW, et al. Use of liquid ventilation with perflubron during extracorporeal membrane oxygenation: chest radiographic appearances. *Radiology.* 194(3): 717–720, 1995.

Jobe A. Surfactant treatment for respiratory distress syndrome. *Resp Care.* 31(6):467–476, 1986.

Short BL. Extracorporeal membrane oxygenation, in GB Avery et al. (eds.) *Neonatology: Pathophysiology and Management of the Newborn.* 4th ed. Philadelphia, PA: J.B. Lippincott Co., 1994.

UNIT FIVE

Advanced and Specialty Care

Remember to breathe. It is after all, the secret of life.
—*Gregory Maguire, A Lion Among Men*

OBJECTIVES

Upon completion of this chapter, the reader should be able to:

1. Describe the levels of NICU's and how each is defined.
2. Define regionalization and the role of transport.
3. Compare and contrast the types of transport, with regard to distances covered, advantages, and disadvantages.
4. Discuss the effects of altitude on PaO_2 and discuss the changes required in F_iO_2 as altitude increases to maintain PaO_2.
5. Describe the effects of altitude on closed air spaces.
6. Describe the skills required by transport personnel.
7. List the equipment needed for transport and describe the modifications required for use during transport.
8. Calculate the duration of oxygen flow with an E and H cylinder when given necessary data.
9. Discuss the preparation required before transporting an infant.
10. Describe four methods to help thermoregulate an infant during transport.
11. Describe the care and transport of the following disorders:
    a. Diaphragmatic hernia
    b. Tracheoesophageal fistula
    c. Omphalocele
    d. Gastroschisis
    e. Meningomyelocele
    f. Cyanotic heart disease

KEY TERMS

Dalton's law	Kling gauze	omphalocele
DeLee suction	maternal thyrotoxicosis	regionalization
gastroschisis	maternal transport	
hypobaric	meningomyelocele	

INTRODUCTION

There are a large number of newborns that require transport to an NICU or other care unit. These neonates have medical and/or surgical problems that require advanced support and care. The term "outborn" has been used to describe these neonates who are cared for in a different facility from where they were born. There is evidence that outcomes improve with expert care and decreased transfer times.[1] Transport requires highly skilled health care personnel and specialized equipment. This chapter will review those skills required for a successful transport.

HISTORY

As neonatal medicine grew increasingly more sophisticated, it became apparent that not every hospital could afford the necessary equipment and personnel or had sufficient births to justify having a NICU. All hospitals that deliver babies, however, must have access to a NICU for those times when a compromised neonate is born.

A possible solution to this problem was presented in a 1976 March of Dimes report *Toward Improving the Outcome of Pregnancy*. This report stratified neonatal care into three levels of complexity along with the recommendation to refer all high-risk patients to those facilities with the resources to care for the patient. This led to a widespread **regionalization** of neonatal care that occurred during the late 1970s and into the 1980s, with one hospital in a specified geographic region providing a level II or level III NICU. The original designation of level I, II, and III NICUs is outlined in Table 21–1.

Table 21–1

ORIGINAL DESIGNATION LEVELS OF NICUs

Level I
- Care for uncomplicated maternity and neonatal cases
- Competent emergency care for unanticipated obstetric or neonatal complications
- Early identification of high-risk maternal and neonatal patients
- Provision of social services and other preventative assistance

Level II
- Total care of uncomplicated maternal and neonatal cases and 75%–90% high-risk patients
- Ability to perform cesarean deliveries with a short start-up time (usually less than 15 minutes)
- In-house obstetric anesthesia with 24-hour coverage

- Ability to provide short-term mechanical ventilation of newborns and therapeutic respiratory care with 24-hour coverage
- 24-hour laboratory, radiology, and blood bank services
- Ability to provide fetal monitoring
- Special nursery for providing care

Level III

- Total care of all maternal and neonatal cases, including all high-risk patients
- 24-hour consultation assistance for hospitals within the region
- Methods and personnel to transport patients from any hospital within region to the level III nursery
- Provisions and personnel to coordinate educational program for the region
- Provides data analysis for the region

In 1993 the March of Dimes Birth Defects Foundation published a follow-up report, *Toward Improving the Outcome of Pregnancy: The 90s and Beyond*. This landmark publication reaffirmed the importance of an integrated system of regionalized care. At that time NICU designations were changed from levels I, II, and III to basic, specialty, and subspecialty, and the criteria for each were expanded.[2] These new definitions were adopted by the American College of Obstetricians and Gynecologists and included in their "Guidelines for Perinatal Care." Despite these new classifications, how they were interpreted and implemented varied dramatically within the United States. In an attempt to clarify the roles of varying levels of NICU's, the American Academy of Pediatrics published a policy, "Levels of Neonatal Care" in 2004.[3] That committee recommended alterations to the NICU classifications and definitions by incorporating data on clinical outcomes, resource allocation and utilization, and service delivery. Their recommendations are shown in Table 21–2.

Since the mid-1980s the number of both neonatologists and NICUs has grown substantially. Despite that trend, there is no evidence to support a lowering of

---

Table 21–2

AAP LEVELS OF NEONATAL CARE

- Level I (basic):
  - Perform neonatal resuscitation, evaluation, and postnatal care of healthy newborns
  - Ability to stabilize newborns at 35 to 37 weeks gestation who remain stable
  - Ability to stabilize newborns less than 35 weeks gestation until transfer for appropriate level facility

continued on the next page

Table 21–2

continued from the previous page

- Level II (specialty):
  - Ability to care for newborns over 35 weeks gestation with physiologic immaturity; who are ill but are expected to stabilize rapidly; non urgent
  - Ability to provide mechanical ventilation for less than 24 hours

- Level III (subspecialty):
  - Ability to provide continuous life support for high risk newborn with critical illness
  - Level IIIA — newborns more than 28 weeks gestation and continuous life support limited to conventional mechanical ventilation
  - Level IIIB — newborns less than 28 weeks gestation needing advanced respiratory care, medical specialists, advanced imaging, urgent
  - Level IIIC — ability to perform surgical repair of critical cardiac functions

Source: Levels of Neonatal Care, Policy Statement from the American Academy of Pediatrics. *Pediatrics.* 130(3):587–597, September 1, 2012.

neonatal mortality with the increase in NICU's.[4] Regionalization allows for a localization of equipment, resources, and experts and avoids costly duplications.

One key element in a successful regionalization effort is a method to transport mothers and neonates from outlying hospitals to the regional center to receive care. Transport allows expert personnel and sophisticated equipment needed to provide the appropriate level of care for the high-risk mother or the compromised neonate. Transport, therefore, is the vital link that connects the rural and smaller hospitals to the advanced care that is found in the NICU.

The major goal of transport is to bring a high-risk mother or a distressed neonate to a tertiary care center in stable condition where advanced care can then be given. Possible indications for transport are listed in Table 21–3.

Table 21–3

COMMON PROBLEMS THAT MAY REQUIRE TRANSPORT

1. Obstetric problems
   a. Premature rupture of the amniotic membranes
   b. Premature labor
   c. Bleeding during the third trimester
   d. Rh incompatibility
   e. Twins, triplets, etc.
   f. Severe maternal eclampsia or preeclampsia
   g. Premature dilation of the cervix
   h. Presence of intrauterine growth retardation with signs of fetal distress

2. Surgical problems
    a. Congenital heart defect
    b. Diaphragmatic hernia
    c. Neural tube defects
    d. Abdominal defects (gastroschisis, etc.)
    e. Hydrocephalus
    f. Maternal problems
        I. Any trauma requiring intensive care
        II. Abdominal or thoracic surgery

3. Medical problems
    a. Severe maternal infection or maternal infection that may affect the fetus or cause premature delivery
    b. Maternal drug overdose
    c. Worsening maternal renal disease
    d. **Maternal thyrotoxicosis**
    e. Class 3 to 4 organic heart disease
    f. Persistent pulmonary hypertension (PPH)

TYPES OF TRANSPORT

There are a variety of ways to transport a neonate in a safe and effective manner. The preferred method is to get the mother to the appropriate care center prior to delivery; however, that is not always possible. In those circumstances, highly trained medical personnel, using specialized equipment are called on to safely and effectively transfer the neonate.

Maternal Transport

The ideal method of transporting a neonate is while it is still in utero, called **maternal transport**. While sophisticated neonatal transport techniques have improved the safety of transporting infants, research shows that in utero transports are safer than postbirth neonatal transports. Morbidity, mortality, and length of hospital intervention remain lower for maternal in utero transportation.[5] The identification of high-risk mothers, using the criteria outlined in Chapter 2, makes it possible to transport the mother still carrying the fetus to the regional center, where both can receive the necessary care.

Unfortunately, not all sick neonates are identified before birth. Many are born in a compromised condition with no indication of their status before birth. This problem necessitates a mechanism of transport that allows the NICU team to be taken to the referring hospital to care for the neonate and then transport the patient back to the NICU. This "portable NICU" is accomplished either by ground, in an ambulance or a customized van, or by air, in a helicopter or fixed-wing aircraft. The means of transport used depends on the location of the NICU and the distances and terrain that need to be covered to access each of the hospitals within the region (Table 21–4).

Table 21–4

MODES OF MATERNAL AND NEONATAL TRANSPORT

Ground
Most efficient within a 25-mile radius of referring hospital.

Advantages:

a. Can be used when there is unavailability of landing sites for a helicopter or fixed-wing aircraft
b. Can be used when inclement weather prevents air travel
c. Usually provides more work area
d. Less vibration and noise than helicopter

Disadvantages:

a. Obstacles on the ground and difficult terrain may tremendously slow the transport.
b. Slowest mode of transport

Helicopter
Most efficient with distances up to 150 miles.

Advantages:

a. Faster mode of transport than ground methods
b. May be faster for shorter distances if ground conditions or terrain make ground transport impractical
c. Does not require a landing strip, can land at or near the hospital

Disadvantages:

a. High noise and vibration levels make assessment and monitoring difficult.
b. May become grounded during inclement weather
c. Small work area
d. Lighting in the patient area after nightfall may interfere with the pilot's vision.
e. Requires highly trained crew
f. Expensive to operate and maintain helicopter
g. Hypobaric effects on patient and equipment

Fixed-wing Aircraft
Most efficient for distances of greater than 150 miles.

Advantages:

a. Able to travel long distances in a short time
b. Less vibration and noise than helicopter
c. Able to travel at higher altitudes, possibly flying over areas of inclement weather or other obstacles

Disadvantages:

a. Must land at an airport, requiring ground transport of the patient between the hospital and aircraft
b. May be grounded in inclement weather
c. Small work area
d. Crew must understand the effects of altitude on the patient
e. Expensive to operate and maintain aircraft
f. Hypobaric effects on patient and equipment

Ground Transport

Under normal circumstances, transports of less than 25 miles are best handled by ground via a critical care ambulance.[6] The advantages of ground transport are that it can be done in more diverse weather conditions, and if difficulties arise during transport that require invasive procedures, the vehicle can be stopped, quieting the vibrations that may hinder the procedure.

The main disadvantage to ground transport is that it is relatively slow, and it may be limited by obstacles such as traffic jams, and natural boundaries. An example of a transport ambulance is shown in Figure 21–1.

Air Transport

There are two primary methods of air transport, helicopter and fixed wing. This section will examine each, along with the advantages and disadvantages.

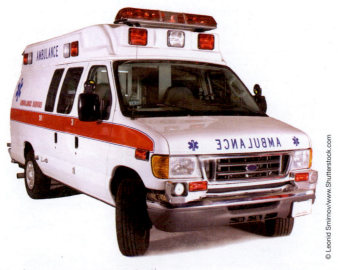

© Leonid Smirnov/www.Shutterstock.com

FIGURE 21–1. Critical care transport ambulance.

Helicopter Air transport by helicopter is normally indicated for distances of up to 150 miles.[6] It is also the preferred method of transport where difficult terrain makes ground transport too time-consuming or even impossible.

The major disadvantage to helicopter transport is the noise level and the vibrations that accompany the ride. The speed of the helicopter, however, makes up for these inconveniences. The main advantage over fixed-wing aircraft is the ability to land at or near the hospital, saving valuable time. Figure 21–2 shows a typical transport helicopter.

Fixed-Wing Aircraft Fixed-wing aircraft are utilized for transports of over 150 miles.[6] These aircraft range from single engine planes to small jets, depending on the distance to be covered. Although the noise level is usually less in a fixed-wing aircraft, the vibrations and turbulence are similar to those of a helicopter.

Obviously, the main advantage to fixed-wing transport is the speed and the distance that can be covered in a short time.

A major disadvantage to air transport is that it is usually confined to acceptable weather conditions. Severe weather, either at the departure point, en route, or at the destination, may make air transport unavailable. Another disadvantage is the lack of space in the aircraft. With two adult personnel, equipment, and the incubator, space is at a premium.

The use of fixed-wing aircraft requires some type of general aviation facility nearby. In some instances, the distance factor may need to be disregarded to allow a helicopter closer access to the hospital.

Considerations for Air Transport Transport in an aircraft requires special attention to the effects of altitude. In particular, one aspect that requires special attention is the effect of altitude on gas pressures. While there is not a precise scale, in general, once altitude exceeds about 8000 feet, the signs of hypoxia begin to develop; however, supplemental oxygen is probably not needed for a healthy person below 12,500 feet.

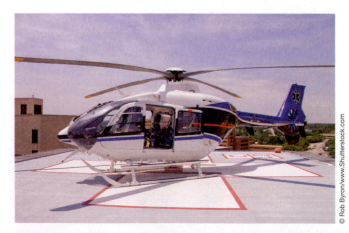

© Rob Byron/www.Shutterstock.com

FIGURE 21–2. Example of a transport helicopter.

Most helicopters fly a few hundred feet above the ground surface, so depending on the part of the country the transport is taking place, altitudes may be well below 8000 feet, or could exceed the 12,500 foot level. As a comparison, the city of Los Angeles is 233 feet above sea level, Oklahoma City is at 1295 feet, and Denver sits at 5430 feet. Fixed-wing aircraft, on the other hand, frequently fly at levels above 12,500 feet. To compensate, the pressure inside the cabin is elevated artificially to approximate an altitude of around 8000 feet.

Dalton's law states that the total pressure of a mixture of gases is the sum of each of the pressures exerted by the individual gases. Thus, we can determine the partial pressure of any gas by knowing what percent it is of the total mixture and by knowing the total pressure of the gas mixture.

The percentage of oxygen is always 20.9% of the total atmospheric gas (21% is used for ease of calculation). Therefore, at any barometric pressure, we can determine the pressure that oxygen is exerting simply by multiplying the barometric pressure by 0.21. As one rises in altitude, the total pressure of the atmosphere decreases; this is known as a **hypobaric** condition. The percent of the gases, however, always remains the same.

At sea level with an average barometric pressure of 760 mmHg, oxygen exerts a pressure of approximately 160 mmHg (760 × 0.21 = 160). At 5000 feet elevation, with an approximate barometric pressure of 640 mmHg, oxygen exerts a pressure of 134 mmHg (640 × 0.21 = 134). It is apparent that, as altitude is increased, the partial pressure of oxygen decreases. The relationship between altitude and environmental PO_2 is illustrated in Table 21–5.

As altitude is increased, it is necessary to increase the percent of oxygen delivered to the patient to maintain the same arterial PO_2. The chart presented in Table 21–6 shows the F_iO_2 required to maintain a constant PaO_2 at increasing altitudes. The value of a transcutaneous monitor or pulse oximeter during transport is apparent, as the F_iO_2 can be titrated up or down as needed to maintain a level PaO_2 or saturation.

A second factor that must be considered regarding hypobaric conditions during air transport is that gas in a closed space expands as the barometric pressure decreases. This is an expression of Boyle's law, where volume varies inversely with pressure. Applying this to the patient, any enclosed volume of gas will expand as altitude is increased. An untreated pneumothorax will expand in the thorax as altitude is increased. Gas that is trapped in the stomach or bowel will also distend and create potential problems. Proper drainage of this free air before lifting off will alleviate most problems.

Seen as insignificant by adults, the effects of acceleration and deceleration need to be considered when transporting any patient, especially the neonatal patient. With the patient lying inline with the aircraft, the forces of acceleration and deceleration may cause significant changes in blood flow. For example, if the head is toward the front of the craft, acceleration may cause blood to be pulled to the lower extremities, reducing blood flow to the brain and cardiopulmonary systems. Conversely, if the head is toward the tail of the craft, acceleration forces may move blood to the head, possibly causing intracranial hemorrhage. One recommendation, is to place the patient parallel to the wings. This may be impractical owing to the limited space and design of the aircraft.[7] In addition, research suggests that the use of specially designed equipment such as pneumatic lifts can reduce acceleration forces.[8]

Table 21–5

THE RELATIONSHIP BETWEEN ALTITUDE AND ENVIRONMENTAL PO$_2$

Altitude	PO$_2$
Sea level	160 mmHg
1000 ft.	155 mmHg
2000 ft.	150 mmHg
3000 ft.	145 mmHg
4000 ft.	140 mmHg
5000 ft.	134 mmHg
6000 ft.	129 mmHg
7000 ft.	124 mmHg
8000 ft.	119 mmHg
9000 ft.	114 mmHg
10,000 ft.	109 mmHg
15,000 ft.	85 mmHg
20,000 ft.	59 mmHg
30,000 ft.	8 mmHg

Other Stressors Transporting patients, especially pediatric and neonatal patients, has a number of other potential stressors that should be recognized and minimized. Stress may induce bradycardia, apnea, and a decrease in oxygen saturation. These stressors include vibration, excessive motion, noise, and possibly hypothermia. While there are practical limitations on what can be done about vibration and noise during transport, such levels inside transport incubators often exceed recommended levels. Furthermore, these and others stressors have been shown to increase morbidity in such patients. Consequently, ways of reducing noise and vibration levels during transportation, such as novel incubator designs and optimal ways to secure such patients, are being investigated.[9] Additionally, it is important to not leave any unsecured equipment inside the incubator that may cause injury during turbulence or while traveling bumpy roads. If noise levels are excessive (60 to 90 dB), hearing protection devices should be provided for the patient. During air transport, outside air temperature drops as altitude is increased. With the change in external temperature, cabin temperature may also fall and create hypothermia in the patient. Constant monitoring of environmental

Table 21-6

F_iO_2 REQUIRED TO MAINTAIN A CONSTANT PAO_2 AT INCREASING ALTITUDE

		Altitude (Feet)									
	Sea Level	2,000	4,000	6,000	8,000	10,000	12,000	14,000	16,000	18,000	20,000
F_iO_2	0.21	0.23	0.24	0.27	0.29	0.31	0.34	0.37	0.41	0.45	0.49
	0.30	0.32	0.35	0.38	0.41	0.45	0.49	0.53	0.59	0.64	0.71
	0.40	0.43	0.47	0.51	0.55	0.60	0.65	0.71	0.78	0.85	0.94
	0.50	0.54	0.58	0.63	0.69	0.75	0.81	0.89	0.98		
	0.60	0.65	0.70	0.76	0.83	0.89	0.98				
	0.70	0.76	0.82	0.89	0.96						
	0.80	0.86	0.94								
	0.90	0.97									
	1.00										

Source: Cloherty JP, Stark AR (eds). *Manual of Neonatal Care.* 4th ed. Philadelphia: Lippincott; 1998. Reproduced with permission.

and patient temperatures help in preventing this stressor. The importance of thermoregulation is discussed later in this chapter.

There are some differing philosophies regarding whether parents should be allowed to accompany the sick neonate or pediatric patient during transport. Often, modes of ground and air transportation have extra seating for passengers but policies on parent-passengers vary widely within the health care transportation environment. The benefits of emotional support for the family and patient, availability of parents for history and consent, and good public relations should be weighed against the potential drawbacks of increased parent and crew anxiety and space limitations.[10]

PERSONNEL

The need for highly skilled, trained personnel on the transport team is obvious. Team members vary from institution to institution and may consist of physicians, respiratory therapists, nurses, paramedics, and emergency medical technicians.

Regardless of which personnel are assigned to the transport team, each must be highly trained to treat and stabilize the sick neonate (Table 21–7). Skills must include placement of IVs, placement of umbilical artery and vein catheters, intubation, and

---

Table 21–7

SKILLS OF THE TRANSPORT TEAM

1. Able to identify maternal and neonatal high-risk factors

2. Trained in all aspects of neonatal resuscitation

3. Trained in specialty skills:
   a. Intubation
   b. Starting IVs
   c. Thermoregulation
   d. Needle aspiration
   e. Mechanical ventilation

4. Able to perform a complete physical assessment and determine gestational age

5. Capable of identifying and treating all types of respiratory distress and its complications

6. Understands and is able to provide emotional and psychosocial support to parents and families

7. Ability to recognize and respond to physiologic effects of transport, particularly hypobaric conditions, noise, and vibration

chest tube placement.[11] A thorough understanding of thermoregulation, oxygenation, ventilation, and management of glucose is also vital.

Transport team members are usually those who have extensive experience in the NICU and are familiar with the treatment of a wide variety of disorders in neonates and high-risk mothers. Extensive training is then done to familiarize each member of the team with the equipment and the special skills that will be required.

NECESSARY EQUIPMENT

Every piece of equipment that is available in the NICU must be available during a transport. The equipment needed for transport is listed in Table 21–8.

This equipment must be carried in a box or bag that is portable and relatively small. Larger equipment, such as the ventilator and tanks, are normally incorporated into the transport incubator.

Table 21–8

EQUIPMENT AND SUPPLIES NEEDED FOR TRANSPORT

Transport incubator

Transport ventilator(s)

Heart rate, blood pressure, and transcutaneous monitors

IV equipment:
   Assorted needles and syringes
   One-half normal saline
   5% D5W
   Ringer's lactate
   25% and 50% dextrose
   Blood administration set

Suction equipment:
   5, 6, 8, and 10 Fr. catheters
   Bulb syringe
   DeLee suction device
   Suction tubing

Thermometer and equipment

Full oxygen and air cylinders

Blood pressure cuff and Doppler device

Stethoscope

continues on the next page

Table 21–8

continued from the previous page

Oxygen analyzer

Resuscitation bag and pressure manometer

Intubation equipment:
>   Laryngoscope handle
>   No. 0 and 1 blade
>   Extra light bulbs
>   Extra batteries, fully charged
>   Magill forceps
>   Endotracheal tubes sizes 2.5, 3.0, 3.5, 4.0, 4.5
>   Tape

CPAP Nasal prongs

Ventilator circuits

Umbilical artery catheterization tray

Blood gas equipment:
>   Blood gas syringes
>   Glass pipettes for collecting capillary samples
>   Stopcocks
>   Heparin flush solution
>   Lancets

Laboratory equipment:
>   Tubes for blood specimens
>   Collection bags for urine
>   Blood culture tubes

Miscellaneous equipment:
>   Appropriate batteries
>   Sterile gloves and floor exam gloves
>   Lubricating ointment
>   Suture materials
>   Scalpels and blades
>   Sterile gowns
>   Oxygen tubing, masks, and cannulas
>   Alcohol swabs
>   Iodophor skin prep solution
>   Kelly clamps
>   Dextrostix
>   Scissors
>   Portable light source
>   Various sizes of gauze sponges
>   Feeding tubes, 5 and 8 Fr.
>   Digital camera and portable printer

Drugs:
  25% albumin
  Dexamethasone
  Naloxone
  Diazepam
  Morphine
  Atropine
  Phenobarbital
  Sodium bicarbonate
  Tolazoline
  Dopamine
  Furosemide
  Epinephrine
  Ampicillin
  Gentamicin
  Kanmycin
  Oxycillin
  Penicillin
  Magnesium sulfate
  Heparin
  Calcium gluconate
  Lidocaine
  Pancuronium
  Phytonadione (Aquamephyton)
  Prostaglandin E
  Albuterol
  Indomethasin
  Racemic Epinephrine
  Surfactant

Self-Supporting Equipment

Any equipment used during a transport must be self-supporting. Thus, it must be battery operated or otherwise able to operate without direct electrical current. Battery-operated equipment should be able to last at least 30 to 45 minutes beyond the expected length of the transport. The ventilator and manual resuscitator should be run from the medical gas cylinders, which require enough cylinders to provide at least 50% more gas than expected use.

The rationale for the excess battery life and gas requirement is that the unexpected must always be anticipated. There could be nothing worse than to have the oxygen run out on a critically ill neonate as the tire to the ambulance is being replaced. Anticipation of potential difficulties will prevent dreaded outcomes.

Determining the Duration of Cylinder Gases

The amount of time left in a medical gas cylinder can be determined. Each cylinder has a known factor that converts the gauge pressure into the liters of gas remaining in the cylinder. By dividing the total liters of gas in the cylinder by the gas flow, the duration of time in minutes can be determined. The equation and cylinder factors are outlined in Table 21–9.

Voltage Converters

Most transport vehicles have voltage inverters that allow the equipment to be plugged into a 120-volt source during the transport, saving battery power. It is also possible to run some equipment from the 12- or 24-volt vehicle system, in which case the internal battery source could also be saved.

Equipment Used during Air Transport

Of special consideration during air transport is that certain monitors may interfere with the aircraft instrumentation. This equipment should be identified and not used during air transport.

Table 21–9

CALCULATION OF CYLINDER DURATION

Cylinder Size	Factor
D	0.16
E	0.28
G	2.41
H	3.14

To calculate the duration of gas flow, use the following equation:

$$\text{duration of flow (minutes)} = \frac{\text{factor} \times \text{gauge pressure (psi)}}{\text{flow rate (L/min)}}$$

For example, an E cylinder with 2000 psi running at 3 LPM:

$$\frac{\text{factor (0.28)} \times \text{gauge pressure (2000)}}{\text{flow rate (3 LPM)}}$$

$$\frac{0.28 \times 2000}{3} = \frac{560}{3} = 186.7 \text{ minutes}$$

Medications

In addition to equipment, there is a host of medications that are commonly administered during neonatal and pediatric transports. Over two thirds of neonatal and pediatric patients are administered some form of medication while being transported. More than one third of such transport patients receive antibiotics, approximately one fourth receive morphine, with about the same number given anticonvulsants. Other classes of medications given during transport include neuromuscular blocking agents, respiratory drugs, inotropes, and sedatives.

The use of different classes of drugs varies by age group. Anticonvulsants are most commonly given to children, sedatives and respiratory medications to infants, and antibiotics to newborns.[12]

INFANT PREPARATION AND TRANSPORTATION

To achieve the goal of transporting the patient to a tertiary center in stable condition, the patient should be stable before being transported. This is accomplished by personnel skilled in resuscitation and stabilization techniques who are present at the delivery. This emphasizes the importance of having personnel trained in resuscitative skills present at every delivery.

Stabilization

Proper stabilization of the neonate includes appropriate medication administration, thermoregulation, oxygenation, ventilation, acid-base balance, proper vascular volume and glucose levels, and stable vital signs.[13] Once stabilization is achieved, the neonate is placed in the transport incubator and connected to the necessary monitors and equipment. The destination hospital is then contacted and advised of the status of the patient.

Following Stabilization

Before leaving, the transport team should have a copy of the patient's chart with all lab data and copies of any x-rays that were taken. The patient is then taken to the mother's room, where the parents are allowed to touch and see their neonate. The procedures for the transport are explained and the parents assured that their neonate will receive the required medical attention. Often a photograph of the infant is taken and left with the parents.

The parents are then asked to sign a release form, consenting to the transport of the neonate. This interaction with the parents is important to help alleviate their fears and concerns. They must be assured that a member of the team will contact them on arrival at the destination and that they are free to call whenever they desire.

The transport team must be sensitive to the parents' needs at this point, because they will often be very frightened and worried.

TRANSPORTATION PROCEDURES

Following the visit with the parents, the patient is taken to the transport vehicle and secured. During the transport the patient is constantly monitored for changes in status. Appropriate care is provided during the transport to maintain stability.

Upon arrival at the regional hospital, the patient is admitted and care is continued as required. A blood gas should be drawn soon after arrival to ensure appropriate oxygenation and ventilation. The parents are then notified of the arrival and the baby's condition.

SPECIAL NEEDS

A majority of neonates requiring transport suffer from lung disease secondary to prematurity and other factors. Besides having lung problems, a premature neonate can be very difficult to thermoregulate, and special attention may be required.

Thermoregulation

To assist with thermoregulation, incubators, warmed IV bags wrapped in a blanket, a cap over the head, a warming blanket, and commercially produced chemical heating pads may all be used.[14] Extreme caution must be exercised on patients with poor perfusion. Burns can develop at even moderate temperatures on these neonates, requiring close attention to temperatures.

In addition, plastic shields and wraps and aluminum foil can be used to reduce radiant and convective heat losses. Minimal handling and opening of incubator doors will also help with the maintenance of a neutral thermal environment.

In recent years, there has been significant improvement in the avoidance of hypothermia and cold stress in infants requiring emergency transport. Adjunct measures, such as continual monitoring of temperature, staff education, and equipment enhancements are largely credited with this improvement. Infants weighing less than 1000 grams account for the largest number of patients experiencing hypothermia.[15]

Diaphragmatic Hernia

Patients requiring surgical intervention will require special attention during transport. The patient with a diaphragmatic hernia should be positioned on his or her side with the head elevated and the affected side of the thorax down, as demonstrated in Figure 21–3.[16] A nasogastric (NG) tube must be in place to evacuate any air that enters the stomach.

The patient should never be bag and mask ventilated, but intubated and ventilated through the ET tube. These procedures help minimize the amount of gastric air distention that further compromises ventilation.

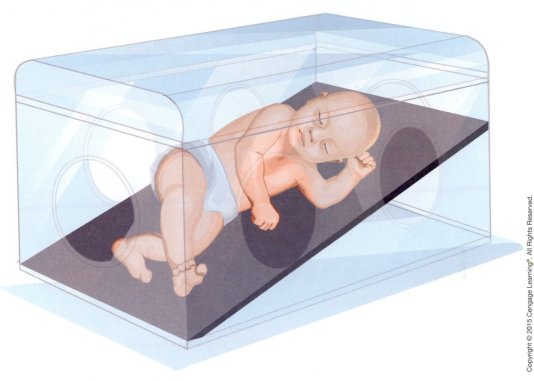

FIGURE 21–3. When transporting a neonate with a diaphragmatic hernia, the head is elevated and the patient is placed with the affected side down (usually the left side).

Tracheoesophageal Fistula

Patients with a tracheoesophageal fistula are transported with their head elevated, a feeding tube placed in the esophageal pouch, which is evacuated regularly to remove the buildup of secretions. If possible, mechanical ventilation should be avoided to avoid distention of the gastrointestinal tract.

Omphalocele and Gastroschisis

Another group of patients who may be difficult to thermoregulate are those with an **omphalocele** or **gastroschisis.** Omphalocele involves the herniation of the intestines directly into the base of the umbilical cord. As shown in Figure 21–4 the organs are covered by a transparent sac.

In gastroschisis, the organs herniate through the abdominal wall, typically to the right of an intact umbilicus. The organs in this defect are not covered by a sac. Figure 21–5.

The primary goals in transporting these patients are to maintain an aseptic environment for the herniated organs, prevent pulmonary aspiration of abdominal contents, prevent excess loss of heat through evaporation, provide respiratory support, and prevent vascular compromise of the organs.[14]

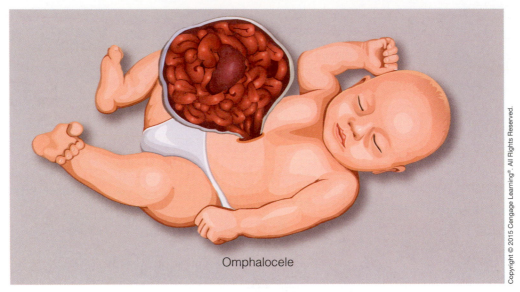

Omphalocele

FIGURE 21–4. Omphalocele.

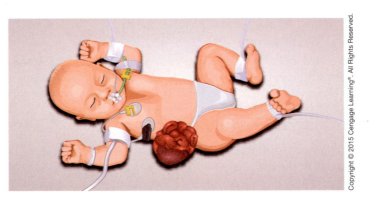

FIGURE 21–5. Gastroschisis.

Preparation of the omphalocele patient before transport requires special precautions. An NG tube is placed and regularly evacuated. The herniated bowel is carefully covered with a layer of warm, sterile, saline-soaked gauze. Antiseptics such as povidone iodine may be added to the gauze. The sac is then wrapped with a layer of dry **Kling gauze** in a figure-eight fashion. No attempt should be made to reduce the defect back into the abdomen. This may damage the intestinal loops, cause an interruption of venous return, and compromise the respiratory status.[14]

Continual monitoring of patient temperature helps maintain thermoregulation. Both evaporative and radiant heat loss from the herniated organs create a major problem. Temperature is maintained by placing the entire lower half of the body in a sterile plastic bag or wrapping the abdomen with clear plastic wrap.[11] The environmental temperature of the incubator is recommended to be kept between 36.5°C and 37.0°C.[14]

Extensive fluid losses, hypovolemic shock, and poor tissue perfusion are seen in many of these patients. To counter these problems, an IV is started in an upper extremity, and fluid replacement is started and kept at two to four times the maintenance range.[14] The upper regions are used for the IV because of the risk of impaired venous return from the lower extremities following dressing and positioning the defect. Broad-spectrum antibiotics such as ampicillin and gentamicin are then started to avert the onset of sepsis.[11]

The patient is then transported with the head elevated. Extreme care must be taken to prevent contamination of the defect and to prevent kinking the intestine.

Meningomyelocele

In the patient with **meningomyelocele**, or spina bifida, extreme care must be taken to avoid contamination of the defect with stool or the environment. If the covering membranes are intact, extreme care must be taken to avoid rupturing them. Covering with sterile saline-soaked gauze and a plastic shield will help protect the defect and maintain thermoregulation.[11] The patient is then transported in the supine position.[17]

Meningomyelocele is shown in Figure 21–6.

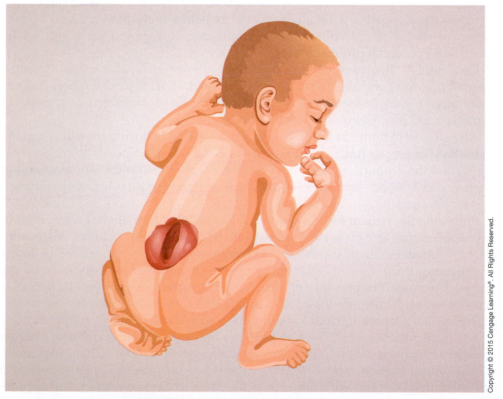

FIGURE 21–6. Meningomyelocele.

Cyanotic Heart Disease

Patients with cyanotic heart diseases may need to be treated with prostaglandin E_1 to maintain the patency of the ductus arteriosus during transport.

SUMMARY

Of all the types of transport, the most desirable is maternal transport, where the high-risk mother is transported before delivery to a tertiary center. Ground transport via an ambulance or specially equipped vehicle is often used when the distance is less than 25 miles, or if weather or other obstacles prevent air transport. Air transport is done via helicopter, usually for distances up to 150 miles, and fixed-wing aircraft for distances greater than 150 miles.

Special considerations are required for air transport. The effect of hypobaric conditions relating to altitude on gas pressures can make a significant impact on patients with air leaks, or air pockets within closed spaces. Additionally, the pressure of oxygen decreases as altitude increases, requiring constant monitoring and adjustment to ensure the patient does not become hypoxemic. Gravitational forces during takeoff and landing may cause alterations in blood flow to the head or vital organs.

Stressors associated with all forms of transport include vibration, excessive movement, noise, and hypothermia. Careful monitoring and securing can help reduce these potential problems.

Personnel on the transport team must be well versed in all aspects of neonatal and maternal care, and able to manage any problem that may arise. These individuals are often highly cross-trained and knowledgeable of the effects of transport on the patient and how to minimize those effects.

All equipment found in the NICU should be available during transport and must be checked for proper function and secured before leaving. Special attention should be afforded the amount of oxygen, to ensure adequate supplies. The possibility of delays and unforeseen problems should be taken into account when determining the necessary supply.

Preparing the patient for transport requires stabilization of vital signs, temperature, blood sugar, acid-base balance, oxygenation, and blood volume. Also, any air leak or trapped air must be treated if a change in altitude is anticipated. All necessary documents must be in order and a visit to the family members must be done prior to departure. The presence of certain defects such as diaphragmatic hernia, tracheoesophageal fistula, omphalocele, meningomyelocele, and cyanotic heart disease require special preparation and handling prior to and during the transport.

The transportation of the high-risk mother or the distressed neonate to a regional center has become a vital part of the health care system. Proper advanced planning, strong communication, and cooperation between hospitals greatly enhances the regionalization concept. With proper coordination, skilled personnel, and appropriate equipment, any neonate should be able to receive the care provided by the modern NICU.

POSTTEST

1. It is January and you are working as a respiratory therapist at a small resort community in the mountains of Colorado and are resuscitating a 28-week gestation neonate. The nearest NICU is over a mountain range with elevations exceeding 13,000 feet and approximately 60 miles away. There is a mountainous road that connects you to the town. Which of the following would not be part of the decision as to the mode of transport for this patient?
   a. the air temperature
   b. weather conditions
   c. how close the NICU is to an airport
   d. availability of a transport team

2. Before departure on a helicopter transport, a neonate's PaO_2 is 65 mmHg. During the flight, the PaO_2 will most likely:
   a. remain the same
   b. decrease
   c. increase
   d. rise initially, then return to baseline

3. Which of the following statements regarding air transport is true?
   a. Trapped air will expand as altitude increases.
   b. Trapped air will decrease in size as altitude increases.
   c. Trapped air in the stomach must not be removed before transport.
   d. As altitude increases, barometric pressure increases.

4. Batteries used to power equipment during a transport should last:
   a. 30 to 45 minutes beyond the expected length of the transport
   b. 10 to 15 minutes beyond the expected length of the transport
   c. 3 to 4 hours
   d. 24 hours

5. How long will an E cylinder of oxygen last with a gauge pressure of 1900 psi running at 5 lpm?
   a. 106 hours
   b. 1 hour 46 minutes
   c. 2 hours 17 minutes
   d. 3 hours

6. Before transporting the neonate to the NICU, the transport team should:
   a. stabilize the infant
   b. contact and advise the NICU
   c. collect all patient chart data
   d. all of the above

7. Of the following, which can help thermoregulate the infant during transport?
   a. warmed IV bags wrapped in a blanket
   b. sprinkling the baby with warm water
   c. blowing warmed oxygen over the baby
   d. placing a small 12-volt heater in the transport incubator

8. Which of the following disorders present the greatest potential thermoregulation problem during transport?
   a. diaphragmatic hernia
   b. gastroschisis
   c. intraventricular hemorrhage
   d. cardiac anomaly

9. To maintain the same PaO_2 for a patient during air transport, hypobaric conditions would generally require what adjustment to the F_iO_2?
   a. decrease
   b. increase
   c. no change
   d. initial decrease then increase

REFERENCES

1. Ohning BL, et al. Transport of the critically ill newborn. Medscape. March 2012
2. Committee on Perinatal Health. *Toward Improving the Outcome of Pregnancy: The 90s and Beyond.* White Plains, NY: March of Dimes Birth Defects Foundation, 1993.
3. American Academy of Pediatrics Levels of Neonatal Care. Committee on Fetus and Newborn. *Pediatrics.* 114(5): 1341–1347, November 1, 2004.
4. Goodman DG, et al The relation between the availability of neonatal intensive care and neonatal mortality. *N Engl J Med.* 346:1538–1544, 2002.
5. Shlossman PA, et al. An analysis of neonatal morbidity in maternal (in utero) and neonatal transports at 24–34 weeks' gestation. *Am J Perinatol.* 14:449–456, 1997.
6. Ohning BL, et al. Transport of the critically ill newborn. Medscape. March 2012.
7. Miller C. The physiologic effects of air transport on the neonate. *Neonatal Network.* 13:7–10, 1994.
8. Peters C, et al. Measuring vibrations of transport stress in premature and newborn infants during incubator transport. *Clin Pediatr* (in German). 209:315–320, 1997.
9. Macnab A, et al. Vibration and noise in pediatric emergency transport vehicles: a potential cause of morbidity. *Aviat Space Environ Med.* 66:212–219, 1995.
10. Lewis MM, et al. Parents as passengers during pediatric transport. *Air Medicine Journal.* 16:38–42, 1997.
11. Cloherty JP, Stark AR (eds). *Manual of Neonatal Care.* 6th ed. Philadelphia: Lippincott, 2011.
12. Kronick JB, et al. Pediatric and neonatal critical care transport: a comparison of therapeutic interventions. *Pediatr Emerg Care.* 12:23–26, 1996.

13. Merenstein GB, Gardner SL. *Handbook of Neonatal Care*. 4th ed. St. Louis: CV Mosby Co, 1998.

14. Richey DA. Transporting the infant with an abdominal wall defect. *Neonatal Network*. 9:53–56, 1990.

15. Bowman ED, Roy RN. Control of temperature during newborn transport: an old problem with new difficulties. *J Paediatr Child Health*. 33:398–401, 1997.

16. Koff PB, Eitzman DV, Nev J. *Neonatal and Pediatric Respiratory Care*. 2nd ed. St. Louis, MO: CV Mosby Co, 1993.

17. Avery GB, Fletcher MA, MacDonald MG. *Pathophysiology and Management of the Newborn*. 5th ed. Philadelphia, PA: JB Lippincott Co, 1999.

BIBLIOGRAPHY AND SUGGESTED READINGS

Fanaroff JM, Fanaroff AA. *Klaus and Fanaroff's Care of the High-Risk Neonate*. 6th ed. Philadelphia: Elsevier Saunders, 2013.

Jaimovich DG, Vidyasagar D. *Handbood of Pediatric and Neonatal Transport Medicine* 2nd ed. Philadelphia, PA: Hanley & Belfus, Inc., 2002.

Riley LE, et al. (eds). *Guidelines for Perinatal Care*. 7th ed. Evanston, IL: American Academy of Pediatrics/American College of Obstetrics and Gynecology, 2012.

CHAPTER 22

Home Care

OBJECTIVES

Upon completion of this chapter, the reader should be able to:

1. Describe the history of modern home care.
2. Identify those factors that make home care preferable over hospital care.
3. Compare and contrast hospital-based, community-based, and bureaucratic home care models.
4. Describe steps in selecting a home care patient.
5. With regard to home ventilator patients, describe each of the following:
   a. Selection of candidates
   b. Preparation for home ventilator care
   c. Selection of a home care ventilator
   d. Training parents and family
6. Describe the equipment and techniques for administering aerosols in the home.
7. Discuss the family training for providing chest physiotherapy and suctioning at home.
8. Define ALTE.
9. Regarding home apnea monitoring, describe each of the following:
   a. Identification of patients for monitoring
   b. Problems associated with home monitoring
10. List the equipment necessary to provide oxygen in the home.
11. Compare and contrast the three methods of home oxygen delivery, including advantages and disadvantages of each.
12. Discuss the role of each of the following in discharge planning:
    a. Case manager
    b. Physician
    c. Respiratory therapist
    d. Nurse
    e. Social worker
    f. Dietician

g. Physical, occupational, and speech therapists

h. Home care company

13. Describe the events and necessary supports involved at the time of discharge.

14. Discuss the effects of home care on the family.

15. Describe why home care sometimes fails and what the respiratory therapist can do to prevent failure.

KEY TERMS

cognitive	metered dose inhaler	spacer
diaphragmatic	(MDI)	turfism
pacemakers	sieve	

INTRODUCTION

It is interesting that as health care has improved in quality over the last century, emphasis is beginning to be placed on care of the patient at home, where it originally started. When dealing with home care of the infant, advancements in technology and equipment have improved patient survival, resulting in many infant patients requiring long-term chronic care. With a shortage of long-term care facilities, a natural choice for this care is the home.

HISTORY OF MODERN HOME CARE

A major advance in home care occurred in the early 1980s when an Iowa parent wanted to take her chronically ill child home. She soon discovered there were no mechanisms in place for the reimbursement of home care. She appealed to then President Reagan for help. The president, seeing the merits of home care, arranged for Iowa authorities to waive Medicaid rules to cover the home care of this patient.

From this case, interest in the care of technology-assisted children surged and was in part responsible for the U.S. Surgeon General's Workshop on Children with Handicaps and Their Families.[1] From this original conference, the groundwork was laid, which resulted in the funding of programs and reports that have given us current models of home care.

An additional concern, further supporting the need for home care, is the effect of the hospital environment on the chronically ill child. It is obvious that the hospital environment does not allow the normal development of family bonds or allow for normal social interactions with siblings, or other children. The long-term effects of this lack of interaction remain unknown, but undoubtedly there are some detrimental aspects. The advantages of home care are outlined in Table 22–1.

Home care allows for more normal family activities to occur. The patient, being in the home environment, is in the constant companionship of those who care for him or her most. The environment is much lower key than that in the hospital with its

Table 22–1

ADVANTAGES OF HOME CARE

1. Normalization of family activities

2. Development of normal parent-sibling and other social relationships

3. Normalization of sleeping, eating, and activity habits for the patient

4. Cost effective

5. Enhances cognitive development

constant noise, alarms, bright lights, and constantly changing personnel. Families are encouraged to send older children to school and even infants should attend special out-of-home programs. The current trend of mainstreaming in school classrooms provides the opportunity for these patients to attend school with "normal" children. The benefits of this are enhanced attention, memory and decision making (**cognitive** skills), and normal psychosocial development.

Controversies Surrounding Home Care

Despite the changes in legislation and the increase in interest in home care, several questions remain unanswered. These include: Which patients are candidates for home care? How is the decision for home care made, and who makes it? Who will help the family and the patient during the transition, and how long will help be provided? These are not easy questions to answer because many complex issues are involved. Possibly the most difficult question to answer is the first, deciding who is a candidate for home care. This is discussed in more detail later in this chapter. While this chapter does not pretend to answer all questions, it does present some rationale on which to base decisions.

HOME CARE MODELS

There are three basic models for pediatric home care described by Aitken: the hospital-based, community-based, and bureaucratic models.[1] We will briefly examine each.

Hospital-Based

As is apparent from the name, this model is located in the hospital, with personnel, financial planning, and care provided by the hospital. The hospital provides all training for those who will be caring for the patient.

The major advantage of this model is the ability of the discharge planning group to maintain some control over the discharge plan. Additionally, the hospital has plenty of human resources in each specialty group to provide support and training.

The major disadvantage to this model is that if outside funding cannot be obtained, the child may remain in the hospital longer, increasing the cost of the hospital stay. The longer hospital stay may also cause the hospital to lose money.

Community-Based

This model is designed to provide all necessary elements of a home care program, using community resources. The organization must hire its own personnel and a board of directors to oversee policies and procedures. Funding is solicited by the board from private sources to ease the burden on families. The community-based model acts as a coordinator between the patient and the hospital in planning the home care.

There are two main advantages to this system. First, the community-based model is better able to determine which available agencies are best suited to handle the needs of the patient and help the parents in their decision. They have the ability to draw from many sources and are not tied to their own resources. Also, by not being supported by a particular hospital, there is less **turfism** between hospitals. Turfism occurs when organizations with seemingly similar goals do not cooperate with each other.

The main disadvantage to this model is the expense involved. In areas of limited human and financial resources, this model may be impractical to operate. There may also be reluctance on the part of the primary care physician to turn over care to another. Finally, personnel involved in this model may have little, if any, control over the discharge planning for the patient.

Bureaucratic

This model integrates home care into an existing public support organization. Structurally, it is similar to the community-based model, but has been absorbed by an established agency to survive financially.

Being a part of an established government agency, this model may be more readily accepted by health care providers. Another advantage is that these agencies often have in place necessary ancillary services, such as nursing services and physical, speech, and occupational therapy. Access to financial resources may be facilitated in this model also.

The main disadvantage to this type of model is that eligibility may be limited to families who are eligible for Medicaid. There also may be a tendency not to use the agency because of a dislike for government bureaucracies. Case managers may be overburdened with the addition of a technology-assisted patient to their heavy load of regular patients.

PATIENT SELECTION

The first step in home care is the selection of appropriate patients who will benefit from home care.

Common Disorders Allowing Home Care

Survivors of respiratory distress syndrome who have developed bronchopulmonary dysplasia probably constitute a majority of ventilator-dependent children. The second category consists of the congenital anomalies, such as diaphragmatic hernia, tracheoesophageal fistula, and esophageal atresia. The third category is the neuromuscular and neurologic diseases. These include myopathies, myelomeningocele, encephalopathy, and infantile botulism. The fourth category consists of patients who have suffered traumatic injuries.

Home Environment

Another factor in patient selection is the home environment and the confidence in the parents to provide the necessary care. The decision to provide home care must be made by the parents. The decision should only be made after the parents have had an extended stay in the hospital.[2]

The parents and all others who will be involved in the care of the infant or child must be willing to sacrifice their time and be willing to dedicate themselves to the care of the infant or child. They should not only be willing, but eager to learn. They must understand the stresses that will come into the family and learn how to deal with them. Parents who do not have these traits may end up not being able to cope with the various situations that arise.

It is the responsibility of the health care team to assist the family in making an informed, responsible decision by reviewing all the alternatives. Home care may not be the best option for every child. It is therefore important to examine all the variables and options before deciding.

HOME CARE OF THE VENTILATOR-DEPENDENT CHILD

Providing home care for the ventilator-dependent patient has become more prevalent. The overall goal should be to select those patients who have the best chance of recovery, or at least who can have an adequate quality of life with home care. The overall objective is to provide an environment that promotes, protects, and supports the physical, cognitive, and social growth and development of the patient.

Patient Selection for Home Ventilator Care

The most difficult patients to select for home care are those requiring long-term mechanical ventilation. Home care of the ventilator-dependent patient presents one of the most gratifying, as well as difficult, situations. On the one hand, the child can leave the confines of the hospital and enjoy the environment of home and family.

On the other hand, the care of the patient places a major stress on the family and they must learn the coping skills needed to deal with their situation.

An assessment of need should be conducted when considering any patient for home mechanical ventilation. The American Association for Respiratory Care's (AARC) clinical practice guideline (CPG) on long-term invasive mechanical ventilation regarding the assessment of need, indicates four primary areas be met:[3]

1. Indications are present and contraindications are absent.
2. The goals of home mechanical ventilation can be met.
3. No continued need for higher level of services exists.
4. Frequent changes in the plan of care will not be needed.

The goals of home mechanical ventilation as stated in the CPG are: To sustain and extend life, to enhance the quality of life, to reduce morbidity, to improve or sustain physical and psychological function of all ventilator assisted individuals (VAIs) and to enhance growth and development in pediatric VAIs, and to provide cost-effective care.

The success of home mechanical ventilation depends largely on the underlying disease. Conditions often linked with long-term ventilator care include neuromuscular disorders and injuries, such as trauma, polio, and muscular dystrophies, thoracic cage deformities such as kyphosis, and pulmonary disorders, such as bronchopulmonary dysplasia (BPD). Typically, the candidate for home ventilator care is one who meets the following criteria outlined by Gilmartin.[4] First, the patient can make no spontaneous effort to breathe or the effort is seriously impaired. Second, the patient has failed several attempts to wean following an acute respiratory failure. Third, the patient's disease causes chronic respiratory failure in which repeated hospital admissions are required or severely limits his or her ability to function. Gilmartin also points out that patients with a primary diagnosis of skeletal disease and/or neuromuscular disease are better candidates for long-term home ventilator care.

Often, the primary disorder is compounded by an underlying disease or disorder, such as chronic cardiopulmonary disease or infection. These secondary conditions must also be considered when home care is contemplated.

Additionally, as cited by the AARC's CPG, indications for ventilation in the home include an inability to be completely weaned from invasive ventilator support and a progression of disease etiology that requires increasing ventilator support. Contraindications to home ventilation are many and include: the presence of a physiologically unstable medical condition requiring a higher level of care or resources than are available in the home. Examples are shown in Table 22–2; the patient's choice not to receive home mechanical ventilation; the lack of an appropriate discharge plan; an unsafe physical environment as determined by the patient's discharge planning team; the presence of fire, health or safety hazards, including unsanitary conditions; inadequate basic utilities (such as heat, air conditioning, or electricity, including adequate amperage and grounding; inadequate resources for care in the home (financial, personnel).

Table 22-2

UNSTABLE MEDICAL CONDITIONS

F_iO_2 requirements > 40%
PEEP > 10 cm H_2O
Lack of mature tracheostomy
Need for continuous invasive monitoring

Preparation for Home Ventilator Care

The preparation to provide home care is initiated when the patient is first admitted to the intensive care unit. From the beginning, parents and family members are familiarized with equipment and the care provided for their infant or child. This initial familiarization paves the way for the family to assume more and more of the care.

Besides being familiar with the machinery, the family must also know how to care for the tracheostomy tube. This can be a frightening and challenging experience for parents and caregivers. An uncuffed tube is preferred for use in the home care setting, to avoid laryngeal and tracheal damage. The patient is also able to vocalize as a small amount of gas is allowed to leak past the tube. Care of the tracheostomy tube, stoma, and secretion removal, must be thoroughly taught to the family and caregivers. Ideally, the use of monitors should be kept to a minimum in the home. Excessive monitors may reduce the observation of the patient by the parents, which is critical in taking care of these patients. Additionally, excess monitors may perpetuate the feeling of having a NICU in the home, taking away the home-like environment. The home should be organized to create a developmentally appropriate atmosphere. The equipment should be organized and arranged in an accessible, safe, and workable manner. The basic equipment required for ventilator home care is listed in Table 22–3.

Selection of a Home Care Ventilator

The selection of a ventilator is made by the discharge team and determined by patient need and availability of equipment. Ideally, the home ventilator should be small, mobile, fairly simple to understand and operate, with built-in alarms to detect disconnects and other possible hazardous situations. In addition, it should have a battery backup, in case of a power outage.

Due to the choice of ventilators available, the following factors should be considered when making a selection:

1. Simplicity, ease of operation, and reliability
2. Wide range of respiratory rates

Table 22–3

EQUIPMENT NEEDED FOR HOME VENTILATOR CARE

Oxygen source (if applicable) with backup cylinder and regulator

Ventilators with patient circuits and humidification device

Alternate power source (i.e., generator or battery with charger)

Self-inflating resuscitation bag

Stationary and AC/DC suction machine

Tracheostomy tube and tracheostomy care items

Pulse oximeter (if indicated)

Sterile water and sterile saline

All necessary disposable items

---

3. Accurate delivery of VT over a wide range of values
4. All modes of ventilation such as assist, assist-control, SIMV, CPAP, and pressure support
5. Adequate humidification
6. Variable or constant flow rates
7. Variety of audible and visual alarms
8. Adjustable pressure relief valve/limit
9. Maximum and minimum pressure capabilities

Pediatric and infant patients present with additional problems that must be considered when making a selection. They require a sensitivity setting that is more sensitive to patient effort. Because infant and pediatric patients have smaller tidal volumes and faster respiratory rates, ventilators must have the ability to deliver these set values. The ventilator must have a quick response time as well as a low internal compliance.[5]

Common home ventilators are listed in Table 22–4, and one is shown in Figure 22–1. Other options for ventilation include **diaphragmatic pacemakers** and negative pressure chest shells. Diaphragmatic pacemakers are surgically implanted and help the respiratory rate by stimulating the phrenic nerve.

Backup ventilation must be made available in the event of a power outage or equipment failure. This is best accomplished with the use of a manual resuscitator attached to an oxygen tank. An additional ventilator also allows the patient to be moved from room to room and prevents the child from being confined to one area in the home.

Table 22-4

HOME VENTILATORS

1. Newport Medical HT50 Home Care Ventilator

2. CareFusion LTV 1200 Ventilator

3. Puritan Bennett Achieva PSO2 Respiratory Medical Ventilator

4. Respironics PLV 100, PLV 102

5. Bear Medical Systems Bear 33

6. Pulmonetic Systems LTV 900, LTV 950

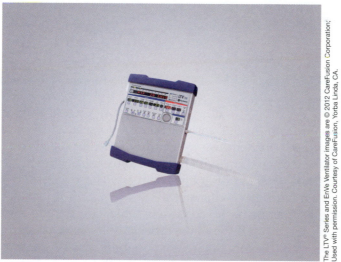

The LTV® Series and EnVe Ventilator images are © 2012 CareFusion Corporation; Used with permission. Courtesy of CareFusion, Yorba Linda, CA.

FIGURE 22-1. An example of a home care ventilator.

Training of Parents and Family

Training of the parents and caregivers in the use of the home ventilator should begin well before the child is ready for discharge. A checklist is often helpful in determining the level of understanding and comprehension of the parents and caregivers. A sample checklist, outlining the training needed to care for the ventilator-dependent child, is shown in Table 22-5. Before discharge can take place, the parents or caregivers must demonstrate competency in these areas by way of return demonstration. The hospital and home care agencies must have documentation attesting to this.

Table 22–5

FAMILY EDUCATION PLAN CHECKLIST

The family, extended family, and any others planning on caring for the patient should be able to demonstrate the following:
- Performance of routine daily care activities
- Ability to adequately provide nutrition to the patient
- Ability to assess the patient's respiratory function
- Performance of correct suctioning, CPT, manual ventilation, and tracheostomy care skills
- Ability to describe signs and symptoms of infection, extubation, and decannulation; airway obstruction; hypoxia; and the appropriate intervention for each
- Ability to describe signs of cardiopulmonary arrest and the proper procedure for performing CPR
- Knowledge of the function of the home ventilator and all associated equipment
- Ability to correctly care for, clean, and store equipment
- Understanding of the dosages and side effects of all medications, and demonstrated ability to administer them

HOME AEROSOL THERAPY

Children may require continuous aerosol therapy to wet and mobilize secretions or may only require intermittent use to reverse bronchospasm. Those who require continuous aerosol are often those with tracheostomy tubes who need supplemental moisture to overcome the effects of dry gas delivery. These aerosols are often heated to provide maximum humidity to the airway.

Two precautions must be observed closely when continuous aerosols are given to a young patient. First, smaller infants, especially those with cardiac defects, are at a risk of fluid overload. Second, there is a possibility that the airway may become burned if the gas temperature is not monitored closely.

Administration of Aerosolized Medications

The administration of aerosolized medications using a hand-held nebulizer may require a compressed gas source. This is provided either by a small electrically powered air compressor or by an air or oxygen cylinder. Another method of medication delivery is an ultrasonic nebulizer specifically made for medication delivery.

The patient, family, and caregivers should all be trained in the proper delivery of aerosolized medications. In addition, they should be taught to recognize medication side effects and when to alter the therapy accordingly.

Another method of delivering aerosolized medications at home is **metered dose inhalers (MDI)**. MDIs are often most effective when delivered using a **spacer** device.

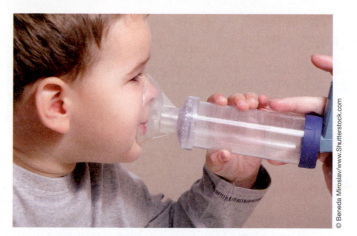

FIGURE 22–2. Use of a spacer and face mask for delivery of aerosolized medications.

Spacers usually require less coordination and may result in better compliance by the patient. Smaller children may be given the medication from an MDI by attaching a mask to the outlet of the spacer, as shown in Figure 22–2, or by using a commercially available spacer supplied with a preattached mask.

CHEST PHYSIOTHERAPY AND SUCTIONING

Many infant patients with chronic lung disorders require chest physiotherapy and suctioning on a long-term basis. Both may be done routinely on patients with a tracheostomy tube to mobilize and remove airway secretions.

Family Instruction

Family and caregivers should be instructed in proper techniques and positioning, and all hazards and potential problems should be covered. Alternative devices to percuss and vibrate the patient should be explained to the family. For example, a small paper cup may be used for percussion and a padded electric toothbrush handle makes an effective vibrator.[6] Percussor cups or palm cups, made of soft vinyl, are available in sizes appropriate for neonatal and pediatric use.

When teaching the family about the pulmonary care of their infant, the respiratory therapist should emphasize the importance of detecting changes in the infant's status that may indicate infection or heart failure. This is best accomplished by establishing a baseline of normal patient status. Once the family is able to identify this baseline information, they can better identify those changes that may indicate infection or heart problems. The family should be instructed to report any changes in status as quickly as possible.

APNEA MONITORING

The use of apnea monitors at home continues to be controversial. With the increased visibility of sudden infant death syndrome (SIDS), home apnea monitoring became very common, with thousands of home monitors placed in the last two decades. The facts, however, show that the presence of these monitors has not lowered the incidence of SIDS.[7]

Identification of Home Apnea Monitoring Patients

To work out some of the controversy surrounding the use of these monitors, the National Institutes of Health (NIH) sponsored the Consensus Development Conference on Infantile Apnea and Home Monitoring in 1986. An important term was defined in this conference, Apparent Life-Threatening Event (ALTE). The conference defined this term as an episode that is frightening to the observer and that is characterized by some combination of apnea (central or occasionally obstructive), color change (usually cyanotic or pallid but occasionally erythematous or plethoric), marked change in muscle tone (usually marked limpness), choking, or "gagging." The conference further recommended that the term ALTE be used instead of "near-miss SIDS."

Several important statements regarding the relationship between apnea and morbidity and mortality are summarized in Table 22–6.

The consensus conference additionally identified a number of features deemed to be desirable for a home apnea monitor. Included are: the ability to store events for later analysis, the ability to detect hypoxemia in addition to detecting hypoventilation, the estimation of tidal volume, and the identification of heart patterns and arrhythmias.[8]

Recommendations made by the conference participants regarding the use of home apnea monitors are listed in Table 22–7.

An important outcome of the conference was a statement that in any circumstances, the use of an apnea monitor cannot guarantee survival.[7]

TABLE 22-6
RELATIONSHIP OF APNEA TO MORBIDITY AND MORTALITY
1. Apnea of prematurity is not a risk factor of SIDS.
2. An ALTE is a risk factor for sudden death.
3. Apnea of prematurity does not per se cause morbidity.
4. An ALTE may be associated with increased morbidity.
5. Infants with a history of ALTE or apnea of prematurity make up only a small portion of SIDS cases.

Table 22-7

RECOMMENDATIONS REGARDING THE USE OF HOME APNEA MONITORS

1. Monitoring is indicated for infants at high risk for sudden death.
   a. Infants with one or more severe ALTE
   b. Symptomatic preterm infants
   c. Siblings of two or more SIDS victims
   d. Infants with conditions such as central hypoventilation

2. Home monitoring is *not* indicated for normal infants.

3. Routine monitoring of asymptomatic preterm infants is not warranted.

4. Pneumograms should not be used to screen for SIDS.

5. The decision to discontinue home monitoring is based on clinical criteria.
   a. Two to three months without significant numbers of alarms or episodes of apnea
   b. Ability to tolerate stress (immunizations, illnesses)

6. The decision-making process with regard to home monitoring is a collaborative enterprise.

7. There should be an adequate support system (medical, technical, psychosocial, and community support).

Problems Associated with Home Apnea Monitoring

A common problem associated with apnea monitors is frequent false alarms that can either keep the family and caregivers continually unsettled or lull them into the "cry wolf" mode where the alarm is either ignored or turned off completely. False alarms may be caused by loose, misapplied, or broken electrodes.

Another potential problem is a lack of compliance in the use of the equipment, especially by teenaged mothers and those in low socioeconomic groups.[7]

OXYGEN THERAPY

The selection of the patient for chronic oxygen therapy is usually based on the inability of the patient to maintain a normal PaO_2 on room air. Documentation of room air PaO_2 is often necessary before third-party payers will pay for home oxygen.

The candidate for home oxygen therapy should be in stable condition with no other major problems at the time of discharge. Home oxygen therapy requires the regular monitoring of PaO_2 or SaO_2 to ensure adequate oxygenation, prevent hyperoxia, and determine possible weaning from the oxygen. This is facilitated by the use of pulse oximeters and transcutaneous monitors.

Family members and all caregivers of the patient on oxygen must be instructed regarding the potential fire hazard associated with its use. The patient should never be near lit cigarettes or any open flame or spark. The parents must understand that the oxygen is not explosive; however combustion is extremely enhanced in an oxygen-enriched environment.

Oxygen Administration Equipment

The equipment used for delivery of oxygen at home includes a nasal cannula, extension tubing, an oxyhood, flowmeter, and humidifier. In most cases, the infant patient will require low-flow oxygen, which is easily provided by a nasal cannula. An oxygen source that can deliver flows of less than 1 L/min should be available because many patients require only fractional amounts of oxygen. This is accomplished by the use of special regulators and flowmeters that deliver $^1/_{16}$ to $^3/_4$ L/min. During naps and at nighttime, an oxyhood may be used to relieve the constant pressure and presence of the cannula on the patient's face. Some type of portable tank should be available to allow movement outside the home. In addition, a full oxygen cylinder should always be available in case of an emergency.

Oxygen Cylinders Oxygen cylinders come in a variety of sizes. The most common sizes for home use are the larger cylinders for the home, and smaller sizes for travel, shown in Figure 22–3.

Cylinders are advantageous for use on the patient with intermittent oxygen requirements. There are, however, several disadvantages to cylinders, which make them a poor choice in most instances. Because of their size and weight, they pose a hazard if they were to fall. They are also relatively expensive for continuous use. A full H cylinder, running at 2 L/min, will only last roughly 2.5 days. A full E cylinder, running at 2 L/min, will only last 5.5 hours.

The amount of time left in a cylinder of gas at any liter flow can be calculated by knowing the cylinder factor, gauge-pressure, and flow rate. (The various cylinder factors and a sample calculation are shown in Table 22–8.)

Obviously, higher flows cause the tank to run out sooner, and lower flows allow a longer use of the tank. Either way, the frequent replacement of tanks becomes expensive and is an ineffective method of delivering continuous home oxygen.

Liquid Systems Liquid oxygen systems use an insulated tank to hold the extremely cold liquid oxygen (Figure 22–4). Liquid home systems allow the liquid oxygen to be siphoned to fill a portable tank or allow the liquid to pass through vaporizer coils, becoming a gas that can then be used by the patient.

The main advantage to a liquid system is that it holds a fairly large quantity of gas. Each liter of liquid oxygen is the equivalent of 860 liters of gas. A 30-liter liquid oxygen tank, running at a constant 2 L/min, will last almost 9 days.

The calculation of time left with a liquid system is based on weight instead of pressure. To calculate the time remaining, one must know the capacity of the

COMMON METRIC EQUIVALENTS (APPROX.)
1 Cubic Foot....7.48 gallons....28.3 liters
1 Gallon...............3.785 liters........0.132 cubic feet
1 Liter....................0.264 gallons....0.035 cubic feet

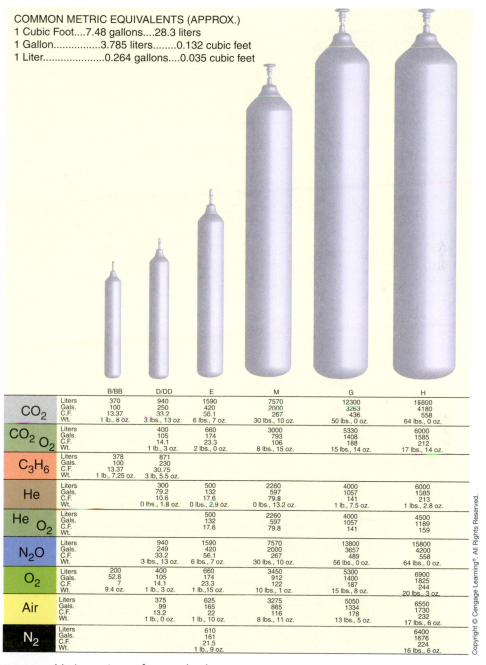

		B/BB	D/DD	E	M	G	H
CO$_2$	Liters	370	940	1590	7570	12300	15800
	Gals.	100	250	420	2000	3263	4180
	C.F.	13.37	33.2	56.1	267	436	558
	Wt.	1 lb., 8 oz.	3 lbs., 13 oz.	6 lbs., 7 oz.	30 lbs., 10 oz.	50 lbs., 0 oz.	64 lbs., 0 oz.
CO$_2$ O$_2$	Liters		400	660	3000	5330	6000
	Gals.		105	174	793	1408	1585
	C.F.		14.1	23.3	106	188	212
	Wt.		1 lb., 3 oz.	2 lbs., 0 oz.	8 lbs., 15 oz.	15 lbs., 14 oz.	17 lbs., 14 oz.
C$_3$H$_6$	Liters	378	871				
	Gals.	100	230				
	C.F.	13.37	30.75				
	Wt.	1 lb., 7.25 oz.	3 lb, 5.5 oz.				
He	Liters		300	500	2260	4000	6000
	Gals.		79.2	132	597	1057	1585
	C.F.		10.6	17.6	79.8	141	213
	Wt.		0 lbs., 1.8 oz.	0 lbs., 2.9 oz.	0 lbs., 13.2 oz.	1 lb., 7.5 oz.	1 lbs., 2.8 oz.
He O$_2$	Liters			500	2260	4000	4500
	Gals.			132	597	1057	1189
	C.F.			17.6	79.8	141	159
	Wt.						
N$_2$O	Liters		940	1590	7570	13800	15800
	Gals.		249	420	2000	3657	4200
	C.F.		33.2	56.1	267	489	558
	Wt.		3 lbs., 13 oz.	6 lbs., 7 oz.	30 lbs., 10 oz.	56 lbs., 0 oz.	64 lbs., 0 oz.
O$_2$	Liters	200	400	660	3450	5300	6900
	Gals.	52.8	105	174	912	1400	1825
	C.F.	7	14.1	23.3	122	187	244
	Wt.	9.4 oz.	1 lb., 3 oz.	1 lb.,15 oz.	10 lbs., 1 oz.	15 lbs., 8 oz.	20 lbs., 3 oz.
Air	Liters		375	625	3275	5050	6550
	Gals.		99	165	865	1334	1730
	C.F.		13.2	22	116	178	232
	Wt.		1 lb., 0 oz.	1 lb., 10 oz.	8 lbs., 11 oz.	13 lbs., 5 oz.	17 lbs., 6 oz.
N$_2$	Liters			610			6400
	Gals.			161			1676
	C.F.			21.5			224
	Wt.			1 lb., 9 oz.			16 lbs., 6 oz.

FIGURE 22–3. Various sizes of gas cylinders.

system and the gauge reading of how much liquid is left. Most liquid oxygen tanks are supplied with a gauge that measures the liquid as being $^3/_4$, $^1/_2$, or $^1/_4$ gone. An example of how to calculate the remaining time in a liquid system is shown in Table 22–9.

Table 22–8

CALCULATION OF CYLINDER DURATION

For each size cylinder there is a factor. Duration is calculated by multiplying the factor by the pressure in the tank, then dividing the product by the rate of flow.

$$\frac{\text{Factor} \times \text{Pressure}}{\text{Flow Rate}}$$

Cylinder Size	Cylinder Factor
D	0.16
E	0.28
H/K	3.14

For example, an E cylinder running at 2 L/min with 1200 psi left in the tank, would be calculated as follows: 0.28 × 1200 psi = 336. Dividing 336 by a flow rate of 2 L/min = 168 minutes. Dividing by 60 minutes will give you 2 hours and 48 minutes of flow left in the tank.

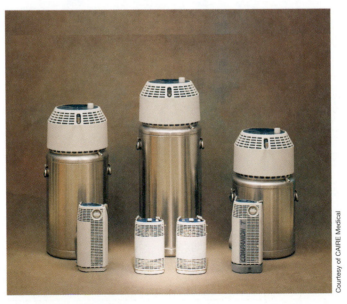

FIGURE 22–4. Liquid oxygen cylinders.

Portable liquid oxygen tanks that are filled from the large tank are used for added mobility. With the small tank, the patient is able to be transported away from the home for short periods.

A disadvantage associated with the use of liquid systems is that the liquid oxygen is continuously evaporating and must be vented to the atmosphere. An unused

Table 22–9

CALCULATION OF LIQUID OXYGEN DURATION

Liquid oxygen weighs 1 pound for every 342 gaseous liters. Therefore, duration of flow in minutes is calculated by multiplying the weight by 342, then dividing the product by the liter flow. A typical liquid oxygen reservoir weighs 70 pounds and at any given flow, the duration can be calculated:

For example, at 2 L/min of flow, the duration of a full reservoir would be calculated as follows:

$70 \times 342 = 23{,}940$ liters of oxygen

Dividing 23,940 liters by a flow rate of 2 L/min = 11,970 minutes of flow. 11,970 divided by 60 minutes results in 199.5 hours of total flow, which is a little over 8 days.

If the tank is $^{3}/_{4}$ full, simply multiply the full weight by 0.75 to find the amount of oxygen left in the reservoir. The duration can then be determined following the above calculation. The same procedure is followed for any reservoir level.

liquid oxygen tank will eventually lose all of its oxygen through evaporation. Because of this, the vented oxygen will create an oxygen-enriched environment, especially if it is in an enclosed space. Continual evaporation also makes it inappropriate when only intermittent oxygen is required. An additional concern is the possibility of frostbite if the unit tips over and liquid oxygen comes into contact with the skin. The modern home liquid oxygen system, however, has very little risk of spilling the liquid oxygen.

When compared to oxygen cylinders, liquid systems are much more cost effective when oxygen must be used continuously.

Oxygen Concentrators

Another method of delivering home oxygen is by an oxygen concentrator (Figure 22–5). The concentrator utilizes a nitrogen **sieve**, which filters the nitrogen out of atmospheric air and typically produces 95% oxygen at 1 to 2 L/min. The highest liter flow available on a concentrator today is 6 L/min.[9]

The percentage of oxygen depends on the liter flow desired, with flows of 1 to 2 L/min delivering the highest oxygen percentage and flows above 2 L/min having a progressively lower oxygen percentage. Oxygen concentrators require electricity to operate and must have a cylinder as a backup in case of a power failure.

Concentrators are generally leased or rented on a monthly basis at a cost far below that of liquid or gas cylinders. For patients requiring low oxygen flows on a continuous basis, the oxygen concentrator is the most cost-effective method of delivering home oxygen.[10] Smaller cylinders are used when the patient needs to travel, because the concentrator is restricted to use in the home environment.

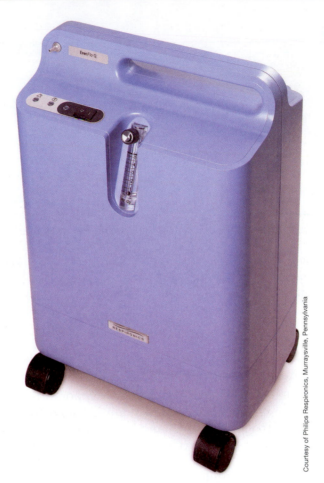

Courtesy of Philips Respironics, Murraysville, Pennsylvania

FIGURE 22-5. Oxygen concentrator.

DISCHARGE PLANNING

Once the patient has met the criteria for potential home care, planning begins for the discharge of the infant or child. Planning must begin well before the actual discharge date to allow adequate time for parent training and preparedness. Discharge planning involves many disciplines, each contributing their expertise to the home care plan of the patient.

Personnel Involved in Discharge Planning

The discharge planning of a patient requires the integration and coordination of several disciplines, each of which is critical in a successful transition.

Case Manager The case manager is usually a certified public health nurse or a certified case management nurse who assesses the patient, family, and home environment and develops a plan of care. The care plan includes all medically necessary services, patient and family strengths and weaknesses, services to be provided by the family, and available community resources.

The case manager coordinates the multitude of services required for the patient and acts as a liaison for the family. Additionally, the case manager monitors and evaluates the quality of care being provided.

Physician The home care physician is a pediatrician experienced in the home management of children. The physician oversees the entire medical care of the infant or child and evaluates the appropriateness and quality of care.

The physician receives information from each of the disciplines and from that determines the time of discharge and the follow-up that will be necessary. The physician should be on call 24 hours a day. As care continues, the physician establishes and then reviews a written home care plan, which specifies the necessary medical care.[11]

The physician should receive reports from the health care providers to assess the on-going care of the infant or child.

Respiratory Therapist The involvement of the respiratory therapist in discharge planning is to determine the respiratory needs of the patient and to train the parents to perform the necessary procedures. If the patient will be on a ventilator, the respiratory therapist helps in the selection of an appropriate ventilator and then teaches the parents the necessary skills to provide ventilator care.

Close attention should be paid to teaching the parents the signs of respiratory distress and infection. The parents should also be taught how to perform CPT, suction, and tracheostomy care.

The parents must gain the confidence to ventilate their baby manually if the need arises, so adequate time must be allowed for practice. If a pulse oximeter is to be used, the parents are instructed in care and placement of the sensor and the setting of alarm limits. They must also be instructed in appropriate measures to take if the alarm limits are violated.

During the training period the parents are gradually allowed to assume the responsibilities that they will be doing at home. The respiratory therapist also develops a plan for eventual weaning off the ventilator, if appropriate, and establishes goals for that accomplishment. For the patient requiring continuous oxygen therapy, the respiratory therapist helps determine the best mode of delivery and then provides the appropriate documentation for the writing of the prescription by the physician.

The parents are taught the signs of hypoxia and how to check for disconnects or blockage in the tubing. They must also be instructed when to order more oxygen so they do not run out.

For patients requiring an apnea monitor, the respiratory therapist helps select an appropriate monitor and then instructs the parents in its use. Of utmost priority is teaching CPR skills to parents, grandparents, and potential babysitters before the infant is discharged. Care must be taken not to frighten the parents into thinking that something disastrous will happen. They must understand that the purpose of all of this training is to prepare them in case the need arises.

Nurse The role of the nurse in the discharge planning is to map out the nursing care that will be required. The nurse teaches the family proper skills in delivering medications, providing hygiene, feeding, dressing changes, and skin care. The nurse also teaches the family assessment skills as required. Home care visits are arranged as needed by the nurse.

The nurse who is involved in discharge planning works very closely with the case manager in follow-up and evaluation of care. Once the infant or child is discharged, the nurse is often the one who actually moves in with the family during the transition to home care.

The home care nurse must be trained in all aspects of the care of the infant or child to handle any emergency that arises.

Social Worker The role of the social worker is to assist the discharge planning by identifying environmental, social, and emotional factors that are of significance. The social worker determines the appropriateness of admission into the home care program and helps develop the child/family psychosocial plan.

Through visits to the family, the social worker provides support and assistance to the family regarding psychosocial and developmental issues. The social worker provides valuable assistance to the family in obtaining financial aid and also serves as the ombudsman for the family.

Dietician The dietician maps out a strategy for the nutritional needs of the infant. Any special diets or supplements are planned and the parents instructed in their use. The dietician closely follows the infant's growth and development and upgrades the diet as needed to meet the ongoing needs of the infant. Close attention is also paid to the caloric intake of the infant. The dietician should be experienced in working with ventilator-dependent infants and understand their special caloric, fluid, and electrolyte needs.

Physical, Occupational, and Speech Therapy Occupational therapy, speech therapy, and physical therapy are involved in the developmental and physical growth of the infant or child. During discharge planning, their plans center on the appropriate social and physical development that should be taking place. Plans are developed that will allow the infant or child to learn skills that are appropriate for his or her age and hopefully prevent an underdevelopment in these skills.

Physical therapy is planned around the needs of the infant or child to gain muscular strength and coordination and reduce the effects of inactivity.

Home Care Company A decision by the discharge planning group regarding the appropriate home care company should be made well before the infant or child is to be discharged. The decision should be based on the needs of the infant or child, the ability of the company to respond quickly to calls, and expert personnel who know and understand the equipment that will be used. The home care company that is chosen should have an on-call respiratory therapist, available 24 hours a day, 7 days a week for any questions or service that may be needed.

The company and their personnel should be involved in the discharge planning as early as possible to assess potential needs and understand the level of care the infant or child will require.

Before the infant or child is discharged, the home care provider assesses the home environment. The home assessment should determine whether there are an appropriate number of properly grounded electrical outlets, appropriate doorway clearance and accessibility, the presence of any hazards such as open flames or sparks, and the presence of a functioning telephone. The room that the patient will be in must have proper ventilation and lighting and be in close proximity to the parents' room. Any recommended changes can then be made prior to discharge of the child. Letters notifying the electric company, telephone company, and local emergency services of life support equipment in the home are sent to establish priority service.

DISCHARGE

The actual day that the patient is discharged will be an emotional day for the parents and family. The health care team must be sure that all the parents' emotional needs will be met. The team informs the parents of support group meeting times and places, possible religious counseling, and counseling for the siblings.

Personnel Needs

The first few days with the child at home may require 24-hour presence of a nurse to provide support as the family becomes accustomed to the new situation. The presence of the health care worker is gradually withdrawn as the family becomes more comfortable with caring for the child. Eventually, the family is left alone to care entirely for their child.

Some patients, because of the nature of their illness or other circumstances, will require regular home visits by a health care worker. The family must understand that they can call for assistance at any time and must be provided with the appropriate telephone numbers. The family will require a lot of support, manifest by frequent phone calls, regular visits, and words of encouragement. They should be invited to participate in family-to-family support groups.

THE EFFECTS OF HOME CARE ON THE FAMILY

A study by McKim indicated that almost half of the mothers of premature infants found the first week to be difficult, even though they were well supported by family and friends.[12]

The effects of home care on the family are numerous. The presence of a sick infant in the home causes major disruptions of family life. The family may feel like they live in an NCIU, with frequent changes of personnel, alarms, and doctor appointments. The sick child becomes the center of the family's life, and attempts to continue with normal activities are often unsuccessful.

The necessity of a live-in nurse brings with it a potential loss of normal interactions and intimacy. The family may be grateful for the care being rendered to their child, but the challenge of having someone live in the home may become a major stumbling block.

The family may become consumed with the care of the infant and the siblings may feel left out and neglected. The relationships among all family members often need to be gradually redefined. The siblings should be included in the care of the infant and made to feel like their brother or sister needs them.

The family may have problems dealing with the health care and financial establishments, adding more stress to the situation. A good case manager and social worker can be of invaluable assistance in these circumstances by providing help to the family in dealing with these establishments.

Another source of potential stress is the impact home care has on the careers of the parents. There may be two opposing feelings: one of guilt for leaving the child home versus one of need for the additional income.[13]

Despite all of the stress that comes from the home care of an infant, most families grow and develop through the experience and handle the stress admirably. Many find that the extraordinary giving and selflessness that is required enhances their love for their child and for the family. The family is bonded tighter by the experience, with family members relying on each other for support and comfort.

Any family who provides home care must receive plenty of empathy and encouragement from the health care team. The success of the home care effort is dependent on a group effort and the combined efforts of all involved.

FAILURE OF HOME CARE

Even with the most well-thought-out and anticipated home care plan, not all home care cases are successful. The most common causes of home care failure should be understood by the health care team in an attempt to avoid them, if possible. A good overview of the reasons for home care failure can be found in Harris.[14]

The most common cause of home care failure is a lack of community and family resources. Signs that the plan is failing include weight loss by the patient, developing skin breakdown and infections, depression of the family, failure to perform treatments, and frequent visits to the emergency department.

Another source of failure is the depletion of the family's financial resources. The consequences of financial depletion include lack of food and transportation and loss of telephone service. The patient may suffer because of the house being too hot in the summer or too cold in the winter.

The emotional depletion of the family occurs when they become financially stressed and physically exhausted. Clues that signal emotional depletion include loss of hope, spirituality, and humor.

Lack of communication among family members, between family and health care workers, and among health care workers may lead to incongruent priorities in the care of the infant. Each participant may have his or her own ideas as to what should be done for the patient. Any mismatch of ideas or priorities should be quickly rendered by opening communication between all involved. In all cases, the opinions and priorities of the family should be preference, with the health care team providing second opinions as necessary.

Although an understanding of these mechanisms for failure may not avert all breakdowns in home care, it may allow the health care team to avoid the most common problems.

SUMMARY

Home care has blossomed in recent years as a viable and often better option to hospitalization. Despite this, questions still remain regarding how to select candidates, how the decision for home care is made, who will help the parents and family, and how long help will be provided.

There are three basic models to providing pediatric home care: 1) hospital based, 2) community based, 3) bureaucratic. Patient selection should be based on the type of patient, the type and severity of the illness, and the home environment. Home ventilator care is possible, assuming certain conditions are in place. They include a mature tracheostomy, F_iO_2 requirements less than 40% no need for invasive monitoring, and an adequate nutritional intake. Several home ventilators are available that are fairly simple to operate, have backup power mechanisms, and alarms to indicate disconnects or ventilator problems.

Home aerosol therapy is often necessary during the home care of respiratory patients. Several companies offer medical compressors that power small volume nebulizers. Portable ultrasonic nebulizers are also available for home use. MDIs are a popular method of delivering aerosolized medicines but require training and coordination to be effective. Patients and their families can also be trained to provide CPT and suctioning at home. Percussors are available for home use, or the patient and family may feel comfortable using hand cupping.

Home apnea monitors have gone from immense popularity to far fewer uses currently. The main reason for the decline in home use is that, despite their use, the incidence of SIDS did not decline. There are, however, a group of patients who stand to benefit from the use of a home apnea monitor. These are patients who have a history of apnea and ALTEs.

Oxygen therapy is becoming more acceptable as a home care treatment. The arrival of oxygen concentrators and liquid oxygen tanks greatly reduced the overall cost and risk associated with long-term oxygen use. Small portable tanks have also made short trips possible.

Discharge planning is a group process and requires the skills of several health care workers. Included in the process are a case manager, physician, respiratory therapist, nurse, social worker, dietician, physical therapy, occupational therapy, speech therapy, and the home care company.

Of great concern with home care is the stress that comes to the family. Proper planning and solid follow-up and support help ease the stress. Because the system is not perfect, home care failures occur. The most common cause of failure is a lack of resources. Other factors include emotional depletion and lack of communication.

Home care of a pediatric or infant patient has many positive aspects and should be encouraged where possible. It is not, however, without some negative aspects. The negative aspects can be minimized by proper preparation of the patient and family. The involvement of many disciplines helps create a successful environment. Anticipation of future problems and needs will help alleviate negative outcomes by allowing proper preparation.

As the role of medicine in our society continues to change, home health care will undoubtedly continue to play a major part.

POSTTEST

1. Which of the following are advantages of home care?
   - I. allows more normal family interaction
   - II. patients get infections less frequently
   - III. cost savings
   - IV. faster recovery from the disease process
     - a. I, III, IV
     - b. I, II, III
     - c. II, II, IV
     - d. III only
2. Which of the following is *not* true regarding the bureaucratic type of home care?
   - a. available to all families
   - b. may be more readily accepted by health care providers
   - c. many ancillary services are already in place
   - d. financial resources may be facilitated
3. Of the following disorders, which is most likely to produce candidates for ventilator home care?
   - a. cardiogenic anomalies
   - b. esophageal atresia
   - c. BPD
   - d. infantile botulism
4. Regarding tracheostomy tubes, which of the following is best suited for home care?
   - a. fenestrated, cuffed tube
   - b. uncuffed, slightly smaller than the trachea
   - c. cuffed, slightly larger than the trachea
   - d. uncuffed, larger than the trachea

5. Which of the following are possible hazards of home aerosol therapy?
   I. tracheal irritation
   II. fluid overload
   III. excessive secretions
   IV. burns
      a. I, II
      b. I, III, IV
      c. III, IV
      d. II, IV
6. Detecting clinical changes that may indicate infection or heart failure requires:
      a. outpatient blood work
      b. frequent examinations by a physician
      c. in-depth training of parents and caregivers
      d. establishing a baseline of normal patient status
7. Which of the following is a common cause of problems with home apnea monitoring?
      a. unfamiliarity with the equipment
      b. interference from radio and television signals
      c. frequent false alarms
      d. the equipment is not indicated
8. The main advantage to liquid oxygen systems is:
      a. they are very inexpensive
      b. they are very lightweight
      c. they hold a large quantity of gas
      d. the delivered oxygen is of a higher purity
9. Which of the following people coordinates home care services and acts as a liaison to the family?
      a. case manager
      b. physician
      c. nurse
      d. social worker
10. Of the following, which is the *least* likely to cause parental stress during home care?
      a. disruption of the family life
      b. the presence of a live-in caretaker
      c. the visual appearance of the infant
      d. constant noise and alarms
11. Which of the following is the *most* common cause of home care failure?
      a. family stress
      b. depletion of family resources
      c. lack of community and family resources
      d. physical exhaustion

REFERENCES

1. Aitken MJ. Matching models to environments: a planning guide to the selection of pediatric home care models. *Home Healthc Nurse.* 7:13–21, 1989.
2. Donar ME. Community care: pediatric home mechanical ventilation. *Holistic Nurs Pract.* 2:68–80, 1988.
3. AARC Clinical Practice Guideline: *Long-Term Invasive Mechanical Ventilation in the Home*—2007 Revision & Update.
4. Gilmartin M. Transition from the intensive care unit to home: patient selection and discharge planning. *Resp Care.* 39:456–480, 1994.
5. *Respiratory Home Care Procedure Manual.* 2nd ed. Pennsylvania Society for Respiratory Care Inc., 1997.
6. Lynch M. Bronchopulmonary dysplasia: management after discharge. *Home Healthc Nurs.* 7:34–40, 1989.
7. Lott D. Home apnea monitoring: an update. *Perinat/Neonat.* 12:223-237, 1988.
8. Consensus Statement: National Institute of Health Consensus Development Conference on Infantile Apnea and Home Monitoring, Sept. 29 to Oct. 1, 1986. *Pediatrics.* 79:292–299, 1987.
9. Wyka K. *Respiratory Care in Alternate Sites.* Albany, NY: Delmar Thomson Learning, 1998.
10. Koff PB, Eitzman DV, Nev J. *Neonatal and Pediatric Respiratory Care.* St. Louis, MO: CV Mosby Co., 1993.
11. Bedore B, Leighton L. Ventilator-dependent children: comprehensive home management. *Caring.* 8:50–52, 54–55, 1989.
12. McKim EM. The difficult first week at home with a premature infant. *Neonatal Network.* 12:72, 1993.
13. Feinberg EA. Family stress in pediatric home care. *Caring.* 4:38, 40–41, 1985.
14. Harris PJ. Sometimes pediatric home care doesn't work. *Am J Nurs.* 88:851–854, 1988.

BIBLIOGRAPHY AND SUGGESTED READINGS

American Association for Respiratory Care. AARC Clinical Practice Guideline: discharge planning for the respiratory care patient. *Respiratory Care.* 40:1308–1312, 1995.

American Association for Respiratory Care. AARC Clinical Practice Guideline: long-term invasive mechanical ventilation in the home. 2007 Revision and Update.

Burton GG, et al. *Respiratory Care. A Guide to Clinical Practice.* 4th ed. Philadelphia, PA: JB Lippincott Co., 1997.

Pierson DJ. Controversies in home respiratory care: conference summary. *Resp Care.* 39:294–308, 1994.

White G. *Equipment Theory for Respiratory Care.* 5th ed. Clifton Park, NY: Cengage Learning, 2015.

CHAPTER 23

Care of the Parents

OBJECTIVES

Upon completion of this chapter, the reader should be able to:

1. Describe the bonding that takes place during each of the following periods:
   a. Pregnancy
   b. Labor and delivery
   c. Home
2. List the factors that cause stress to the parents following delivery of a sick neonate.
3. Describe the following environmental factors and their role in creating stress in the parents:
   a. Appearance of the neonate
   b. Staff communications
   c. Alteration of parental roles
4. Compare and contrast maternal and paternal stress as it relates to the above factors.
5. Describe how the respiratory therapist can reduce stress factors for the parents.
6. Define grief.
7. Describe each stage of grief and its accompanying clinical signs and symptoms.
8. Describe how the respiratory therapist can help the parents through each stage of grief.

KEY TERMS

anticipatory grief	lethargy	pessimism
bonding	optimism	psychosocial
empathetic		

INTRODUCTION

One very important area of concern that has risen from the rapid advance of neonatology, and one that is frequently overlooked, is caring for the family of the sick neonate. An essential part of the work of any neonatal practitioner is addressing the psychological needs of each family member. Although not intended to be all inclusive, this chapter takes a brief look at the bonding process, the grieving process, and how the respiratory therapist can help the family cope.

BONDING

The intense attachment that is developed between a baby and its parents is called bonding. For most, bonding occurs quickly and for others, it may take a little longer. It is now generally accepted that bonding takes place over time. Understanding the process will help the parents and loved ones make this important adaptation.

Bonding During Pregnancy

The **bonding** of parent to child begins with the anticipation of the child (Table 23–1). Upon discovering that pregnancy has begun the family begins preparations for the new addition. The nursery is prepared, furniture and bedding are purchased. The family begins to imagine what the child will look like, guessing its sex and thinking of potential names. They dream of the future and the happiness the newborn will bring to them. The first sounds of the heartbeat and the first signs of movement

---

Table 23–1

STEPS OF BONDING AND ATTACHMENT

1. Planning of the pregnancy

2. Confirmation of the pregnancy

3. Acceptance of the pregnancy

4. Feeling the first fetal movements

5. Acceptance of the fetus as an individual

6. Labor and subsequent birth of the infant

7. Seeing the infant for the first time

8. Touching the infant

9. Taking care of the infant

further increase expectations and heighten the excitement, because the baby is now an individual, no longer an imagined being.

As pregnancy continues, the mother is made continuously aware of the fetus's presence, as the physical discomfort of the pregnancy begins to weigh on her. The father, although not physically involved in the pregnancy, may find himself worrying about his wife and the baby. As the pregnancy advances, the lifestyle of the family changes. The mother is not able to do those things that she could previously do, and plans may be altered and changed.

Even though not present, the fetus is making a significant impact on the life of the family. It is already developing a personality, and the family finds itself laughing at the internal gyrations, hiccoughs, and limb stretches.

Bonding During Labor and Delivery

The onset of labor presents an emotional and psychological crisis for the family. The long-awaited time has finally arrived. All the difficulties encountered during the pregnancy and the anticipation is rewarded by the birth of a healthy infant. Everyone present is in an excited and anticipatory state; however, labor is also a time of physiologic crisis for the mother. She must endure tremendous pain and discomfort, for the most part, alone.

Birth of the infant brings tears, kisses, and joy to the family. The sound of a healthy cry and the presence of all fingers and toes and no defects bring a sigh of relief. Bonding now begins at an advanced level. The neonate, before now only seen in the imagination, is now held by the family. The initial touching and eye contact is an important part of the bonding process. The parents spend the first hours encouraging their neonate to look at them and having the newborn grasp their fingers. In addition to the psychological benefits of skin-to-skin contact between the parent and the infant, research suggests that physiological improvements in respiratory rates and pattern, heart rate, and oxyhemoglobin may also be promoted.[1]

During this time shortly following the delivery, the neonate is identified as having characteristics similar to the parents and other family members. This inspection is important and serves to allow the parents and family to accept the infant as a part of the family.

Bonding at Home

Arrival at home brings a new lifestyle to the family (Figure 23–1). The first few months are filled with frequent awakenings at night and other adaptations. The infant is totally dependent on the parents for his or her welfare. This is a time of tremendous growth in the maturity of the family and in their love for the new infant. The love and bonding that develop continue to increase as the infant grows.

Thus, bonding has taken place from the moment that the pregnancy was planned and continues throughout the life of the child. Any disruption of these normal bonding events can cause an emotional and psychological crisis for the family. It is during these times that the health care worker must be aware of the needs of the family and be able to address those needs appropriately.

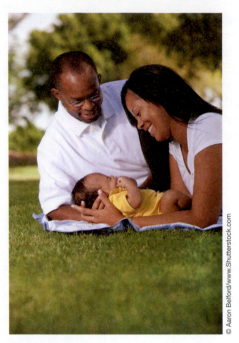

FIGURE 23–1. Bonding with the newborn.

CAUSES OF PARENTAL STRESS

The premature delivery of a neonate produces many stressors on the family. The sudden disruption of the pregnancy is a grief-producing occurrence that must be dealt with by the family. A review by Obeidat et al.[2] showed that parents with an infant in the NICU experience depression, anxiety, stress, and loss of control, and they vacillate between feelings of inclusion and exclusion related to the provision of health care to their neonate Additionally, several environmental stressors have been identified with which the family must also deal.

In the event of a premature delivery or other birth crisis, what should have been a happy, joyful time has become a major stress-inducing experience for the family. It is during this time and in the days and weeks to follow that the NICU team must be aware of the emotional and psychological needs of the family. By understanding the factors that create stress and individually assessing each neonate and their family with regard to such stress, the respiratory therapist can help reduce those factors through an individualized approach to care and family dynamics. Following a discussion of stress factors, we will examine the stages of grief, which the family commonly passes through following a birth crisis.

Identifying Stress Factors

Three sources of stress have been identified: 1) *personal and family background factors,* 2) *situational conditions,* and 3) *environmental stimuli.*[3] Personal and family background factors are the past and present experiences, beliefs, and attitudes that the family brings to the crisis. Situational conditions are threats to normal family behavior and interaction that occur following the birth of an ill neonate. A major situational condition is the presence of a language and/or cultural barrier. An excellent review of language and cultural differences has been produced by Santa Clara University.[4] The final factors, environmental stimuli, arisen from both the **psychosocial** and physical environment of the NICU3[2] The psychosocial environment relates to one's ability to interact and develop within a social setting. Our focus will be on these environmental factors.

Environmental Stress Factors

The entire environment of the NICU creates varying degrees of stress on the family. The physical separation from the newborn, the heat, noise and alarms, abundance of high-tech equipment, crowds of medical personnel, and the sight of other critically ill neonates may overwhelm the parents. In fact, research has shown that parental anxiety levels can reach near-panic levels initially.[5] Other research has found that 28% of the mothers of critically ill neonates reported clinically significant psychological distress compared to 10% of the general population.[6]

Appearance of the Neonate The appearance and behavior of the neonate are another source of stress for the parents and family. Their newborn does not look like they had imagined.

The shock produced by the visual appearance of the newborn is often difficult to get over. In addition, the tangle of wires and tubing attached to their newborn furthers the shock. The preemie may have gelatinous skin with numerous bruises and abrasions from delivery. Neonates may also be subject to potentially painful procedures. Preparation of the parents for these sights will help reduce the visual shock.

High-Tech/Impersonal Environment An additional source of stress can be the high-tech, impersonal appearance of the NICU. Initially, many parents find the NICU appearance shocking and intimidating. Equipment with wiring, tubing, and blinking lights looks frightening. These factors combined with audible alarms can be unnerving to parents, who themselves may be adversely affected by sensory overload and a sense of alienation.[7]

Staff Communication Another source of environmental stress is the communication, or lack thereof, between staff and family. As much as possible, the parents should be involved in the care of the neonate. They should be involved in decision making and not simply told what will happen next.

Alteration of Parental Role A final source of environmental stress is the alteration of the parental role in the care of the neonate. The family takes on a subordinate role, and often may feel as though they are spectators only, without any control over outcomes. This is often magnified by the thoughtless treatment of parents by respiratory therapists as though they are outsiders.

Maternal versus Paternal Stress

Research has shown that the mothers of critically ill neonates have a more adverse reaction to the NICU environment than the fathers.

An interesting study done by Perehudoff sampled the reactions of fathers and mothers to various NICU environmental stressors.[3] The study indicates that mothers and fathers perceived environmental stress differently, and that overall the mother was more stressed than the father. Mothers indicated that parental role alteration was the highest source of stress, followed by NICU sights and sounds, the neonate's appearance and behaviors, and, finally, staff communications and relations.

In contrast, fathers indicated that the highest degree of stress was caused by the sights and sounds, followed by parental role alteration. The final two stressors were the same in fathers as in the mothers.

Another study performed by Shields-Poe and colleagues supported some of the findings described above and found that other factors also affected parental stress levels such as where and when the parents first saw their infant.[8]

Other Stressors

In addition to the environmental stressors, other factors have been shown to contribute to parental stress. Increased tendency toward trait-anxiety and a strong desire for the pregnancy resulted in higher stress levels for parents of NICU patients.[8] Other research indicates that additional parental stressors may be related to siblings' reaction to the NICU experience and disruption from the daily family routine.[9]

IMPLICATIONS FOR THE RESPIRATORY THERAPIST

An understanding of the environmental stress factors will aid the respiratory therapist in helping the parents and family cope with the multitude of stressors. Allowing the parents opportunities to care for their neonate may help reduce the alteration of their parental role (Figure 23–2).

The shock of the sights and sounds of the NICU can be lessened by explaining to the parents in advance what they will see and what to expect. Pictures of premature infants will allow the parents and family to prepare for what their neonate will look like. It is important to emphasize that their baby looks perfectly normal for its gestational age. The parents must be assured that their baby looks exactly like it should. Cultural and religious considerations should also be identified early and respected to avoid additional stress for the family.

Finally, good communication between staff members and family will greatly lessen stress by instilling in the parents some degree of participation and control. The parents must feel comfortable to call whenever they desire to get an update on their baby's status. The staff should avoid phrases such as "he's stable" or "there's no change in her status." Instead, the parents should be informed of current ventilator settings, weight gains or losses, and the rationale for any change in medications

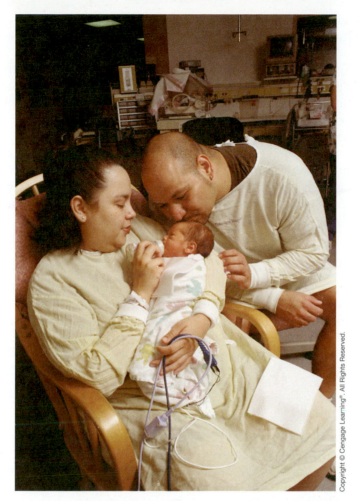

FIGURE 23–2. Parents should be encouraged to care for their baby in the NICU.

or treatments should be explained to the parents. The staff should encourage the parents to share their feelings and frustrations openly, always being **empathetic** toward their difficult situation. Empathy differs from sympathy in that it recognizes the emotions being experienced by another person. Support-group participation by parents should also be encouraged.

UNDERSTANDING GRIEF

Grief has been defined as "an abiding and pervasive sense of sadness that over-whelms us when we are separated from a person, place, or object important to our emotional life."[10] Unless one has experienced grief, it is unlikely that person truly understands what a grieving person is feeling. An unfortunate consequence of this lack of understanding is the tendency to ignore the symptoms and needs of one who is grieving.

The birth of an ill neonate is a situation that produces grief in the parents and family members. Critical illness or death of an infant or child is one of the greatest stresses that a parent can experience. The anticipation that the baby may not survive further enhances the grief.[11] An understanding of what occurs during the grieving period will help respiratory therapists provide the necessary support and will enable them to better empathize with and tolerate the behavior of the family. It is also important for the respiratory therapist to recognize individual differences in each person's grieving process. The respiratory therapist should try to empathize and not get defensive if parents manifest feelings of anger, frustration, and self-pity toward them.

Anticipatory Grief

Death does not necessarily have to occur for grief to be present. **Anticipatory grief** occurs when the death of a love one appears likely.[10] This is often the type of grief that parents and family members of a critically ill neonate experience. A person undergoing anticipatory grief passes through the same stages as if death had actually occurred. They require the same amount of support and assistance as any other grieving person.[10]

Stages of Grief

A pioneer in the development of grief stages was Elisabeth Kübler-Ross.[12] Studies done on the dying revealed that grieving is a process that occurs in an inexact pattern. Each phase represents the dominant feelings or processes that are occurring. The phases are not limited to any time frame, nor does every grieving person pass through each stage to the same degree. These are merely presented to allow some insight into what the parents of an ill infant may be experiencing. The stages presented here follow the pattern offered by Weizman and Kamm.[13]

Shock: The First Stage of Grief The initial emotion felt by the parents is one of shock, denial, and disbelief. No matter how prepared the family may think they are for the delivery, no one is ever totally ready for the shock that accompanies a premature delivery. It often occurs during the time in the pregnancy when the mother is still bonding with the infant. The mother is in the process of undergoing not only a physical change, but also a psychological change as the pregnancy advances. The pregnancy has usually progressed far enough to allow the family to accept the infant as an individual, but not to the point where they are emotionally ready for the delivery.

The premature delivery causes a type of psychological dislocation to take place. As previously mentioned, the initial shock is intensified by several environmental factors, such as the sight of the neonate and the high-tech environment of the NICU.

Confusion Included in the feeling of shock is an overwhelming sense of confusion. There is a feeling of not knowing what to do or who to turn to. Time may become distorted, and memory of the events surrounding the birth of the neonate may be cloudy.

Denial Another phase of shock is denial. Denial is an attempt to shield oneself from the pain and impact of the event. Denial may present itself subtly or openly by the parents. They may refuse to believe what is told them by the physician and may even go so far as to look for another "specialist" to take care of their infant.

Denial may take one of two contrasting patterns. Some parents may feel that, regardless of what they are being told, their infant will be all right. On the other extreme, they may believe that the situation is hopeless, regardless of what they are told. In these instances, parents may exhibit a reluctance to see, touch, or hold their infant.[14]

Parents often tend to be more negative (**pessimistic**) than positive (**optimistic**) about their infant's condition. Pessimism is that unfortunate state of mind where the anticipation of undesirable outcomes becomes the primary thought. This pessimism may be fostered by overly negative reports from the health care team. Whereas it is never justified to give unrealistic hope to the family, it is equally damaging to be overly gloomy in the prognosis. The odds are weighted heavily in the infant's favor in most NICUs, so a cautious optimism may be more helpful to the parents than a continual negative outlook.

The NICU team must work together when talking to the family. It is not uncommon for one team member to report that the infant is doing better, only to have another claim that the infant is the same or worse than before. Such mixed signals cause the parents to lose faith in the team and possibly wonder if anyone really knows what they are talking about. Discussions with the family regarding the overall status of their infant may best be handled by the attending neonatologist.

Bargaining Bargaining is an attempt to find a magical solution by promising anything in return for a healthy infant. Promises such as "I will be the perfect parent" and "I'll never do anything wrong again" are common pleas.

Bargaining often had deep religious overtones. Promises are made to God that the person will do whatever is required, if God will only heal their child. Bargaining is like denial, in that it is a temporary release from reality that allows the person to feel as if they have some control over what is happening. It allows the person more time to acquire the needed strength to face the problem.

Isolation An attempt to become isolated from the entire situation is often seen next in grieving people. The isolation may be an attempt to be protected from further emotional damage. The person may feel that no one understands, causing them to withdraw from the situation.

The health care team should make every effort to close the gap of isolation, to stay in contact with the family, encourage their presence in the NICU, and consider support-group referral.

Undoing: The Second Stage of Grief During this stage, the person attempts to undo what has happened so life can return to what it was. There may be thoughts of what should have or could have been done to prevent the premature birth. Thoughts such as these are an attempt to undo what has happened in the mind of the parent.

Guilt A common feeling during the undoing stage is that of guilt. In an attempt to undo the situation, the mother may become obsessed with the idea that something she did, or did not do, caused the premature birth. The parents may feel that they have some sort of physical defect that caused the birth. The mother often feels that she is at fault for the crisis.

The NICU team must be careful to in no way reinforce this idea. The family, and especially the mother, must understand that nothing she did, or did not do, caused the premature delivery. Some may feel that the early birth is a punishment for something they did. The fixation of blame is a natural human tendency, even if it is upon oneself. Positive reinforcement by the NICU team will help to minimize the guilt that may be present.

Anger: The Third Stage of Grief Many families undergoing a crisis may at some point become angry. Anger is directed in many ways and toward many people. Anger may be directed at the health care team, whom the parents may see as ghouls whose only desire is to inflict further pain on their infant. They may vent their anger on anyone who is present. The expression of anger is an attempt to affix blame for the crisis on someone or something.

Threats of lawsuits may be directed at the nurse for starting an IV or at the respiratory therapist for obtaining a heel stick blood gas. Anger is often directed toward God, with the family wondering why He would allow such a thing to happen to them. The mother may be angry at those who have normal babies, or at every pregnant woman.

Parents and families may even blame each other for the premature birth. The father may blame the mother for not quitting work or for some other action that he views as causing the premature birth. The family may even express anger toward the infant for being born early. The in-laws may accuse the son-in-law of not earning enough money to allow their daughter to quit work while pregnant.

Regardless of where the anger is directed, the respiratory therapist must understand that it is a natural part of the grieving process and must be patient with the family. One must always keep in mind that the expression of anger is essential in the grieving process.

Sadness: The Fourth Stage of Grief When the reality of the event finally begins to sink in, an overwhelming feeling of sadness occurs. Parents may feel like life is not worth living without their baby. They express extreme disappointment and hopelessness in their situation. This stage is possibly the most painful stage of grief, one in which the family requires much love and support.

Avoidance of Sadness To avoid the profound sadness of this stage, the parents may engage in a bustle of activity, so they will not have time to feel sad. They may withhold and suppress feelings of sadness by refusing to cry or talk about the situation. During this time, the health care worker must encourage the parents to express their sadness and talk openly about their disappointment. Suppressing the feeling only brings anger and a prolongation of the sadness. Only when the feelings of anger and sadness are relieved are the parents able to continue their emotional recovery.

Depression Continued feelings of guilt and the inability to express anger may lead to depression. Depression is often characterized by a loss of appetite, lack of sleep, and overall **lethargy**. The person becomes withdrawn and unresponsive. In addition, the mother may suffer a normal postpartum depression, which is heaped on the previous depression.

Physical exhaustion from lack of sleep further complicates the depression. The person suffering from severe depression may need to be treated with medications to induce sleep and help with the feelings of hopelessness. As always, continual support by the NICU team is invaluable. The mother must understand that she is not a failure. Severe extended depression requires immediate attention and should never be passed off as being just a part of the grieving process.

Integration: The Fifth Stage of Grief As a person slowly passes through each stage of grief, there is a gradual accomplishment of integration.

Acceptance An important milestone in integration is acceptance. The time will finally arrive when the parents accept the crisis and begin to handle it in a constructive way. It may arrive quickly, or may be delayed, but eventually comes. Acceptance comes when the family becomes familiar with the surroundings in the NICU.

The parents have adapted to the dramatic change in their lifestyle, and visiting their sick baby is now a part of their routine. They know and trust the health care team and understand what is happening to their infant. They are involved in the care of the infant and hold it as often as possible. Once acceptance occurs, the parents of infants with a favorable NICU outcome can now look forward to the day the baby is released with anticipation and happiness.

In situations where the infant dies, it will take a considerable amount of time before acceptance occurs. Often in such situations, pictures are taken of the baby to aid in the grieving and acceptance process. Professional counseling and bereavement support groups often benefit the parents and family of the deceased infant.

Grieving and the Respiratory Therapist Death is a reality in the NICU setting and can significantly add to the respiratory therapist's job stress. Research reveals that respiratory therapists often experience feelings of helplessness, intense sorrow, chronic fatigue, and irritability when an infant dies. It is important for respiratory therapists to first acknowledge such feelings. Communication with coworkers, counseling professionals, and friends and family is often helpful in this grieving process.[15]

SUMMARY

An understanding of the stages of grief will help the respiratory therapist to accept and be empathetic toward parental behaviors. With this enhanced understanding in hand, the respiratory therapist can help address parental grief by appropriately sharing information with parents to avoid a sense of abandonment. Additionally, they can also assist parents in the grieving process by being sensitive to cultural and religious issues and taking an overall empathetic approach to family interaction and patient care.[16] Grieving often involves feelings of shock, denial, anger, and bargaining, which are necessary in that they allow time to accept the crisis in small, manageable doses. The stages discussed may not occur in order, and some may not occur at all.

Members of the family may go through stages at different speeds and be at different levels of understanding, making communication among them difficult. The mother, because of her deeper feelings toward the infant, often suffers more severely than the father during the various stages.

The intensity of emotions will vary among family members. Some persons may accept the crisis from the beginning, while others withdraw and want nothing to do with the neonate. Although the parents have reached acceptance of the initial crisis, they may go through each stage again with each new setback.

The parents should be encouraged to have frequent contact with their infant. This tends to hasten the acceptance of the child. The family must be informed of the various types of equipment being used and why it is being used. Daily updates are vital and help the family to adapt to the situation. Counselors who are experts in dealing with crisis should be involved with the family from the beginning.

Parents should be encouraged to express emotions and seek help in dealing with those emotions. Positive reinforcement by members of the health care team is vital in supporting the parents during these difficult trials. Programs may also be developed for the siblings to help them understand what is happening to their brother or sister.

Even with an understanding of the grief process, it is still impossible to know how the family is feeling at any one moment. It is at those times that a hug or a shoulder to cry on are the best things that the health care worker can offer.

POSTTEST

1. Parent-to-child bonding begins:
    a. with the anticipation of the child
    b. at the first signs of life
    c. during the last trimester of pregnancy
    d. during delivery

2. Which of the following are potential sources of stress for the parents of sick neonates?
    I. personal and family background
    II. physiological compromise
    III. ethical judgments
    IV. situational conditions
    V. environmental stimuli
        a. I, III, IV
        b. II, III
        c. III only
        d. I, IV, V

3. Studies have shown that the highest source of stress in mothers of sick neonates is:
    a. the appearance of the neonate
    b. alteration of the parental role
    c. NICU sights and sounds
    d. staff communications

4. When the death of a loved one appears likely, grief felt by the family is termed:
    a. contemplatory
    b. expectant
    c. anticipatory
    d. envisioning

5. The first stage of grief includes which of the following?
    I. shock
    II. confusion
    III. denial
    IV. guilt
    V. isolation
        a. I, III, IV
        b. I, V
        c. I, II, III, IV, V
        d. I, II, III, V

6. Sadness and its avoidance are found in which stage of grief?
    a. stage I
    b. stage II
    c. stage III
    d. stage IV

7. A visit to the NICU prior to delivery of a high-risk infant may reduce which of the following stages of grief?
    a. denial
    b. anger
    c. guilt
    d. shock

8. The human tendency to affix blame on someone or something generally produces:
   a. anger
   b. guilt
   c. shock
   d. acceptance

9. The family member who begins making promises is in the phase of:
   a. denial
   b. acceptance
   c. bargaining
   d. anger

10. When the family becomes familiar with the NICU surroundings and personnel and begins involving themselves in the care of the infant, they have entered the stage of:
    a. denial
    b. bargaining
    c. anger
    d. acceptance

11. Parents and family members may best be helped through grief by which of the following?
    I. constant encouragement
    II. explanations of the care being given
    III. allowing involvement in the care of the infant
    IV. leaving them alone
    V. recommending professional help
    a. II, III, V
    b. I, II, III
    c. I, II, III, V
    d. I, III, V

12. The respiratory therapist can help reduce the stress level of parents of critically ill neonates by doing all of the following *except*:
    a. displaying empathy toward the family
    b. communicating as openly as practical with the parents
    c. support-group referral
    d. being pessimistic so as not to get the parents' hopes up

REFERENCES

1. Cleary GM, et al. Skin-to-skin parental contact with fragile preterm infants. *J Am Osteopath Assoc.* 97:457–460, 1997.
2. Obeidat HM, et al. The parental experience of having an infant in the newborn intensive care unit. *J Perinat Educ.* 18(3):23–29, Summer, 2009.

3. Perehudoff B. Parents' perceptions of environmental stressors in the special care nursery. *Neonatal Network.* 9:39–44.

4. Peterson-Iyer KA. Difficult birth: Navigating language and cultural differences. http://www.scu.edu/ethics/practicing/focusareas/medical/culturally-competent-care/difficult-birth.html.

5. Huckabay LM, Tilem-Kessler D. Patterns of parental stress in PICU emergency admission. *Dimensions in Critical Care Nursing.* 18:36–42, 1999.

6. Meyer EC, et al. Psychological distress in mothers of pre-term infants. *J Dev Behav Pediatr.* 16:412–417, 1995.

7. Jamsa K, Jamsa T. Technology in neonatal intensive care—a study on parents' experiences. *Technol Health Care.* 6:225–230, 1998.

8. Shields-Poe D, Pinelli J. Varibles associated with parental stress in neonatal intensive care units. *Neonatal Network.* 16:29–37, 1997.

9. Haines C, et al. A comparison of the stressors experienced by parents of intubated and non-intubated children. *J Adv Nurs.* 21:350–355, 1995.

10. Doyle P. *Grief Counseling and Sudden Death: A Manual and Guide.* Springfield, IL: Charles C Thomas, 1980.

11. Kenner C, Lott JW. Parent transition after discharge from the NICU. *Neonatal Network.* 9:31–37, 1990.

12. Kübler-Ross E. *On Death and Dying.* New York, NY: The Macmillan Co., 1969.

13. Weizman SG, Kamm P. *About Mourning: Support and Guidance for the Bereaved.* New York, NY: Human Sciences Press Inc., 1985.

14. Lundqvist A, Nilstun N. Neonatal death and parents' grief. Experience, behaviour and attitudes of Swedish nurses. *Scandinavian Journal of Caring Sciences.* 12:246–250, 1998.

15. Downey V, et al. Dying babies and associated stress in NICU nurses. *Neonatal Network.* 14:41–46, 1995.

16. Sahler OJ, et al. Medical education about end-of-life care in the pediatric setting: principles, challenges, and opportunities. *Pediatrics 105.* 3(pt 1):575–584, 2000.

BIBLIOGRAPHY AND SUGGESTED READINGS

Arnold JH, Gemma PB. *A Child Dies. A Portrait of Family Grief.* Philadelphia, PA: Charles Press, 1994.

Carter BS, Levetown M. *Paliative Care for Infants, Children, and Adolescents: A Practical Handbook.* Baltimore, MD: Johns Hopkins University Press, 2004.

Donnelly K. *Recovering from the Loss of a Child.* San Jose, CA: iUniverse, 2001.

Finkbeiner AK. *After the Death of a Child: Living with Loss Through the Years.* Baltimore, MD: Johns Hopkins University Press, 1998.

Humphery GM. *Counselling for Grief and Bereavement.* Los Angeles, CA: SAGE Publications Ltd., 2008.

Keogh MJ. *As Much Time as it Takes: A Guide for the Bereaved, Their Family and Friends* Newburyport, MA: Hampton Roads Publishing Co., 2005.

Kumar, SM. *Grieving Mindfully*. Oakland, CA: New Harbinger Publications, 2005.

Obeidat HM et.al. The parental experience of having an infant in the newborn intensive care unit. *J Perinat Educ.* 18(3):23–29, Summer, 2009.

Peterson-Iyer K. *A Difficult Birth: Navigating Language and Cultural Differences.* http://www.scu.edu/ethics/practicing/focusareas/medical/culturally-competent-care/difficult-birth.html.

Worden JW. *Grief Counseling and Grief Therapy.* Springer Publishing Co., 2009.

APPENDIX A

Laboratory and Clinical Proficiency Check-Offs

Bag and Mask Ventilation
Performance Evaluation

Student Name: _____   Date: _____

Instructor Name: _____

TASK:	PEER	LAB	CLINICAL
1. Obtain equipment			
a. stethoscope	☐	☐	☐
b. resuscitation bag, with reservoir if self-inflating	☐	☐	☐
c. pressure manometer and tubing	☐	☐	☐
d. properly fitting mask	☐	☐	☐
2. Observe universal precautions, including washing hands	☐	☐	☐
3. Check bag for proper function			
a. occlude bag opening	☐	☐	☐
b. fill bag with gas	☐	☐	☐
c. compress bag	☐	☐	☐
d. check for leaks	☐	☐	☐
e. measure 20 to 40 cm H_2O pressure	☐	☐	☐
f. check function of pop-off valve	☐	☐	☐
4. Position the patient: head slightly tilted	☐	☐	☐
5. Position the mask over mouth and nose with a proper seal	☐	☐	☐
6. Ventilate the patient			
a. watch for chest rise	☐	☐	☐
b. rate of 40–60 breaths per minute	☐	☐	☐
c. appropriate inspriatory pressures	☐	☐	☐
d. insert nasogastric tube if manual ventilation lasts longer than 2 minutes	☐	☐	☐
7. Auscultate lungs	☐	☐	☐
8. Continue ventilation until			
a. spontaneous effort is adequate	☐	☐	☐
b. patient is intubated and placed on ventilator	☐	☐	☐

	PEER	LAB	CLINICAL
9. Leave the patient area clean and safe	☐	☐	☐
10. Wash hands before leaving the room	☐	☐	☐
11. Document and monitor oxygenation and ventilation	☐	☐	☐

***Upon completion of check-off, student should be able to perform the task with no prompting.

Completion Dates & Signatures:

Date Peer _____   Signature: _____

Date Lab _____   Signature: _____

Date Clinical _____   Signature: _____

Capillary Heel Stick
Performance Evaluation

Student Name: _____   Date: _____

Instructor Name: _____

TASK:	PEER	LAB	CLINICAL
1. Heel Prep			
a. obtain heated cloth or chemical warmer	☐	☐	☐
b. select appropriate heel location	☐	☐	☐
c. wrap foot in cloth/warmer	☐	☐	☐
d. allow heel to warm 5–7 minutes	☐	☐	☐
2. Observe universal precautions, including washing hands	☐	☐	☐
3. Obtain Equipment			
a. small lancet	☐	☐	☐
b. alcohol swab or sterile saline wipe	☐	☐	☐
c. Betadine swab	☐	☐	☐
d. heparinized capillary tube	☐	☐	☐
e. metal flea and magnet	☐	☐	☐
f. sterile gauze	☐	☐	☐
g. rubber caps	☐	☐	☐
h. blood gas data label	☐	☐	☐
4. Prepare equipment			
a. open swabs	☐	☐	☐
b. open lancet	☐	☐	☐
5. Perform procedure			
a. completely unwrap heel	☐	☐	☐
b. wipe heel w/ alcohol swab or saline wipe	☐	☐	☐
c. stick heel in appropriate location	☐	☐	☐
d. fill capillary tube w/ sample	☐	☐	☐
e. wipe site with alcohol swab or saline wipe after obtaining sample	☐	☐	☐
f. hold pressure w/ gauze until bleeding stops	☐	☐	☐
g. secure gauze with tape/band-aid	☐	☐	☐

	PEER	LAB	CLINICAL
6. Insert flea and cap each end of the tube	☐	☐	☐
7. Mix sample with flea and magnet	☐	☐	☐
8. Leave the patient area clean and safe			
9. Wash hands before leaving the room	☐	☐	☐
10. Document results in patient chart	☐	☐	☐

***Upon completion of check-off, student should be able to perform the task with no prompting.

Completion Dates & Signatures:

Date Peer _____   Signature: _____

Date Lab _____   Signature: _____

Date Clinical _____   Signature: _____

Chest Physiotherapy
Performance Evaluation

Student Name: _____   Date: _____

Instructor Name: _____

TASK:	PEER	LAB	CLINICAL
1. Review chart			
a. check order	☐	☐	☐
b. contraindications	☐	☐	☐
c. secretions	☐	☐	☐
d. pathophysiology of the lung disease	☐	☐	☐
e. patient condition	☐	☐	☐
f. past response to therapy	☐	☐	☐
g. current chest x-ray	☐	☐	☐
2. Observe universal precautions, including washing hands	☐	☐	☐
3. Obtain required equipment			
a. stethoscope	☐	☐	☐
b. percussor/vibrator	☐	☐	☐
c. resuscitation bag and mask	☐	☐	☐
d. suction equipment	☐	☐	☐
4. Identify the patient	☐	☐	☐
5. Assess vital signs			
a. breath sounds	☐	☐	☐
b. pulse	☐	☐	☐
c. respiratory rate and effort	☐	☐	☐
d. color	☐	☐	☐
e. oxygenation status	☐	☐	☐
6. Place patient in appropriate position for secretion drainage and removal	☐	☐	☐

	PEER	LAB	CLINICAL
7. Appropriately percuss/vibrate patient chest wall			
a. correct equipment	☐	☐	☐
b. appropriate rate and rhythm	☐	☐	☐
c. appropriate striking force	☐	☐	☐
d. percuss within anatomic boundaries	☐	☐	☐
e. appropriate duration	☐	☐	☐
8. Leave the patient area clean and safe	☐	☐	☐
9. Return patient to desired position	☐	☐	☐
10. Reassess vital signs	☐	☐	☐
11. Appropriately suction the patient	☐	☐	☐
12. Wash hands before leaving the room	☐	☐	☐
13. Document equipment, data, results and observations	☐	☐	☐
14. Monitor appropriately	☐	☐	☐

***Upon completion of check-off, student should be able to perform the task with no prompting.

Completion Dates & Signatures:

Date Peer _____   Signature: _____

Date Lab _____   Signature: _____

Date Clinical _____   Signature: _____

Chest X-Ray Interpretation Performance Evaluation

Student Name: _____   Date: _____

Instructor Name: _____

TASK:	PEER	LAB	CLINICAL
1. Systematically examine the x-ray			
a. check identification tag	☐	☐	☐
b. orient to right and left	☐	☐	☐
c. determine exposure	☐	☐	☐
d. identify artifact	☐	☐	☐
e. determine patient position	☐	☐	☐
f. determine if inspiratory or expiratory	☐	☐	☐
g. examine the diaphragm	☐	☐	☐
h. examine the abdomen	☐	☐	☐
i. determine the proper position of the UAC and UVC	☐	☐	☐
j. examine the cardiac silhouette	☐	☐	☐
k. examine the lung hilum	☐	☐	☐
l. examine the trachea	☐	☐	☐
m. determine the position of the endotracheal tube	☐	☐	☐
n. examine the bronchus and the lung tissue	☐	☐	☐
2. Determine possible lung pathology present	☐	☐	☐
3. Suggest appropriate treatment or changes	☐	☐	☐
4. Document appropriate findings in patient chart	☐	☐	☐

***Upon completion of check-off, student should be able to perform the task with no prompting.

Completion Dates & Signatures:

Date Peer _____   Signature: _____

Date Lab _____   Signature: _____

Date Clinical _____   Signature: _____

Endotracheal Suctioning Performance Evaluation

Student Name: _____   Date: _____

Instructor Name: _____

TASK:	PEER	LAB	CLINICAL
1. Verify physician's order	☐	☐	☐
2. Prepare equipment	☐	☐	☐
a. appropriate-sized catheter	☐	☐	☐
b. adjust vacuum pressure accordingly to patient size (newborn vs. pediatric)	☐	☐	☐
c. prepare resuscitation bag and mask			
d. sterile saline	☐	☐	☐
3. Observe universal precautions, including washing hands	☐	☐	☐
4. Assess patient			
a. auscultate chest	☐	☐	☐
b. observe baseline vitals	☐	☐	☐
5. Perform procedure			
a. hyperoxgenate as needed	☐	☐	☐
b. aseptically open suction kit	☐	☐	☐
c. aseptically place sterile gloves	☐	☐	☐
d. attach catheter to suction tubing	☐	☐	☐
e. insert catheter into endotracheal tube without applying suction and advance to predetermined depth	☐	☐	☐
f. reconnect ventilator or manually ventilate for 4 to 5 breaths. Total time patient is disconnected from vent should not exceed 15 seconds.	☐	☐	☐
g. monitor and treat bradycardia/hypoxia	☐	☐	☐
h. instill saline if needed	☐	☐	☐
i. repeat as necessary	☐	☐	☐
j. clear line with remaining saline	☐	☐	☐
k. resume ventilation for patient	☐	☐	☐
6. Document the procedure in the patient chart	☐	☐	☐

	PEER	LAB	CLINICAL
7. Leave the patient area clean and safe	☐	☐	☐
8. Wash hands before leaving the room	☐	☐	☐
9. Monitor appropriately	☐	☐	☐

***Upon completion of check-off, student should be able to perform the task with no prompting.

Completion Dates & Signatures:

Date Peer _____   Signature: _____

Date Lab _____   Signature: _____

Date Clinical _____   Signature: _____

Intubation
Performance Evaluation

Student Name: _____ Date: _____

Instructor Name: _____

TASK:	PEER	LAB	CLINICAL
1. State indications for intubation	☐	☐	☐
2. Obtain equipment	☐	☐	☐
a. stethoscope	☐	☐	☐
b. tape	☐	☐	☐
c. appropriate size endotracheal tubes and stylet	☐	☐	☐
d. appropriate size laryngoscope blades (check function)	☐	☐	☐
e. manual resuscitation bag (check function)	☐	☐	☐
f. scissors	☐	☐	☐
g. oxygen blender	☐	☐	☐
h. shoulder roll	☐	☐	☐
3. Observe universal precautions, including washing hands	☐	☐	☐
4. Position patient	☐	☐	☐
5. Hyperoxygentate the patient	☐	☐	☐
6. Perform the procedure			
a. insert blade into mouth w/ laryngoscope in left hand	☐	☐	☐
b. advance blade to base of tongue	☐	☐	☐
c. lift blade up	☐	☐	☐
d. suction if needed	☐	☐	☐
e. visualize the epiglottis, advance blade over epiglottis	☐	☐	☐
f. gently lift epiglottis and visualize vocal cords	☐	☐	☐
g. insert ETT into the trachea the appropriate distance	☐	☐	☐
h. remove blade and stylet	☐	☐	☐
7. Re-oxygenate and auscultate for bilateral breath sounds	☐	☐	☐
8. Secure the tube with tape or securing device	☐	☐	☐
9. Obtain chest x-ray to confirm tube placement	☐	☐	☐
10. Document pertinent information in patient chart	☐	☐	☐

	PEER	LAB	CLINICAL
11. Leave the patient area clean and safe	☐	☐	☐
12. Wash hands before leaving the room	☐	☐	☐
13. Monitor appropriately	☐	☐	☐

***Upon completion of check-off, student should be able to perform the task with no prompting.

Completion Dates & Signatures:

Date Peer _____   Signature: _____

Date Lab _____   Signature: _____

Date Clinical _____   Signature: _____

Nasal CPAP
Performance Evaluation

Student Name: _____   Date: _____

Instructor Name: _____

TASK:	PEER	LAB	CLINICAL
1. Obtain equipment			
a. nasal prongs or nasal mask	☐	☐	☐
b. necessary tubing	☐	☐	☐
c. temperature probe	☐	☐	☐
d. oxygen blender	☐	☐	☐
e. humidifier and heater w/ sterile water	☐	☐	☐
f. water trap	☐	☐	☐
g. device to create CPAP	☐	☐	☐
h. pressure manometer	☐	☐	☐
i. oxygen analyzer	☐	☐	☐
j. low-pressure alarm	☐	☐	☐
k. sterile water w/ 25% acetic acid	☐	☐	☐
2. Observe universal precautions, including washing hands	☐	☐	☐
3. Prepare equipment			
a. connect blender flow meter to humidifier inlet	☐	☐	☐
b. fill humidifier with sterile water	☐	☐	☐
c. connect tubing to humidifier outlet	☐	☐	☐
d. place water trap in tubing	☐	☐	☐
e. connect insp. and exp. tubing to nasal prongs	☐	☐	☐
f. attach CPAP valve or submerge exp. tubing into sterile water w/ 25% acetic acid	☐	☐	☐
g. attach manometer to circuit/check pressure	☐	☐	☐
h. place nasal prongs onto patient	☐	☐	☐
5. Evaluate			
a. proper bubbling	☐	☐	☐
b. proper placement/position	☐	☐	☐
c. proper pressure	☐	☐	☐

	PEER	LAB	CLINICAL
d. analyzed F_iO_2	☐	☐	☐
e. circuit temperatures	☐	☐	☐
f. humidifier and water level	☐	☐	☐
6. Charting			
a. breath sounds and work of breathing	☐	☐	☐
b. sputum volume, color, consistency	☐	☐	☐
c. blood gas results	☐	☐	☐
d. oxygen saturation	☐	☐	☐
7. Report			
a. changes in status	☐	☐	☐
b. adverse reactions	☐	☐	☐
c. unusual findings	☐	☐	☐
8. Leave the patient area clean and safe	☐	☐	☐
9. Wash hands before leaving the room	☐	☐	☐
10. Monitor appropriately	☐	☐	☐

***Upon completion of check-off, student should be able to perform the task with no prompting.

Completion Dates & Signatures:

Date Peer _____   Signature: _____

Date Lab _____   Signature: _____

Date Clinical _____   Signature: _____

Nasopharyngeal Suctioning Performance Evaluation

Student Name: _____   Date: _____

Instructor Name: _____

TASK:	PEER	LAB	CLINICAL
1. Verify physician's order	☐	☐	☐
2. Prepare equipment	☐	☐	☐
a. select the appropriate sized catheter	☐	☐	☐
b. adjust vacuum pressure according to patient size (newborn or pediatric)	☐	☐	☐
c. prepare resuscitation bag and mask	☐	☐	☐
d. sterile saline	☐	☐	☐
3. Observe universal precautions, including washing hands	☐	☐	☐
4. Assess patient			
a. auscultate chest	☐	☐	☐
b. observe baseline vitals	☐	☐	☐
5. Perform procedure			
a. hyperoxygenate as needed	☐	☐	☐
b. open suction kit	☐	☐	☐
c. place sterile gloves	☐	☐	☐
d. attach catheter to suction tubing	☐	☐	☐
e. moisten catheter tip with water soluble lubricant	☐	☐	☐
f. insert catheter into nares, applying gentle upward, backward pressure until the nasopharynx is reached	☐	☐	☐
g. apply intermittent suction while withdrawing catheter	☐	☐	☐
h. monitor and treat bradycardia/hypoxia	☐	☐	☐
i. repeat as necessary	☐	☐	☐
j. clear line with remaining saline	☐	☐	☐
6. Document the procedure and pertinent information	☐	☐	☐
7. Leave the patient area clean and safe	☐	☐	☐

	PEER	LAB	CLINICAL
8. Wash hands before leaving the room	☐	☐	☐
9. Monitor appropriately	☐	☐	☐

***Upon completion of check-off, student should be able to perform the task with no prompting.

Completion Dates & Signatures:

Date Peer _____   Signature: _____

Date Lab _____   Signature: _____

Date Clinical _____   Signature: _____

Orogastric Catheter Placement
Performance Evaluation

Student Name: _____   Date: _____

Instructor Name: _____

TASK:	PEER	LAB	CLINICAL
1. Prepare equipment			
a. stethoscope	☐	☐	☐
b. tape	☐	☐	☐
c. appropriate size catheter	☐	☐	☐
d. manual resuscitation bag	☐	☐	☐
e. 20 cc syringe	☐	☐	☐
2. Observe universal precautions, including washing hands	☐	☐	☐
3. Prepare patient			
a. auscultate chest	☐	☐	☐
b. hyperoxygenate as needed	☐	☐	☐
c. observe baseline vitals	☐	☐	☐
4. Perform procedure	☐	☐	☐
a. measure length of catheter	☐	☐	☐
b. insert the catheter through mouth to desired depth	☐	☐	☐
c. attach a 20 cc syringe	☐	☐	☐
d. gently remove gastric contents	☐	☐	☐
e. remove syringe from catheter, leave open	☐	☐	☐
f. tape/secure catheter to infants cheek	☐	☐	☐
5. Document pertinent information in patient chart	☐	☐	☐
6. Leave the patient area clean and safe	☐	☐	☐
7. Wash hands before leaving the room	☐	☐	☐
8. Monitor appropriately	☐	☐	☐

***Upon completion of check-off, student should be able to perform the task with no prompting.

Completion Dates & Signatures:

Date Peer _____   Signature: _____

Date Lab _____   Signature: _____

Date Clinical _____   Signature: _____

Oropharyngeal Suctioning Performance Evaluation

Student Name: _____   Date: _____

Instructor Name: _____

TASK:	PEER	LAB	CLINICAL
1. Verify physician's order	☐	☐	☐
2. Prepare equipment	☐	☐	☐
a. appropriate sized catheter	☐	☐	☐
b. adjust vacuum pressure accordingly to patient size	☐	☐	☐
c. prepare resuscitation bag and mask	☐	☐	☐
d. sterile saline	☐	☐	☐
3. Observe universal precautions, including washing hands	☐	☐	☐
4. Assess patient			
a. auscultate chest	☐	☐	☐
b. observe baseline vitals	☐	☐	☐
5. Perform procedure			
a. hyperoxygenate as needed	☐	☐	☐
b. open suction kit	☐	☐	☐
c. place sterile gloves	☐	☐	☐
d. attach catheter to suction tubing	☐	☐	☐
e. moisten catheter tip with saline	☐	☐	☐
f. insert catheter through mouth to the oropharynx	☐	☐	☐
g. apply intermittent suction and withdraw catheter	☐	☐	☐
h. monitor and treat bradycardia/hypoxia	☐	☐	☐
i. repeat as necessary	☐	☐	☐
j. clear line with remaining saline	☐	☐	☐
6. Document the procedure and pertinent information	☐	☐	☐
7. Leave the patient area clean and safe	☐	☐	☐
8. Wash hands before leaving the room	☐	☐	☐
9. Monitor appropriately	☐	☐	☐

***Upon completion of check-off, student should be able to perform the task with no prompting.

Completion Dates & Signatures:

Date Peer _____   Signature: _____

Date Lab _____   Signature: _____

Date Clinical _____   Signature: _____

Oxygen Administration via Cannula or Mask
Performance Evaluation

Student Name: _____   Date: _____

Instructor Name: _____

TASK:	PEER	LAB	CLINICAL
1. Verify physician's order	☐	☐	☐
2. Observe universal precautions and hand washing	☐	☐	☐
3. Obtain required equipment			
a. oxygen flow meter	☐	☐	☐
b. humidifier, sterile water	☐	☐	☐
c. oxygen blender	☐	☐	☐
d. oxygen connecting tubing	☐	☐	☐
e. oxygen administration device	☐	☐	☐
f. "No Smoking" sign	☐	☐	☐
4. Identify the patient	☐	☐	☐
5. Adjust the device to the ordered level	☐	☐	☐
6. Apply the device to the patient	☐	☐	☐
7. Confirm F_iO_2 as appropriate	☐	☐	☐
8. Assess vital signs			
a. breath sounds	☐	☐	☐
b. pulse	☐	☐	☐
c. respiratory rate and effort	☐	☐	☐
d. color	☐	☐	☐
9. Dispose of excess equipment	☐	☐	☐
10. Leave the patient area clean and safe	☐	☐	☐
11. Wash hands before leaving the room	☐	☐	☐
12. Document equipment, concentration, and liter flow	☐	☐	☐
13. Monitor appropriately	☐	☐	☐

***Upon completion of check-off, student should be able to perform the task with no prompting.

Completion Dates & Signatures:

Date Peer _____   Signature: _____

Date Lab _____   Signature: _____

Date Clinical _____   Signature: _____

Oxygen Hood Therapy Performance Evaluation

Student Name: _____   Date: _____

Instructor Name: _____

TASK:	PEER	LAB	CLINICAL
1. Verify physician's order	☐	☐	☐
2. Observe universal precautions and hand washing	☐	☐	☐
3. Obtain required equipment	☐	☐	☐
a. oxygen flow meter	☐	☐	☐
b. humidifier w/ heater, sterile water	☐	☐	☐
c. oxygen blender	☐	☐	☐
d. appropriate size hood	☐	☐	☐
e. oxygen analyzer	☐	☐	☐
f. water trap	☐	☐	☐
g. thermometer probe	☐	☐	☐
h. connecting tubing	☐	☐	☐
i. "No Smoking" sign	☐	☐	☐
4. Identify the patient	☐	☐	☐
5. Connect blender to gas outlet and attach flow meter	☐	☐	☐
6. Connect blended flow meter to humidifier	☐	☐	☐
7. Connect aerosol tubing from humidifier to hood	☐	☐	☐
8. Place water trap in line	☐	☐	☐
9. Position hood next to infant	☐	☐	☐
10. Insert thermometer probe	☐	☐	☐
11. Set desired F_iO_2, flow, and temperature	☐	☐	☐
12. Analyze F_iO_2	☐	☐	☐
13. Check temperature	☐	☐	☐
14. Place infant in hood	☐	☐	☐

	PEER	LAB	CLINICAL
15. Assess vital signs			
a. breath sounds	☐	☐	☐
b. pulse	☐	☐	☐
c. respiratory rate and effort	☐	☐	☐
d. color	☐	☐	☐
16. Dispose of excess equipment	☐	☐	☐
17. Leave the patient area clean and safe	☐	☐	☐
18. Wash hands before leaving the room	☐	☐	☐
19. Document procedure and assessment	☐	☐	☐
20. Monitor appropriately	☐	☐	☐

***Upon completion of check-off, student should be able to perform the task with no prompting.

Completion Dates & Signatures:

Date Peer _____   Signature: _____

Date Lab _____   Signature: _____

Date Clinical _____   Signature: _____

Physical Assessment Performance Evaluation

Student Name: _____   Date: _____

Instructor Name: _____

TASK:	PEER	LAB	CLINICAL
1. Observe universal precautions and hand washing	☐	☐	☐
2. Visually inspect the neonate			
a. overall appearance	☐	☐	☐
b. proportions and posture	☐	☐	☐
c. head	☐	☐	☐
d. chest	☐	☐	☐
e. extremities	☐	☐	☐
f. lanugo	☐	☐	☐
3. Head-to-toe assessment			
I. Head			
a. fontanelles	☐	☐	☐
b. ears	☐	☐	☐
c. nose	☐	☐	☐
d. mouth	☐	☐	☐
e. neck	☐	☐	☐
II. Thorax			
a. skin	☐	☐	☐
b. breasts	☐	☐	☐
c. lungs	☐	☐	☐
d. heart	☐	☐	☐
III. Abdomen	☐	☐	☐
IV. Genitalia	☐	☐	☐
V. Extremities	☐	☐	☐
a. sole creases	☐	☐	☐
b. pulses	☐	☐	☐
4. Determine gestational age from preceding assessment	☐	☐	☐

	PEER	LAB	CLINICAL
5. Return patient to bed and position	☐	☐	☐
6. Document results and observations	☐	☐	☐
7. Leave the patient area clean and safe	☐	☐	☐
8. Wash hands before leaving the room	☐	☐	☐
9. Monitor appropriately	☐	☐	☐

***Upon completion of check-off, student should be able to perform the task with no prompting.

Completion Dates & Signatures:

Date Peer _____   Signature: _____

Date Lab _____   Signature: _____

Date Clinical _____   Signature: _____

Pulse Oximeter
Performance Evaluation

Student Name: _____　Date: _____

Instructor Name: _____

TASK:	PEER	LAB	CLINICAL
1. Verify physician's order	☐	☐	☐
2. Observe universal precautions and hand washing	☐	☐	☐
3. Obtain required equipment			
a. monitor	☐	☐	☐
b. probe	☐	☐	☐
c. device to secure probe	☐	☐	☐
4. Identify the patient	☐	☐	☐
5. Select proper site on patient	☐	☐	☐
6. Attach the oximeter probe on patient	☐	☐	☐
a. secure with Coban or restraint	☐	☐	☐
b. set alarm limits	☐	☐	☐
7. Monitor the oximeter	☐	☐	☐
a. pulse and heart rate correlate	☐	☐	☐
b. continued proper positioning	☐	☐	☐
c. O_2 saturation maintained at desired level	☐	☐	☐
8. Change probe site per protocol	☐	☐	☐
9. Assess vital signs			
a. breath sounds	☐	☐	☐
b. pulse	☐	☐	☐
c. respiratory rate and effort	☐	☐	☐
d. color	☐	☐	☐
10. Dispose of excess equipment	☐	☐	☐
11. Leave the patient area clean and safe	☐	☐	☐
12. Wash hands before leaving the room	☐	☐	☐

	PEER	LAB	CLINICAL
13. Document appropriate data in the patient chart.	☐	☐	☐
14. Monitor appropriately	☐	☐	☐

***Upon completion of check-off, student should be able to perform the task with no prompting.

Completion Dates & Signatures:

Date Peer _____   Signature: _____

Date Lab _____   Signature: _____

Date Clinical _____   Signature: _____

Ventilator Circuit Change Performance Evaluation

Student Name: _____ Date: _____

Instructor Name: _____

TASK:	PEER	LAB	CLINICAL
1. Wash hands	☐	☐	☐
2. Obtain required equipment			
a. patient circuit	☐	☐	☐
b. humidifier equipment	☐	☐	☐
c. sterile water	☐	☐	☐
d. stethoscope	☐	☐	☐
e. resuscitation bag	☐	☐	☐
f. eye protection	☐	☐	☐
3. Prepare new circuit	☐	☐	☐
a. turn off heater	☐	☐	☐
b. remove used humidifier and replace w/ new one	☐	☐	☐
c. place new inspiratory line to humidifier outlet	☐	☐	☐
d. place expiratory line near expiratory valve	☐	☐	☐
e. place patient connection near patient head	☐	☐	☐
f. place pressure monitor near pressure monitor	☐	☐	☐
4. Change circuit			
a. assistant to manually ventilate patient	☐	☐	☐
b. disconnect old tubing and replace w/ new tubing	☐	☐	☐
c. attach new expiratory line	☐	☐	☐
d. attach pressure tubing to pressure monitor	☐	☐	☐
5. Occlude patient connection and verify pressure	☐	☐	☐
6. Attach new circuit to patient			
Verify patient ventilation			
a. auscultate	☐	☐	☐
b. chest excursion	☐	☐	☐
c. O_2 saturation	☐	☐	☐

	PEER	LAB	CLINICAL
7. Dispose of dirty equipment properly	☐	☐	☐
8. Perform a complete vent check	☐	☐	☐
9. Leave the patient area clean and safe	☐	☐	☐
10. Wash hands before leaving the room	☐	☐	☐
11. Document equipment and procedure	☐	☐	☐
12. Monitor appropriately	☐	☐	☐

***Upon completion of check-off, student should be able to perform the task with no prompting.

Completion Dates & Signatures:

Date Peer _____   Signature: _____

Date Lab _____   Signature: _____

Date Clinical _____   Signature: _____

Ventilator Monitoring Performance Evaluation

Student Name: _____   Date: _____

Instructor Name: _____

TASK:	PEER	LAB	CLINICAL
1. Obtain equipment			
a. stethoscope	☐	☐	☐
b. oxygen analyzer	☐	☐	☐
c. suction equipment	☐	☐	☐
2. Observe universal precautions and hand washing	☐	☐	☐
3. Assess patient			
a. confirm correct patient	☐	☐	☐
b. appearance	☐	☐	☐
c. chest excursion	☐	☐	☐
d. check heart rate	☐	☐	☐
4. Auscultate and suction if necessary	☐	☐	☐
5. Evaluate:			
a. mode of ventilation	☐	☐	☐
b. respiratory rate (patient and ventilator)	☐	☐	☐
c. peak inspiratory pressure	☐	☐	☐
d. PEEP	☐	☐	☐
e. inspiratory time or DPP	☐	☐	☐
f. I:E ratio	☐	☐	☐
g. peak flow	☐	☐	☐
h. set and delivered volumes	☐	☐	☐
i. set and delivered pressures	☐	☐	☐
j. compliance	☐	☐	☐
k. analyzed F_iO_2	☐	☐	☐
l. circuit temperatures	☐	☐	☐
m. humidifier and water level	☐	☐	☐

	PEER	LAB	CLINICAL
n. vent alarms and monitor alarms	☐	☐	☐
o. endotracheal tube position	☐	☐	☐
p. TCM or pulse ox readings	☐	☐	☐

6. Charting

	PEER	LAB	CLINICAL
a. breath sounds	☐	☐	☐
b. sputum volume, color, consistency	☐	☐	☐
c. blood gas results	☐	☐	☐
d. pertinent information and ventilator changes	☐	☐	☐

7. Report

	PEER	LAB	CLINICAL
a. changes in status	☐	☐	☐
b. adverse reactions	☐	☐	☐
c. unusual findings	☐	☐	☐
8. Leave the patient area clean and safe	☐	☐	☐
9. Wash hands before leaving the room	☐	☐	☐
10. Monitor appropriately	☐	☐	☐

***Upon completion of check-off, student should be able to perform the task with no prompting.

Completion Dates & Signatures:

Date Peer _____   Signature: _____

Date Lab _____   Signature: _____

Date Clinical _____   Signature: _____

Ventilator Parameter Change Performance Evaluation

Student Name: _____   Date: _____

Instructor Name: _____

TASK:	PEER	LAB	CLINICAL
1. Verify physician's order	☐	☐	☐
2. Observe universal precautions, including washing hands	☐	☐	☐
3. Assess acid/base and oxygenation status from ABG or TCM	☐	☐	☐
4. Evaluate current ventilator settings	☐	☐	☐
5. Determine all possible ventilator changes to normalize ABG	☐	☐	☐
6. Select appropriate ventilator changes	☐	☐	☐
7. Discuss potential complications	☐	☐	☐
7. Make appropriate ventilator changes	☐	☐	☐
8. Follow up changes on TCM and/or ABG	☐	☐	☐
9. Leave the patient area clean and safe	☐	☐	☐
10. Wash hands before leaving the room	☐	☐	☐
11. Document changes in patient chart	☐	☐	☐
12. Monitor appropriately	☐	☐	☐

***Upon completion of check-off, student should be able to perform the task with no prompting.

Completion Dates & Signatures:

Date Peer _____   Signature: _____

Date Lab _____   Signature: _____

Date Clinical _____   Signature: _____

Ventilator Setup
Performance Evaluation

Student Name: _____   Date: _____

Instructor Name: _____

TASK:	PEER	LAB	CLINICAL
1. Verify physician's order	☐	☐	☐
2. Observe universal precautions and hand washing	☐	☐	☐
3. Obtain required equipment	☐	☐	☐
a. circuit	☐	☐	☐
b. humidifier equipment	☐	☐	☐
c. temperature probes	☐	☐	☐
d. bacterial filter	☐	☐	☐
e. sterile water	☐	☐	☐
4. Connect equipment to ventilator	☐	☐	☐
a. place bacterial filter between ventilator and humidifier inlet	☐	☐	☐
b. place humidifier on heating unit and set temperature	☐	☐	☐
c. connect inspiratory line to humidifier outlet and expiratory line to exhalation valve	☐	☐	☐
d. connect temperature probes	☐	☐	☐
e. connect pressure line to patient "Y"	☐	☐	☐
6. Set initial parameters	☐	☐	☐
7. Test equipment			
a. alarm function	☐	☐	☐
b. check system for leaks	☐	☐	☐
8. Dispose of excess equipment	☐	☐	☐
9. Cover with protective bag	☐	☐	☐

***Upon completion of check-off, student should be able to perform the task with no prompting.

Completion Dates & Signatures:

Date Peer _____   Signature: _____

Date Lab _____   Signature: _____

Date Clinical _____   Signature: _____

APPENDIX B

Strategies to Prepare for the Neonatal/Pediatric Speciality Examination

GENERAL TEST-TAKING STRATEGIES

As you probably already know, there is no such thing as a perfect test. Every test you have ever taken will include areas that you feel are clear and fair and other areas that seem vague and obscure. Because it is impossible to prepare for exactly what will be on the Neonatal/Pediatric Respiratory Care Specialty Examination, the best preparation is to understand some general strategies in test taking. By following these strategies, the practitioner will be better prepared for any examination. Before examining each strategy, it must be understood that it *is* possible to learn how to take tests.

Tests measure two things: your knowledge and your test-taking skills. Test-taking is just like any other skill in that it can be improved with practice.

EFFECTIVE PREPARATION

The first step in effective preparation is to *begin early*. In fact, it is never too early to begin studying for the examination. If you have not already started, start today. Before you actually begin studying, you must know *what* to study. This study guide has been designed to do exactly that, to point out what to study in order to prepare for the Neonatal/Pediatric Specialty Examination.

The next important step is to *study regularly*. Just like exercise, studying is most effective when you do it on a regular basis. A successful test taker is one who does not "cram" at the last minute. It is important to deliberately structure your time. Schedule a certain starting and stopping time. Set aside a certain time of day when you will study. Plan to study in an environment that is free from distractions. The amount of time is not as important as the environment. You can accomplish more in 15 minutes in a quiet, comfortable environment than studying for one hour in an environment with frequent disruptions and noise.

Ideally, the studying should be done in the same location and at the same time each day. Start with the most difficult areas first. It is the tendency of most people to work on the easy areas first and putting off the harder areas for later. Resist that temptation and work on the harder areas first.

If you are going to be studying for an hour or more, be sure to take 5- to 10-minute breaks at regular intervals. Do not study until you are exhausted and then take a break. Taking a break every 30 minutes or so will help to keep you fresh. During the breaks, stand up and move around, do some relaxation exercises and massage your neck and other tense areas. Never try to study when you are tired.

If you begin your studying early on, you will eventually reach the point where you feel you understand the material. When you reach this point, continue to study! It is beneficial to be *overprepared* when taking an examination. However, this is true only to a certain point. As a general rule, study for an additional 25% of the time you have spent thus far.

Another important strategy in examination preparation is to review tests that are similar to the one you will be taking. Understanding the types of questions in the Neonatal/Pediatric Specialty Examination and practicing the thought processes involved will be a tremendous help in your preparation. It is recommended that you become well acquainted with the test format by taking the free practice exam offered on the NBRC website (http://www.nbrc.org/Pages/NPS.aspx). When reviewing and taking the sample examination, duplicate the testing environment as much as possible. Take the sample examination using the same rules and regulations set down in the NBRC guidelines. Duplicate and use the supplied answer sheet. Mark your answers by filling in the bubble by the correct response with a pencil. Follow the time limit constraints. Get used to sitting and taking the practice examination in a 3-hour session. Do not use a calculator or notes, because you will not have these available during the actual examination. By duplicating the conditions during practice examinations, your comfort level will increase before taking the actual examination, and your chances of successfully passing will increase.

Next, *organize* your studying. It is best to start by getting an overview of the material. For this examination, it may be best to break the test into general areas such as the three content areas, or even break it into smaller areas. As you review the chosen area, make note of the general ideas and themes. If you are studying from a textbook, highlight the main concepts and ideas. Writing notes will help reinforce the concepts in your memory.

The last step in examination preparation is to *review* your notes and material on a regular basis. Reviewing helps you to recall those areas previously studied and greatly enhances retention of the material.

ENVIRONMENTAL VARIABLES

Almost everyone suffers from some degree of anxiety when taking an examination. Although stress cannot always be eliminated altogether, there are several things that can be done to lower the level of stress.

First, following the examination preparation steps outlined above will reduce the stress caused by entering the examination unprepared. One of the biggest stress producers is the feeling of being unprepared for what is on the examination. Proper preparation will greatly reduce this stress.

Stress is also reduced by entering the examination well rested and healthy. For this reason, it is unwise to cram the night before. Save the night before the test to relax and get to bed early. Arise early enough to arrive at the testing center at least 30 minutes before the examination is scheduled to start. A hurried morning, or an unexpected delay in transit will only serve to increase anxiety. The more calm, cool, and collected you are when you begin the examination, the better you will do. Do not take a tranquilizer or other drug; doing so interfere with your judgment or make you drowsy. Wear comfortable clothing, particularly in layers. This way you can adjust your own comfort level in the room by removing or adding a layer of clothing. Anything you can do to increase your comfort level will enhance your chances of success.

Although it is often impossible to avoid sickness, it is never too early to begin a regime of regular exercise. Physical well-being can tremendously enhance the ability to perform well on the examination. Some light exercise just before the examination will help you to relax and loosen up tense muscles. Perhaps a brisk walk around the testing center would be possible before entering to take the examination.

During the examination, stop regularly to stretch your muscles, take a few deep breaths, close your eyes, and relax for just a few moments. This will help you stay fresh and avoid the fatigue that often accompanies long stretches of intense concentration.

DAY OF THE EXAM

Plan your time in advance to arrive at the assessment center 15 minutes prior to your scheduled exam time. You will need two forms of identification, including at least one of the following: drivers license with a photograph, state identification with a photograph, passport, or military identification card with a photograph. A second form of ID must display your name and signature. Personal items are not allowed in the testing center. Wallets, keys, cell phones, and personal communication devices must be locked in a soft locker, provided at the testing center. Make yourself aware of the examination restrictions as any misconduct could result in dismissal from the testing center.

USE OF YOUR TIME DURING THE EXAMINATION

For the Neonatal/Pediatric Respiratory Care Specialty Examination, you will be given three hours to complete 140 multiple-choice questions (120 scored items and 20 pretest items). In order to complete the examination within the allotted time period, it will be necessary to allocate your time wisely.

For this examination, if every question were allotted the same amount of time, you would have 1 minute and 12 seconds for each question. However, you will find that some questions can be answered much quicker and some will take longer to answer. The key is not to spend too much time on any one question. If you are spending too much time on a question, or you do not know the answer, circle it and return to it later. By circling the answer and coming back, there may be a question further into the examination that stimulates your thought process and will allow you to answer the previous question. If you elect to do this, take care when placing your responses on the answer sheet so as not to get succeeding answers in the wrong place. Periodically check the time and assess how well you are using the time. For example, by 30 minutes into the examination, you should be near question number 25, at one hour question number 50, and so on.

It may prove helpful to write any equations down before beginning the examination in the front of the booklet. This technique frees your mind from the stress of trying to recall the information when fatigue has set in and makes recall more difficult.

When you have reached the end of the examination, return to those questions you had circled and spend the remaining time answering them.

ANSWERING QUESTIONS WHEN YOU DO NOT KNOW THE ANSWER

The question always arises what to do with those questions in which the answer is not known. Is it best to leave it unanswered, or to simply guess? The answer to that question is that it is always better to guess than to leave the question unanswered. Instead of randomly choosing an answer, there is a strategy for guessing that will improve your chance of getting the correct answer.

First, it cannot be emphasized strongly enough to thoroughly understand the question before attempting to answer the question. Look for words, such as not, never, always, will, which may change the nature of the question. Do not read anything into the question. Let us use the following question as an example.

Table B–1

PREPARATION FOR THE EXAMINATION

A. Content
   1. Start early
   2. Know what to study
   3. Study regularly
      a. schedule a start and stop time
      b. plan a consistent time
      c. have a regular study area
   4. Study the most difficult areas first
   5. Take breaks at regular intervals
   6. Be overprepared rather than underprepared
   7. Review tests that are similar to the target test
      a. duplicate the expected testing conditions
   8. Organize your study
      a. start with an overview
      b. divide material into content areas
      c. make copious notes
   9. Review notes and materials regularly
B. Environmental Variables
   1. Decrease stress
      a. be prepared
      b. be rested
      c. relax
   2. Arrive early
      a. do relaxation exercises
      b. have proper materials
      c. wear comfortable, layered clothing

1. A neonate is being ventilated at a peak inspiratory pressure PIP of 30 cm H_2O, with a PEEP of 5 cm H_2O at a rate of 40 breaths per minute and an FiO_2 of 0.40. The transcutaneous oxygen monitor is reading a PaO_2 of 45 mmHg. Which of the following would you recommend?
   a. Increase the PIP to 35 cm H_2O
   b. Increase the PEEP to 7 cm H_2O
   c. Increase the temperature of the incubator
   d. Increase the FiO_2 to 0.50

If the candidate were to read into the question, any of the choices could be viable answers. For example, if the patient has RDS, we could justify increasing the PIP. However, the question does not tell us about breath sounds or chest excursion or even that the patient has RDS. Again, if the patient is being exposed to cold stress, it may be appropriate to increase the temperature of the incubator. The question does not tell us that the patient is cold and therefore we cannot justify increasing the temperature. These are examples of reading into the question more information than is given.

Once you feel you understand the question, examine each choice carefully. What you will try to do is to eliminate as many of the choices as possible to improve your odds of choosing the correct answer. For example, if you are given four choices, there is a 25% chance that you will guess correctly. If you can rule out one of the choices, the odds increase to 33%. If you can rule out two of the choices, the odds become 50%.

If none of the choices can be eliminated, go with your first impression. Although this is a poor method of answering a question, often one of the choices will "feel" right. If all else fails, guess. Item c is the most frequent correct answer on may multiple-choice exams. If you have already eliminated choice c, then b becomes the most likely choice. This strategy is only to be used as a "last ditch" effort. Once the choice is made, do not second guess and continue changing the answer. This is true of the test in general. Once an answer has been chosen, do not change it unless you are certain the wrong choice was made.

In summary, read the question carefully until you understand what is wanted. Answer only what is asked, do not answer what you *think* should have been asked. Do not jump to any conclusions after reading the question and watch for key words in the question that may change the meaning of the question.

NBRC CANDIDATE HANDBOOK

The NBRC has developed an exhaustive handbook (https://www.nbrc.org/NPSDocs/NBRC%20Candidate%20Handbook.pdf) to help candidates prepare for the credentialing exams, including the Neonatal/Pediatric Specialty Examination. The handbook reviews and details all of the admission and examination policies and information about the content of the exams. It is highly recommended that you review the handbook carefully and familiarize yourself with all information contained therein.

PRACTICE EXAMS AND STUDY GUIDES

As previously mentioned, the NBRC provides a free practice examination for the Neonatal/Pediatric Specialty Examination (https://www.nbrc.org/Pages/NPS.aspx). The practice exam is web-based and closely simulates an actual examination. This exam is to be used as a self-evaluation tool and familiarize you with the software used to administer the examination. Additionally, several vendors provide seminars and reviews to help prepare for the exam. Examples of those include the following:

Kettering National Seminars (http://www.ketteringseminars.com/)
Lindsey Jones (http://lindsey-jones.com/)
Mometrix Test Preparation (http://www.mo-media.com/nps/)
Test Prep Review (http://www.testprepreview.com/nps.htm)

Selected Average Laboratory Values

AVERAGE BLOOD CHEMISTRY VALUES FOR TERM INFANTS

ION	BIRTH	24 HOURS	48 HOURS
Sodium, mmol/L	147	145	149
Potassium, mmol/L	7.8	6.3	5.9
Calcium, mg/dL	9.3	7.8	7.9
Chloride, mmol/L	103	103	103
Glucose, mg/dL	73	63	59

AVERAGE BLOOD CHEMISTRY VALUES FOR LOW BIRTH WEIGHT INFANTS

ION	<1000 g	1001–1500 g	1501–2000 g
Sodium, mmol/L	138	133	135
Potassium, mmol/L	6.4	6.0	5.4
Chloride, mmol/L	100	101	105

AVERAGE HEMATOLOGIC VALUES

	BIRTH	1 MONTH	5 YEARS	10 YEARS
Hematocrit	54	40	40	40
Hemoglobin gm/dL	14–24	11–17	12.5–15	13–15.5
Platelets	140–300,000/mm^3	200–470,000/mm^3	150–450,000/mm^3	150–500,000
Red blood count	4.8–7.1 million/mm^3		4.2–6.2 million/mm^3	4.2–5.6 million/mm^3
White blood count	9000–30,000/mm^3	5000–19,500/mm^3	5000–10,000/mm^3	4–10.5 mm^3
Absolute Neutrophil Count (mean range x10^3)	11	3.8	3.8	4.4
Lymphocytes (Absolute)	2.5–10.5	1.8–9.9	1–5.5	1–3.5
Total bilirubin	0.1–5.8 mg/dL	0.2–1.2 mg/dL	0.2–1.2 mg/dL	0.2–1.2 mg/dL

APPENDIX D

Charts of Average Vital Signs

AVERAGE PREMATURE NEONATAL BLOOD PRESSURE

WEIGHT	SYSTOLIC (mmHg)	DIASTOLIC (mmHg)
750 g	34–54	14–34
1000 g	39–59	16–36
1500 g	40–61	19–39
3000 g	51–72	27–46

NORMAL PEDIATRIC VITAL SIGNS

AGE	PULSE RATE	
	MALES	FEMALES
0–12 months	132–138	123–129
5 years	78–85	78–85
10 years	66–71	68–70
15 years	60–63	64–67

RESPIRATORY RATE

AGE	MALES	FEMALES
0–12 months	30–32	29–31
5 years	22	21
10 years	19	19
15 years	18	18

BLOOD PRESSURE

AGE	SYSTOLIC	DIASTOLIC
0–12 months	80 +/− 16	46 +/− 16
5 years	94 +/− 14	55 +/− 9
10 years	107 +/− 16	57 +/− 9
15 years	118 +/− 19	60 +/− 10

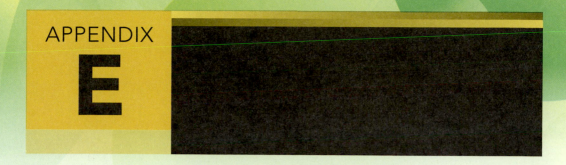

CONVERSION CHART: POUNDS AND OUNCES TO GRAMS

POUNDS

		0	1	2	3	4	5	6	7	8	9	10	11
	0	0	454	907	1361	1814	2268	2272	3175	3629	4082	4536	4990
	1	28	482	936	1389	1843	2296	2750	3203	3657	4111	4564	5018
	2	57	510	964	1417	1871	2325	2778	3232	3685	4139	4593	5046
	3	85	539	992	1446	1899	2353	2807	3260	3714	4167	4621	5075
	4	113	567	1021	1474	1928	2381	2835	3289	3742	4196	4649	5103
	5	142	595	1049	1503	1956	2410	2863	3317	3770	4224	4678	5131
O	6	6	170	624	1077	1531	1984	2438	2892	3345	3799	4552	4706
U	7	198	652	1106	1559	2013	2466	2920	3374	3827	4281	4734	5188
N	8	227	680	1134	1588	2041	2495	2948	3402	3856	4309	4763	5216
C	9	255	709	1162	1616	2070	2523	2977	3430	3884	4337	4791	5245
E	10	283	737	1191	1644	2098	2551	3005	2459	3912	4366	4819	5273
S	11	312	765	1219	1673	2126	2580	3033	3487	3941	4394	4848	5301
	12	340	794	1247	1701	2155	2608	3062	3515	3969	4423	4876	5330
	13	369	822	1276	1729	2183	2637	3090	3544	3997	4451	4904	5358
	14	397	850	1304	1758	2211	2665	3118	3572	4026	4479	4933	5386
	15	425	879	1332	1786	2240	2693	3147	3600	4054	4508	4961	5415

Pounds = weight in grams/454

Grams = weight in pounds × 454

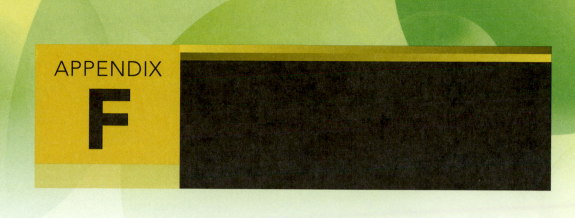

CONVERSION CHART: FAHRENHEIT TO CELSIUS

°F	°C	°F	°C
95.0	35.0	99.6	37.6
95.2	35.1	99.8	37.7
95.4	35.2	100.0	37.8
95.6	35.3	100.2	37.9
95.8	35.4	100.4	38.0
96.0	35.6	100.6	38.1
96.2	35.7	100.8	38.2
96.4	35.8	101.0	38.3
96.6	35.9	101.2	38.4
96.8	36.0	101.4	38.6
97.0	36.1	101.6	38.7
97.2	36.2	101.8	38.8
97.4	36.3	102.0	38.9
97.6	36.4	102.2	39.0
97.8	36.6	102.4	39.1
98.0	36.7	102.6	39.2
98.2	36.8	102.8	39.3
98.4	36.9	103.0	39.4
98.6	37.0	103.2	39.6
98.9	37.1	103.4	39.7
99.0	37.2	103.6	39.8
99.2	37.3	103.8	39.9
99.4	37.4	104.0	40.0

$$°C = [(°F - 32) \times 5]/9$$
$$°F = [(°C \times 9)/5 + 32$$

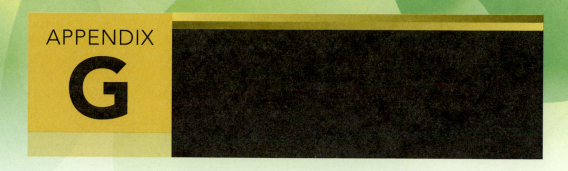

APPENDIX

G

CONVERSION CHART: FRENCH TO MILLIMETERS AND INCHES

FRENCH SIZE	DIAMETER	
	(mm)	(INCHES)
1	1/2	0.013
2	2/3	0.026
3	1	0.039
4	1 1/3	0.052
5	1 2/3	0.065
6	2	0.078
7	2 1/3	0.091
8	2 2/3	0.104
9	3	0.118
10	3 1/3	0.131
11	3 2/3	0.144
12	4	0.157
13	4 1/3	0.170
14	4 2/3	0.183
15	5	0.196
16	5 1/3	0.209
17	5 2/3	0.233
18	6	0.236
19	6 1/3	0.249
20	6 2/3	0.262

Copyright © Cengage Learning®. All Rights Reserved.

CONVERSION CHART: INCHES TO CENTIMETERS

INCHES	CENTIMETERS
¼	0.635
½	0.026
1	2.54
2	5.08
3	7.62
4	10.16
5	12.70
10	25.40
11	27.94
12	30.48
13	33.02
14	35.56
15	38.10
16	40.64
17	43.18
18	45.72
19	48.26
20	50.80
21	53.34
22	55.88
23	58.42
24	60.96

Inches = centimeters/2.54

Centimeters = inches × 2.54

Physical Growth Chart

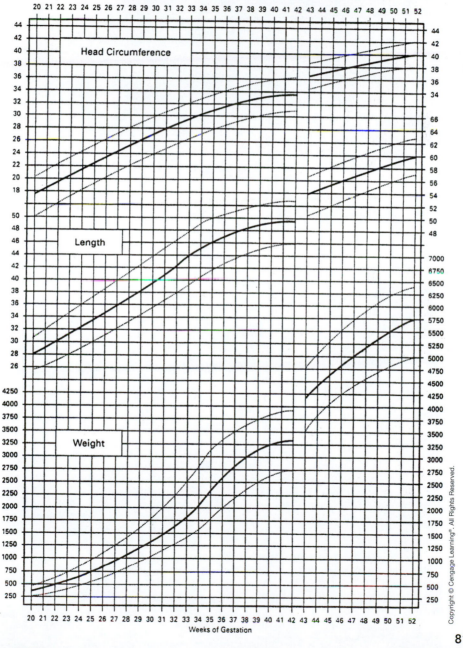

Weeks of Gestation

Glossary

abruptio placentae The abnormal separation of the normally implanted placenta from the uterus in a pregnancy of 20 weeks or more, occurring before the delivery of the fetus.

acrocyanosis A condition in the newborn characterized by a cyanotic discoloration of the hands and feet. Also known as peripheral acrocyanosis of the newborn.

active transport The movement of molecules across a cell membrane by means of a chemical activity, allowing the passage of large molecules, which would normally be unable to pass.

acute lung injury (ALI) Lung injury that follows an acute traumatic event such as inhalation of a noxious gas, injury to the thorax, or hypoperfusion.

adaptive support ventilation (ASV) A mode of ventilation that helps determine appropriate ventilator settings, based upon the patient's respiratory mechanics.

adsorption The binding or adhesion of molecules or particles to a surface.

afterload The resistance against which the left ventricle must eject its blood volume during systole. Afterload is created by the volume of blood already in the vascular system and the resistance of the vessel walls.

air bronchogram The visualization of the air-filled bronchus on a chest radiograph. Normally not seen, it is visible when consolidated or atelectatic lung tissue behind the bronchus creates a white background on the radiograph against which the air-filled bronchus can be visualized. Additionally, it may indicate a dilation of the bronchus secondary to distal consolidation or atelectasis.

air leak syndrome Air leak syndrome includes pulmonary interstitial emphysema, pneumothorax, pneumomediastinum, pneumopericardium, pneumoperitoneum, subcutaneous emphysema, and systemic air embolism. These can occur individually or in combination.

airway pressure release ventilation (APRV) An alternative mode for mechanical ventilation; however, it had not gained popularity until recently as an effective safe alternative for difficult-to-oxygenate patients with acute lung injury/acute respiratory distress syndrome (ALI/ARDS). APRV has many appealing features applicable to our current understanding of ALI/ARDS treatment, such as minimizing ventilator-induced lung injury (VILI) using lung protective strategies.

alae nasi The external border located at the opening to the nasal passages. Being cartilaginous, it normally maintains the patency of the nasal openings during spontaneous ventilation.

alpha-fetoprotein (AFP) A protein normally synthesized by the liver, yolk sac, and GI tract of the fetus. Elevated levels of AFP in the amniotic fluid help in the diagnosis of neural tube defects such as spina bifida.

amblyopia A dimness of sight especially in one eye without apparent change in the eye structures—called also lazy eye, lazy-eye blindness.

amniocentesis A procedure in which a small amount of amniotic fluid is removed from the uterus. The needle used to extract the fluid is guided by ultrasound to locate a suitable pocket of fluid. The amniotic fluid is then analyzed for numerous fetal genetic defects and for fetal maturity.

amnioinfusion A method of thinning thick meconium that has passed into the amniotic fluid by the instillation of fluid into the amniotic cavity.

amnion The membrane that covers the fetal side of the placenta, the outer covering of the umbilical cord, and the entire internal surface of the uterus.

anaerobic Pertaining to the absence of oxygen.

anencephaly A genetically transmitted defect in which the brain and spinal cord are absent, the cranium remains open, and the vertebral canal remains a groove.

anticipatory grief Grief brought on by the anticipation of a traumatic event, such as the death of a loved one.

anuria Absence of or defective urine excretion.

aponeurosis Any of the broad flat sheets of dense fibrous collagenous connective tissue that cover, invest, and form the terminations and attachments of various muscles.

asphyxia Severe hypoxia, which leads to hypoxemia, hypercapnia, acidosis, and eventual death if not corrected.

assist/control (a/c) A mode of mechanical ventilation in which the ventilator provides a positive pressure breath for each spontaneous breath initiated by the patient.

assisted spontaneous breathing (ASB) A mode of ventilation that integrates intrinsic feedback mechanisms to help prevent ventilator-induced lung injury, and improve synchrony between the ventilator and the patient's demand.

attention deficit hyperactivity disorder (ADHD) One of the most common childhood brain disorders that can continue through adolescence and adulthood. Symptoms include difficulty staying focused and paying attention, **difficulty controlling behavior, and hyperactivity (overactivity).**

autism spectrum disorder A group of developmental brain disorders. The term "spectrum" refers to the wide range of symptoms, skills, and levels of impairment, or disability, that children with ASD can have.

automode One of the modes of ventilation that allows for a smooth transition from controlled ventilation to supported ventilation when the patient begins to spontaneously trigger breaths.

autosomal-recessive trait A pattern of inheritance in which the transmission of a recessive gene results in a carrier state if the person is heterozygous for the trait, and in an infected state if the person is homozygous for the trait.

azoospermia A lack of spermatozoa in the semen.

balloon septostomy (Rashkind procedure) The enlargement of an opening in the cardiac septum between the right and left atria. It is done under anesthesia by passing a deflated balloon attached to a cardiac catheter through the foramen ovale into the left atrium. The balloon is then inflated and pulled through the foramen ovale to enlarge its opening.

baroreceptor A cluster of pressure-sensitive nerve endings found in the alls of the atria, the vena cava, the aortic arch, and the carotid sinus. Stretching of the nerves results in stimulation of central reflex mechanisms leading to vasodilation or constriction.

Battle's sign Bruising over the mastoid process, as a result of extravasation of blood along the path of the posterior auricular artery. It is an indication of a fracture of the middle cranial fossa of the skull, and may suggest underlying brain trauma.

beta-lactam A group of antibiotics (penicillins and cephalosporins) that inhibit bacterial cell wall synthesis.

bias flow The rate of continuous flow of humidified blended gas through the patient circuit during high-frequency ventilation.

biphasic Part of a mode of ventilation in which a pressure control mode of ventilation is combined with an inverse inspiratory to expiratory ratio.

blastocyst The form of fetal embryologic development that follows development of the morula. It is a spherical mass of cells having a central, fluid-filled cavity called the blastocoele and surrounded by two layers of the cells: the triphoblast, which becomes the placenta, and the embryoblast, which becomes the embryo.

blastoderm The layer of cells forming the wall of the blastocyst. It gives rise to the primary germ layers, the endoderm, mesoderm, and ectoderm.

blastomere One of the two cells which develops in the first division of the fertilized ovum. The blastomere divides and subdivides to become the morula.

bonding The attachment process that occurs between an infant and parents beginning with the planning of the baby. Bonding is initially stronger in the mother until delivery, when the father begins a strong bonding process.

breech Abnormal fetal delivery in which the fetus emerges feet, knees, or buttocks first.

bronchiolitis obliterans organizing pneumonia (BOOP) A rare lung condition in which the bronchioles and alveoli become inflamed with connective tissue.

brown fat A type of fat found in newborns. Due to its unique thermogenic activity, brown fat is a unique source of heat energy for the newborn.

bulimia nervosa An eating disorder characterized by binge eating and purging, or consuming a large amount of food in a short amount of time followed by an attempt to rid oneself of the food consumed (purging), typically by vomiting, taking a laxative, diuretic, or stimulant, and/or excessive exercise, because of an extensive concern for body weight.

calcaneus The heel bone.

caput succedaneum A localized pitting edema found in the scalp of a newborn that may overlie the sutures of the skull. It is the result of pressure from the cervix on the fetal head. Usually not dangerous, it disappears within the first few days of life.

chemoreceptor A sensory nerve stimulated by chemical stimuli such as CO_2 and H^+ ion concentration. Chemoreceptors located in the carotid artery detect changes in $PaCO_2$ and signal the central respiratory center to increase or decrease ventilation.

chief complaint A concise statement describing the symptom, problem, condition, diagnosis, or other factor that is the reason for a medical encounter.

child In law, a person 14 years of age and under. In medicine, a term used to describe a patient between infancy and youth.

choana The funnel-shaped opening between the posterior nares and the nasopharynx.

choanal atresia A congenital anomaly in which a membranous or bony occlusion blocks the choana. Choanal atresia is caused by the failure of the nasopharyngeal septum to rupture during embryologic development.

chorionic villi The tiny vascular fibrils on the surface of the placenta that infiltrate the endometrium of the uterus. They form the point at which maternal and fetal blood exchange nutrients and blood gases.

choroid plexus Tangled masses of tiny blood vessels found in the third, lateral, and fourth brain ventricles.

conditional variable The conditions that must exist for initiating a sigh breath, or a mandatory breath during synchronized intermittent mandatory ventilation (SIMV).

cognitive That which pertains to the mental processes of comprehension, judgment, memory, and reasoning.

color flow mapping The use of color images with ultrasound, which enables the technician to observe the direction of blood flow. Often used to visualize blood flow through the ductus arteriosus or other heart defect.

compliance The measurement of the distensibility of the lung, measured by the lung volume produced per unit of pressure change.

conductive (conduction) The transfer of heat from a warmer object in direct contact with a cooler object.

conjugate A biological event in which two substances are joined together for various metabolic functions.

contrecoup An injury occurring on the side of an organ opposite to the side on which a blow or impact is received.

control variable A ventilator parameter that does not change when compliance or resistance changes.

convective The transfer of heat from a warm object to cooler air circulating over or around the object.

costophrenic angle The angle at the bottom of the lung where the diaphragm and the chest wall meet as seen on a chest radiograph.

cotyledon One of the visible segments on the maternal surface of the placenta containing the fetal vessels, chorionic villi, and the intervillous space.

coup An injury occurring on the side of an organ on which a blow or impact is received.

crackle Formerly called "rales," crackles are described as fine bubbling sounds heard on auscultation of the lungs caused by air entering fluid-filled alveolus and distal airways.

Crigler-Najjar syndrome A congenital, familial, autosomal abnormality in which glucuronyl transferase is deficient or absent. Characterized by nonhemolytic jaundice, an accumulation of unconjugated bilirubin, and severe disorders of the central nervous system.

cryotherapy A treatment that uses cold as a destructive medium, usually liquid nitrogen.

Dalton's law A law of physics stating that the sum of the pressure exerted by a mixture of gases is equal to the total of the partial pressures exerted by each gas if they were separated. $P_B = P_1 + P_2 + P_3 \ldots$.

decerebrate As relating to posture, the extension and internal rotation of the arms and the extension of the legs with the feet in forced plantar flexion. This type of posturing usually means there has been severe damage to the brain.

decorticate As relating to posture, the rigid flexion of the upper extremities at the wrists and elbows. The legs may also be in a flexed position. Decorticate posture is a sign of damage to the nerve pathway between the brain and spinal cord. Its presence is typically not as serious as decerebrate posturing.

decubitus A recumbent or horizontal position. For example, a lateral decubitus that is lying on one side.

DeLee suction A suction device in which the clinician supplies the suction to the catheter. Any debris is collected in a small collection tube, protecting the clinician from inhaling materials.

densities Relating to the shades of gray seen on a radiograph. Substances that absorb x-rays result in a white density. Substances that absorb little or no x-rays result in a dark density.

diaphragmatic pacemaker An electrode that stimulates the diaphragm to contract. The electrode is maintained by an electronic controller on which the operator determines the rate and strength of contraction.

dichotomy A division or separation into two or more parts.

differential diagnosis (DDx) A systematic diagnostic method used to identify the presence of an entity where multiple alternatives are possible. A process of elimination or at least of obtaining information that shrinks the "probabilities" of candidate conditions to negligible levels.

diffusion time During mechanical ventilation, the length of time that the inspired gas is in contact with the alveoli.

dilatation The widening of the cervix during labor measured during vaginal examination, expressed in cm or finger breadth. Full dilatation of the cervix is 10 cm.

dipalmitoyl phosphatidylcholine (DPPC) The major phospholipid compound found in pulmonary surfactant.

disseminated Widespread or scattered.

disseminated intravascular coagulation (DIC) A grave coagulopathy that results from the overstimulation of the body's clotting and anticlotting processes in response to disease or injury.

doll's eye reflex A normal response in newborn infants is for the eyes to remain stationary as the head is rotated from side to side. This reflex is abnormal in adults. *See also* Oculocephalic.

Doppler The change in frequency when a sound is emitted by an object moving toward or away from an observer. In Doppler scanning, ultrasonic waves are reflected from a moving structure such as the heart to yield information on the structure.

driving pressure The gradient between two pressures that causes a gas or substance to move from the area of higher pressure to the area of lower pressure. The larger the difference between the two pressures, the higher the driving pressure.

ductus arteriosus The vascular channel that connects the pulmonary artery to the descending aorta in fetal circulation.

ductus venosus The vascular channel in the fetal circulation that passes through the liver and connects the umbilical vein to the inferior vena cava.

duoPAP A mode of ventilation in which support alternates between two preset positive pressure levels. The patient can breathe spontaneously at either pressure level. Spontaneous breaths are also synchronized as the pressures shift from low pressure to high pressure.

dyscrasias An abnormal blood or bone marrow condition, such as aplastic anemia or Rh incompatibility.

dystocia A pathologic or difficult labor.

ectoderm The outermost of the three primary germ layers found in the developing embryo. The ectoderm gives rise to the nervous system, eyes, ears, epidermis, and mucous membranes.

effacement The shortening of the vaginal part of the cervix and the thinning of its walls during labor. Effacement is expressed as a percentage of full effacement, which is 100%.

elastic The ability of a tissue to return to its original shape and size following a deforming stress being placed on it.

electromyography A procedure to test and record the intrinsic electric activity in a skeletal muscle. This is done by applying electrodes to the skin and observing the electrical activity on an oscilloscope.

embryo In human development, the early stages of growth and differentiation that is characterized by cleavage, the laying down of fundamental tissues, and the formation of primitive organs and organ systems. The term covers the time of implantation to the end of the eighth week after conception.

emesis To expel the contents of the stomach through the esophagus and out the mouth.

empathetic The ability to recognize and share the emotions and feelings of another and to understand the meaning of that person's behavior.

encephalocele A protrusion of the brain through a congenital defect in the skull.

endoderm The innermost of the germ layers found in the developing embryo. From the endoderm arise the epithelium of the respiratory tract, the GI tract, the urinary tract, pharynx, tonsils, and thyroid gland.

engagement The fixation of the presenting part of the fetus in the maternal pelvis. Engagement occurs when the presenting part is level with the ischial spines of the maternal pelvis.

enteral Pertaining to the intestines, often associated with feedings or medications.

enzyme-linked immunosorbent assay (ELISA) A laboratory test used to detect specific antigens or antibodies, using enzyme-labeled immunoreactants and a solid-phase binding support such as a test tube. It is commonly used in the diagnosis of the AIDS infection.

epistaxis Bleeding from the nose due to a variety of causes.

Erb's point The third intercostal space on the left sternal border where the second heart sound is best auscultated.

erythroblastosis fetalis A type of hemolytic anemia that occurs in newborns as a result of maternal-fetal blood group incompatibility involving the Rh factor and the ABO blood groups.

estriol A naturally occurring human estrogen found in high concentrations in urine. Its level in the maternal urine may be used to ascertain the proper function of the placenta.

evaporative As relates to the loss of heat through the changing of water to vapor on the surface of the skin.

excoriation The act of abrading or wearing off the skin. Typically limited to the epidermal layer.

external thermal gradient (ETG) The difference in temperature between the external environment and the patient's skin temperature.

extravasation A passage of blood, serum, or lymph into the interstitial spaces of the tissue.

extrinsic Developing or having its origin outside the body.

facilitated diffusion The movement of ions or molecules through the cell membrane by the interaction with a carrier protein that aids in their passage. This is probably done by binding chemically with the ion or molecule and shuttling it through the membrane.

fertilization The union of male and female gametes to form a zygote from which the embryo develops.

fetus Term used to describe the developing human from around two months after conception to birth.

flow-inflating bag A manual resuscitation bag that is inflated by the flow of oxygen and is not self-inflating.

Fontan procedure A surgical treatment of hypoplastic left heart syndrome in which the main pulmonary artery and the right atrium are connected.

fontanelle The space on a newborn's cranium between the cranial bones, covered by a tough membrane.

foramen ovale An opening in the septum separating the atria of the heart found in fetal circulation.

full ventilatory support A mode of ventilation which provides all of the required minute ventilation for a patient.

functional residual capacity (FRC) The volume of gas remaining in the lungs following a normal exhalation.

fundus As relating to the uterus, the end opposite the cervix.

galactosemia An inherited, autosomal recessive disorder of galactose metabolism, characterized by a deficiency of the enzyme galactose-l-phosphate uridyl transferase. Hepatosplenomegaly, cataracts, and mental retardation often develop.

gastroschisis A congenital defect characterized by an incomplete closure of the abdominal wall with protrusion of the viscera.

germinal matrix An area of profuse vascularization in the developing fetal brain located adjacent to the walls of the ventricles.

global developmental delay A significant delay in two or more developmental domains: gross and fine motor, speech and language, cognition, personal and social development, or activities of daily living.

glucagon A hormone produced by the alpha cells found in the islets of Langerhans that stimulates the conversion of glycogen to glucose by the liver.

glucocorticoid A class of steroid hormones that bind to the glucocorticoid receptor at the cellular level and regulate glucose metabolism.

gravida A pregnant woman—often used in combination with a number or figure to indicate the number of pregnancies a woman has had.

growing fracture Also known as a craniocerebral erosion or leptomeningeal cyst due to the usual development of a cystic mass filled with cerebrospinal fluid, this is a rare complication of head injury, usually associated with linear skull fractures of the parietal bone in children under age 3.

guaiac A wood resin used on a reagent strip to test for the presence of blood in the stool or urine.

hematoma A mass of, usually clotted, blood that forms in a tissue, organ, or body space as a result of a broken blood vessel.

hemotympanum The presence of blood in the tympanic cavity of the middle ear, often the result of basilar skull fracture.

hilum The depression where the blood vessels, nerves, and bronchus enters the lungs.

human placental lactogen (HPL) A placental hormone that may be deficient in certain abnormalities of pregnancy.

hydrocephaly A pathologic condition characterized by an abnormal accumulation of cerebrospinal fluid within the cranial vault, resulting in dilation of the ventricles.

hydrocyanic acid An aqueous solution of hydrogen cyanide (HCN), which is a poisonous weak acid and is used chiefly in fumigating and in organic synthesis. When inhaled, it is chemically changed into cyanide, which prevents the uptake of oxygen from the blood by the tissues and rapidly leads to death.

hydrolysis The chemical alteration or decomposition of a compound with water.

hydrophobic The property of repelling water molecules.

hydrops fetalis The massive accumulation of fluid in the fetus or newborn often in association with erythroblastosis fetalis. Effusions of the pericardial, pleural, and peritoneal spaces also occur.

hydroscopic The property of taking on water molecules.

hyperalimentation The administration of a nutritionally adequate hypertonic solution consisting of glucose, protein hydrolysates, minerals, and vitamins through an indwelling catheter usually in the superior vena cava. Also called total parenteral nutrition, or TPN.

hyperlucency As pertaining to a radiograph, that area which is very dark, indicating an accumulation of air or gas.

hyperosmolar Pertaining to an increased concentration of osmotically active components such as electrolytes and proteins.

hyperpnea A deep, labored, or rapid respiration.

hypobaric Less than atmospheric pressure.

hypoplastic Any organ or tissue that is underdeveloped.

hypotonia Having a smaller concentration of solute-to-solution ratio than that found in intravascular or interstitial fluids.

hypoxic-ischemic encephalopathy A serious injury to the infant brain in which death of brain cells occurs secondary to hypoxemia or diminished cerebral blood perfusion accompanying systemic hypotension.

hypoventilation A reduction in ventilation that results in an increase in carbon dioxide in the blood.

immunoglobulin Any one of five distinct antibodies present in the serum and external secretions of the body.

independent lung ventilation (ILV) The anatomical separation of the right and left lungs that isolates a diseased lung from contaminating the non-diseased lung. Ventilation is then provided to only one lung.

infant Typically a baby in the first year of life.

inotropic That which pertains to the strength or force of muscular contractions.

intervillous space The space located between the chorionic villi of the placenta. The intervillous space acts as a reservoir for maternal arterial blood, which exchanges nutrients and waste with the fetal blood.

internal thermal gradient (ITG) The difference in temperature between the core of the body and the skin surface.

intraosseous Situated within, occurring within, or administered by entering a bone such as a resuscitative fluid or medication.

intratemporal Relating to the channels within the temporal bone. The facial nerve travels a complex course through the temporal bone and is very susceptible to injury when the temporal bone is involved.

intrinsic Originating within the body.

intussusception The prolapse of one segment of bowel into the lumen of another segment.

kernicterus An abnormal toxic level of bilirubin that accumulates in the tissues of the central nervous system, sometimes causing severe degenerative disorders.

Kling gauze A brand name of wrapping gauze that comes in variable widths and lengths. Normally used to wrap around limbs and extremities.

lanugo Soft, downy hair that covers the normal fetus from approximately the fifth gestational month until term, at which point it is nearly gone.

lavage The process of instilling a sterile solution into an organ, including the trachea, in order to wash or to loosen secretions.

lethargy The state of being indifferent, apathetic, or sluggish.

leukotrienes A class of biologically active compounds that occur naturally in leukocytes. Leukotrienes produce inflammatory and allergic reactions.

logarithm The exponent that indicates the power to which a number must be raised to produce a given number. For example, in the formula $B^2 = X$, 2 is the logarithm of X.

Lucey Driscol syndrome A syndrome possibly passed as an autosomal recessive trait characterized by inhibited uridine disphosphate glucuronosyl transferase and leading to rapidly progressive jaundice and kernicterus.

mainstream nebulizer A nebulizer designed to be used inline with the flow of inspired gas. In a mainstream nebulizer, the aerosol is created inline with the flow of gas, which then carries the aerosol to the patient.

malignant hyperthermia Any elevated temperature of the body as that occurring in heatstroke or excessive fever.

mammalian dive reflex A reflex that is triggered specifically by cold water contacting the face which optimizes respiration to allow staying underwater for extended periods of time. Typically blood is shunted from the skin's surface to the core of the body.

mandatory minute ventilation (MMV) A mode of ventilation in that ensures the patient receives the set minute volume despite fluctuating spontaneous breathing levels.

mAs/kVp Abbreviation for milliampere seconds/kilovolt. Used to determine the necessary energy for exposing a radiograph.

maternal transport Moving a high-risk pregnant patient to a referral hospital prior to delivery.

meconium A thick, dark green, sticky material that collects in the intestines of the fetus and becomes the material expelled during the first bowel movements. It is composed of intestinal secretions, amniotic fluid, and intrauterine debris.

meninges The membranes that envelop the central nervous system.

meningomyelocele A saclike protrusion of either the cerebral or spinal meninges through a congenital defect in the skull or in the vertebral column, which forms a cyst filled with cerebrospinal fluid.

mesoderm The middle of the three germ layers found in the developing embryo. The mesoderm forms the bones, connective tissues, muscles, blood, vascular, and lymphatic tissues.

metered dose inhaler (MDI) A small canister containing a prescribed drug that releases a specific dose of aerosolized drug when activated.

methemoglobinemia A condition in which a type of hemoglobin is formed from blood, hemoglobin, or oxyhemoglobin by oxidation, and that differs from hemoglobin in containing ferric iron and in being unable to combine reversibly with molecular oxygen.

micrognathia Also called Pierre-Robin syndrome, a congenital underdevelopment of the mandible that may cause upper airway obstruction from the tongue falling back into the oropharynx.

mode of ventilation When mechanical ventilation is provided, the method of support that is used to ventilate the patient.

morula The clump of blastomeres formed by the dividing fertilized ovum.

multigravida A woman who has been pregnant more than once.

murmur As relating to heart sounds, a low-pitched fluttering or humming heard just before, during, or after the normal heart sounds.

muscarinic Pertaining to that which stimulates the receptors of the postganglionic parasympathetic receptors.

myelomeningocele Spina bifida in which neural tissue of the spinal cord and the investing meninges protrude from the spinal column forming a sac under the skin.

narrow complex tachycardia An elevated heart rate (above 100/minute) in which the electrical signal originates in the atria and passes forward through the atrioventricular (AV) node.

near drowning Indicates a patient who almost died from not being able to breathe (suffocating) under water.

necrotizing enterocolitis An acute inflammation of the bowel that occurs primarily in preterm or neonates of low birthweight. Bacterial invasion of the intestinal wall may lead to perforation and peritonitis.

necrotizing tracheobronchitis A localized area of tissue damage and death in the trachea and bronchi caused by the continual contact of pulsed gas delivered during high-frequency jet ventilation.

neonate An infant less than a month old.

neurocranium The portion of the skull that encloses and protects the brain.

neutrally adjusted ventilator assist (NAVA) A mode of ventilation that uses monitoring of the electrical activity of the diaphragm (EDI) to determine asynchrony of ventilation support and patient effort.

obtundation The use of a drug to soothe or deaden pain in order to reduce patient anxiety and discomfort. Often done by reducing the consciousness level of the patient.

occult Being hidden from view or difficult to observe.

oculocephalic (reflex) A reflex used to test the integrity of the brainstem. The head is quickly moved from side to side. Failure of the eyes to lag properly or to assume the midline position indicates a lesion on the ipsilateral side at the level of the brainstem.

oligohydramnios An abnormally small amount of or the absence of amniotic fluid.

omphalocele A congenital herniation of the intra-abdominal viscera through the abdominal wall near the umbilicus.

open lung tool (OLT) Available on the Maquet Servo-i ventilator, this is a tool that follows breath-by-breath ventilation parameters, including dynamic compliance.

opening pressure The amount of pressure needed to open and expand the alveoli.

optimism A belief or disposition that everything will work out for the best.

ora serrata The zigzag margin found in the retina of the eye.

otorrhea A discharge from the external ear.

ototoxic Referring to a substance having a harmful effect on the eighth cranial nerve or on the organs of hearing and balance.

ovum The female germ cell extruded from the ovary at ovulation.

oxidation A reaction in which either the oxygen content of a compound is increased or the positive valence of a compound or radical is increased because of a loss of electrons.

pallor The absence of normal color in the skin or an unnatural paleness to the skin.

paradoxical Any situation or occurrence in which the outcome is the opposite of what is expected.

parenteral Pertaining to the uptake of substances or medications by any route other than the digestive tract.

parity The number of times a female has given birth, counting multiple births as one and usually including stillbirths.

partial ventilatory support Those modes of mechanical ventilation indicated for patients who are capable of maintaining all or part of their minute ventilation spontaneously.

parturition The action or process of giving birth.

pericranium The external periosteum of the skull.

periosteum The membrane of connective tissue that covers all bones except at the articular surfaces.

periventricular leukomalacia The neuropathologic consequence of a generalized reduction in cerebral blood flow in the premature infant resulting in necrosis of the periventricular white matter.

persistent fetal circulation A condition in which blood flow continues following the fetal pattern after delivery. The shunts involved include the ductus arteriosus and the foramen ovale.

pessimism The tendency to always view the grim side of every situation.

petichiae Small purple or red spots on the skin resulting from minute hemorrhages within the dermal or submucosal layers.

pharmacokinetics The study of all aspects of drug use on the body to include routes of absorption and excretion, duration and action, and biotransformation.

pheochromocytoma A chronic hypertension caused by a vascular tumor of the adrenal medulla or sympathetic paraganglia. It is characterized by hypersecretion of epinephrine and norepinephrine.

phosphatidylglycerol (PG) One of the minor acidic phospholipids found in surfactant. Its presence in amniotic fluid signals the maturity of the fetal lungs.

phospholipid One of a class of compounds containing phosphoric acid, fatty acids, and a nitrogenous base. Phospholipids are found in many living cells.

pica An abnormal craving for and eating of substances (as chalk, ashes, or dirt) not normally eaten that occurs in nutritional deficiency states.

pinna The cartilaginous portion of the external ear.

placenta previa An abnormal implantation of the placenta near to or covering the cervical opening.

pleural effusion An abnormal accumulation of fluid between the lung and the pleural lining. The fluid is either a transudate, which is a relatively protein-free fluid extruded from a tissue, or an exudate, which is a fluid high in protein that has escaped from the blood vasculature.

pneumotachograph An instrument that measures the velocity of expired gas flows.

polyhydramnios A condition of excessive amounts of amniotic fluid, usually more than 2000 ml.

posthemorrhagic hydrocephalus The abnormal accumulation of cerebrospinal fluid in the ventricles caused by blockage and obstruction that results from residual adhesions from the initial disease process.

preeclampsia An abnormal condition occurring during pregnancy in which the maternal blood pressure elevates after week 24 of gestation. Hypertension is accompanied by proteinuria and edema. The etiology remains unknown.

pressure-controlled ventilation A mode of mechanical ventilation in which inspiratory pressure remains constant when compliance or resistance changes.

pressure regulated volume control (PRVC) A dual mode of ventilation that requires a set tidal volume, minute volume, and respiratory rate. The ventilator can detect the level of pressure necessary to deliver the set volume, and it can adjust to provide the least amount of pressure to achieve the set volume.

primary apnea A cessation of breathing with accompanying bradycardia that follows the onset of asphyxia in the fetus.

primigravida An woman pregnant for the first time.

prolapse The failing or sliding of an organ from its normal position.

proportional pressure support (PPS) An optional setting on the Drager Evita XL ventilator that is intended for differentiated proportional support of spontaneous breathing with pathological compliance and/or resistance.

pseudocholinesterase A nonspecific cholinesterase that hydrolyses noncholine esters as well as acetylcholine.

pseudocysts A space or cavity containing a gas or liquid that does not have a lining membrane.

psychosocial Pertaining to a combination of psychologic and social factors.

purpura Any of several hemorrhagic states characterized by patches of purplish discoloration resulting from extravasation of blood into the skin and mucous membranes.

pyrogen A fever-producing substance.

raccoon eyes Periorbital ecchymosis that is a sign of basal skull fracture, a craniotomy that ruptured the meninges, or (rarely) certain cancers.

radiant The transfer of heat from a warm object to a cooler object not in direct contact by the emission of heat rays.

radiopaque A substance or object that does not allow the passage of x-rays. The result is a white area on the exposed film. Often used to assess the location of catheters and tubes in the body.

rapid eye movement (REM) A stage of sleep characterized by the rapid and random movement of the eyes.

rapid shallow breathing index (RSBI) The ratio of respiratory frequency to tidal volume used as a tool to help wean patients off from mechanical ventilation.

rebound effect The sudden contraction, swelling, or edema that follows the effects of a bronchodilatory or vasodilatory drug.

reconcentration The concept that a nebulized drug becomes higher in concentration as the fluid level diminishes. This is caused by a combination of evaporation of the diluent and the baffling of larger aerosol particles, which fall back into the solution and eventually make the drug concentration higher.

red reflex The reddish-orange reflection of light from the eye's retina that is observed when using an ophthalmoscope.

reduction The addition of hydrogen to a substance, the removal of oxygen from a substance, or a decrease in the valence of the electronegative part of a compound.

reflux An abnormal backward flow of fluid as in stomach fluids flowing up the esophagus.

regionalization The organization of health care delivery within a geographic region that ensures availability of all hospital services to the population residing within the region and avoiding costly duplication.

resistance The opposition to flow offered by the walls of the airways or of the blood vessels. Resistance is increased as the diameter of the vessel or airway is decreased.

reticulogranular A cloudy or hazy appearance of the lung fields seen on a chest radiograph of a patient with respiratory distress.

rhonchi Abnormal breath sounds heard during auscultation caused by the airway being obstructed with secretions, muscular spasm, or external pressure. The sounds are described as a snore or rumbling, are more pronounced during exhalation, and usually clear with coughing.

rugae Ridges or folds of skin found in the stomach and on the mature male scrotum.

rule of nines A standardized method used to quickly assess how much body surface area (BSA) has been burned on a patient.

scaphoid A sunken anterior abdominal wall.

scoliosis A lateral curvature of the spine.

secondary apnea A cessation of breathing accompanied by bradycardia and hypotension that follows extended asphyxia in the fetus or newborn. Spontaneous respirations will not occur again unless the infant is mechanically ventilated and the asphyxia reversed.

secondary drowning syndrome Pulmonary edema and resulting asphyxia, resulting from hypoxia and increased permeability of pulmonary capillaries occurring in a patient who has been immersed in water and aspirated some of it.

self-inflating bag A manual resuscitation bag that inflates following each compression whether or not there is gas flow into the bag.

septum primum An embryologic structure in the developing heart, which eventually becomes the atrial and ventricular septum.

servo-controlled A device that utilizes a feedback loop for control. An example is a home thermostat, which measures the temperature and triggers the furnace when the temperature drops below the set level. As the temperature rises above the set level, the thermostat stops the furnace.

sieve A filter or mesh screen that only allows the passage of particles smaller than the openings in the filter or mesh.

simple diffusion The movement of fluids or particles from an area of higher concentration to an area of lower concentration through a semipermeable membrane following brownian movement.

sinus venosus The embryologic structure in the fetal heart that eventually becomes the inferior and superior vena cava and a portion of the right atrium.

sodium-potassium exchange resin (Kayexalate) A resin-containing solution administered via enema in which sodium ions are released from the solution and replaced by potassium ions in the intestines. Used to treat hyperkalemia.

spacer A device placed between the discharge port of a metered dose inhaler and the patient's mouth. Used to allow better distribution of the nebulized particles in the patient's tracheobronchial tree.

spectrophotometric infrared analysis The measurement of different species of hemoglobin in a blood sample by determining the amount of infrared light absorbed.

sphingomyelin A type of sphingolipid found in steady quantities in amniotic fluid. Compared with the concentration of lecithin, it is a part of the determination of lung maturation during the L/S ratio test.

static attraction The attraction of two tissues or objects that is maintained by a thin fluid layer between the two tissues or objects. An example is the attraction between the visceral and parietal pleura of the lungs and thorax.

stations The level of the biparietal plane of the fetal head in relation to the level of the ischial spines on the maternal pelvis measured in negative cm above the spines and positive cm below the spines.

strabismus The inability of one eye to attain binocular vision with the other because of imbalance of the muscles of the eyeball.

stratum corneum The outermost layer of the skin composed of dead cells converted to keratin.

subglottic Situated or occurring below the glottis.

supine Lying on the back.

surfactant A combination of lipoproteins found in mature alveoli that reduce the surface tension of the pulmonary fluids.

synchronized intermittent mandatory ventilation (SIMV) A mode of ventilation that allows the ventilator to sense a patient's own breathing and permit spontaneous breathing between mechanical ventilations while assuring sufficient mandatory breaths should the patient's own **rate fall below a preset value.**

synchronized intermittent positive pressure ventilation (SIPPV) A form of synchronous ventilation in which baby triggers/initiates the breath while ventilator does the work of breathing.

systolic ejection clicks An extra heart sound heard during mid- to late systole having a click-like quality. A frequent cause of ejection clicks is prolapse of the mitral valve.

Tanner scale A scale of physical and sexual development in children, adolescents and adults.

T-piece resuscitator A lightweight, stand alone resuscitator unit made by Fisher & Paykel Healthcare.

teratogen Any substance or agent that interferes with normal fetal development and causes one or more developmental abnormalities in the fetus.

thermoneutral zone That point at which the basal rate of heat production is in equilibrium with the rate of heat loss to the external environment.

thermoregulation The maintenance or regulation of body temperature within a normal range.

thoracic gas volume The volume of gas in the thorax as measured by a body plethysmograph. Thoracic gas volumes include gas that may or may not be in free communication with the airways.

thrombocytopenia An abnormal reduction in the number of blood platelets. It is often a result of destruction of erythroid tissue in bone marrow or an immune response to a drug.

thumb technique A technique of providing chest compression during CPR by placing both thumbs on the lower third of the infant's sternum with the fingers cradled around the infant's back and chest.

thymus The primary central gland of the lymphatic system located in the mediastinum and extending superiorly into the neck to the lower edge of the thyroid gland.

thyrotoxicosis A disorder characterized by an enlarged thyroid gland, exophthalmos, and hyperthyroidism of unknown origin. Also called Graves' disease.

time-cycled pressure limited (TCPL) A mode of ventilation in which the PIP is set and the volume that results from the delivered pressure is variable according to compliance.

titrate The addition or administration of definite amounts of a solution or drug until a given endpoint or sign is achieved.

tocodynamometer An instrument used to measure the force of uterine contractions.

tocolysis Uterine relaxation resulting in a postponement of labor.

tonic posturing An abnormal sign of brain dysfunction in which some or all skeletal muscles remain in a contracted state.

TORCH An acronym that describes a group of pathological agents that cause similar symptoms in newborns and that include especially a toxoplasma (*Toxoplasma gonii*), cytomegalovirus, herpes simplex virus, and the togavirus causing German measles.

trabeculae A small tissue element in the form of a small beam, strut, or rod, generally having a mechanical function and usually composed of dense collagenous tissue.

transillumination The use of a high-intensity light passing through body tissues for the purpose of examining a structure interposed between the observer and the light source.

Transition Passage from one state or stage to another.

Trendelenburg A position in which the head is lower than the body and legs. Often used during chest physiotherapy to aid in bronchial drainage.

trophoblast The layer of tissue that forms the wall of the blastocyst in the early stages of embryologic development.

truncus arteriosus The embryologic structure of the developing heart, which becomes the aorta and pulmonary artery.

turfism The claiming of a geographic or territorial region as belonging to an individual or organization.

turgor The normal resiliency of the skin, which is a result of the outward pressure of the cells and interstitial fluid.

ultrafiltration The act of filtering large molecules from small molecules by creating a pressure gradient across a filter containing small pores.

unstressed volume The volume of gas in the lungs when the thorax is at its resting level.

updraft nebulizer An aerosol-creating device in which the aerosol must exit the nebulizer in order to enter the inspiratory stream of gas going to the patient. Also called a side-stream nebulizer.

vaso-obliteration The destruction of the retinal vasculature in the first stages of retinopathy of prematurity. In response to hyperoxia and other factors, the vessels may permanently constrict and become necrotic.

venoarterial Removal of the blood from a large vein and returning the blood to an artery. When used with ECLS, the blood is often removed from the right atrium and returned to the aorta.

venovenous Removal of the blood from a vein and returning the blood to a vein.

ventricular-peritoneal shunt A surgically created passageway in which the cerebrospinal fluid is diverted through a plastic tube to the abdominal cavity where it is absorbed. Used to drain excess amounts of fluid from the brain in hydrocephalus.

ventriculostomy A surgically created opening that allows cerebrospinal fluid to drain from the ventricles of the brain to the cistera magna. Also known as the Torkildsen procedure.

vernix An off-white, cheese-like substance that covers the skin of the fetus and newborn. It is composed of sebaceous gland secretions, lanugo, and epithelial cells. It aids in thermoregulation and in the delivery of the fetus by facilitating the passage through the birth canal.

vigorous The act of being carried out forcefully and energetically.

viscosity The thickness, density, and stickiness of a fluid. A viscous fluid is thicker and denser than a nonviscous fluid.

volume-controlled ventilation A mode of mechanical ventilation in which as compliance or resistance changes in the lung, volume does not change but pressure changes.

volume control plus (VC+) A mode of ventilation in which an inspiratory time and a target tidal volume are set and a test breath is delivered to the patient. The delivered breath incorporates a decelerating flow and a plateau in order to determine lung compliance. The ventilator will adjust subsequent breaths depending on whether they were greater or smaller than the target volume.

volume guarantee (VG) A dual mode of ventilation in which the PIP is set as is a minimum tidal volume. The breath delivered is a pressure control breath, but if the minimum volume is not reached, the breath delivery type may switch to a volume breath in order to deliver the minimum volume set.

Western blot A laboratory test used to detect the presence of antibodies to specific antigens. It is thought to be more reliable than the ELISA test and is often used to verify the results of the ELISA test.

wheeze A form of rhonchus that has the sound of a high-pitched whistle or a musical quality. Often heard over areas of airway constriction or obstruction.

Index